Ways of Living

Ways of Living

Adaptive Strategies for Special Needs

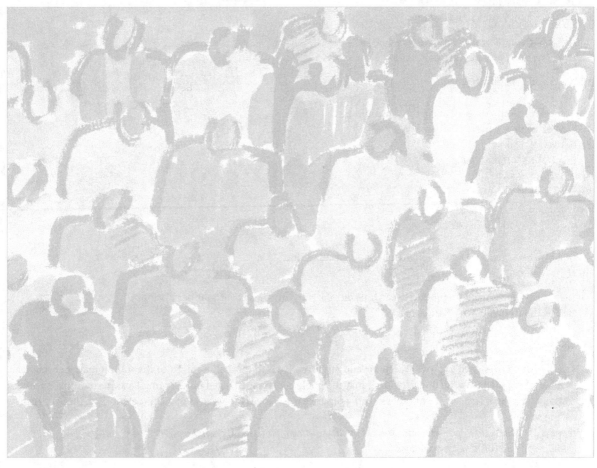

EDITED BY

CHARLES H. CHRISTIANSEN, EdD, OTR, OT(C), FAOTA
KATHLEEN M. MATUSKA, MPH, OTR/L

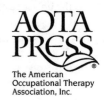

AOTA PRESS

The American
Occupational Therapy
Association, Inc.

Mission Statement

The American Occupational Therapy Association advances the quality, availability, use, and support of occupational therapy through standard-setting, advocacy, education, and research on behalf of its members and the public.

AOTA Staff

Karen C. Carey, CAE, Associate Executive Director, Membership, Marketing, and Communications
Audrey Rothstein, CAE, Group Leader, Communications

Chris Davis, Managing Editor, AOTA Press
Barbara Dickson, Production Editor

Robert A. Sacheli, Manager, Creative Services
Sarah E. Ely, Book Production Coordinator

Marge Wasson, Marketing Manager

The American Occupational Therapy Association, Inc.
4720 Montgomery Lane
Bethesda, MD 20814
Phone: 301-652-AOTA (2682)
TDD: 800-377-8555
Fax: 301-652-7711
www.aota.org
To order: 1-877-404-AOTA (2682)

Disclaimers

This publication is designed to provide accurate and authoritative information in regard to the subject matter covered. It is sold or distributed with the understanding that the publisher is not engaged in rendering legal, accounting, or other professional service. If legal advice or other expert assistance is required, the services of a competent professional person should be sought.
—*From the Declaration of Principles jointly adopted by the American Bar Association and a*
 Committee of Publishers and Associations

It is the objective of The American Occupational Therapy Association to be a forum for free expression and interchange of ideas. The opinions expressed by the contributors to this work are their own and not necessarily those of either the editors or The American Occupational Therapy Association.

ISBN: 1-56900-192-8

Library of Congress Control Number: 2004106221

Design by Sarah E. Ely
Printed by Victor Graphics, Baltimore, MD

Contents

List of Tables, Figures, Boxes, Case Studies, and Appendixes

Foreword

How we spend our days is, of course,
how we spend our lives.

—ANNIE DILLARD

Ways of Living eloquently describes how people spend their days and lives and the adaptive strategies that enable performance of everyday activities of life. This text helps us appreciate the very personal nature of these activities and the complex influences of health conditions and the environment on performance. These two ideas are the foundation of occupational therapy practice.

Ways of Living helps us understand how activities shape a person's unique identity and how variation in style and performance is part of the meaning of activity. If you have any doubt about these ideas, try some people-watching in a restaurant or shopping mall and notice the individuality in grooming, dressing, eating, and sexual expression. This variation offers clues about an individual's culture, class, vocation, interests, and tastes. It supports the importance of person-centered approaches in occupational therapy.

Occupational therapy practitioners observe the effects of other factors on performance, too. Health conditions and environmental barriers influence performance of everyday activities. This knowledge of health and environment make occupational therapy practitioners uniquely prepared to put the puzzle pieces of person, environment, and activities or occupations into a coherent whole. That is, by understanding an individual's perspective on activities and how certain health conditions or environments or disabilities influence performance, we are able to address the life goals of the person.

This third edition of *Ways of Living* expands beyond self-care strategies to include a broader array of activities and occupations. This important revision gives the text broader applications and relevance for individual and classroom learning. Charles H. Christiansen, Kathleen M. Matuska, and the outstanding contributors to *Ways of Living* have provided a wealth of information and a dose of professional perspective that are a wonderful resource for occupational therapy practice. *Ways of Living* will become a valuable addition to our professional libraries and will help us realize our professional goal—to help people spend their days as they want to spend their lives.

—Julie Bass Haugen, PhD, OTR/L, FAOTA
Professor and Chair
Department of Occupational Science
*   and Occupational Therapy*
College of St. Catherine
St. Paul, MN

Reference

Dillard, A. (1989). *The writing life*. New York: Harper & Row.

Preface to the Third Edition

Recent developments in science and technology are changing the world quickly. When the first edition of this book was published in 1994 by the American Occupational Therapy Association (AOTA), the World Wide Web and Internet were not known to most people. And, although occupational therapy was experiencing some significant changes (accompanied by a phenomenal growth in the number of academic programs in the United States), for the most part those changes reflected a continuation of known trends from the 1980s.

One notable exception is the emergence of occupational science. Since the seminal papers introducing occupational science as an academic discipline were published in the early 1990s there has been tremendous growth in the science of occupation. From the beginning, it was the intent that occupational science would guide research and inform practice. A claim can be made that the practice of occupational therapy has already been influenced greatly by occupational science. Of course, the science is still in its infancy, but the worldwide interest in understanding people as occupational beings is striking, and many of the papers and topics of discourse at occupational science conferences are truly breathtaking in the significance they hold for occupational therapy. We think they have already begun to change practice.

Another striking development during the past decade has been the emergence of the World Health Organization's (WHO) *International Classification of Functioning, Disability, and Health* (ICF; WHO, 2001). The conceptual framework underlying the ICF is so compatible with the philosophy, principles, and models of occupational therapy practice that this widely discussed way of thinking about people and health will surely enable the field to play a more significant role in policy discussions about health and disability throughout the world. The ICF makes it clear that health enables activity and participation and that activity and participation are vital to human well-being.

Each of these events also has influenced the third edition of this book. The emergence of occupational science and the more lifestyle-oriented emphasis of the ICF have made it apparent that a book focusing only on interventions for self-care is too narrow to be of significant value to students or practitioners. As a consequence, this new edition asked authors to broaden their scope to include the range of occupational areas beyond self-care or basic activities of daily living. The book uses the occupational areas and terminology of the *Occupational Therapy Practice Framework* adopted by the AOTA in 2002 to describe practice and is guided by the concepts inherent in the ICF. In addition, readers will find many references to concepts and research from occupational science.

Appreciation is extended to Charles Hayden, editorial assistant, for his usual loyal, committed, and diligent work; to Judy Wolf and Jay Tanet for administrative support; and to Brian Berlin and Jenifer Buyten for photographic assistance. We also thank Carolyn Baum, PhD, OTR/L, FAOTA, and Amy Heinz, OTR, for academic assistance. Finally, we salute the staff at AOTA Press, especially Chris Davis and Barbara Dickson, who have provided dependable support and constant encouragement during the accelerated timeline for completion of this edition.

—*Charles H. Christiansen, EdD, OTR, OT(C), FAOTA*
George T. Bryan Distinguished Professor and Dean
School of Allied Health Sciences
University of Texas Medical Branch at Galveston

—*Kathleen M. Matuska, MPH, OTR/L*
Associate Professor and Graduate Program Director
Department of Occupational Science &
Occupational Therapy
College of St. Catherine
St. Paul, MN

References

American Occupational Therapy Association. (2002). Occupational therapy practice framework: Domain and process. *American Journal of Occupational Therapy, 56,* 609–639.

World Health Organization. (2001). *International classification of functioning, disability, and health.* Geneva: Author.

About the Contributors

Beatriz C. Abreu, PhD, OTR, FAOTA, is director of occupational therapy at the Transitional Learning Community at Galveston and clinical professor at the University of Texas Medical Branch at Galveston. She earned her undergraduate degree in occupational therapy at the University of Puerto Rico, her MA in psychology from the New School for Social Research, and her PhD in occupational therapy from New York University. Abreu is an educator and master clinician who has been honored for her contributions to brain injury rehabilitation. Her professional publications include articles, chapters, research reports, and guidelines for practice in occupational therapy. She has delivered invited presentations in neurorehabilitation throughout the United States, Canada, South America, Japan, China, and Italy.

Diane J. Atkins, OTR, FISPO, specializes in rehabilitation of upper-extremity amputees, particularly those with bilateral limb loss, as well as those requiring myoelectric componentry. Her experience includes serving as coordinator of the Amputee Program at the Institute for Rehabilitation and Research in Houston, Texas, and assistant professor in the Department of Physical Medicine and Rehabilitation at Baylor College of Medicine in Houston. She speaks and teaches to professional audiences throughout the United States, Canada, Europe, South America, Australia, and the Far East. She is a board member and fellow of the International Society of Prosthetics and Orthotics and an honorary member of the American Academy of Orthotics and Prosthetics. Atkins is the co-editor and author of *Comprehensive Management of the Upper-Limb Amputee* (1989). She also authored a chapter in *Atlas of Limb Prosthetics: Surgical and Prosthetic Principles* (2nd ed.,1992) and co-edited *Functional Restoration of Adults and Children With Upper Extremity Amputation* (2004).

Catherine L. Backman, PhD, OT(C), is associate professor at the School of Rehabilitation Sciences, University of British Columbia, and research scientist at the Arthritis Research Centre of Canada, Vancouver.

Karin J. Barnes, PhD, OTR, is associate professor in the Occupational Therapy Department at the University of Texas Health Science Center at San Antonio. She teaches pediatric occupational therapy and research courses to graduate occupational therapy students. Her research interests include children with developmental disabilities, school system occupational therapy, hand-skill development, sensory-processing disorders, and activities of daily living of children with disabilities.

Margie Benge, BS, OTR, is director of Triangle Therapy Services, LLC, providing occupational therapy services in rural Ohio. She has taught as a part-time faculty member at Sinclair Community College in Dayton, Ohio. Her current practice specializes in pediatrics, incorporating hippotherapy and animal-assisted therapy in a natural setting.

Jane Case-Smith, EdD, OT/L, FAOTA, is professor in the Division of Occupational Therapy at Ohio State University. She teaches pediatric occupational therapy and research courses to undergraduate and graduate students. Her research has been primarily in the areas of infant and preschooler motor development. Case-Smith has edited numerous books on occupational therapy practice with children and has presented internationally on pediatric assessment, early intervention, and hand-skill development.

Margaret A. Christenson, MPH, OTR, FAOTA, is president of Lifease, Inc., the developer of EASE®3.2 software and LivAbility, an online questionnaire. The software generates reports that provide customized ideas and products for safety, convenience, and independence in the home setting. Christenson is a frequent seminar leader and has spoken to numerous consumer and professional groups on how to adapt the living environment to compensate for age-related changes and how to incorporate universal design. She is a consultant to organizations, architects, interior designers, and long-term-care administrators and has written many articles, books, and other materials on these topics. Christenson was Minnesota Occupational Therapist of the Year, is a past chair of the Gerontology Special Interest Section of the American Occupational Therapy Association, and the AOTA delegate to the most recent White House Conference on Aging.

Charles H. Christiansen, EdD, OTR, OT(C), FAOTA, is dean and George T. Bryan Distinguished Professor at the University of Texas School of Allied Health Sciences in Galveston. He has been involved in the education of rehabilitation providers for the past 25 years and is an active researcher with an interest in lifestyle and health, occupational science, and functional assessment. Christiansen is a fellow of the American Occupational Therapy Association and a member of the Canadian Association of Occupational Therapists. He is the founding editor of *OTJR: Occupation, Participation, and Health* and the author and editor of several textbooks in occupational therapy.

Sandra Fletchall, OTR, CHT, MPA, occupational therapist and certified hand therapist, has specialized in occupational therapy of clients with amputations, burns, and complex fractures for the past 29 years, providing services to people with catastrophic injuries in a variety of settings. Fletchall currently works in private practice with clients who have needs ranging from acute care to return to work; her practice includes home and work assessments and functional assessments. She also coordinates an amputee clinic specializing in injured workers. Fletchall has received several awards for outstanding practice and leadership from the Tennessee Occupational Therapy Association and an award from the University of Tennessee (Memphis) for teaching. In 2000 she received the American Occupational Therapy Association Recognition of Achievement Award for advancements in burn and prosthetic rehabilitation. Fletchall is the author of numerous journal articles on burns, amputations, and prosthetics.

Gelya Frank, PhD, is associate professor in the Department of Occupational Science and Occupational Therapy at the University of Southern California. A cultural anthropologist and founding member of the discipline of occupational science at USC, she is known for her work involving life histories and life stories. Her most recent book, *Venus on Wheels: A Cultural Biography* (2000), documents 20 years of collaborative research on the life of an American woman born without arms and legs.

Susan L. Garber, MA, OTR, FAOTA, FACRM, is professor in the Department of Physical Medicine and Rehabilitation, Baylor College of Medicine, and a research health scientist at the Michael E. DeBakey Veterans Affairs Medical Center in Houston, Texas. She received a BS in occupational therapy from Columbia University and a MA in occupational therapy education from Texas Woman's University. Garber has been the principal investigator or co-investigator on 30 funded projects. She has served on two clinical practice guideline development panels under the auspices of the Agency for Health Care Policy and Research and was chairperson of two development panels working on clinical practice guidelines for the prevention and treatment of pressure ulcers for people with spinal cord injury, sponsored by the Paralyzed Veterans of America. Garber is the site principal investigator on the merit review

project Assisted Movement Neuro-Rehabilitation: VA Multi-Site Trial and the principal investigator on the multisite project Preventing Pressure Ulcers in Veterans with spinal cord injury, sponsored by the Department of Veterans Affairs Health Services Research and Development Service. She has authored or co-authored 28 peer-reviewed papers, more than 18 abstracts, and 14 book chapters.

Don Golembiewski, MA, is director of the outreach program of the Hadley School for the Blind of Winnetka, Illinois. Previously he served as the coordinator of the Wisconsin Independent Living for Older Blind Individuals program and participated in the direct itinerant rehabilitation teaching program, providing services to blind adults in a nine-county area in Wisconsin. Golembiewski received a master's degree in blind rehabilitation from Western Michigan University in 1977 and has held a number of leadership positions in his field. He is past president of the Madison, Wisconsin, Central Lions Club and a preceptor for occupational therapy students at the University of Wisconsin–Madison. He has worked collaboratively with Northern Colorado University, Mississippi State University, the State of Colorado Services for the Blind, Northern Illinois University, and the American Foundation for the Blind. He is a co-author of *Coping With Low Vision* (1993).

Theresa L. Gregorio-Torres, MA, OTR, is senior therapist for Ultra Staff, Inc., which provides occupational therapy services at the Institute for Rehabilitation and Research (TIRR), TIRR Out-Patient Services, and TIRR Challenge Program in Houston. She also is an instructor in the Department of Physical Medicine and Rehabilitation at Baylor College of Medicine. She received her BS from the University of Louisiana at Monroe and her MA in occupational therapy education and occupational therapy ergonomics certificate from Texas Woman's University in Houston. Gregorio-Torres worked at TIRR for more than 23 years. She currently represents the American Occupational Therapy Association on the Consortium for Spinal Cord Medicine Clinical Practice Guidelines of the Paralyzed Veterans of America. Her other interests include assistive technology evaluation and prescription. She has co-authored six papers, three monographs, and one book.

Kristine Haertl, PhD, OTR/L, is full-time faculty member in the Department of Occupational Science and Occupational Therapy at the College of St. Catherine in St. Paul, Minnesota. Haertl received her doctoral degree in health psychology from Capella University. Her clinical expertise includes areas of psychiatric, cognitive, and sensory integration occupational therapy practice. She has a small private practice, is a community practitioner, and is a quality consultant for the federal Head Start programs. Haertl's research interests include the effects of environmental design, program development, and meaningful occupations on client success and quality of life.

Carol Haertlein, PhD, MS, BS, is associate professor of occupational therapy at the University of Wisconsin–Milwaukee, chair of the Occupational Therapy Department, and a scientist with the Center for Addiction and Behavioral Health Research. She is a fellow of the American Occupational Therapy Association and a former member of the AOTA Commission on Education. Her current scholarly interests include the examination of community success for people with serious mental illness (in collaboration with Virginia Stoffel), falls prevention for community-dwelling older adults, and the reduction and prevention of college student drinking.

Judith A. Jenkins, MA, OTR, is senior occupational therapist on the rehabilitation unit at the University of Texas MD Anderson Cancer Center. She earned her undergraduate degree in occupational therapy at Western Michigan University and her master's degree in occupational therapy from Texas Women's University. Her experience as a clinician includes working in acute care, inpatient rehabilitation, outpatient rehabilitation, and work hardening. Jenkins is a member of the American Occupational Therapy Association and the Texas Occupational Therapy Association.

Patricia LaVesser, PhD, OTR/L, is instructor in the program in occupational therapy at Washington University Medical School, St. Louis, Missouri. She received her doctoral degree in social work from Washington University. Her clinical expertise includes early intervention and school-based practice. Currently, she is developing research projects with community occupational therapy clinicians and parents to study the effectiveness of intervention for children who are identified as having autism, pervasive developmental disorders, and sensory-processing problems or who may be at risk for the development of such problems.

Kathleen M. Matuska, MPH, OTR/L, is associate professor and graduate program director at the College of St. Catherine, St. Paul, Minnesota. She has more than 20 years of experience as an occupational therapist providing direct service and consultation in a variety of settings and 10 years of experience in undergraduate and graduate education. Matuska is

author and project director of several community-based service-learning grants and co-investigator of past and current research in multiple sclerosis with Virgil Mathiowetz. She is treasurer of the Society for the Study of Occupation, USA. She is the author of several journal articles and book chapters.

Kerri Morgan, MSOT, OTR/L, is instructor in the program in occupational therapy at Washington University Medical School, St. Louis, Missouri, and the research lab manager for the social participation, environment, and assistive technology research laboratory. Her job responsibilities include teaching the assistive technology class to second-year graduate occupational therapy students and managing several grants from a variety of funding sources, including the Centers for Disease Control and Prevention and the National Institute of Disability and Rehabilitation Research. Morgan is a consultant for two local independent-living centers, where she performs state assessments to determine the eligibility of people with disabilities for the personal assistance service program.

Penelope A. Moyers, EdD, OTR, FAOTA, is dean and professor, School of Occupational Therapy, University of Indianapolis, Indiana.

Margaret A. Perkinson, PhD, is research associate in anthropology and psychology at Washington University, St. Louis, Missouri. She received her doctoral degree in human development and aging, with a concentration in medical anthropology, from the University of California, San Francisco. Her research interests include family caregiving for older adults in the community and in nursing homes, friendship patterns and community development in continuing care retirement communities and naturally occurring retirement communities, driving and dementia, and physical activity and dementia.

Monica Perlmutter, MA, OTR/L, is instructor in the program in occupational therapy at Washington University Medical School, St. Louis, Missouri, and lead occupational therapist for the program's in-home and low-vision services. Academic responsibilities include teaching in the problem-based learning curriculum and in related practice courses. Her research interests currently focus on measurement of the occupational performance of older adults with vision loss and of people with Parkinson's disease who have undergone deep brain stimulation implantation.

Janet L. Poole, PhD, OTR/L, FAOTA, is associate professor and graduate program coordinator, Occupational Therapy Graduate Program, Department of

Orthopaedics, University of New Mexico, Albuquerque.

Sandra Utley Reeves, OTR/L, is an occupational therapist with more than 20 years of experience treating burn patients at two university medical centers. She is currently at Shands Hospital at the University of Florida in Gainesville.

Roger O. Smith, PhD, OT, FAOTA, is professor of occupational therapy and director of the Rehabilitation Research Design and Disability Center at the University of Wisconsin–Milwaukee. He has authored American Occupational Therapy Association Self-Study/Self-Paced Course lessons, including two on technology related to occupational therapy, and has written and presented widely on outcomes and technology-related topics. Smith's doctoral work was based on industrial engineering and bridged technology and disability areas. His master's work was in health sciences, and his undergraduate work focused on psychology and communication. Smith has directed several assistive technology training grants and funded research studies that investigate methods of outcomes measurement.

Martha E. Snell, PhD, is professor of education at the Curry School of Education at the University of Virginia, where she directs the graduate programs in severe disabilities and early childhood special education. A proponent of an interdisciplinary and collaborative team approach for serving children and adults with disabilities, Snell often teams with occupational therapists and other personnel to prepare teachers through course work and supervised field experiences. Her research interests include instructional methods for students with severe disabilities and inclusion of students with disabilities in general education.

Carol Stein, MA, OTR/L, is chief of occupational therapy of the Greater Los Angeles Veterans Administration Healthcare System facilities. A founding member of the discipline of occupational science at the University of Southern California, she has 25 years of experience as an occupational therapist.

Virginia C. Stoffel, MS, BS, is associate professor of occupational therapy at the University of Wisconsin–Milwaukee, coordinates the graduate program, and is a scientist and core leader for the Center for Addiction and Behavioral Health Research, which is also located at the University of Wisconsin–Milwaukee. She is past chair of the American Occupational Therapy Association's Mental Health Special Interest Section, a fellow of AOTA, and a member of the AOTA Specialties Board. Stoffel's clinical experiences have been in mental health and substance abuse intervention programs. She has been involved in several federally funded projects, including Project MATCH (funded by the National Institute in Alcohol Abuse and Alcoholism), and Project ARRIVE (funded by the National Institute on Mental Health). She and Carol Haertlein also have been the recipients of grant funding from the American Occupational Therapy Foundation, AOTA, and the Wisconsin Occupational Therapy Association's Research Fund.

Laura K. Vogtle, PhD, OTR/L, ATP, is associate professor and interim chair in the Department of Occupational Therapy and director of the Post Professional Master's Program in occupational therapy at the University of Alabama at Birmingham. Prior to completing her doctorate in program evaluation, she was a pediatric clinician for 23 years. She recently has become involved in research regarding aging in adults with developmental disabilities. She participates in transdisciplinary team teaching and is a strong supporter of collaborative intervention for children and adults with disabilities. Her research interests include outcomes research and the use of social context in occupational therapy treatment.

Mary Ellen Young, PhD, CRC, is assistant professor in the Department of Rehabilitation Counseling at the College of Health Professions. She was previously assistant professor in the Department of Physical Medicine and Rehabilitation at Baylor College of Medicine. Young has authored or co-authored more than 20 peer-reviewed publications and has given more than 50 professional presentations. She served as co-investigator for a study on sexuality of women with physical disabilities at the Center for Research on Women With Disabilities. Young's research interests can be broadly defined as the study of adaptation to disability, especially catastrophic injury or chronic illness. Specific topics of interest in addition to sexuality include vocational outcomes, community integration, substance abuse, cultural diversity and minority issues, and abuse and violence in the lives of people with disabilities.

Chapter 1

The Importance of Everyday Activities

CHARLES H. CHRISTIANSEN, EdD, OTR, OT(C), FAOTA

KATHLEEN M. MATUSKA, MPH, OTR/L

KEY TERMS

ADL

engagement

IADL

ICF

identity

leisure

narrative

occupational deprivation

occupational disruption

participation

play

quality of life

social role

spiritual

stigma

work

OBJECTIVES

Upon completion of this chapter, the reader will be able to

- Identify the major occupational areas or categories of daily activity,
- Define stigma,
- Explain how activities contribute to identity building,
- Identify threats to well-being associated with restricted engagement in activities,
- Define occupational disruption and occupational deprivation, and
- Provide examples of activities associated with well-being.

This chapter is about the activities people do every day and why they are important to well-being. Being well involves more than simply feeling good: It involves both health and the way people feel about themselves and their lives. Occupational therapy was established because people recognized that participation in daily activities both enables and reflects a person's state of well-being. In other words, what a person is doing and how he or she is doing it can often provide many clues about who that person is and how he or she is feeling, both emotionally and physically. What people do during a typical day often serves as a window on their well-being.

Most people go about their daily routines without thinking too much about their daily activities or what they are doing at any given moment. If a special event, person, or situation requires actions that differ from ordinary day-to-day activities, however, people usually pay more attention to those activities. Such events, including new or broken relationships, unexpected surprises, promotions at work, birthdays, weddings, funerals, graduation ceremonies, and natural disasters, typically are accompanied by noteworthy emotional states: anxiety, fear, surprise, anger, sadness, gratitude, frustration, or joy (Klinger, 1998).

The emotions associated with activities serve many purposes. They arouse our senses and get our attention, enable us to adapt to challenging or threatening circumstances, motivate us to take further action, add color and beauty to our lives, and provide signals to help us communicate and adjust our behaviors in social situations. When emotions accompany actions, those actions often become meaningful (Bruner, 1990); that is, they become connected with other experiences we have had, and through those connections we "make sense of them." Stated another way, our activities, in the context of our life stories, give our lives meaning.

This chapter discusses the importance of everyday activities to well-being. It is organized into three sections. The first section discusses the categories of activity that make up a typical day. The next section discusses the personal and social significance of everyday activities and emphasizes the importance of daily activities to quality of life, personhood, identity, and social roles. The final section explores threats to participation in everyday activities, including disabilities, disfigurement, stigma, social policy, attitudes, and environmental barriers (which are described as forms of occupational deprivation and disruption). The chapter concludes with a review of recent studies that support the importance of activities to quality of life and well-being.

Defining and Describing Categories of Everyday Activities

Behavioral scientists have tried various approaches to describing or grouping activities according to their characteristics, yet no universal set of categories has been adopted. It is difficult to categorize an activity without knowing more about where and when it is performed, the people with whom it is performed, and the purposes that underlie it (Christiansen, 1994; Christiansen & Townsend, 2004). For example, the game of golf can be played by professional athletes to earn a living or by amateurs as a type of weekly recreation. Moreover, golf is often used as a means for promoting business transactions. Is golf a leisure activity or a work activity—or both? The answer depends on the intended goals of the participants and the context of the experience.

An activity's *context* consists of the various aspects of the situation in which it takes place. For example, waiting is a common activity. Consider two contexts in which people are waiting. In the first, a woman waits in a dentist's office for a procedure that will be uncomfortable and, perhaps, painful. Her emotions are ambivalent. On the one hand, she wants to get the procedure over with and get on with her day. On the other hand, she dislikes sitting in the chair and having her mouth serve as the source of shrill sounds and unpleasant vibrations.

In the second example of waiting, a woman waits at the airport for her lover after a long absence. She cannot wait to embrace and experience the joy of being together once again. Her anticipation is full of happy expectation. The waiting period is both agonizing and pleasant because it connects previous joyful memories with an anticipated joyful experience.

In these two examples, the experiences of the same activity are vastly different because of the places, people involved, anticipated outcomes, and meaning of the situations. Many characteristics of situations can influence the context and meaning of an activity and the emotions associated with it.

People do not always do exactly what they want to do because they have requirements, obligations, and expectations that influence how they use their time. Aas (1980) proposed that activities be classified according to whether they represent endeavors that are necessary (e.g., sleeping and eating), contracted (e.g., paid work or school), committed (e.g., child care, housekeeping, meal preparation, and shopping), or free time (i.e., activities chosen during the time remaining after attending to necessary, committed, and contracted activities). Time-use researchers have adopted certain conventions for their research, as depicted in the categories shown in Table 1.1. Note that these categories differ from those typically used to describe everyday activities by occupational therapists and occupational therapy assistants.

Everyday Activities as Viewed Within Occupational Therapy

Occupational therapy practitioners typically divide activities of daily living into several broad categories, which include activities for earning a living; those related to leisure and recreation; and activities related to personal care and self-maintenance, including rest and sleep. The American Occupational Therapy Association (AOTA) groups activities into categories, including ADL, IADL, work, education, play, leisure, and social participation (AOTA, 2002). In Table 1.2, notice how those categories compare with those used in national studies of time use and depicted in Table 1.1. The sections that follow explain in greater detail the specific activities and characteristics that define these categories.

Basic Activities of Daily Living

Activities at home and in the community designed to enable basic survival and well-being are sometimes referred to as *activities of daily living* (ADL). They include activities related to basic personal care (such as toileting, bathing, grooming, and dressing), eating, using the telephone, managing medications, and sexual expression.

Although not listed in most descriptions of basic ADL, sleep and its associated routines can also be considered a self-care activity. Sleep constitutes nearly one third of each day in the lives of typical working adults (Aronoff, 1991). In addition to the time it consumes, sleep is an obligatory occupation that is necessary for health and may have other purposes. Research has shown relationships between activity (including social involvement) and the quality and quantity of sleep (Ohayon, Zulley, Guilleminault, Smirne, & Priest, 2001).

Instrumental Activities of Daily Living

In the late 1960s, M. Powell Lawton, a gerontologist, recognized that living independently in the community requires a level of competence that enables the accomplishment of tasks beyond those of basic self-care (Lawton, 1971). He termed these complex tasks *instrumental activities of daily living* (IADL). Recently, IADL also have been referred to as *extended activities of daily living* (EADL; Christiansen, in press). Activities in this category include care of others, care of pets, child rearing, use of communication devices (such as the telephone or telecommu-

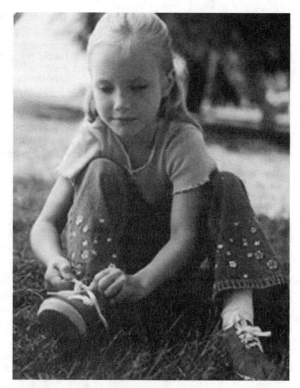

Figure 1.1. Dressing is one specific activity within the occupational area known as activities of daily living. Dressing independently as a child (and as an adult) is important for demonstrating self-reliance. Image © PhotoDisc, Inc.

nication device for the deaf), community mobility, financial management, health management and maintenance, home establishment and management, meal preparation and cleanup, safety and emergency responses, and shopping.

ADL and IADL are a foundation for survival and for participation in the community. Research has shown that self-maintenance activities consume about 10% to 15% of the average able-bodied person's waking day (Szalai, 1972). People with disabilities and older people require a slightly higher proportion of time to accomplish self-maintenance activities (Lawton, 1990; McKinnon, 1992; Yelin, Lubeck, Holman, & Epstein, 1987).

Work

Work includes activities needed to engage in paid employment or volunteer activities. This category includes employment-related activities (such as job seeking and acquisition), job performance, retirement-related activities, and exploration and participation in volunteerism. Time-use scientists recognize that work occurs both in and outside the home. When scientists want to distinguish between the

Table 1.1. Time-Use Categories From the International Classification of Activities for Time-Use Statistics

01	Work for organizations	Paid work for corporations, government, nonprofits
02–05	Household work	Primary production Nonprimary production Construction Services for income
06	Unpaid domestic services	Preparing and serving food Cleaning house and surroundings Clothes care Household management Shopping Travel related to these activities
07	Unpaid caregiving services	Care of children and adults Travel related to these activities
08	Community services	Voluntary and obligatory services for members of the community Travel related to these activities
09	Learning	Attendance of classes at all levels of instruction, including preprimary, primary, vocational Higher education and literacy classes Travel related to learning activities
10	Socializing and community participation	Socializing, communicating, and participating in community events Travel related to these activities
11	Attending/visiting cultural, entertainment, and sports events/venues	Visiting cultural events or venues, exhibitions Watching shows, movies Visiting parks, gardens, zoos Visiting amusement centers, fairs, festivals, circus Watching sports events Travel to and from these places
12	Hobbies, games, and other pastime activities	Active participation in arts, music, theatre, dance Engaging in technical hobbies such as collecting stamps, coins, trading cards, computing, crafts Playing games Taking courses related to hobbies Travel related to these activities
13	Indoor and outdoor sports participation	Active participation in indoor and outdoor sports Coaching, training Looking for gym, exercise program, trainer Assembling and readying sports equipment Taking courses related to sports
14	Mass media	Reading (not related to work, learning) Listening to radio or other audio devices Use of computer technology not strictly for work, learning, household management, or shopping Going to the library for leisure Travel to and from places for these purposes
15	Personal care and maintenance	Activities required by the individual in relation to meeting biological needs Performing own personal and health care and maintenance or receiving this type of care Activities in relation to spiritual/religious care Doing nothing, resting, relaxing Meditating, thinking, planning

Note. Adapted from G. Bediako and J. Vanek, April 22–25, 1998, presented at the International Conference on Time Use, Luneburg, Germany. From the United Nations draft International Classification for Time-Use © 2000 United Nations. Reprinted with permission, from http://unstats.un.org, "Methods and Classifications."

Table 1.2. Terminology for Activities of Daily Living From the *Occupational Therapy Practice Framework*

Areas of Occupation	Specific Activities Within the Area	Definition
Activities of Daily Living (ADL): Activities that are oriented toward taking care of one's own body	Bathing, showering	Obtaining and using supplies; soaping, rinsing, and drying body parts; maintaining bathing position; and transferring to and from bathing positions
	Bowel and bladder management	Includes complete intentional control of bowel movements and urinary bladder and, if necessary, use of equipment or agents for bladder control
	Dressing	Selecting clothing and accessories appropriate to time of day, weather, and occasion; obtaining clothing from storage area; dressing and undressing in a sequential fashion; fastening and adjusting clothing and shoes; and applying and removing personal devices, prostheses, or orthoses
	Eating	The ability to keep and manipulate food or fluids in the mouth and swallow it
	Feeding	The process of setting up, arranging, and bringing food or fluids from the plate or cup to the mouth
	Functional mobility	Moving from one position or place to another (during performance of everyday activities), such as in-bed mobility, wheelchair mobility, transfers (wheelchair, bed, car, tub, toilet, tub or shower, chair, floor); performing functional ambulation and transporting objects
	Personal device care	Using, cleaning, and maintaining personal care items, such as hearing aids, contact lenses, glasses, orthotics, prosthetics, adaptive equipment, and contraceptive and sexual devices
	Personal hygiene and grooming	Obtaining and using supplies; removing body hair (use of razors, tweezers, lotions, etc.); applying and removing cosmetics; washing, drying, combing, styling, brushing, and trimming hair; caring for nails (hands and feet); caring for skin, ears, eyes, and nose; applying deodorant; cleaning mouth; brushing and flossing teeth; or removing, cleaning, and reinserting dental orthotics and prosthetics
	Sexual activity	Engagement in activities that result in sexual satisfaction
	Sleep-rest	A period of inactivity in which one may or may not suspend consciousness
	Toilet hygiene	Obtaining and using supplies; clothing management; maintaining toileting position; transferring to and from toileting position; cleaning body; and caring for menstrual and continence needs (including catheters, colostomies, and suppository management)

Continued

Table 1.2. *Continued*

Areas of Occupation	Specific Activities Within the Area	Definition
Instrumental Activities of Daily Living (IADL): Activities that are oriented toward interacting with the environment and that are often complex—generally optional in nature (i.e., may be delegated to another)	Care of others (including selecting and supervising caregivers)	Arranging, supervising, or providing the care for others
	Care of pets	Arranging, supervising, or providing the care for pets and service animals
	Child rearing	Providing the care and supervision to support the developmental needs of a child
	Communication device use	Using equipment or systems such as writing equipment, telephones, typewriters, computers, communication boards, call lights, emergency systems, braille writers, telecommunication devices for the deaf, and augmentative communication systems to send and receive information
	Community mobility	Moving self in the community and using public or private transportation, such as driving or accessing buses, taxicabs, or other public transportation systems
	Financial management	Using fiscal resources, including alternate methods of financial transaction and planning and using finances with long-term and short-term goals
	Health management and maintenance	Developing, managing, and maintaining routines for health and wellness promotion, such as physical fitness, nutrition, decreasing health risk behaviors, and medication routines
	Home establishment and management	Obtaining and maintaining personal and household possessions and environment (e.g., home, yard, garden, appliances, vehicles), including maintaining and repairing personal possessions (clothing and household items) and knowing how to seek help or whom to contact
	Meal preparation and clean up	Planning, preparing, and serving well-balanced, nutritional meals and cleaning up food and utensils after meals
	Safety procedures and emergency responses	Knowing and performing preventive procedures to maintain a safe environment as well as recognizing sudden, unexpected hazardous situations and initiating emergency action to reduce the threat to health and safety
	Shopping	Preparing shopping lists (grocery and other); selecting and purchasing items; selecting method of payment; and completing money transactions

Continued

Table 1.2. *Continued*

Areas of Occupation	Specific Activities Within the Area	Definition
Education: Includes activities needed for being a student and participating in a learning environment	Formal educational participation	Including the categories of academic (e.g., math, reading, working on a degree); nonacademic (e.g., recess, lunchroom, hallway); extracurricular (e.g., sports, band, cheerleading, dances); and vocational (prevocational and vocational) participation
	Exploration of informal personal educational needs or interests (beyond formal education)	Identifying topics and methods for obtaining topic-related information or skills
	Informal personal education participation	Participating in classes, programs, and activities that provide instruction or training in identified areas of interest
Work: Includes activities needed for engaging in remunerative employment or volunteer activities	Employment interests and pursuits	Identifying and selecting work opportunities based on personal assets, limitations, likes, and dislikes relative to work
	Employment seeking and acquisition	Identifying job opportunities, completing and submitting appropriate application materials, preparing for interviews, participating in interviews and following up afterward, discussing job benefits, and finalizing negotiations
	Job performance	Including work habits, for example, attendance, punctuality, appropriate relationships with coworkers and supervisors, completion of assigned work, and compliance with the norms of the work setting
	Retirement preparation and adjustment	Determining aptitudes, developing interests and skills, and selecting appropriate avocational pursuits
	Volunteer exploration	Determining community causes, organizations, or opportunities for unpaid "work" in relationship to personal skills, interests, location, and time available
	Volunteer participation	Performing unpaid "work" activities for the benefit of identified selected causes, organizations, or facilities
Play: Any spontaneous or organized activity that provides enjoyment, entertainment, amusement, or diversion	Play exploration	Identifying appropriate play activities, which can include exploration play, practice play, pretend play, games with rules, constructive play, and symbolic play
	Play participation	Participating in play; maintaining a balance of play with other areas of occupation; and obtaining, using, and maintaining toys, equipment, and supplies appropriately
Leisure	Leisure exploration Leisure participation	
Social Participation	Community participation Family participation Peer–friend participation	

Note: From "Occupational therapy practice framework: Domain and process," by American Occupational Therapy Association, 2002, *American Journal of Occupational Therapy, 56*, pp. 609–639. Copyright © 2002 by the American Occupational Therapy Association. Reprinted with permission.

work of maintaining households and that of earning a living, they refer to the latter category as *paid work*. Places of employment typically consist of groups of people who gain more than income for their time there. Even in factories where wages are based on piecework (i.e., a fixed amount for each item manufactured or completed), a set of relationships develops among those sharing time there that fulfills human needs for socialization and esteem. Regular work schedules also impose a temporal order on lives, so that the structure of the day and week becomes part of a person's habit patterns (Zerubavel, 1981, 1985, 1989).

Volunteerism consists of contributing one's time and talent toward an area of interest that benefits society or a specific group. Although it is generally accepted that public volunteerism fosters goodwill and trust in groups and in societies by promoting social capital, it also is said to offer the benefit of participation to great numbers of people; in so doing, it provides opportunities for learning and relationship building (Brudner & Kellough, 2000).

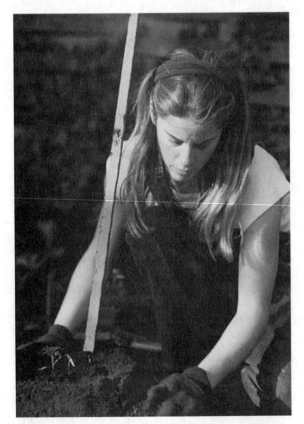

Figure 1.2. Volunteer work provides important opportunities for learning and building relationships, whether during young adulthood, middle age, or the later stages of life.
Photo © PhotoDisc, Inc.

Volunteerism enables a person to contribute knowledge and skills for the benefit of others without obligation and with minimal social expectation beyond altruism and earnest effort.

Education

Education includes activities needed for being a student and participating in a learning environment. This category of activity includes formal and informal educational participation and involves sensory and cognitive processing. Although formal and informal education occurs throughout life, formal education in developed countries typically constitutes a major portion of time use during a typical week for children and adolescents.

Play

Play can be defined as "any spontaneous or organized activity that provides enjoyment, entertainment, amusement, or diversion" (Parham & Fazio, 1997, p. 252). Another definition of play suggests that activities in this category are selected for amusement, recreation, diversion, sport, or frolic (Christiansen, in press). Brian Sutton-Smith (2001), one of the world's foremost scholars on play, noted that play is almost impossible to define because it is so ambiguous. He observed that many categories of play have been named in the scholarly literature, including celebrations, rituals, contests, risky play, vicarious or audience play, mind play, solitary play, and informal social play; each category includes multiple types of activities. No theory of play has yet been widely adopted, although theorists generally accept that play serves important learning and adaptation functions, contributes to variety and diversity in human activity, and provides an outlet for self-expression. Johan Huizinga (1950) suggested that play is fundamental to culture; it is contained within defined space and time and pursued without necessity, and with a mood of enthusiasm or rapture and absorption appropriate to the occasion or setting.

Leisure

Leisure can be defined as "a nonobligatory activity that is intrinsically motivated and engaged in during discretionary time, that is, time not committed to obligatory occupations such as work, self-care, or sleep" (Parham & Fazio, 1997, p. 250). As with play, leisure activities are freely chosen. Stebbins (1997) identified two broad categories of leisure: (1) *serious leisure*, which consists of activities that involve significant personal effort or commitment, such as hobbies, volunteerism, and self-development; and (2) *casual leisure*, which consists of activities that are

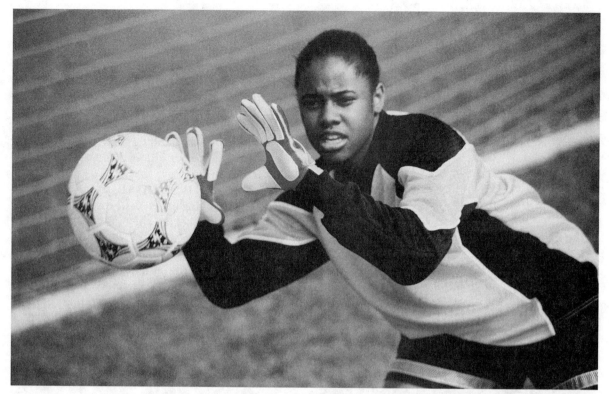

Figure 1.3. Team sports such as soccer exemplify the importance of play. During play, the simultaneous enjoyment, absorption, challenge, and mastery can help meet many human needs. Image © PhotoDisc, Inc.

pleasurable, are of short duration, are intrinsically rewarding, and require little effort, such as relaxation, watching television, going to plays or sporting events, and conversing with friends.

Recent theories suggest that leisure fulfills important psychological needs, including agency (or acting with purpose), novelty, belongingness, service, sensual enjoyment, cognitive stimulation, self-expression, creativity, competition, vicarious competition, and relaxation (Tinsley, 1995). Holmberg, Rosen, and Holland (1990) set forth a personality theory that provides a practical link between personality types and preferences for engagement in leisure activity. They suggested that personality traits cluster into six major categories and that people in each category tend to find certain types of leisure activities appealing, depending on individual traits. Recent research supports the idea that leisure participation during periods of unemployment can help meet needs related to engagement and participation (Waters & Moore, 2002).

Social Participation

Finally, an important area of occupation identified in the occupational therapy literature is social participation. This category encompasses activities associated with organized patterns of behavior that are characteristic and expected of anyone who interacts with others within a given social system. Social participation includes community-based activities that result in successful interaction at the community level as well as activities that help fulfill required or desired familial or friendship roles. This category also includes activities at different levels of intimacy, including sexual activity.

Social participation is an extremely important area of occupation for several reasons. First, because our understanding of the world is socially constructed and roles are learned vicariously through observing others, social relationships are instrumental to the creation of an understanding about what to do, when to do it, and why we do it. Second, social relationships give us feedback about our own behavior that is necessary for learning about ourselves. The feedback gained from social relationships is essential for the development of self-concept and self-awareness and, ultimately, our sense of self, or *identity*.

Daily Round of Activities

The activities performed in a usual day, sometimes called the "round" of activities, often follow a de-

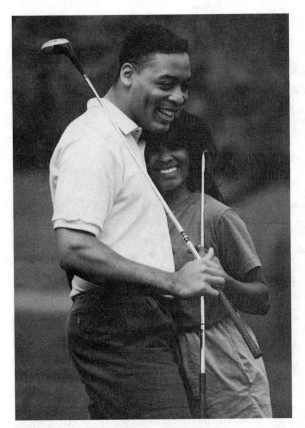

Figure 1.4. Leisure activities can fill many needs, such as belongingness, relaxation, and competition. Studies show that leisure involvement can be important in coping with the stress associated with unemployment. Image © PhotoDisc, Inc.

evolved as group-living, culture-bearing, and symbol-using animals. Individuals, whether in committees or communities, vary in their acceptance by and influence within a group. This place in the group can be referred to as a person's *social standing*. Within any particular group, one's social standing may change. Therefore, a person with a lower level status within a work setting might offset his or her social standing there by participating as an active leader or officer of the neighborhood association.

According to Hogan (1983), social standing influences daily living in two basic ways. First, because people are social beings, they must get along with others. Second, because social standing matters, much of individual well-being requires an ability to compete successfully and to gain standing in a group—that is, to have satisfactory and rewarding relationships with others. Social acceptance makes it possible for people to gain valuable knowledge and assistance in meeting life's demands. Relationships with other members of a group create obligations and opportunities for participation in shared activities, some of which foster interdependence and group well-being.

In considering the typical activities in which a person participates in a given week, it is easy to identify social activities that build relationships between people and within groups. Strolling through any park or green space on a sunny afternoon, one is certain to observe people walking and enjoying

fined sequence that is influenced by social customs, routines, habits, and natural rest and activity cycles. Although the sequence of activities may vary by age and culture, the amount of time devoted to various categories of activity is remarkably consistent across cultures. Engagement in specific activities at any given time is a reflection of personality and motivation; it also reflects a person's needs, values, and opportunities as provided by both time and place. The following section considers how everyday activities provide personal meaning and significance in a social context.

Personal and Social Significance of Everyday Activities

Psychologist Robert Hogan (Hogan, 1983; Hogan, Jones, & Cheek 1985; Hogan & Sloan, 1991) has provided a basis for understanding the importance of everyday activities in his theory of personality. Hogan's research starts with the fact that humans

---

Box 1.1. Learning Activity— How Do You Spend Your Time?

For the next week, keep a log of how you spend your time. Use a daily planner or a grid on which you have plotted spaces in 24 hourly increments. At the end of the week, total the number of hours you have spent in the following categories:

- Self-care (eating, bathing, grooming, dressing)
- Instrumental activities (shopping, cleaning, food preparation, laundry)
- Sleep
- Paid work
- Education
- Leisure activities you choose.

Divide the total in each category by 168 (the total number of hours in a week) to calculate the percentage of time spent in each category. Compare your percentages with those described in studies of working adults.

nature together, jogging or cycling in groups, or playing competitive sports. What purposes do jogging and cycling serve? What are the individual or group purposes behind competitive sports or timed races? Certainly, one can readily identify both social and individual motives in many leisure and work activities. Even early self-care activities have an important social purpose. Our grooming and dressing as we prepare for the day are heavily influenced by our social roles and the expectations that accompany them. For example, we tend to pay more attention to our hair styling and attire when we have to attend an important meeting.

The ability to achieve and maintain standing in social groups requires a social identity. Hogan (1983) noted that people spend a good deal of time developing, negotiating, repairing, enhancing, and defending who they are and would like to be. Clearly, personal identity is achieved mainly through activities, and people engage in a large proportion of activities as an expression of self, as manifested through the type of activity, the people with whom the activity is accomplished, and how the activity is conducted (McAdams, 1993). Sociologist Erving Goffman (1959) suggested that the issue of how activities are carried out can be fundamental to *self-presentation,* a term describing how people attempt to influence the perceptions of others during interactions. Goffman's research showed clearly that performance of an activity while unobserved is much different from performance of the same activity while others are present. The style of engagement can be drastically different, depending on the relationship of the person doing the activity to others who are present. Much of our knowledge about "how to do in public" comes from learning through observation, a process that is sometimes called *vicarious learning.*

Hogan (1983) claimed that the basis for social interaction occurs through roles (e.g., spouse, parent, friend, or colleague), each of which carries different behavioral expectations defined by the group (whether friends, family, workplace, or social organization). Individual differences in the extent to which people can successfully fulfill their roles account for variations in influence and popularity, which over time take on a more enduring quality, known as *reputation.*

Importance of Activities to Identity

We make sense of our lives through the activities that form our life stories. The activities in which we participate contribute to our sense of self (McAdams, 1993), or *identity*—that is, who we are.

Many theorists agree that the formation of an acceptable identity is central to how a person understands one's life. Understanding who we are requires social interaction, and the daily activities we choose shape how others perceive us. For example, Christiansen (1999) proposed that activity choice and engagement are required to create an identity, which in turn provides a context for creating meaning. By demonstrating competence and the ability to perform valued social roles responsibly, people establish themselves as accepted and valued members of groups. Similarly, psychologist Jerome Bruner (1990), in his well-regarded book *Acts of Meaning*, suggested that the creation of meaning occurs through engagement in activities that become part of a person's autobiography or personal narrative.

Scholars use the term *narrative* to describe personal or life-related stories. The central idea behind narrative is that people understand themselves and their lives through accounts that have central figures (ourselves), beginnings, middles, current situations, and future chapters. According to Mancuso and Sarbin (1985), any slice of life, when carefully considered, is interpreted and experienced as part of a story. In speaking of the influence of narrative in self-identity, Polkinghorne (1988) wrote the following:

> We achieve our personal identities and self-concept through the use of, and make our existence into a whole by understanding it as an expression of a single unfolding and developing story. We are in the middle of our stories and cannot be sure how they will end; we are constantly having to revise the plot as new events are added to our lives. Self, then, is not a static thing or a substance, but a configuring of personal events into an historical unity, which includes not only what one has been but also anticipations of what one will be. (p. 150)

Psychologist Dan McAdams of Northwestern University has devoted his career to studying the identities central to life stories (McAdams, 1993, 1999). Among his many interesting findings is the observation that many stories have common themes and that those central themes often pertain to developing relationships with others or demonstrating one's competence through achieving important goals. McAdams's research has shown that stories in which people view themselves as overcoming adversity to achieve success are associated with perceived well-being, whereas stories in which lives take an unfortunate turn for the worse and a person fails to realize his or her dreams are associated with depression and lower affect (McAuley & Katula, 1998). Note that developing relationships with others and demonstrating competence through the achievement of goals valued by self or others occur through participation in everyday activities.

How Personal Life Stories Motivate People to Engage in Activities

Because people interpret their lives as stories, they also live them as stories that have many possible endings. The possible future chapters and endings for stories involve many anticipated selves. These possible selves influence the choices people make and the behaviors they exhibit on a daily basis. People are motivated to become like people they want to be (e.g., wealthy, successful, or popular) and to avoid becoming like people they do not want to be (e.g., unpopular, unattractive, or unhealthy). Studies by psychologist Hazel Markus and her colleagues have shown that the images of possible selves provide important motivation to perform roles in ways that enhance people's social standing and views of themselves (Markus & Nurius, 1986). Clearly, then, engaging in activities is important to people because doing so enables the shaping of identity and the expression of self. Because activities are the principal means by which needs are met, it is hardly surprising that activity engagement reflects goals and is viewed by the World Health Organization (WHO) as fundamental to well-being and quality of life.

WHO View of the Importance of Everyday Activities

The WHO published a system for classifying illness and disease as they influence human function, the *International Classification of Functioning, Disability, and Health* (ICF; WHO, 2001). The ICF acknowledges that function, or participation in valued activities, represents an interaction between a person and an environmental context; in doing so, it recognizes that illness may limit participation in activities or performance of social roles (Table 1.3).

The ICF is a classification of health and health-related domains. It helps us describe changes in body function and structure, what people with a health condition can do in a standard environment (i.e., their level of capacity), and what they actually do in their usual environment (i.e., their level of performance):

> ICF puts the notions of "health" and "disability" in a new light. It acknowledges that every human being can experience a decrement in health and thereby experience some disability. This is not something that happens to

only a minority of humanity. ICF thus "mainstreams" the experience of disability and recognizes it as a universal human experience. By shifting the focus from cause to impact it places all health conditions on an equal footing, allowing them to be compared using a common metric—the ruler of health and disability. (WHO, 2002, p. 3)

This description of the ICF emphasizes that what matters to people when they have health problems is the manner in which such problems interfere with their participation in valued activities. The ability to participate fully in everyday life activities is a quality-of-life issue that has a profound effect on individual satisfaction and well-being (Christiansen, Backman, Little, & Nguyen, 1999).

The WHO (1995) defines *quality of life* as "a person's perception of his or her life as viewed in the context of goals, expectations, standards, and concerns (WHOQOL Group, 1995, p. 1405). Quality of life is thus a broad concept that is influenced in a complex way by the following individual factors:

- Physical health
- Psychological state
- Level of independence
- Environmental features
- Social relationships
- Personal beliefs (including spirituality).

The first four factors (i.e., the factors that enable participation) are often barriers to participation in activities and therefore represent the kinds of concerns typically addressed by occupational therapy. The remainder of this chapter, however, focuses on how the factors that enable participation influence the last two factors: social relationships and meaning. Participation in occupations is more than just passing time; it is the process through which people express their identities and create meaning in their lives.

Illness and Disability as Participation Restrictions

We expect to be able to pursue our goals and participate in the world around us through our actions and activities. We seldom anticipate that our pursuits will be interrupted by unforeseen events, as they can be when we become isolated from opportunity, restricted from participation by environmental circumstances, or experience illness and disability.

In 1977, Tristram Englehardt Jr., a physician and medical philosopher, published a paper in

Table 1.3. Structure and Classification Definitions From the *International Classification of Functioning, Disability, and Health*

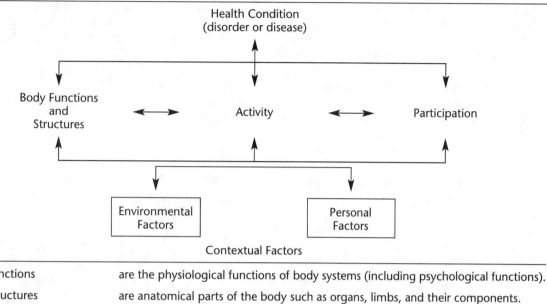

Body functions	are the physiological functions of body systems (including psychological functions).
Body structures	are anatomical parts of the body such as organs, limbs, and their components.
Impairments	are problems in body function or structure such as a significant deviation or loss.
Activity	is the execution of a task or action.
Participation	is involvement in a life situation.
Activity limitations	are difficulties a person may have in executing activities.
Contextual factors	include personal factors and environmental factors that influence health and functioning.
Personal factors	are internal influences on functioning and disability. These include gender, age, coping styles, social background, education, profession, past and current experience, overall behavior pattern, character, and other factors that influence how disability is experienced by the individual. These factors are not classified in ICF because of the wide social and cultural variation that influences these factors.
Environmental factors	make up the physical, social, and attitudinal environment in which people live and conduct their lives. These include: products and technology, the natural environment and human-made changes to the environment, support and relationships, attitudes, services.
Participation restrictions	are problems an individual may experience in involvement in life situations.

Note. Adapted from *The International Classification of Functioning, Disability, and Health,* by the World Health Organization, 2001, Geneva, Switzerland: Author. Copyright © 2001 by the World Health Organization. Used with permission.

which he observed, "Humans are healthy or diseased in terms of the activities open to them or denied them" (p. 667). His statement deserves further explanation.

Some illnesses, such as the common cold, are nuisances because of the discomfort and inconvenience they cause. People with colds may miss a day or two from their typical activities, but such inconveniences are temporary disruptions. In comparison, catastrophic illnesses and injuries, such as spinal paralysis or traumatic brain injury, result in the permanent disruption of the daily occupations that make up lives (Whiteford, 2004).

When disastrous health problems occur—often in an instant—people do not comprehend what has happened to them. Medical diagnoses such as "cerebral infarct" or "spinal cord lesion" are not part of most people's everyday language and are not readily understood. Patients and families typically want health care professionals to provide a practical explanation related to engagement in daily activities. Questions such as "Will I be able to ride my horse again?" or "Can I play the piano when I recover?" become the means for understanding the conditions because people's activities define their lives and who they are. In contrast to short-term illness and disability, extended disruptions become *deprivations* in that they deprive people of participating in the activities that allow them to define who they are and gain meaning.

When people are first confronted with a disabling condition that will result in permanent disability, they seldom ask whether they will be able to perform everyday activities such as eating without assistance or going to the toilet. Able-bodied people take these ordinary acts of self-maintenance for granted to such an extent that their basic place in everyday life is not apparent. It is only when their performance becomes difficult or impossible that their importance becomes evident. Indeed, people with disabilities who write about their own experiences typically comment on the unexpected challenges presented by their inability to perform routine daily tasks such as dressing and bathing.

In the following excerpt from *The Body Silent*, anthropologist Robert Murphy provides an account of the effects of a spinal tumor that progressively diminished his ability to live without assistance from others:

> I was quite self-sufficient back in that stage of my disability. I could dress my upper body, though I never did master pants and shoes, and I took care of most of my personal needs. I shaved, brushed my teeth, sponge bathed most of my body, and I used the toilet without assistance. Yolanda would go off to work every day, leaving lunch in the refrigerator, and I would fend for myself. I even managed to reheat coffee. The only time that I required help was in getting dressed in the morning and undressed at night. (2001, p. 62)

The abnormal cells that caused Murphy's tumor created gradual paralysis, which eventually cost him his life. Murphy experienced his condition not as a series of biological events but as a progressive barrier to performing the daily tasks he had previously taken for granted. When his inability to walk and his lack of arm strength and coordination limited his ability to participate in everyday activities at home and in the community, he recognized that his very identity as a college professor, husband, and father was threatened.

Murphy was unique in the sense that he had unusual insight into his situation and was able to continue for many years in his role as a professor despite his physical limitations. In another sense, however, his situation provides a typical example of the powerful consequences of being unable to participate in daily activities as a result of functional limitations involving thinking, feeling, or moving. Those consequences included a change in his life story and a threat to his identity, which he struggled hard to maintain even as his functional skills disintegrated.

Box 1.2. Spinal Cord Injury— Sudden Life Transition

Actor Christopher Reeve, who became famous in the movie *Superman*, is a notable example of a man who has experienced the traumatic life change of a spinal cord injury. His life changed dramatically in 1995 at the age of 42 after the horse he was riding in a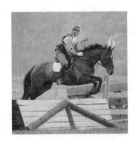

Photograph © Terri Miller. Used with permission.

competition balked at jumping a short fence. Because his hands were tangled in the reins, Christopher landed on his head, causing an injury to his spinal cord and permanent paralysis involving most of his body. Reeve remains active in various causes, including a drive to find a cure for paralysis. He has written a book entitled *Still Me (A Life)*, in which he talks about the importance of social relationships in bringing meaning to his life. The following excerpt from his book illustrates this:

> When a catastrophe happens it's easy to feel so sorry for yourself that you can't even see anybody around you. But the way out is through your relationships. The way out of that misery or obsession is to focus more on what your little boy needs or what your teenagers need or what other people around you need. It's very hard to do, and often you have to force yourself. But that is the answer to the dilemma of being frozen—at least it's the answer I found. (Reeve, 1998, p.14)

Activity Engagement and Threats to Identity

Sometimes, because of serious illness, disease, or injury, people are unable to return to their previous living situations and must make new sense of who they are and will become. Their identities change because their ability to perform important roles as parents, spouses, or workers may be reduced. Occupational therapists may be in daily contact with people whose self-identities are in transition (Mattingly & Fleming, 1993).

People with spinal cord injuries offer dramatic examples of how people experience abrupt role transitions. Patients with spinal cord injuries are often young, active men in excellent physical condition who were skiing or swimming in one instant and paralyzed for life in the next. During their rehabilitation, they encounter considerable anxiety regarding their roles as desirable marital partners, productive members of the workforce, and accepted members of their peer groups (Zejdlik, 1992).

Role transitions take place in other ways: In fact, they are a normal part of life. Everyone,

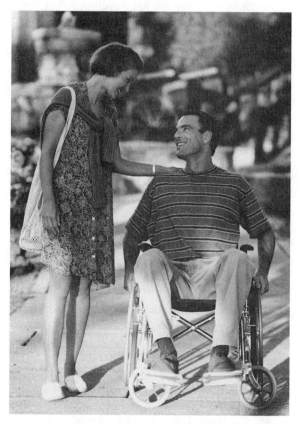

Figure 1.5. Social participation is thought to be important to the development of a personal identity, or a person's sense of self. When participation is restricted, this represents a threat to identity. Image © PhotoDisc, Inc.

whether disabled or not, must confront transitions because their circumstances and abilities change. For example, the aging process leads to a series of role changes at predictable stages in life. As young adults, people move from being students to being workers; they often marry and become parents. Later, parents may become grandparents.

As life progresses, physical and sensory skills decline and activities change. As the capacity for self-reliance declines, people may be placed in situations in which choice and control are limited (e.g., institutions and medical facilities), and their sense of self as competent members of society becomes diminished. During these life changes, acts that were previously viewed as ordinary or routine become symbols of competency. Thus, retaining or relearning the ability to perform tasks of self-maintenance, such as dressing without assistance, becomes a means of fostering self-identity.

People are expected to remain self-reliant unless they are incapable of caring for themselves. In society, people are typically excused from social obligations only when they are ill or otherwise incapable of performing their roles and responsibilities. Consider the idea of the "sick role." As described by Parsons (1951), the sick role is a transitional state in which people are exempt from typical role responsibilities during their recovery from an illness. Thus, when we have the flu, people excuse us from our everyday obligations. We are permitted to miss work or school, and most deadlines are extended automatically. This "exemption," however, requires that we take steps to facilitate our recovery, such as limiting our social activities and seeking medical attention if appropriate.

Unfortunately, when people become old or disabled, they are often seen as being in the sick role. Consequently, they risk being assigned a permanently diminished standing because they are exempt from engaging in valued social roles. According to Goffman (1963), they have become the victims of stigma because they are no longer seen as people who are capable of fulfilling their roles.

Stigma

Stigma describes a social situation in which a person is devalued because he or she cannot meet expected behavior in performing his or her role. Goffman (1963) portrayed all interaction as consisting of *crediting* or *discrediting* role performances. A discrediting role performance can result from any number of behaviors that are different from those expected within a given social situation. For example, Goffman noted that behaviors such as yawning, stuttering, or appearing nervous or self-conscious; problems with balance or muscular control; or lack of control of one's emotions can diminish the credibility of a person during a social encounter. Because people with physical or emotional disorders may be unable to control some behaviors that would be expected in a given situation, their performances can become discrediting. Thus, to avoid social stigma a person with obvious disabilities must learn to manage the impressions he or she conveys during social interaction.

Disfigurement

Stigma also can result from appearing to be different as a result of bodily disfigurement. Disfigurement refers to any physical abnormality that is sufficiently unusual as to be easily noticeable. Adolescents and young adults are frequently self-conscious about facial blemishes or acne because they believe it detracts from their appearance and places them at a disadvantage socially. Likewise, people with severe scarring, amputations, or other noticeable physical conditions that mark them as atypical have concerns about how those conditions affect the manner in which they will be accepted by others. A very bad haircut can be seen as spoiling one's appearance, but it can be corrected. A permanent condition is more of a problem, and although efforts may be made to disguise or hide such disfiguration, the psychological harm of feeling stigmatized is a disadvantage.

The movie *Elephant Man* (Cornfeld, Sanger, & Lynch, 1980) portrays the life of John Merrick, an Englishman with a severely disfiguring condition resulting in grotesque skin growths. In the 19th century, it was not unusual for people with disfigurements to be treated as "freaks" and placed in carnival sideshows by unscrupulous profiteers who sought to capitalize on the curiosity of the public. Befriended by a compassionate London physician, Frederick Treves, Merrick began to change his view of himself as the result of his acceptance by others.

Disability may result in a changed body image, which in turn may change both a person's view of self and others' views of him or her. The following excerpt from the book *Able Lives* (Morris, 1988), written to document the experiences of women with spinal cord injuries, illustrates this reality:

> One of the hardest parts of becoming disabled is acceptance of, and living with, a changed body image. Our body shape and the aids we use (a wheelchair or crutches) are the visible signs of disability. Appearance plays a very important part in interaction with other peo-

ple. What is more, women face an additional problem in that our physical attractiveness is generally the way our femininity and sexuality are measured by other people. (p. 160)

Thus, as the excerpt reveals, acceptance by others also requires maintaining expected standards of dress and appearance. People are expected to present themselves according to social norms, and appearance and dress have been shown to influence perceptions of status and competence (e.g., Ware & Williams, 1975).

The ability to manage basic self-care tasks is a fundamental prerequisite for successful social interaction for the able-bodied person, and it is no less important for the person with a disability. Overcoming stigma and regaining an acceptable social identity may be the most significant challenge confronting people with disabilities. Stigma presents a formidable social barrier and limits participation in other activities necessary for well-being.

Attitudinal Barriers to Participation

In recent years, people with conditions that limit their participation in society, rehabilitation professionals, and social activists have banded together to influence legislation and social policy. Part of their efforts stem from a recognition that language influences thoughts and attitudes (Bruce & Christiansen, 1988), so they have worked hard to introduce new terminology in medicine, law, and everyday language that does not perpetuate outdated views. The term *disablement* is preferred over the terms *disability* and *handicap* because it is intended to convey a view that a person's ability to participate in society reflects a circumstance based on a combination of factors, including body structure and function; attitudes; social policies; and physical structures in the built environment, such as buildings, vehicles, and streets, not just a person's physical impairment.

Occupational Deprivation and Disruption

As stated earlier, attitudes; policies; and environmental features, such as the design of objects, equipment, furniture, buildings, and even streets and parks, can combine with functional deficits to interfere with engagement in valued activities. That interference can lead to *occupational disruption* and *deprivation,* terms that have been introduced into the occupational science and occupational therapy literature to describe conditions that limit activity engagement (Whiteford, 2000, 2004). Occupational disruption is a temporary condition of being restricted from participation in necessary or meaningful occupations; it may be caused by illness, temporary relocation, or temporary unemployment (Stone, 2003). Most people experience occupational disruption at one time or another and find ways to cope with these temporary modifications of lifestyle and routine without significant lasting consequence.

In contrast, occupational deprivation involves prolonged exclusion from engaging in occupations that are necessary or meaningful. Conditions leading to deprivation are outside the control of the individual and may include geographic isolation, incarceration, or functional disability. Occupational therapy personnel can provide valuable assistance to help ameliorate the restrictions on participation brought about by occupational deprivation.

Studies of Participation and Well-Being

Social participation involves engagement in activities that are meaningful in life; its importance to well-being and quality of life has been demonstrated in recent research involving people with and without functional performance deficits. Many of the studies involving people with disabilities illustrate that functional ability is often not a significant determinant of either participation or well-being. For example, recent studies of people with spinal cord injury have found that life satisfaction is most

---

Box 1.3. Learning Activity

Imagine, for a disturbing moment, what life would be like if you were suddenly paralyzed from a spinal cord injury and had to depend on the assistance of others for your basic and instrumental activities of daily living. Rank the following concerns you would imagine having in those circumstances from 1–10 (most concern to you = 1, least concern = 10). Do you imagine that people differ in their concerns? What personal and contextual factors might explain those differences?

_____ Being employed
_____ Maintaining friendships
_____ Being an acceptable mate or spouse
_____ Being accepted by others
_____ Pursuing favorite hobbies
_____ Driving
_____ Traveling outside the community
_____ Being able to live in a comfortable environment
_____ Learning new ways of living
_____ Being able to have and care for children

---

influenced by role performance and the extent of participation in everyday activities and is not significantly influenced by degree of impairment or disability (Boschen, Tonack, & Gargaro, 2003; Dijkers, 1999; Fuhrer, Rintala, Hart, Clearman, & Young, 1992; LoBello et al., 2003). A prospective study of a large group of people with traumatic brain injury similarly concluded that factors associated with engagement in valued activities in the community predicted life satisfaction (Corrigan, Bogner, Mysiw, Clinchot, & Fugate, 2001).

Studies of people without disabilities have also shown that engagement in valued activities is related to higher levels of perceived well-being (happiness) and life satisfaction. For example, a longitudinal study of seniors in Manitoba, Canada, found that happiness, along with functional ability and mortality, was directly related to activity level (Menec, 2003). Of particular interest is the finding that different activities were associated with different outcomes. Engagement in social and productive activities was predictive of happiness, functional ability, and life span, whereas engagement in solitary activities, such as hobbies requiring careful handwork, was predictive of only happiness. The author concluded that social and productive activities may provide physiological benefits related to function and longevity; solitary activities may provide important psychological benefits that help engender a positive sense of well-being. The results are consistent with findings that engagement in social and high-demand leisure activities were associated with higher physical health scores, whereas engagement in low-demand leisure activities was associated with higher mental health scores (Everard, Lach, Fisher, & Baum, 2000). Everard (1999) found that the reasons for participation in activities also influenced well-being. Activities engaged in for social purposes predicted better well-being than activities pursued simply to pass time. This finding seems to support the important link between social relationships, activity, and identity described earlier in this chapter.

The potential importance of meaningful leisure activity was demonstrated in an interesting study by Waters and Moore (2002). The researchers asked samples of employed and unemployed people to report on their unmet needs, moods, and participation in leisure activities. Unemployed participants engaged in social leisure activities less and solitary activities more than employed particants; they reported higher levels of depression, lower self-esteem, and greater unmet needs than the employed. The meaning attained through social and

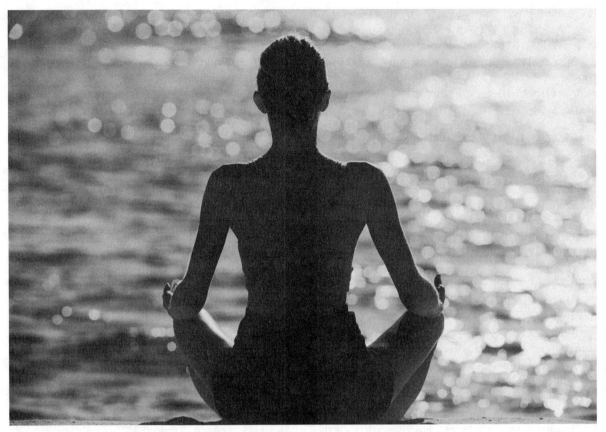

Figure 1.6. Studies have shown that engagement in occupation is important to health and well-being.

solitary leisure activities acted to reduce but not completely alleviate perceived feelings of deprivation and, thus, psychological distress in unemployed participants. Among the employed study participants, however, only social leisure had an impact on perceived deprivation and psychological health. The findings suggest that participation in leisure activities that are meaningful, rather than simply frequent, may be a constructive and readily achievable coping response during unemployment.

Other studies have shown that access to the environment through transportation and mobility is a significant factor in life satisfaction in people with disabilities because access enables opportunities for participation and engagement in valued activities. Studies of adolescents with severe burns (Barnum, Snyder, Rapoff, Mani, & Thompson, 1998), of children and adolescents with spina bifida (Appleton et al., 1997), of people with spinal cord injury (Elliott & Shewchuck, 1995; McColl & Skinner, 1995), and of adult men recovering from heart attacks (Sullivan, LaCroix, Russo, & Katon, 1998) support the importance of these factors in promoting adjustment and positive affect.

Summary

Enabling engagement in activity is an important and worthwhile goal for occupational therapy. Daily activities are part of the ordinary round of human time use; engagement in daily and other activities is necessary for well-being and quality of life. Humans are social and depend on others for understanding themselves, and activities help them construct meaning within the context of their life stories. Threats to activity engagement and social participation include occupational disruption and deprivation, of which disability is a major example. Occupational therapists can do much to promote or enable engagement in activities, thereby contributing to health, life satisfaction, and well-being for people whose function is compromised as well as for those who wish to remain active and healthy during the later stages of their lives. Recent research supports the assertions made in the chapter.

Study Questions

1. Why should sleep be considered an ADL?
2. Describe how IADL differ from BADL.

3. Describe the social importance of everyday activities.
4. How do activities contribute to identity building?
5. Discuss potential threats to identity associated with illness and injury.
6. Contrast the concepts of occupational deprivation and occupational disruption.
7. What types of activity seem to contribute most to perceived well-being?

References

Aas, D. (1980). *Designs for large scale time use studies of the 24 hour day. It's about time.* Sofia, Bulgaria: Institute of Sociology at the Bulgarian Academy of Science.

American Occupational Therapy Association. (2002). Occupational therapy practice framework: Domain and process. *American Journal of Occupational Therapy, 56,* 609–639.

Appleton, P. L., Ellis, N. C., Minchom, P. E., Lawson, V., Boell, V., & Jones, P. (1997). Depressive symptoms and self concept in young people with spina bifida. *Journal of Pediatric Psychology, 22*(5), 707–722.

Aronoff, M. S. (1991). *Sleep and its secrets: The river of crystal light.* Los Angeles: Insight Books.

Barnum, D. D., Snyder, C. R., Rapoff, M. A., Mani, M. M., & Thompson, R. (1998). Hope and social support in the psychological adjustment of children who have survived burn injuries and their matched controls. *Children's Health Care, 27*(1), 15–30.

Boschen, K. A., Tonack, M., & Gargaro, J. (2003). Long-term adjustment and community reintegration following spinal cord injury. *International Journal of Rehabilitation Research, 26*(3), 157–162.

Brudner, J., & Kellough, K. (2000). Volunteers in state government: Involvement, management and benefits. *Nonprofit and Voluntary Sector Quarterly, 29*(1), 111–130.

Bruce, M. A., & Christiansen, C. H. (1988). The issue is: Advocacy in word as well as deed. *American Journal of Occupational Therapy, 42,* 189–191.

Bruner, J. (1990). *Acts of meaning.* Cambridge, MA: Harvard University Press.

Christiansen, C. (1994). Classifications and study in occupation: A review and discussion of taxonomies. *Journal of Occupational Science, 2*(3), 3–21.

Christiansen, C. H. (1999). Occupation as identity: An essay on competence, coherence, and the creation of meaning. *American Journal of Occupational Therapy, 53*(6), 547–558.

Christiansen, C. H. (in press). Functional evaluation and management of self care and other activities of daily living. In J. DeLisa & B. Gans (Eds.), *Rehabilitation medicine: Principles and practice* (4th ed.). Philadelphia: Lippincott Williams & Wilkins.

Christiansen, C. H., Backman, C., Little, B. R., & Nguyen, A. (1999). Occupations and well-being: A study of personal projects. *American Journal of Occupational Therapy, 53*(1), 91–100.

Christiansen, C., & Townsend, E. (2004). An introduction to occupation. In C. Christiansen & E. Townsend (Eds.), *Introduction to occupation: The art and science of living* (pp. 1–28). Upper Saddle River, NJ: Prentice Hall.

Cornfeld, S., & Sanger, J. (Producers), & Lynch, D. (Director). (1980). *The elephant man* [Motion picture]. England: Brooksfilms.

Corrigan, J. D., Bogner, J. A., Mysiw, W., Clinchot, D., & Fugate, L. (2001). Life satisfaction after traumatic brain injury. *Journal of Head Trauma Rehabilitation, 6,* 543–554.

Dijkers, M. (1999). Correlates of life satisfaction among persons with spinal cord injury. *Archives of Physical Medicine and Rehabilitation, 80*(8), 867–876.

Elliott, T., & Shewchuck, R. (1995). Social support and leisure activities following severe physical disability: Testing the mediating effects of depression. *Basic and Applied Social Psychology, 16*(4), 471–487.

Englehardt, H. T. (1977). Defining occupational therapy: The meaning of therapy and the virtues of occupation. *American Journal of Occupational Therapy, 31*(10), 666–672.

Everard, K. (1999). The relationship between reasons for activity and older adult well being. *Journal of Applied Gerontology, 18*(3), 325–340.

Everard, K. M., Lach, H. W., Fisher, E. B., & Baum, M. C. (2000). Relationship of activity and social support to the functional health of older adults. *Journal of Gerontology: Psychological Sciences, 55,* S208–S212.

Fuhrer, M. J., Rintala, D. H., Hart, K. A., Clearman, R., & Young, M. E. (1992). Relationship of life satisfaction to impairment, disability, and handicap among persons with spinal cord injury living in the community. *Archives of Physical Medicine and Rehabilitation, 73,* 552–557.

Goffman, E. (1959). *The presentation of self in everyday life.* New York: Doubleday.

Goffman, E. (1963). *Stigma: Notes on the management of a spoiled identity.* Englewood Cliffs, NJ: Prentice Hall.

Hogan, R. (1983). A socioanalytic theory of personality. In M. M. Page (Ed.), *Nebraska Symposium on Motivation* (pp. 55–90). Lincoln: University of Nebraska Press.

Hogan, R., Jones, W. H., & Cheek, J. M. (1985). Socioanalytic theory: An alternative to armadillo psychology. In B. R. Schlenker (Ed.), *The self and social life* (pp. 175–201). New York: McGraw-Hill.

Hogan, R., & Sloan, T. (1991). Socioanalytic foundations for personality psychology, *Perspectives in Personality, 3*(Part B), 1–15.

Holmberg, K., Rosen, D., & Holland, J. L. (1990). *The leisure activities finder.* Odessa, FL: Psychological Assessment Resources.

Huizinga, J. (1950). *Homo ludens: A study of the play element in culture.* Boston: Beacon Press.

Klinger, E. (1998). The search for meaning in evolutionary perspective and its clinical implications. In P. T. P. Wong & P. S. Fry (Eds.), *The human quest for meaning* (pp. 27–50). Mahwah, NJ: Erlbaum.

Lawton, M. P. (1971). The functional assessment of elderly people. *Journal of the American Geriatric Society, 19*(6), 465–481.

Lawton, M. P. (1990). Age and the performance of home tasks. *Human Factors, 32*(5), 527–536.

LoBello, S. G., Underhil, A. T., Valentine, P. V., Stroud, T. P., Bartolucci, A. A., & Fine, P. R. (2003). Social integration and life and family satisfaction in survivors of injury at 5 years postinjury. *Journal of Rehabilitation Research and Development, 40*(4), 293–300.

Mancuso, J. C., & Sarbin, T. R. (1985). The self narrative in the enactment of roles. In T. R. Sarbin & K. E. Schiebe (Eds.), *Studies in social identity* (pp. 233–253). New York: Praeger.

Markus, H., & Nurius, P. (1986). Possible selves. *American Psychologist, 41,* 954–969.

Mattingly, C., & Fleming, M. (1993). *Clinical reasoning: Forms of inquiry in a therapeutic practice.* Philadelphia: F. A. Davis.

McAdams, D. P. (1993). *The stories we live by: Personal myths and the making of the self.* New York: Guilford.

McAdams, D. P. (1999). Personal narratives and the life story. In L. A. Pervin & O. P. John (Eds.), *Handbook of personality: Theory and research* (pp. 478–500). New York: Guilford.

McAuley, J., & Katula, J. (1998). Physical activity interventions in the elderly: Influence on physical health and psychological function. In G. Schulz, G. Maddox, & P. Lawton (Eds.), *Interventions research with older adults: Annual review of gerontology and geriatrics* (18th ed., pp. 111–155). New York: Springer.

McColl, M., & Skinner, H. (1995). Assessing inter- and intrapersonal resources: Social support and coping among adults with a disability. *Disability and Rehabilitation, 17*(1), 24–34.

McKinnon, A. L. (1992). Time use for self care, productivity and leisure among elderly Canadians. *Canadian Journal of Occupational Therapy, 59*(2), 102–110.

Menec, V. H. (2003). The relation between everyday activities and successful aging: A 6-year longitudinal study. *Journal of Gerontology, 58*(2), S74–S82.

Morris, J. A. (Ed.). (1988). *Able lives.* London: The Women's Press.

Murphy, R. (2001). *The body silent.* New York: Norton.

Ohayon, M. M., Zulley, J., Guilleminault, C., Smirne, S., & Priest, R. G. (2001). How age and daytime activities are related to insomnia in the general population: Consequences for older people. *Journal of Gerontology, 49*(4), 360–366.

Parham, L. D., & Fazio, L. S. (1997). *Play in occupational therapy for children.* St. Louis, MO: Mosby.

Parsons, T. (1951). *The social system.* London: Routledge & Kegan Paul.

Polkinghorne, D. (1988). *Narrative knowing and the human sciences.* Albany: State University of New York Press.

Reeve, C. (1998). *Still me (A life).* New York: Ballantine.

Stebbins, R. A. (1997). Casual leisure: A conceptual statement. *Leisure Studies, 16,* 17–25.

Stone, S. (2003). Workers without work: Injured workers and well-being. *Journal of Occupational Science, 10*(1), 7–13.

Sullivan, M. D., LaCroix, A. Z., Russo, J., & Katon, W. J. (1998). Self-efficacy and self-reported functional status in coronary heart disease: A six-month perspective study. *Psychosomatic Medicine, 60,* 473–478.

Sutton-Smith, B. (2001). *The ambiguity of play.* Cambridge, MA: Harvard University Press.

Szalai, A. (Ed.). (1972). *The use of time.* The Hague: Mouton.

Tinsley, H. (1995). Psychological benefits of leisure participation: A taxonomy of leisure activities based on their need-gratifying properties. *Journal of Counseling Psychology, 42,* 123–132.

Ware, J. E., Jr., & Williams R. G. (1975). The Dr. Fox effect: A study of lecturer effectiveness and ratings of instruction. *Journal of Medical Education, 50,* 149–156.

Waters, L., & Moore, K. (2002). Reducing latent deprivation during unemployment: The role of meaningful leisure activity. *Journal of Occupational and Organizational Psychology, 75*(1), 15–32.

Whiteford, G. (2000). Occupational deprivation: Global challenge in the new millennium. *British Journal of Occupational Therapy, 64*(5), 200–210.

Whiteford, G. (2004). When people cannot participate: Occupational deprivation. In C. Christiansen & E. Townsend (Eds.), *Introduction to occupation: The art and science of living* (pp. 221–242). Upper Saddle River, NJ: Prentice Hall.

World Health Organization. (1995). *WHOQOL: Measuring quality of life.* Geneva: Author.

World Health Organization. (2001). *International classification of functioning, disability and health. ICIDH-2.* Geneva: Author.

World Health Organization. (2002). *Towards a common language for functioning, disability and health.* Geneva: Author.

WHOQOL Group. (1995). The world health organization quality of life assessment (WHOQOL): Position paper from the World Health Organization. *Social Science and Medicine, 41*(10), 1403–1409.

Yelin, E., Lubeck, D., Holman, H., & Epstein, W. (1987). The impact of rheumatoid arthritis and osteoarthritis: The activities of patients with rheumatoid arthritis and osteoarthritis compared to controls. *Journal of Rheumatology, 14*(4), 710–717.

Zejdlik, C. (1992). *Management of spinal cord injury* (2nd ed.). Boston: Jones and Bartlett.

Zerubavel, E. (1981). *Hidden rhythms: Schedules and calendars in social life.* Chicago: University of Chicago Press.

Zerubavel, E. (1985). The harmonics of timekeeping. In E. Zerubavel (Ed.), *The seven day circle: The history and meaning of the week* (pp. 61–106). New York: Free Press.

Zerubavel, E. (1989). *The seven day circle: The history and meaning of the week.* Chicago: University of Chicago Press.

Chapter 2

The Meaning of Self-Care Occupations

GELYA FRANK, PHD

CAROL STEIN, MA, OTR/L

KEY TERMS

activity limitation

aesthetic anxiety

compassion

disability

division of labor

environmental factors

existential anxiety

health condition

illness

impairment

infantilization

performance failure

personal factors

reciprocity

sick role

stigma

stigma symbols

OBJECTIVES

Upon completion of this chapter, the reader will be able to

- Define illness and disability from the standpoint of activity and social participation;
- Explain how being able to do basic activities of daily living independently can influence a person's feelings about self-concept;
- Understand how basic activities of daily living, such as eating, grooming, and toileting, have important social and cultural meanings;
- Discuss how occupational therapists can help clients discover new and better ways to care for themselves;
- Describe how institutional care can objectify the lives of the residents and become a source of alienation; and
- Understand the social importance of meals.

Daily activities are laden with personal meaning, but when they are described in purely technical terms, they become impersonal. For example, occupational therapists use words such as "toileting," "grooming," and "feeding" to refer to components of an area of occupational performance known as *activities of daily living* (ADL). This stark, impersonal, and technical language strips away the rich meanings that the body and its functions take on in our culture and offends most occupational therapists worthy of their professional title.

The biological sciences consider using the bathroom, combing hair, putting on clothes, and eating as objective events; they may describe them, for example, as a set of muscle movements. But when someone suffers a stroke or spinal cord injury or becomes the parent of a child with a birth defect, he or she quickly discovers worlds of significance packed into even the simplest self-care activities. When occupational therapists speak to people about their self-care, they need a language that fits their clients' experiences.

Defining Symptoms in Occupational Terms

Health condition refers to a disease, disorder, or injury as defined by medical science. Social scientists use *illness* to refer to a person's experience of that disorder or suffering (Eisenberg, 1977). Medical anthropologist Arthur Kleinman (1988) coined the term *illness problems* to refer to the practical problems that affect one's ability to perform one's usual daily activities; the World Health Organization (WHO) uses the term *activity limitations* to mean the same thing (WHO, 2002). Illness problems are a key part of the way we give meaning to the group of problems that arise because of our disease:

> Illness problems are the principal difficulties that symptoms and disability create in our lives. For example, we may be unable to walk up our stairs to our bedroom. Or we may experience distracting low back pain while we sit at work. Headaches may make it impossible to focus on homework assignments or housework, leading to failure and frustration. Or there may be impotence that leads to divorce. (Kleinman, 1988, p. 4)

Kleinman (1988) suggested that health care providers have a better chance of giving meaningful care when they gain an understanding of a patient's illness experience or activity limitation. Chronic illnesses, he noted, swing back and forth between good and bad times. Knowing how a backache limits a patient, for example, can enable a health care provider to help that person deal with feelings and practical problems that make the bad times worse. Thus, according to Kleinman, medical care for people with chronic illnesses should include (1) "empathic witnessing of the experience of suffering" and (2) "practical coping with the major psychosocial crises that occur from time to time" (p. 10). Occupational therapists are well qualified professionally to carry out this prescription.

Self-Care Experiences— The Importance of "Self"

Adults' personal accounts of their own illnesses or of parenting children with chronic illnesses and disabilities illustrate the personal side of self-care activities. The body's failure to perform activities once taken for granted threatens the sense of self (Corbin & Strauss, 1988). In all stories, a defining moment separates the experience of the disability from an earlier, sweeter time that can never be recaptured.

Agnes de Mille, dancer and choreographer, first noticed symptoms of the stroke she suffered when her hand did not work to sign a contract. In her 70s at the time, de Mille saw this performance failure as a threat to her lifetime identity: "Please do something fast," she told her doctor, "because I've got to be on the stage in one hour delivering a very difficult lecture and I've never been late for anything in the theater in my life" (de Mille, 1981, pp. 21–22).

People who become disabled often say that their bodies or some body parts become alien to them. Sometimes parts of their bodies even seem dead. "Half of me was imprisoned in the other half," wrote de Mille (1981, p. 57) about the weeks immediately after her stroke. Six months later, she felt as though her whole self were split in two: "My right arm, my right leg, that whole side of my body gone. I was to be two bodies, one of them not my friend, alien. And must I drag this creature about with me, this Siamese horror, forever? Forever not my friend? Very likely" (de Mille, 1981, p. 219).

Nine months after a modified radical mastectomy for breast cancer, poet Audre Lorde expressed a similar feeling—the longing for a past self who could perform daily activities effortlessly. Lorde wrote, "I must be content to see how really little I can do and still do it with an open heart. I can never accept this, like I can't accept that turning my life around is so hard, eating differently, sleeping differently, moving differently, being differently. . . . I want the old me, bad as before" (Lorde, 1980, pp. 11–12).

In moments when the body performs better, the old sense of self may return. Like those of the women above, Robert F. Murphy's (1987) personal history was "divided radically into two parts: pre-wheelchair and post-wheelchair," but his return to the lecture halls of Columbia University, even in a wheelchair, meant a return to his former self: "Hey, it's the same old me inside this body!" (p. 81).

It is rarely possible to recover the "same old me" without re-evaluating one's identity. Social psychologists working with clients in rehabilitation say that "adjustment" to disability requires accentuating the positive—one's remaining assets—and turning away from the negatives—what is missing (Wright, 1983). Efforts to reconstruct one's personal identity after chronic illness and disability may be called *biographical work* (Corbin & Strauss, 1988).

The struggles detailed in the narratives of this chapter show how participation restrictions (formerly called "handicaps") interfere with the daily activities of each of these people and the importance they attributed to overcoming them. For example, de Mille, who finally managed to get to the toilet in the night using a three-pronged cane without falling or bumping herself, wrote, "My trip to the bathroom in privacy and decency meant more to me than a rave notice in the [New York] *Times*" (1981, p. 167).

"Unspeakable Practices"—Toileting

The ability to go to the toilet is closely entwined with one's identity. An illustration of this principle comes from the experience of Irving Kenneth Zola, a sociologist, who lived at Het Dorp, a planned independent living community in the Netherlands for people with physical disabilities, for a week as a participant observer and spokesperson for the independent living movement (Zola, 1982). During his stay, Zola decided to use a wheelchair for the first time in decades to report how, from his new position in a wheelchair, he handled the "unspeakable practices" of urinating and defecating. It was an experience that led him to reevaluate the part disability played in his identity.

Getting off the wheelchair and onto the toilet, sitting on the toilet, and getting back onto the wheelchair, Zola realized two things: First, the bathroom's barrier-free design made this process work more easily than he remembered it. Using the grab bar, he was able to raise himself from the toilet despite his weak stomach muscles and legs. He became aware of how unnecessary his previous difficulties in going to the bathroom had been. Second, Zola

felt uncomfortable using the toilet from a seated position. He felt that a man of his age ought to urinate standing up. With his permission, readers may follow him into the bathroom on the morning of Friday, May 26, 1972:

Two difficulties did remain. For lack of a better term I call the first one "cultural" and the second "psychosocial." As a Western man I had been trained to urinate standing with both feet firmly planted on the ground. Thus, to sit and urinate took some getting used to. This did, however, provide a side benefit. Standing I had always needed one hand free to steady myself. Sitting at least made it a more relaxed activity. My second problem was more "psychosocial." Before leaving the bathroom I tried to think if I had "to go" again. Once more I was reduced to the status of a child as I recalled parental admonitions to the effect, "We are starting on a trip so you better use the toilet now." I did the same thing with my own children. What were the toilet facilities like elsewhere in the Village? Would they be as easy to negotiate as the one in my room? (Zola, 1982, pp. 65–66)

Zola's story shows how the ability and willingness to adapt behavior—even in the most private situations—may hinge on unspoken cultural rules defining social identity. His ability to step back and observe his reactions helped him. Such critical thinking can help other people with disabilities make choices about what works for them.

Architectural Barriers and Special Equipment

In Zola's case, barriers that he had experienced previously when manipulating a wheelchair were not present in the bathrooms at Het Dorp; the environment there promoted a positive identity. Murphy (1987), writing about his progressive paralysis as a result of a spinal cord tumor, showed how the physical environment can affect the meaning of symptoms, thereby affecting identity. The tumor made it difficult for him to climb the stairs, but the bedrooms and his study were on the second floor. Murphy became confined to the first floor of his two-story suburban home. He had considered getting a stairway lift, but the cost was so high that it would have been cheaper to buy a new home. All discussion about getting Murphy up to the second floor ended one day in 1977 when his son and his son's friend carried him upstairs. Murphy discovered that the bathrooms would have to be torn up to make them accessible. That was the last time he saw the second floor of his house. As it turned out, Murphy's paralysis soon worsened to the point that he would not have been able to get to and from the lift and his wheelchairs anyway.

Murphy moved permanently to the family room on the first floor, to which a half bathroom was added. This event marked Murphy's change in status within the family and in society. His choice of activities and the quality of his life became increasingly dictated by the demands of his self-care and the nature of his own house as well as that of cars, motels, restaurants, and doorways in the world around him. He lamented the loss of his ability to move spontaneously, which resulted in the loss of aspects of his self:

> I could go nowhere without a driver, usually Yolanda [Murphy's wife] or Bob [his son], and every trip entailed logistics. If we wanted to eat at a restaurant or go to the movies, we had to call first to make sure there were no steps. And if we wanted to stay at a motel, we had to measure the width of the bathroom door, for my wheelchair is twenty-six inches wide. Whenever we traveled, we needed equipment. Aside from the wheelchair, we had to transport the walker, bedpan, urinal, and assorted accessories. As my condition worsened, the list grew longer. Gone were the days when we would give in to a sudden urge to go somewhere or do something. But gone also were the days when I could wander into the kitchen for a snack or outside for a breath of fresh air. This loss of spontaneity invaded my entire assessment of time. It rigidified my short-range perspectives and introduced a calculating quality into an existence that formerly had been pleasantly disordered. (Murphy, 1987, p. 76)

Home Care, Family Dynamics, and Rehabilitation Policy

A separate meaning to self-care exists for the caretaker. Within marriages, or with people who live together, the couple typically works together to manage activity limitations (Corbin & Strauss, 1988). For example, a husband may help perform the self-care activities of his wife. Consequently, how the recipient of care experiences eating, dressing, and going to the bathroom will be colored by the experiences of the caretaker.

Often the division of labor in the family becomes unbalanced when a spouse or children take care of another family member's basic needs. Feelings of exhaustion, depression, anxiety, self-pity, and resentment are common. Caretakers often feel guilty about their reactions. In a study about couples managing chronic illness at home, one woman described her exhaustion over the physical work she did to help her husband:

> All night long he would say, "Get me water, put me on the commode." I would tell K., "Let me sleep; let me rest. I don't mind waiting on you hand and foot during the day, but at night let me sleep". . . . He got out of bed one night and urinated all over the floor. I had to get up and clean him up and put him back to bed. I didn't realize he was taking up so much of my energy. That twenty-four hour stuff was getting to me . . . . After he died, I was so exhausted. . . . I am still. . . . God was good to me in a way. Had [my husband] been sick any longer, it would have broken me physically and financially. (Corbin & Strauss, 1988, pp. 293–294)

Women, whether or not they work outside the home, are still responsible for most of the caring for family members with chronic illnesses and disabilities (Abel & Nelson, 1990). Studies show that wives more commonly remain married to and help with the self-care duties of their husbands with chronic illness or disability than the reverse (Asch & Fine, 1988).

When men help their wives or children with self-care activities, they experience the same pressures, of course. As traditional gender roles give way to more equal sharing of household tasks, more research is needed to show how men learn to provide primary care needs (Hochschild, 1989). Traditional gender roles still govern men's behavior, however; for example, read how one older man explained his resentment in the role of caregiver for his wife:

> I am a bundle of nerves because I can't get out and play handball anymore. I have to give up my sex life. I am a healthy physical man. It is a toughie. You can't masturbate at seventy-three; it isn't going to do you any good. I'll be honest with you, there isn't a dame that I miss when I go out shopping or anywhere. . . . Sometimes I get impatient. She pushes me pretty hard in the morning: "I want my cereal. You didn't do this." I say, "Give me a chance. If you were in the hospital, you would have three or four attendants." I lift her out of the bed onto the commode. I have to make sure of the catheter. I say, "Honey, I only have two legs, two arms, and one mind." I can't afford to have someone living here full time. I would have to mortgage my house. Some of the bills I have received from the doctors are unbeliev-

able. It has been a year now and I am still paying on some. . . . She gets depressed and so do I. . . . Some of my friends are going to Reno on a bus. I wish I could climb on the bus and go with them. (Corbin & Strauss, 1988, p. 296)

Josh Greenfeld, father of a child with emotional disabilities, wrote about his fear that he always will have to take care of his son Noah's bathroom problems. Greenfield's fears about the future magnified the unpleasantness of his present situation:

What a night! Noah was up all of it. Two urinations, two b.m.'s, four diaper changes in all. And the period in between, he bounced and jumped and chirped.

Obviously Noah isn't making much headway; he has become more and more lax in his toilet training. And when I project, all I see is a sleepy life of never-ending diaper changing for us all. (Greenfeld, 1972, pp. 106–107)

Excessive responsibility as a parent caused Helen Featherstone's outrage when a practitioner suggested a small addition to her son Jody's home program. It was recommended that she brush Jody's teeth three times per day for 5 min with an electric toothbrush to counteract gum overgrowth caused by his antiseizure medication. Featherstone, mother of three children, was handling so many demands already that she exploded:

Jody, I thought, is blind, cerebral-palsied, and retarded. We do his physical therapy daily and work with him on sounds and communication. We feed him each meal on our laps, bottle him, change him, bathe him, dry him, put him in a body cast to sleep, launder his bed linens daily, and go through a variety of routines designed to minimize his miseries and enhance his joys and his development. (All this in addition to trying to care for and enjoy our other young children and making time for each other and our careers.) Now you tell me that I should spend fifteen minutes every day on something that Jody will hate, an activity that will not help him to walk or even defecate, but one that is directed at the health of his gums. This activity is not for a finite time but forever. It is not guaranteed to make the overgrowth go away but may retard it. Well, it's too much. Where is that fifteen minutes going to come from? What am I supposed to give up? Taking the kids to the park? Reading a bedtime story to my eldest? Washing the breakfast dishes? Sorting the laundry? Grading students' papers? Sleeping? Because there is no time in my life that hasn't been

spoken for, and for every fifteen-minute activity that is added, one has to be taken away. (Featherstone, 1980, pp. 77–78)

People who receive their care at home often are highly aware of the sacrifices their families make for them and try to avoid demanding too much. While visiting the independent living community at Het Dorp, Zola found that the residents frequently mentioned how much freer they felt there for this reason. Such comments triggered a childhood memory for Zola: He remembered trying to avoid bothering his parents, partly because he disliked feeling guilty and childish because he could not take care of himself:

I recalled the experience of confinement at home after my accident. As much as my parents assured me of their love, I could not help but feel that I was a burden. So gradually I tried to adjust: to eat, to sleep, to defecate when it was convenient for them. They never asked for that adjustment, but I knew that if I made them stay up later, or get out of bed to fetch something, I would feel not only more like a little child, but guilty for making demands! (Zola, 1982, p. 126)

The recipient and caretaker shape the meaning of health care, but it is, in an important sense, also shaped by public policy (Fisher & Tronto, 1990; Strauss & Corbin, 1988). Access to health insurance; insurance coverage for rehabilitation services; and the availability and quality of nursing homes, attendant care, and respite care all contribute to the meaning of self-care within relationships between caregivers and the family members for whom they care.

Hospitals and Institutional Care

If the receiver's healthy idea of self-care is turned negative by a relative caretaker's attitude, imagine what happens in a hospital, the "physician's workshop," a factory for the sick (Rosenberg, 1987). The standard procedures of the hospital depersonalize patients. Hospital patients depend on strangers for their care. Routines dictate not only when to eat, comb hair, or wash but also, on occasion, when to go to the bathroom.

If dinner is scheduled for 4:30 p.m., as it was on a floor in which I once spent two months, then that's when you eat. And if your bowels don't move often enough to suit the nursing staff, laxatives are the answer. The infamous routine that demands that all temperatures be taken at 6:00 a.m. is well known to all who have been patients. I even spent five weeks on one floor where I was bathed at 5:30 every morning because the daytime nurses were too busy to do it. (Murphy, 1987, pp. 20–21)

Arnold Beisser was hospitalized for 3 years beginning in 1950 after becoming paralyzed by polio. His alienation from his own failed body—"[I was] more like a sack of flour than a human being" (1989, p. 21)—grew worse because of depersonalized care. Beisser spent every moment of the first year and a half on his back in an iron lung. A young man in his mid-20s who had been a national tennis champion and was a medical school graduate, he could no longer perform bladder and bowel functions that used to be automatic, even though he felt the urges. He had to depend on strangers to help him:

> Intermittently people would open one or another of the portholes of my new metal skin and invade my private space. They would enter the most personal and private parts of me as they reached inside to move a leg or arm, or insert a needle or a bedpan. There was not even the pretense that my new space belonged to me, and entry beneath my new metal skin was at the discretion of others. (Beisser, 1989, p. 18)

Beisser's body boundary was now the iron lung; his head, which remained outside the machine, was the only part of him that was recognizably human. Lying on his back, vulnerable, Beisser viewed the people who approached him as attackers:

> I would often see their shadows before I saw them. They came at me from above like great condors, diving toward my exposed soft parts. People would capriciously and suddenly enter my most private spaces to do what was "best" for me. Since they did not ask my permission before doing things to me, they were like hostile invasions, and I felt violated. (p. 23)

Beisser discovered that nurses and technicians treated his body as an object. He would become enraged to find that they had made judgments for him, assuming that they knew whether he felt hot or cold. But he quickly learned to smile patiently and to explain to his nurses why he might need the blanket despite their perception that he did not: He dared not express his anger for fear of being punished by being ignored or handled roughly:

> You cannot get mad in hospitals. If you do, you may be in trouble. The next time you call for something, there may be a long delay in the nurses' response, or no response at all. There is always more than enough for the nurses to do in hospitals, so some things come

first and some are left unattended. Angry patients come last. (p. 19)

People who must depend on others for help with bowel and bladder functions are sometimes treated like infants. Beisser realized that he was seen as a baby. Some of his caregivers were concerned with controlling an unruly child or with nurturing a helpless infant:

> Nurses and attendants often talked to me as if I were a baby. If I became soiled through no fault of my own, they were likely to say, "Naughty, naughty," or "You've been a bad boy." Some people were so perplexed that they simply fled in despair. None of these attitudes helped clarify my confusion about how I thought of myself. (p. 22)

Note that these examples occurred almost 15 years ago. Today, saying such things as "You've been a bad boy" to a patient under these conditions would be considered verbal abuse, which is not to be tolerated.

Beisser's survival needs were "just a job" for some of his caregivers. A nurse or attendant might leave him suspended midair in a lift or in some other awkward position when the schedule called for her to go on a coffee break. Getting help while the nurses changed their work shift was impossible, no matter how urgent the problem. Beisser felt completely humiliated by these heartless helpers, to whom he gave such nicknames as "Leona the Late," "Ed the Reluctant," and "Ivan the Terrible." He felt robbed of his sense of himself as a person and made to feel like "an undeserving outsider" (Beisser, 1989, p. 37).

Beisser had a completely different set of experiences, however, with several helpers on the hospital staff who had compassion for his situation and treated his needs as more important than their own. With them, he learned about the life-enhancing effects of care that is generously given and felt "returned from exile" and "a pariah forgiven for his crime" (Beisser, 1989, p. 38). It had been dehumanizing to have to worry about his basic needs. Simply knowing that compassionate and willing helpers were present made it possible for Beisser to relax and tolerate otherwise unbearable physical sensations:

> Getting enough air, being able to go to the bathroom when necessary, having enough food and rest are urgent needs, and I could do none of these elemental things for myself. When those needs were not met, I could not be compassionate to someone else. There is no opportunity for higher levels of human function when you are short of air, and all that you can think of is getting the next

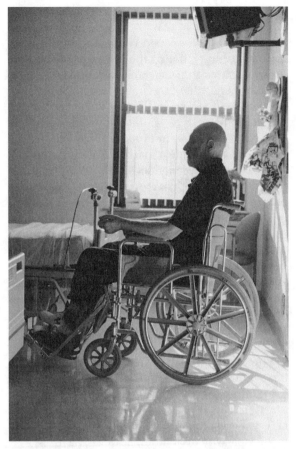

Figure 2.1. Often, the presence of a disability can result in stigma, creating feelings of isolation and social rejection. Image © Photodisc, Inc.

breath. I am not good for anything else unless these needs are met. But here is the remarkable thing. The urgency with which I experience my needs depends on the confidence I have that they can be met, whether they are or not. They are not so urgent when I am surrounded by people who willingly help me if called upon. (p. 39)

Feeding, Eating, and Dining

The body's failure to perform, barriers in the physical environment, the lack of helpers, and institutional routines also affect the meaning of eating. Eating and going to the bathroom have profoundly different social meanings, but when the body cannot perform either of these tasks, even our friends and relatives can become disgusted—and their reactions increase our own shame. Excretion is the most private and unseen activity. When others witness our difficulty with going to the bathroom, we are filled with a profound shame. Irish author Christo-

pher Nolan wrote about his "agony" as a 15-year-old schoolboy trying to sit through a science lesson and control his bowels after a dose of laxative. Born with cerebral palsy, he was used to asking for help except in going to the bathroom: "He knew he cast roles of responsibility on his fresh-faced friends, but bringing him to the toilet was a chore he would never ask them to do for him" (Nolan, 1987, p. 117).

In contrast, eating is the most social of activities. Ideally, meals are shared. Partaking of food together means being involved in social relations, being a recognizable member of the human community and of family life. When we foul our clothing or our table, we lose that recognition.

Murphy's inability to feed himself, a kind of performance failure, resulted in frustration and anger not because he would go hungry, but because he had lost an essential mark of his human identity:

> A paralytic may struggle to walk and become enraged when he cannot move his leg. Or a quadriplegic may pick up a cup of coffee with stiffened hands and drop it on his lap, precipitating an angry outburst. I had to give up spaghetti because I could no longer twirl it on my fork, and dinner would end for me in a sloppy mess. This would so upset me that I would lose my appetite. (Murphy, 1987, pp. 106–107)

Feeding Oneself—Shame and Pride

Diane DeVries, a woman born in 1950 without legs and with short arm stumps (Frank, 2000), suggested that people with disabilities may experience deep shame about not being able to eat normally in public. Despite having no forearms or hands, DeVries imposed strict standards of table behavior on herself and others who had disabilities similar to her own:

> Whatever I did, like feed myself, drink, I was able to do it without any sloppiness. You know, I've even seen a girl at camp with no arms that bent down and lapped her food up like a dog. . . . And I knew her. And I went up to her and said, "Why in the hell do you do that?" And I said, "They asked if you wanted a feeder or your arms on. You could have done either one, but you had to do that." She said, "Well, it was easy for me." To me that was gross. She finally started wearing arms, and she started feeding herself. But that to me was just stupid, because people wouldn't even want to eat at the same table as her. (Frank, 1986, p. 209)

DeVries was proud of her own ability to eat and drink by herself without making a mess (Frank, 1986). Eating without help, like controlling one's bowel and bladder, is an important developmental milestone. Children with disabilities may never develop a healthy sense of self and gain the acceptance of others unless they find or are taught alternative socially acceptable ways of eating and going to the bathroom (Gliedman & Roth, 1980).

DeVries's discovery of a way to feed herself, using her above-elbow stumps, became an important foundation for developing a sense of herself as a competent person:

> I have been [feeding myself] for so long that I cannot recall when I took my first independent mouthful of food. According to Irene [Diane's mother], this memorable event occurred one morning when she left me sitting in my highchair before a bowl of cereal, as she went to prepare dishwater over at the sink. When she returned I was balancing a spoonful of food on the rim of the bowl, and by applying pressure to the spoon's handle, I was able to raise the food-laden spoon high enough for it and my mouth to meet. I was about three years old. (DeVries, 1992, p. 112)

Food Choices—Preferences and Limitations

Getting food into one's mouth or adjusting to being fed by others can be extremely upsetting. But it is just as threatening to discover that a disability demands that you eat different food. A person developing a metabolic disorder, such as diabetes, will find the need to change his or her eating habits a life-and-death struggle. In fact, in a study of social factors contributing to the deaths of 40 patients on dialysis, researchers found that 11 deaths classified as due to cardiac arrest could be reclassified as resulting from eating restricted food, such as potato chips and beer, and ignoring restrictions on the intake of fluids (Plough, 1986; Plough & Salem, 1982). Some people would rather risk dying than change their choice of comfort foods.

Hospitals schedule meals without considering patient preferences, and at times they provide nutrition in forms that are unpalatable. When Anne Finger was in the hospital to give birth, the carton of milk she was given repelled her as much as the plastic meal. From her viewpoint as a lactose-intolerant woman, the routine institutional meal was inedible:

> My breakfast tray arrives. Since I am on a liquid diet, I get a carton of milk—which I can't drink because I am lactose intolerant—a plastic container of reconstituted orange juice, a cup of beef broth and a square of red Jell-O on

a white plastic plate. I drink the orange juice. (Finger, 1990, p. 123)

We are what we eat. In Western countries in the late 19th century, during the Industrial Revolution, fleshy bodies signified wealth and health. Even in the 1950s and 1960s, the "meat-and-potatoes" man was a man of means. But by the late 20th century, the ideal body type and food preferences had changed. Abstention from food, along with a slim, "hard" body, became a marker of status in the advanced capitalist economies (Bordo, 1990). Within a few decades, the meat-and-potatoes man had become a dying ideal and a dying breed. Popular media highlighted the rise of eating disorders, such as bulimia and anorexia, which probably have always existed but suddenly acquired new social meanings (Bell, 1985).

What we eat reflects our social standing. A man who buys pizza and beer on a date may be viewed differently from one who buys filet mignon and cabernet sauvignon, depending on the context. Sometimes the identification with the food we eat is so strong as to become a definition: "I am vegetarian" or "I keep kosher." People delight and take pride in eating spicy Szechwan, Indian, Thai, or Mexican food, or they may need to eat Oreo cookies at least once a day.

People with disabilities, however, have less freedom and choice than other people in defining themselves with food because of low income, lack of mobility, and lack of public access. A Louis Harris and Associates (1986) survey indicated that in the United States, people with disabilities shopped or ate out much less than their nondisabled counterparts. People with disabilities were three times more likely never to eat in restaurants than people without disabilities. Up to 13% of people with disabilities never shopped for groceries, compared with only 2% of the nondisabled population.

Compared with most Americans, a disproportionate number of people with disabilities and chronic illnesses are poor. They cannot afford to eat at expensive restaurants or buy a wide range of foods. Such conditions are especially severe for those who are homeless, mentally ill, or both; those who are elderly or housebound; and those who have developmental disabilities or mental illness and live in board-and-care facilities.

Meals as the Enactment of Social Relationships

Providing, preparing, and sharing food are important bricks in the foundation of social life. Every society distinguishes between foods that are edible and inedible and defines proper eating behavior. Every culture celebrates birthdays, coming-of-age ceremonies, and anniversaries by sharing food across households. Almost all holidays, whether secular or religious, involve some kind of feasting or fasting. In churches, mosques, and temples, food symbolizes the holiest of states, whether eaten in communion with one's fellow worshippers or offered as a sacrifice to one's God or ancestors.

Food is necessary to the survival of both man and animals, but for people to feel human, they must be able to participate in the social relations surrounding food. Consider, for example, the act of dining. de Mille (1981) wrote, "The dining room is concerned, of course, with food and therefore had been the focal point of my life as a child. It was the place of family interchanges" (p. 197). Although she claimed that the dining room was a focal point for food, she goes on to talk not about bread and soup, or pheasant and soufflés, but about the faces, manners, and emotions associated with the changing roles of the family members who have sat in the various seats.

For de Mille's 32nd wedding anniversary, which occurred 1 month after her stroke, her husband, Walter, brought together a party at the hospital of the people she loved, including her son, Jonathan. It brought back memories of many happy celebrations in the past and gave de Mille the sense that she could overcome her disability. Evidently, the food provided at the party was there more for symbolic purposes than for nutritional value:

> The celebration was topped by the hospital's present, a great big beautiful wedding cake, very rich and delicious. (The wedding cake Walter and Jonathan had brought was later given to the nurses.) And I knew that my friends and Walter were glad that I was alive, glad for me, glad for Walter. Glad for what I was beginning to be able to do. And there was happiness there because I was going to live. And we had toasts, many of them. They did. I had only a thimbleful of the champagne. (de Mille, 1981, p. 79)

The celebration strengthened de Mille's determination to recover. At 8:00 p.m. she found herself in bed; her husband leaned over the pillow. She whispered, "I'm going to live. I'm going to make it. I'll be out of here soon" (de Mille, 1981, p. 80).

Robert Murphy, Diane DeVries, and others whose voices are heard in the passages quoted earlier all describe how important the ability to eat was to their sense of dignity, but having an enjoyable family meal sometimes means giving up the goal of independent self-feeding that occupational therapists encourage in their clients. The mother of a small child who is blind continued to spoon-feed her child to preserve quality of life for her family:

> Rosalyn Gibson . . . told the group that she still spoon-fed her blind three-year-old because the alternatives created such chaos. Meanwhile, the teachers encouraged Nancy to feed herself at school and urged Rosalyn to follow their lead. . . . They spoke of time saved in the long run. Rosalyn thought about the family meals ruined by flying food and recrimination, and the long hours of clean-up. (Featherstone, 1980, p. 29)

Similarly, if occupational therapist Esther Huecker was to succeed in getting Timmy, who was totally dependent on intravenous feeding, to eat, she had to engage him in a social relationship. Her task was to get Timmy to enjoy food despite his unfamiliarity with hunger and reluctance to put objects in his mouth. Her lure was her own participation in the experience of getting to know food. After months of treatment, a successful meal became like a "dance" between them:

> His mother had saved his food tray so that we could have dinner together. We began our usual rituals. He brushed his teeth, washed his face, opened all of the containers, and began to smell and name what was on his plate. Timmy picked up a green bean and dipped it into the gravy to lick. I talked about putting gravy on his potatoes, but there was no hole to keep it from spilling. He gingerly poked a hole with his finger and licked the potatoes. He helped to mince some chicken in a grinder and then took small tastes from a spoon. The meal felt like a well-choreographed dance. I could anticipate his needs and prepare him for his risk-taking actions. His success generated more risk-taking. After exploring and tasting everything on his tray several times, Timmy announced he was "all done." Picking him up from the high chair, I felt exhilarated that the experience had been so satisfying. Timmy put his arms around my neck and gave me a kiss, something that had never occurred in a spontaneous moment. (Frank, Huecker, Segal, Forwell, & Bagatell, 1991, p. 258)

Murphy wrote that when people cannot reciprocate—cannot help their helpers get and eat food—they feel devalued; they lose self-respect. He describes two young women living together in a wheelchair-adapted apartment in a retirement housing project, whose creative solution to feeding problems challenged that potential devaluation:

> One is a spinal cord-damaged quadriplegic with good upper body strength, although she has considerable atrophy of the hands. The other has cerebral palsy; she has moderate speech impairment and very limited arm and hand use. Both women use wheelchairs. Nevertheless, they both completed college, where they lived in dorms, and now were sharing an apartment. Each had a van, and the two did their own cooking and shopping, taking care of all their needs. The woman with cerebral palsy was unable to hold and use eating implements, so she was hand-fed by the other. (Murphy, 1987, pp. 201–202)

In the mutual relationship of these two women, one helping the other takes place within a larger context of give and take. Together they appear to transform one's "feeding" the other into dining together. In occupational therapy, even when the immediate (short-term) treatment goal is focused narrowly on helping a person get food to his or her mouth with built-up utensils, eating remains an expression of social membership, cultural values, and personal preferences. The ultimate goal of treatment is to enable the client to participate in all of these activities.

Grooming and Dressing as Self-Expression

Grooming and dressing are often affected by chronic health conditions or disability. Yet clothing, hairstyle, figure, jewelry, and cosmetics are important markers of a person's social identity because they tend to display a person's gender, age, grade, occupation, status, ethnicity, and class (Storm, 1987). Changes in personal appearance send a message that the person's place in society has changed.

Hospital gowns, bedclothes, and slippers worn as regular daytime attire, and wheelchairs or other adaptive equipment announce, "Here is a sick person!" Uncombed hair and strong body odors, at least in mainstream North American culture, mark a person as an outsider, someone on the margins of society. They are "stigma symbols" (Goffman, 1963) that suggest that the person is not competent to participate in society.

The term *stigma* refers to negative judgments about (1) minority ethnic and racial groups, (2) morally disapproved behaviors, or (3) physical differences caused by chronic illnesses or disabilities

(Goffman, 1963). To escape from being stigmatized, immigrants might hide their strangeness by learning the language of the new country. In the same way, people with chronic illnesses or disabilities may often hide aspects of their appearance that could be "discredited" and try to "pass" as normal.

Chronic illnesses and disabilities are likely to stigmatize someone only when they become obvious to others. Although grooming and dressing reveal information that can improve one's social identity, they also can conceal information that would otherwise be socially damaging. Gaining control over and maintaining one's appearance can help improve the definition of a disability for oneself and others.

Stigma and Deviance Disavowal

Young people learn to view themselves in terms of the reactions they get from others (Mead, 1934). The horrified glance of a mother or father caught contemplating a life of caregiving slavery can destroy a child's self-image, but sometimes a parent who sees

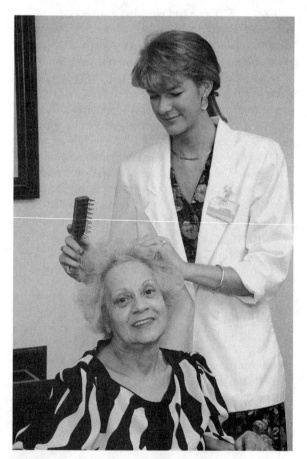

Figure 2.2. For many people with chronic illnesses, grooming and dressing are an important means of self-expression. Image © Photodisc, Inc.

value beyond a disability can improve the young person's image of self as well. The autobiography of Jane Addams, a leader of the settlement movement during the Progressive Era (ca. 1890–1920) and co-founder of Hull House in Chicago, where one of the first occupational therapy courses was taught, provides a famous example. Although Addams was born with a spinal deformity, her father's supportive view helped the girl develop a sense of self-worth:

> As a child, Jane Addams imagined herself to be a grotesque outsider: "I prayed with all my heart that the ugly, pigeon-toed little girl, whose crooked back obliged her to walk with her head held very much upon one side, would never be pointed out to the visitors as the daughter of this fine man." The tender gallantry of Mr. Addams bowing to his little girl and tipping his "high and shining silk hat" in public recognition, a charming fairy-tale picture the older autobiographer remembers with abiding gratitude, prevents a morbid self-hatred from festering in her mind. She could, at least inwardly, hold her head high. (Leibowitz, 1989, p. 119)

When people with disabilities and chronic illnesses cannot hide their difference, they, like Jane Addams, depend on positive evaluations made by others. Even when those judgments are negative, though, they do not have to accept them. Instead, they can act to influence how they are seen and treated. They may vigorously reject the sick role (Parsons, 1951). Being sick temporarily excuses them from work but at the cost of a loss of full social status and control over their situations until declared well by a doctor. For chronically ill or disabled people, the sick role threatens to become a permanent trap.

Some members of the independent living and disability rights movement resist this trap by becoming militant. They make a point of showing off their "stigma symbols" to protest stereotypes of social inferiority and to combat discrimination. Like gays and lesbians, members of Black and other ethnic activist groups, and feminists, movement activists have achieved changes in laws, policies, and social awareness by displaying their disabilities in public (Berkowitz, 1987).

People who do not have a father like Jane Addams's or the heart for public display can make clever use of fashion to avoid being stigmatized. The clothing, makeup, and hairstyles of a particular period create a language or cultural code that people use to communicate information about themselves (Barthes, 1967; Sahlins, 1976). Like everyone else, people with disabilities use clothing and cosmetics to conceal, distract from, or compensate for a defect (Kaiser, Freeman, & Wingate, 1990). After her stroke, de Mille used all three strategies:

> I bought Chinese suits with long coats and the brace was hidden in my pants [concealment] and I was told I looked very smart. . . indulging myself with the loveliest tunics and Indian Benares silk pants of contrasting or complementary tones and little colored slippers [deflecting attention]. The more decrepit my body, the more dashing my dress [compensation]—plain but très gai, très daring. Another flag went up the mast to signal my recovering and making my new life a happy one. (1981, p. 223)

Poet and essayist Nancy Mairs (1987, 1989) also described selecting clothes because she could manage to button them. Diagnosed with multiple sclerosis at about age 30, Mairs lost some of her ability to groom and dress herself: "With only one usable hand, I have to select my clothing with care not so much for style as for ease of ingress and egress, and even so, dressing can be laborious. I can no longer do fine stitchery, pick up babies, play the piano, braid my hair" (1989, p. 121).

But Mairs managed to dress in a way that controls our impression of her: The photo of Mairs (1989) on the dust jacket of her memoir *Remembering the Bone House* shows an attractive woman. Mairs is dressed in a simple shift. Her straight hair, cut to chin length, and the tilt of her shoulders draw attention to Mairs's incisive yet kind, dark eyes and generous mouth. A touch of cosmetics (nail polish and lipstick) and a bit of jewelry (long earrings, a wide bangle bracelet, a glimpse of narrow gold chains about her neck and wrist, plain gold wedding ring) adds to the effect of a woman in the mainstream. Sensuality and elegance (rather than plainness or disability) are communicated in this portrait.

Not all people can or want to invest themselves or their resources in grooming and dress. But grooming and dress—or the lack of it—nevertheless serve expressive functions, as in the case of Billy, who was born with multiple handicaps, was dependent on a ventilator, and was fed through a gastrostomy tube (Pierce & Frank, 1992). Occupational therapist Doris Pierce wrote, "When Billy was dressed in his first baby outfit, his oldest brother, who had refused to see Billy since his first visit, stayed with him all day" (Pierce & Frank, p. 974). In her field notes, Pierce recorded the brother's comment, "He looks like a real baby!"

Finally, the display of stigmatizing behaviors may be self-protective or involuntary in certain circumstances. Anthropologist Paul Koegel (1987) wrote about homeless mentally ill women in Los Angeles:

> Were they chronically mentally ill or were they simply reacting very sanely to the enormous stress of an insane situation? Was the fact that they wore four pairs of pants during the summer a reflection of an inability to properly identify weather-appropriate clothing or was it a highly conscious strategy aimed at frustrating potential rapists? . . . Was their poor hygiene the result of poor self-management skills or their restricted access to sinks and showers? (p. 30)

Occupational therapist Sandra Greene (1992), who studied a day shelter for women in the Los Angeles area, found a wide range of strategies related to grooming and dress among its homeless clients. A few women were able to maintain a normal appearance and took pride in their personal cleanliness and dress; some rented storage spaces to protect their clothing from theft. They were aware that carrying suitcases or bundles of possessions marked them as homeless. For others, just taking a shower was important, even when they made no attempt in their dress to conceal their homelessness:

> For women who value passing as a non-homeless woman, the availability of a place to keep clean is extremely important so that they don't "look like one of these filthy women." For some women who do not seem to take steps to pass as a non-homeless woman, this service is still considered important and is often mentioned as one of the services they like to use at the shelter. (Greene, 1992, p. 168)

Resisting Cultural Stereotypes of Beauty, Fashion, and Sexuality

Stigma is always relative to the dominant values of a particular culture. Anthropologist Nora Groce (1985) studied the population on Martha's Vineyard, where there had been, since the early 17th century, a high incidence of hereditary deafness due to the small gene pool and frequent intermarriage of families on the island. She discovered that hearing impairments were not stigmatized there:

> I thought to ask Gale what the hearing people in town had thought of the deaf people.
>
> "Oh," he said, "they didn't think anything about them, they were just like everyone else."

> "But how did people communicate with them, by writing everything down?"
>
> "No," said Gale, surprised that I should ask such an obvious question, "You see, everyone here spoke sign language."
>
> "You mean the deaf people's families and such?" I inquired.
>
> "Sure," Gale replied, as he wandered into the kitchen to refill his glass and find some more matches, "and everybody else in town, too, used to speak it, my mother did, everybody." (Grace, 1985, pp. 2–3)

Writers in the disabilities rights movement are challenging mainstream stereotypes of beauty and sexuality in society. Research shows that people tend to attribute positive personal characteristics to those who are physically attractive and negative characteristics to those who are seen as abnormal or different (Kaiser et al., 1990). Negative stereotypes of men and women with disabilities have been perpetuated in television and films, fiction, and drama (Kent, 1987; Longmore, 1987).

Political scientist Harlan Hahn (1988), a polio survivor, posed the question, "Can disability be beautiful?" Hahn suggested that when confronted with disability, people without disabilities tend to experience an "existential" anxiety (i.e., the projected threat of the loss of physical capabilities) and an "aesthetic" anxiety (i.e., fear of others whose traits are perceived as disturbing or unpleasant). His historical research indicates, however, that Western cultures have eroticized as well as stigmatized people with physical differences. Although it is rarely openly acknowledged, Hahn argued, people with disabilities in art and literature often have been portrayed with a certain sexual appeal.

Hahn urged people with disabilities to speak out as cultural critics of rigid, conformist ideals of the body beautiful. The culturally shared "language" of grooming and dress provides a vocabulary to do so. Some students with disabilities, for example, wear T-shirts with mottos and humorous slogans that display their social uniqueness and suggest a desire for more attention from society. Examples include, "I'm no quad; I'm just tired of walking"; "High level quads do it with a 'joy stick'"; "I'm accessible"; and "If I prove I'm better, will you admit I'm equal?" (Kaiser et al., 1990, p. 42).

DeVries has made choices since childhood about her grooming and dress (Frank, 2000). She accepted cultural ideals of attractiveness *and* challenged negative stereotypes about the handicapped. As a child, DeVries wore shift dresses over a three-wheeled "scooter" used with a crutch. During puberty, she decided that the scooter was strange-looking and decided to use an electric wheelchair instead.

Although any piece of adaptive equipment may be a "stigma symbol," a wheelchair was more appropriate for DeVries than was her three-wheeled scooter, especially at the county rehabilitation facility, where she then lived among teenagers and young adults with disabilities. A member of a peer culture of disability, she modeled herself after a young woman with a spinal cord injury who encouraged her to use her female assets to look "together." For DeVries, this choice had the following meaning:

> To go around in whatever you're in, your wheelchair, or your braces, or whatever, and not look clumsy. It's not looking "self-assured" either. I keep wanting to say that, but I don't think that's the word. I mean, people are already looking at you. You know, any crip's going to be looked at. But at least if they look at you, at least they'll say: "Wow, look at that person in the wheelchair. Hey, but you know, not too bad!" (Frank, 1986, p. 208)

Some people with amputations choose to wear long sleeves or full skirts to cover their missing limbs:

> I get a different response from people when I wear short sleeves so I very seldom wear short sleeves. It camouflages my disability (missing arm) when I wear long sleeves.
>
> Because of my amputation at the hip, I prefer dresses without a waist or gathering at the bodice of the dress. Dresses that flare out more at the tail are more attractive. (Kaiser et al., 1990, p. 39)

DeVries, however, prefers to wear close-fitting clothes that accentuate her assets. Displaying what she *does* have has been a better strategy for her than attempting to conceal her multiple limb deficiencies:

> Like when I was a kid, I hated wearing skirts and dresses, because with a skirt you could notice even more that there are legs missing than when you wore shorts and a top. Shorts and a top fitted your body and that made the fact that no legs were there not look so bad. (Frank, 1986, p. 209)

Overcoming Barriers to Self-Expression

The choices that people with disabilities make to show who they are often run afoul of the helpers—family members, professionals, and attendants—they depend on. A fine line exists between help and control. When she was a young teenager, DeVries liked dresses with narrow straps that she could slip into by herself and allowed her the greatest freedom of movement. Some members of her rehabilitation team did not like her choices, however, and challenged her right to determine what was appropriate dress:

> Diane prefers wearing spaghetti strap or other low cut sun dresses because she feels less encumbered and can also undress more easily. Those present felt that this is somewhat unattractive and possibly disturbing. It has been suggested to the family that she wear unbuttoned bolero jackets over the dresses but this has not been carried through. The subject of Diane's appearance to those present and to those around her was discussed at length. This seems to be a definite problem. Some felt that the cart [which Diane uses for mobility] is disturbing to behold. Some felt that they prefer seeing her with the prosthesis and others dissented. This area might be explored further as this seems to be a somewhat problematic area. (Frank, 1986, p. 207)

DeVries suggested that people with handicaps learn to say no and to stay in control of their grooming and dress when helped by another:

> Like me, I would never wear a skirt, a long skirt, like they used to. I've even seen some people with no arms wearing long sleeves pinned up or rolled clumsily so they're this fat. You can find a lot of clothes that fit you. It's not hard. If they have someone take care of them, they won't tell them: "No. I want my hair this way." They'll just let them do it. That's dumb. It's your body. They're helping you out. (Frank, 1986, p. 210)

At conventions of Little People of America, a self-help organization for people of profound short stature, one of the best-attended events is the annual fashion show (Ablon, 1984). Although most little people can wear children's clothing with minor alterations and children's shoes, children's styles are inappropriate for mature people. The fashion show displays clothing made specifically for little people as well as adult-size clothing that has been adapted with major alterations. Women model elegant suits, dresses, and sportswear, whereas men usually model formal suits. Little People of America members also attend sewing workshops and patronize representatives of tailoring firms who fit them and take custom orders. Women sometimes order shoes from Hong Kong, where average sizes are smaller than in the United States.

Claiming control over one's appearance, self-expression, and social identity can be a positive experience. Ernestine Amani Patterson (1985) wrote that she had an intense desire to wear her hair braided in cornrows, African style, with colorful beads and tinkling bells, but her blindness limited her from doing her hair herself. After beauticians and others discouraged her, a woman from Liberia, owner of "a most exotic African artifacts shop" finally gratified her desire. By insisting on cornrows, Patterson rejected the isolating stigma of blindness and claimed her identity as a "Black sister":

> Of course, people are still the same inevitable and specific in their cruelty: "Your hair is pretty," or "Your dress is pretty." The lines between womanhood and blindness are never supposed to meet. And with Blackness on top of that, what must people be seeing! And although I seldom hear: "You are looking nice," I am not the same, even if they are. Since that Saturday in the shop with the wooden floor and squeaky steps, where the heater had to be turned on against the chilly morning, I have always looked forward to the bus ride and short walk there. Mrs. Younger [her Liberian friend] has not only increased her clientele, other girlfriends of hers from Africa help out with the hair. So it's lovely talking to all of them. And since most of these women are used to me now, we relate as Black sisters. And though this was not a first step in my growth, mine is actually a case wherein the style of my hair altered the shape of my head within. How many women can say that with satisfaction about any beauty treatment they try? (Patterson, 1985, p. 243)

Summary

Self-care is not simply an objective routine. Every disability challenges not only the body but also the human being who relates to the family, the friends, the helpers, and others who move in the society of which he or she is a part. These challenges are what the chronic health conditions and disability mean to the person enduring it. Once survival needs are met, the narratives of people with chronic illnesses and disabilities show that the key problems caused by impairments are *occupational*. That is, the activity limitations caused by the performance failures of the body prevent people from engaging in the customary activities that fill their lives and give them meaning. Personal identity and social relations are at stake in even the most simple activities of self-care; the

ability or inability to perform those activities can result in basic self-esteem or profound shame.

Occupational therapists can help people with disabilities by recognizing that self-care occupations are deeply meaningful. People must cope with feelings of frustration when their ability to perform daily activities breaks down. They experience anger and depression over their loss of control and being helpless and dependent on others. They feel distress and guilt about the necessary reorganization of family relations that their illness has caused.

People with chronic illnesses and disabilities need access to basic health care through adequate insurance, rehabilitation services, attendant care, respite care, adaptive equipment, employment opportunities, and income supports. Such resources must be provided by an enlightened social policy. In each area, compassionate caregivers can make an important difference in the quality of life for the person with a chronic illness or disability.

People adapt to disability over time. Their attitudes toward their disabilities—the meanings they attach to them—depend partly on where they stand on the rehabilitation path, because attitudes change. Caregivers' attitudes can change, too. The ability to reevaluate cultural rules about "the right way" to do things can make impairments less handicapping and less stigmatizing. With experience and time, a concerned practitioner can learn to handle clients in ways that enhance, rather than limit, personal and social identity.

Acknowledgment

The writing of this chapter was supported in part by a 3-year grant from the American Occupational Therapy Foundation to the Department of Occupational Therapy at the University of Southern California. The author's discussion of Arnold Beisser's autobiography closely follows an insightful analysis on models of occupational therapy practice given by Elizabeth Yerxa, EdD, LHD, OTR, FAOTA, in 1991. The authors wish to acknowledge their debt to Dr. Yerxa for directing scholarly attention in the field of occupational therapy to the impact of disability-related experiences on individual identity and dignity.

Study Questions

1. Explain the difference between illness and disease as understood or experienced by patients or clients.
2. How do the body's performance failures affect a person's sense of self?

3. Identify some of the meanings associated with toileting, eating, and grooming.

4. How does the setting in which an activity or occupation occurs influence its meaning?

5. Describe possible occupational therapy interventions that can help a client avoid stigmatization.

6. Consider potential strategies for assisting clients with expressing their sense of control and selfhood in performing basic ADL. Explain why identifying such strategies is important.

References

Abel, E. K., & Nelson, M. (1990). Circles of care: An introductory essay. In E. K. Abel & M. K. Nelson (Eds.), *Circles of care: Work and identity in women's lives* (pp. 4–34). Albany: State University of New York Press.

Ablon, J. (1984). *Little people in America: The social dimensions of dwarfism.* New York: Praeger.

Asch, A., & Fine, M. (1988). Introduction: Beyond pedestals. In M. Fine & A. Asch (Eds.), *Women with disabilities: Essays in psychology, culture, and politics* (pp. 1–37). Philadelphia: Temple University Press.

Barthes, R. (1967). *Système de la mode* [System of style]. Paris: Seuil.

Beisser, A. R. (1989). *Flying without wings: Personal reflections on being disabled.* New York: Doubleday.

Bell, R. (1985). *Holy anorexia.* Chicago: University of Chicago Press.

Berkowitz, E. D. (1987). *Disabled policy: America's programs for the handicapped.* New York: Cambridge University Press.

Bordo, S. (1990). Reading the slender body. In M. Jacobus, E. F. Keller, & S. Shuttleworth (Eds.), *Body/politics: Women and the discourses of science* (pp. 83–112). New York: Routledge & Kegan Paul.

Corbin, J. M., & Strauss, A. (1988). *Unending work and care: Managing chronic illness at home.* San Francisco: Jossey-Bass.

de Mille, A. (1981). *Reprieve: A memoir.* New York: Doubleday.

DeVries, D. (1992). *Autobiography.* Unpublished manuscript.

Eisenberg, L. (1977). Disease and illness: Distinctions between professional and popular ideas of sickness. *Culture, Medicine, and Psychiatry, 1,* 9–23.

Featherstone, H. (1980). *A difference in the family: Living with a disabled child.* New York: Penguin.

Finger, A. (1990). *Past due: A story of disability, pregnancy and birth.* Seattle, WA: Seal Press.

Fisher, B., & Tronto, J. (1990). Toward a feminist theory of caring. In E. K. Abel & M. K. Nelson (Eds.), *Circles of care: Work and identity in women's lives* (pp. 35–62). Albany: State University of New York Press.

Frank, G. (1986). On embodiment: A case study of congenital limb deficiency in American culture. *Culture, Medicine, and Psychiatry, 10,* 189–219.

Frank, G. (2000). *Venus on wheels: A cultural biography.* Berkeley: University of California Press.

Frank, G., Huecker, E., Segal, R., Forwell, S., & Bagatell, N. (1991). Assessment and treatment of a pediatric patient in chronic care: Ethnographic methods applied to occupational therapy practice. *American Journal of Occupational Therapy, 45,* 252–263.

Gliedman, J., & Roth, W. (1980). *The unexpected minority: Handicapped children in America.* New York: Harcourt Brace Jovanovich.

Goffman, E. (1963). *Stigma: Notes on the management of spoiled identity.* Englewood Cliffs, NJ: Prentice Hall.

Greene, S. L. (1992). *An ethnographic study of homeless mentally ill women: Adaptive strategies, needs and services.* Unpublished master's thesis, University of Southern California, Los Angeles.

Greenfeld, J. (1972). *A child called Noah.* New York: Holt, Rinehart & Winston.

Groce, N. E. (1985). *Everyone here spoke sign language: Hereditary deafness on Martha's Vineyard.* Cambridge, MA: Harvard University Press.

Hahn, H. (1988). Can disability be beautiful? *Social Policy, 18,* 26–32.

Hochschild, A. (1989). *The second shift: Working parents and the revolution at home.* New York: Viking Press.

Kaiser, S. B., Freeman, C. M., & Wingate, S. B. (1990). Stigmata and negotiated outcomes: Management of appearance by persons with physical disabilities. In M. Nagler (Ed.), *Perspectives on disability* (pp. 33–45). Palo Alto, CA: Health Markets Research. (Reprinted from *Deviant Behavior, 6,* 205–224)

Kent, D. (1987). Disabled women: Portraits in fiction and drama. In A. Gartner & T. Joe (Eds.), *Images of the disabled, disabling images* (pp. 47–63). New York: Praeger.

Kleinman, A. (1988). *The illness narratives: Suffering, healing, and the human condition.* New York: Basic.

Koegel, P. (1987). Ethnographic perspectives on homeless and homeless mentally ill women. In P. Koegel (Ed.), *Proceedings of a two-day workshop sponsored by the Division of Education and Service Systems Liaison.* Bethesda, MD: National Institute of Mental Health.

Leibowitz, H. (1989). The sheltering self: Jane Addams's *Twenty Years at Hull-House.* In *Fabricating lives: Explorations in American autobiography* (pp. 115–156). New York: Knopf.

Longmore, P. K. (1987). Screening stereotypes: Images of disabled people in television and motion pictures. In A. Gartner & T. Joe (Eds.), *Images of the disabled, disabling images* (pp. 65–78). New York: Praeger.

Lorde, A. (1980). *The cancer journals.* San Francisco: Spinsters Ink.

Louis Harris and Associates. (1986). *The ICD survey of disabled Americans: Bringing disabled Americans into the mainstream.* New York: International Center for the Disabled.

Mairs, N. (1987). On being a cripple. In M. Saxton & F. Howe (Eds.), *With wings: An anthology of literature by and about women with disabilities* (pp. 118–127). New York: Feminist Press.

Mairs, N. (1989). *Remembering the bone house: An erotics of place and space.* New York: Harper & Row.

Mead, G. H. (1934). *Mind, self, and society: From the standpoint of a social behaviorist.* Chicago: University of Chicago Press.

Murphy, R. F. (1987). *The body silent.* New York: Henry Holt.

Nolan, C. (1987). *Under the eye of the clock: The life story of Christopher Nolan.* New York: St. Martin's.

Parsons, T. (1951). Illness and the role of the physician: A sociological perspective. *American Journal of Orthopsychiatry, 21,* 452–460.

Patterson, E. A. (1985). Glimpse into transformation. In S. E. Browne, D. Connors, & N. Stern (Eds.), *With the power of each breath: A disabled women's anthology* (pp. 240–243). Pittsburgh, PA: Cleis Press.

Pierce, D., & Frank, G. (1992). A mother's work: Feminist perspectives on family-centered care. *American Journal of Occupational Therapy, 46,* 972–980.

Plough, A. L. (1986). *Borrowed time: Artificial organs and the politics of extending lives.* Philadelphia: Temple University Press.

Plough, A. L., & Salem, S. R. (1982). Social and contextual factors in the analysis of mortality in end-stage renal disease patients. *American Journal of Public Health, 72,* 1293–1295.

Rosenberg, C. E. (1987). *The care of strangers: The rise of American's hospital system.* New York: Basic.

Sahlins, M. (1976). La pensée bourgeoise: Western society as culture. In M. Sahlwins (Ed.), *Culture and practical reason* (pp. 166–204). Chicago: University of Chicago Press.

Storm, P. (1987). *Functions of dress: Tool of culture and the individual.* Englewood Cliffs, NJ: Prentice Hall.

Strauss, A., & Corbin, J. M. (1988). *Shaping a new health care system: The explosion of chronic illness as a catalyst for change.* San Francisco: Jossey-Bass.

World Health Organization. (2002). *Towards a common language for functioning, disability and health.* Geneva: Author.

Wright, B. A. (1983). *Physical disability: A psychosocial approach* (2nd ed.). New York: Harper & Row.

Zola, I. K. (1982). *Missing pieces: A chronicle of living with a disability.* Philadelphia: Temple University Press.

Chapter 3

Evaluation to Plan Intervention

CHARLES H. CHRISTIANSEN, EdD, OTR, OT(C), FAOTA

KEY TERMS

analysis of occupational
   performance

assessment

correlation

evaluation

norms

occupational profile

Rasch analysis

reliability

stability

standardized

validity

OBJECTIVES

Upon completion of this chapter, the reader will be able to

- Describe the basic purposes of evaluation and assessment;
- List questions appropriate to the development of an occupational profile;
- Understand the meaning of "performance contexts";
- Identify important characteristics of assessment instruments;
- Appreciate the relationship between target outcomes and assessment selection;
- Describe the purposes and characteristics of selected assessment instruments suitable for measuring occupational performance in activities of daily living, independent activities of daily living, play, leisure, work and education, environmental contexts, and social participation; and
- Understand how informal and formal assessment methods are used in combination during the analysis of occupational performance.

Evaluation is the process of understanding through information gathering and analysis for the purpose of setting goals for service delivery or intervention. Services can be delivered to individuals, groups (such as school-based classes or families), or populations (members of organizations or communities). This chapter focuses on evaluation of individual clients and the settings in which they engage in the occupations of life.

Overview of the Evaluation Process

The evaluation process consists of the formal and informal collection of useful information (sometimes called data) from multiple sources. Informal data collection includes casual observation, interactions with the clients or people in the client's life, and general knowledge of communities and situations. Formal data collection usually involves assessment tools. These, too, incorporate observation and interaction by occupational therapy personnel or by other professionals.

Occupational therapy evaluation is a dynamic, two-part process. It relies on informal and formal observation methods to develop an occupational profile of the client and assess his or her occupational performance (Figure 3.1).

Ideally, the evaluation process emphasizes data reflecting the performance of activities in natural contexts. Doing so provides a more representative in-

dication of strengths and weaknesses of contextual (situational) factors, person-related factors, and activity-related factors. A complete evaluation attends to performance issues in all areas that affect the person's ability to engage in occupations and in activities. The evaluation process gathers information on performance skills, performance patterns, and the context or situational factors that influence performance, as well as activity demands and client factors.

When the occupational therapist gathers information on performance skills, his or her attention is directed to specific features of doing (such as bending or choosing) rather than the underlying body functions or capacities that support those acts, such as joint range of motion or motivation. A client demonstrates a performance skill when the demands of an activity (which include such aspects as necessary objects, space, sequencing, required actions, required body functions, and structures) and the contexts of the activity (the cultural, physical location, social, personal, spiritual, temporal, and virtual factors) come together during the performance of that activity (what needs to be done). The client, the demands of the activity, and the contexts of the activity combine as factors that influence occupational performance.

Development of the Occupational Profile

As a first step in the evaluation process, the client must be understood through development of an oc-

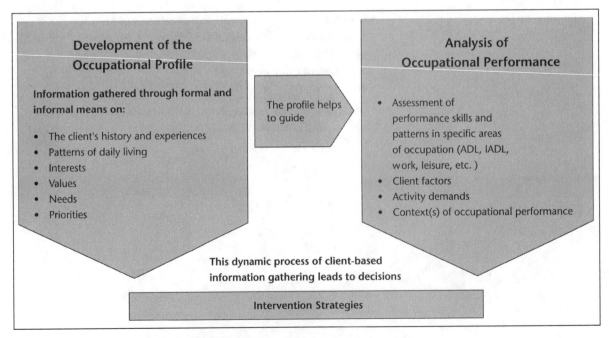

Figure 3.1. A summary of the evaluation process.

cupational profile (American Occupational Therapy Association, 2002). The occupational profile provides a summary of the client's identity and occupational history and his or her priorities, interests, values, and needs. The intent is to understand the client as an occupational being from his or her perspective to provide client-centered care. The following questions are germane to this part of the evaluation:

- Who is the client?
- What life experiences and previous patterns of activities have been meaningful?
- What areas of occupation are important to the client?
- What contexts support engagement in desired occupations?
- What contexts present obstacles, barriers, or conditions that inhibit engagement?
- What are the client's current concerns? Why are services being sought?
- What outcomes are expected from occupational therapy?

The occupational profile helps the therapist formulate an "occupational" view of the client, which in turn enables the development of a working hypothesis concerning identified problem areas. The therapist forms a preliminary evaluation of the client's strengths and weaknesses and the causes of the client's occupational performance problems. The therapist's impressions must be tested through the use of assessment tools and strategies: the analysis of occupational performance.

Analysis of Occupational Performance

The analysis of occupational performance involves determining a client's ability to carry out the activities of daily living (ADL) in the various areas of occupation. It requires the identification of performance skills and patterns and aspects of occupational engagement that affect those skills and patterns. The process helps identify facilitators of and barriers to performance. Occupational performance evaluation requires an appreciation of the complex nature of occupational performance: Therapists must recognize that occupational performance involves a dynamic interaction among skills, activity demands, client factors, and contexts. Information from the occupational profile guides the therapist in identifying specific areas needing evaluation and selecting specific assessment tools. The therapists' particular conceptual frames of reference will predispose him or her to specific, theoretically consistent tools or approaches.

The therapist can use several factors to determine the suitability of a particular scale (Box 3.1). It is important to base the evaluation on the client's needs and circumstances, understand the relationship between performance of everyday activities and the elements of skill, and appreciate the difference between assessments based on self-reports versus those based on observation of actual performance (Finlayson, Havens, Holm, & Van Denend, 2003; Rogers et al., 2003).

Evaluation often is biased toward using standardized assessment tools. A standardized tool is one that has well-defined procedures for administration and scoring. Some tools are based on normative data gathered from sample populations. A limitation of standardized instruments is that one set of items and procedures must be used for all clients and situations. Standardized instruments do not have items that represent all situations. Additionally, instruments that provide normative data may have little meaning within specific contexts because the norm provides information on a statistically derived "typical situation and client," which may resemble but does not accurately describe any specific situation or client. Moreover, a long list of every possible task would be impractical and would make it difficult to compare the efficacy of treatment approaches across large numbers of clients.

The therapist can gain valuable information that contributes to a client's evaluation during informal observation and interactions, particularly during structured interviews. The development of the occupational profile yields important information that informs the selection of assessment instruments and helps validate findings from standardized assessment tools. Both standardized and nonstandardized approaches have a place in assessing occupational function.

Some assessment approaches are based on the reports of clients or family members, which often are used in following up on clients after discharge or termination of care. Studies of self-report instruments have shown that what clients or those living with them say they can do may not always match their actual day-to-day performance. A client may be capable of doing a defined task under certain circumstances or on an occasional basis, but not on a regular basis. It is important to determine a person's consistent level of function, which can be done reliably and validly only in the person's day-to-day living environment (Christiansen, 2004).

A client's ability to perform everyday activities is influenced by the demands of the activity, the context(s) of action, and client factors. The client's

Box 3.1. Selecting Assessment Instruments

Researchers consider numerous characteristics when developing an instrument to measure any aspect of occupational performance. These include

- The scope of tasks addressed by the instrument,
- The instrument's sensitivity to changes in the client,
- The reliability of the assessment procedures,
- The validity of the instrument,
- The nature of resulting data, and
- The feasibility of the assessment instrument.

Some instruments cover a broad range of functional tasks; others limit themselves to a few self-care tasks. The extent to which instruments address each self-care task or assess the client's level of function also varies. For example, one instrument may evaluate the task of dressing using a single item that refers to the complete task, and another instrument may use several items to address the task's component parts, such as putting on socks, fastening shirt buttons, and so forth.

An instrument's sensitivity reflects the degree to which it detects small changes in the client. Sensitivity is particularly important in measuring the effects of intervention. An instrument that lacks sensitivity will fail to indicate small gains in the client's ability to perform self-care tasks.

The procedures for administering and scoring the instrument must be stated clearly in the test manual or protocol. Reliable procedures will yield consistent scores or descriptors from one assessment period to another and among assessments given by different individuals.

Validity relates to what behaviors the assessment instrument measures and how well it does so. A test that is valid in one situation may not be valid in different or changed circumstances. For example, a test of mobility that was developed for ambulatory subjects may be unsuitable for assessing mobility in wheelchair users. In this example, the content validity is not precisely determined by a statistical calculation; rather, it is a judgment call made by the potential test user. How well a test measures what it purports to measure may be more precisely measured by comparing performance on the test with the results of another instrument already considered to be an accurate indicator of the behavior of interest. If two tests measure the same thing, a person's performance using the first measure should relate to their performance on the second. The comparison often is expressed as a correlation coefficient, indicating the extent of relationship between two instruments.

A completed assessment instrument may provide a detailed profile that describes the client's self-care ability, or it may result in a single code or numerical value that represents a measure of overall function. Instruments may be descriptive or evaluative, and the purpose of the assessment directs the type of data collected. Useful evaluative instruments quantify function, the assumption being that the numerical score will change as the subject's performance changes. A single overall score for something as complex as self-care is misleading, however, so caution is advised when interpreting a global score that represents the sum of several subtests. Most assessment instruments for adults are designed to yield scores that allow practitioners to measure change or compare performance to normative data. Some tests have a developmental focus, so that the resulting data indicate the subject's performance in relation to a developmental continuum.

The training, equipment, and time required to administer the assessment all influence the usefulness of the instrument in any given setting.

Assessment instruments that are suitable for program evaluation and research purposes will have similar desirable characteristics. Comprehensiveness, accuracy, sensitivity to change, and feasibility are just some of the characteristics to be considered before making a choice.

general health and physical abilities, mental and emotional states, living environment, and relationships with others can influence his or her performance of tasks in any occupational area. Understanding the relative influence of those factors on a given client's performance helps the therapist consider all the barriers to function during intervention planning. Ideally, clients should be assessed in environments that represent their everyday living situations (Rogers & Holm, 1994). Effective evaluations are always individualized and capture the uniqueness of the client. This book includes a case study that illustrates how the various components of the evaluation process, including the development of the occupational profile, the analysis of occupational performance, and the assessment of contexts, provide the basis for identifying intervention needs and formulating goals for intervention (Box 3.2). The case study continues in Chapter 4 to illustrate how evaluation leads to the planning of interventions that are described for various conditions reviewed in this book.

The rest of this chapter identifies and discusses specific assessment tools for analysis of occupational performance. A comprehensive review of all available tools in each occupational area is beyond the scope of this chapter; therefore, the intent is to provide examples of scales that are widely used by occupational therapists or other professionals in each occupational area. Before using any instrument, it is important for professionals to gather as much information as possible on its procedures, strengths, limitations, and, of course, reliability and validity. Information can be gained from the professional literature and (for published tests) by consulting recent editions of the *Mental Measurements Yearbook* or *Tests in Print,* available in printed form or online through the Buros Institute.

Assessment of ADL

The literature provides many instruments and recommendations for evaluating performance of ADL (Christiansen, 2004). The challenge for occupational therapists is to develop effective strategies for determining clients' basic ADL performance by selecting the most appropriate instruments. During the 1970s, new instruments proliferated. Some of these new instruments were hastily constructed; few of them were well-standardized, validated, or based in theory (McDowell & Newell, 1996). Fortunately, the number of newly developed tools has slowed in recent years, and greater attention has been given to the consistent use of fewer, higher quality tools (McDowell & Newell, 1996). Therapists have come to appreciate that it is important to use only instruments with documented reliability and evidence of validity.

When a therapist evaluates a client, he or she makes several important decisions based on the person's ability to safely and independently perform ADL. It is important to remember that independent performance does not always equate with safe performance (Rogers, Holm, Beach, Schulz, & Starz, 2001). When an individual cannot eat, bathe, or dress independently, some type of personal assistance usually is required. The person's occupational roles and social and physical environments may change. Evaluation of ADL may lead to determinations about whether care or assistance may be necessary and the degree of care or assistance required. These determinations contribute to decisions regarding discharge from care settings into long-term care, skilled nursing, or supported home care environments.

Selected Measures of BADL

Several specific instruments evaluate everyday tasks that are sometimes called basic activities of daily living (BADL). BADL typically include bathing or showering, bowel and bladder management, dressing, eating, feeding, functional mobility, personal device care, personal hygiene and grooming, sexual activity, sleep and rest, and toilet hygiene. Instruments that assess other types of ADL and combined or global instruments are discussed in separate sections later in the chapter. Instruments in this section are presented in the order of their development and appearance in the literature. An attempt has been made to include those scales most widely used in the United States and in the international community.

Barthel Index

In 1965, Mahoney and Barthel published a weighted scale for measuring basic ADL with chronically disabled patients (Mahoney & Barthel, 1965). The Barthel Index includes 10 items: feeding, transfers, personal grooming and hygiene, bathing, toileting, walking, negotiating stairs, and controlling the bowel and bladder. Items are scored differentially according to a weighted scoring system that assigns points based on independent or assisted performance. For example, a person who needs assistance in eating would receive 5 points, whereas a person who eats independently would be awarded 10 points. A patient with a maximum score of 100 points is defined as continent, able to eat and dress independently, walk at least a block, and climb and descend stairs. The authors were careful to note that a maximum score did not necessarily signify independence because this instrument does not assess important tasks such as cooking, housekeeping, and socialization.

Several versions of the Barthel Index appear in the literature, and this scale may be the most widely studied and used self-care scale in the world. Studies have shown that the scale has acceptable psychometric properties, including that it is sensitive to change over time, it is a significant predictor of rehabilitation outcome, and it relates significantly with other measures of patient status. Shortened versions of the Barthel Index (BI-3 and BI-5) have shown evidence of satisfactory psychometric characteristics and predictive validity acceptable for use in outcome measurement (Ellul, Watkins, & Barer, 1998; Hsueh, Huang, Chen, Jush, & Hsieh, 2000). A mailed, self-report version also has been reported in the literature (Gompertz, Pound, & Ebrahim, 1994).

Box 3.2. Case Study of Irene: Example of Information Gathered for an Occupational Therapy Evaluation

Occupational Profile
(Gathered from interview)

Irene is a 52-year-old divorced woman who was diagnosed with multiple sclerosis 20 years ago. Until a recent exacerbation of her symptoms, Irene lived alone in an apartment and was independent in all areas of self-care, including driving. Disabling fatigue forced her to quit her job several years ago. Irene has been very active in her church, attending weekly services and the women's club. She loves to go to movies and restaurants and has averaged about two social outings per week, accompanying either her daughter or a friend. She loves to read.

Irene's usual pattern has been to sleep until about 8:00 a.m. She does most of her housework and errands on rising in the morning, when she has the most energy and feels the best. After the work is done, she either goes to a church activity or takes a half-mile walk before lunch. Typically she feels exhausted by the afternoon and naps for 2 or 3 hours. She generally spends evenings reading or watching TV, with occasional outings.

Irene recently experienced an exacerbation of her symptoms, including double vision, left-sided weakness and numbness, and cognitive problems. All of Irene's symptoms worsen with fatigue.

Analysis of Occupational Performance
(Gathered from the Canadian Occupational Performance Measure [COPM] and Activity Card Sort and from observation during the interview)

1. Irene now struggles more with dressing and bathing because these tasks take her longer and are more fatiguing. Although she can complete the tasks, she finds it easier to bathe less frequently and to wear the same clothes for several days without removing them at night.
2. She has not been cooking. Instead, she depends on eating the food her daughter brings over. She reports that she can cook, but it takes too much effort.
3. Irene's daughter has been doing the laundry.
4. She has not been driving because of her double vision. Therefore, she depends on her daughter for delivering groceries and doing her banking.
5. She has stopped going to the church group meetings and is too fatigued for outings in the evening.
6. Reading has become difficult, especially in the evening.
7. Irene spends most of her day listening to the TV, sleeping, and talking with friends on the telephone.

Assessment of Client Factors
(Gathered from manual muscle testing, sensory testing, and interview)

1. Irene's left arm and hand are weak. She has grade 3/5 muscle strength throughout, and her maximal grip was 10 pounds.
2. She can discriminate sensations on her arm and hand but reports a feeling of tingling in the fingers and forearm.
3. Irene's vision is best in the morning; her vision worsens as the day progresses. At times she can see the TV well enough to watch it, but later in the day she cannot see well enough to read.
4. She has short-term memory problems that worsen with fatigue.
5. She reports her level of fatigue as severe.
6. She admits to feeling depressed.

Assessment of Performance Contexts
(Gathered from observation in her home and interviews with Irene and her daughter)

1. Irene's apartment is small, and she keeps it clutter-free and minimally furnished. The building's laundry room is three doors down on the same, first-story level as the apartment. She has a wheeled laundry cart.
2. Irene's bathroom has a combination tub and shower. She had grab bars installed several years ago as a precaution against falling.
3. She wears knit, stretchy clothes for ease and comfort.
4. Irene's apartment is well lit for reading and other tasks.
5. Her daughter works during the day but has been coming over two or three nights a week to take care of miscellaneous housework and to bring several meals.
6. Her friends at the church have been calling her on the telephone and some have volunteered to pick her up to attend group meetings, but she has declined their offers.
7. Irene's daughter is very concerned about her mother's apparent lack of interest in bathing, dressing, hygiene, and household tasks. She believes Irene is forgetting things more often and that she sleeps too much. The daughter is unable to take her mother to her church groups during the day, and she is very concerned about Irene's limited social activity. She has a family of her own and finds it very difficult to attend to all her mother's needs.

Note: This case study continues in Chapter 4 with a discussion of Irene's goals and the intervention planning her therapist completes in collaboration with her.

The initial Barthel Index score was found to be the most reliable predictor of final rehabilitation outcome in a study of survivors of stroke conducted by Hertanu and colleagues (Hertanu, Demopoulos, Yang, Calhoun, & Fenigstein, 1984). The Barthel Index also has been found to correlate significantly with type of discharge and shorter length of stay for patients with cerebrovascular accidents (CVA; Granger, Hamilton, Gresham, & Kramer, 1989; Wylie & White, 1964), with independent living outcomes for patients with spinal cord injuries (De-Jong, Branch, & Corcoran, 1996), and with participation of young adults with disabilities (Bent, Jones, Molloy, Chamberlain, & Tennant, 2001).

The Extended Barthel Index (EBI) was subsequently developed to address perceived limitations of the Functional Independence Measure (FIM™) and existing Barthel Index by adding items for comprehension, expression, social interaction, problem solving, memory/learning/orientation, and vision/neglect (Prosiegel et al., 1996). One study showed that the EBI is a reliable, valid, and practical instrument that is sensitive to changes over time. Because of the manner in which the new items are administered, rater training is necessary. Time required to administer the EBI was described as significantly shorter than the time needed to administer the FIM™. (The FIM is discussed further in the section on combined measures for adults. FIM is a trademark of the Uniform Data System for Medical Rehabilitation, a division of UB Foundation Activities, Inc.)

Katz Index of Independence in ADL

The Katz Index of Independence in ADL was originally developed to study results of treatment and prognosis in elderly people and people with chronic illness (S. Katz, Ford, Moskowitz, Jackson, & Jaffe, 1963). Development of the index was based on observations of a large number of activities performed by patients following hip fracture (S. Katz, Downs, Cash, & Grotz, 1970).

The index evaluates a patient's functional independence in six areas: bathing, dressing, going to the toilet, transfers, continence, and feeding. Using three descriptors for rating independence in each of the six subscales, the rater applies specific rating criteria to derive an overall grade of independence. Depending on the determined level of independence, a patient is graded as A, B, C, D, E, F, G, or Other. A patient graded as "A" would be functioning independently in all six rated functions, whereas a patient graded as "G" would be dependent in all rated functions. Patients graded as "Other" are dependent in at least two functions but not classifiable as C, D, E, or F. Through observations over a defined period of time, the observer determines whether the patient is assisted or whether the patient functions on his or her own when performing the six activities. Assistance is graded as "active personal assistance," "directive assistance," or "supervision."

Studies have demonstrated that scoring in the Katz Index of Independence in ADL reflects an ordered pattern, meaning that someone who was able to perform a given activity independently at higher levels would be able to perform all activities performed by people graded at lower levels. This hierarchical structure correctly classifies the functional ability of patients 86% of the time and reflects a desirable property of scalability (Guttman, 1950). The Katz Index of Independence in ADL has been used as a tool to accumulate information about clients with many types of conditions. In addition to its high coefficients scalability, it also has demonstrated good interrater reliability (Brorsson & Asberg, 1984).

Combined Measures of ADL/IADL for Adults

A few global measures combine items that assess BADL with items that measure instrumental activities of daily living (IADL). Scales in this category include the FIM, the Performance Assessment of Self Care Skills (PASS), and the Canadian Occupational Performance Measure (COPM).

Functional Independence Measure

The FIM was developed by a task force of the American Congress of Rehabilitation Medicine and the American Academy of Physical Medicine and Rehabilitation, which met to develop a reliable and valid instrument that could be used to document the severity of disability and the outcomes of rehabilitation treatment as part of a uniform data system (Hamilton, Granger, Sherwin, Zielezny, & Tashman, 1987).

The FIM organizes 18 items for measurement in six categories, as follows:

- Self-care (eating, grooming, bathing, upper body dressing, lower body dressing, and toileting);
- Sphincter control (bowel and bladder management);
- Mobility (transfers for toilet, tub, or shower and bed, chair, or wheelchair);
- Locomotion (walking, wheelchair, and stairs);
- Communication, including comprehension and expression; and
- Social cognition (social interaction, problem solving, and memory).

Using the FIM, therapists grade patients' functional independence on each item according to a 7-point scale in which a score of 7 indicates complete independence and a score of 1 indicates complete dependence (Figure 3.2).

In 1995, the Centers for Medicare and Medicaid Services (CMS) of the United States government contracted to use the FIM as the basis for the rehabilitation prospective payment system and to use the FIM as part of a new patient assessment tool known as the Inpatient Rehabilitation Facility–Patient Admission and Information Report (IRF-PAI). Uniform Data System has developed a mastery test for medical rehabilitation to encourage consistency among FIM users (Granger, Deutsch, & Linn, 1998).

Several studies reviewed in a meta-analysis have shown that the FIM is a reliable instrument (Ottenbacher, Hsu, Granger, & Fiedler, 1996).

Since the inception of the FIM, many validity studies have demonstrated that the scale has concurrent predictive, and construct validity (Christiansen, 2004b). Studies also have compared various modes of test administration, including interviews, telephone reports, and direct observation (Karamehmetoglu et al., 1997). These studies suggest that the FIM retains acceptable reliability under different conditions of administration.

The FIM does have limitations, however. The FIM was found to have acceptable scalability only when broken down into two parts that treat the 13 motor and 5 cognitive items as separate subscales. Ceiling effects, in which scores tend to cluster at the high end of the scale, also have been reported (Hall et al., 1996). These characteristics limit the scale's usefulness in measuring change within groups.

An adaptation of the FIM, the Self-Reported Functional Measure, quantifies the ability of patients to care for themselves when they enter rehabilitation treatment and to chart their own progress until they are discharged into the community or to another facility (Hoenig, Hoff, McIntyre, & Branch, 2001). Recent studies of the Self-Reported Functional Measure show that the instrument predicts inpatient hospitalization but not outpatient health care use (Hoenig et al., 2001) and that it can also predict caregiver hours (Samsa, Hoenig, & Branch, 2001).

Performance Assessment of Self-Care Skills (PASS)

The PASS (Version 3.1) is a criterion-referenced instrument designed to evaluate independent living capacity in adults. It has been used with both healthy and disabled adults (Holm & Rogers, 1999). The PASS has been used for planning interventions and for documenting changes over time.

The 26 items in the PASS scale address functional mobility, personal care, and home management. Tasks in three performance areas—independence, safety, and outcome—receive independent scores on a 4-point scale that ranges from 0, indi-

---

Motor Items

Self-Care
  A. Eating
  B. Grooming
  C. Bathing
  D. Dressing upper body
  E. Dressing lower body
  F. Toileting
Sphincter Control
  G. Bladder management
  H. Bowel management
Transfer
  I. Bed, chair, wheelchair
  J. Toilet
  K. Tub, shower
Locomotion
  L. Walk, wheelchair
  M. Stairs

Cognitive Items

Communication
  N. Comprehension
  O. Expression
Social Cognition
  P. Social interaction
  Q. Problem solving
  R. Memory

Levels of Scoring

Independence
  7 = Complete independence (timely, safely)
  6 = Modified independence (device)
Modified Independence
  5 = Supervision
  4 = Minimal assistance (subject 75%+)
  3 = Moderate assistance (subject 50%+)
Complete Dependence
  2 = Maximal assistance (subject 25%+)
  1 = Total assistance (subject 0%+)

Legend: An administration protocol is used for guidance in evaluating a patient's performance in completing the tasks or movements required under each item category. Based on observed performance, the patient is assigned a score from 1–7, and the scores on each item are summed to yield a total score. This score represents the patients' level of independence in the activities of daily living evaluated at the time of scale administration.

Figure 3.2. Components of the Functional Independence Measure.

cating dysfunction, to 3, indicating function. Each task is broken down into subtasks, which allows the evaluator to pinpoint the specific aspects of performance that may be problematic. The PASS scale also documents the amount of assistance needed to complete tasks, thus providing a guide for quantifying the caregiving support necessary for the client.

The PASS is based on four established functional assessment tools for seniors. Its reliability, as measured through estimates of internal consistency, test–retest, and interrater consistency, has been reported at .80 and above (Rogers, Holm, Goldstein, McCue, & Nussbaum, 1994). The PASS has been used with a wide range of clients, including people without health problems and people with many types of diagnoses having functional sequelae, such as traumatic brain injury, multiple sclerosis, spinal cord injury, arthritis, CVA, macular degeneration, and depression (Rogers & Holm, 2000; Rogers et al., 2001, 2003). The scale can discriminate among clients on the basis of their ability to perform complex tasks and by the severity of their conditions, and studies have shown additional evidence of its convergent validity (Rogers et al., 1994; Rogers & Holm, 2000).

Canadian Occupational Performance Measure (COPM)

The COPM is an outcome measure that was developed in consultation with the Department of National Health and Welfare and the Canadian Association of Occupational Therapy (Law et al., 1990; Pollock, 1993). The COPM includes roles and role expectations from within the client's living environment using a semi-structured, individualized interview approach (Pollock, 1993).

The COPM focuses primarily on activities related to self-care, productivity, and leisure but also can be used to assess a client's specific ability limitations. The COPM was developed to help therapists establish functional performance goals based on a client's perceptions of need and to provide an objective measure of change in specific problem areas.

A caretaker may complete the scale if the client is unable to do so. The COPM considers the client's views of the importance of each activity and the client's satisfaction with his or her performance. The instrument takes into account client roles and role expectations and, in focusing on the client's own environments and priorities, ensures that contextual factors are considered in the assessment process.

The COPM can be used to measure outcomes across a broad range of situations and clients. Ad-

ministration requires a five-step process using a semi-structured interview conducted by the therapist together with the client or caregiver. The steps are

1. Problem identification and definition,
2. Initial assessment,
3. Occupational therapy intervention,
4. Reassessment, and
5. Calculation of change scores.

Completing the scale requires about 30 to 40 min. During administration, problems are identified and defined jointly by the therapist, the client, and appropriate caregivers. After activities of concern are identified, the client is asked to rate the importance of each activity on a scale of 1 to 10. These ratings are for information and not considered in the determination of client change. The client or caregiver must then rate the client's ability to perform the specified activities and his or her satisfaction with performance using the same 10 point scale. These scores are then compared over time. The scale yields two scores, one for performance and the other for satisfaction.

An extensive pilot study of the COPM involved administration in several countries, including New Zealand, Greece, and Great Britain (Law et al., 1994). The scale has since been translated and used in several additional countries. Early findings indicated that the average change scores for performance and satisfaction were approximately 1.5 times the standard deviation of the scores, indicating sensitivity of the instrument to perceived changes in occupational performance by clients. Some reports have indicated that clients occasionally experience difficulty with self-rating their performance (Bodiam, 1999), and the suitability of the measure for use with clients demonstrating cognitive or affective problems has been questioned. Recent studies have not substantiated these concerns, however (Chesworth, Duffy, Hodnett, & Knight, 2002).

Studies have reported high reliability for both performance and satisfaction scores (Sewell & Singh, 2001). Validity studies have been equally encouraging. Trombly and colleagues studied goal achievement by adults with traumatic brain injury and found that client perceptions of progress as measured by the COPM were accompanied by improved scores on scales of independent living and social participation (Trombly, Radomski, & Davis, 1998). A comparative study of rehabilitation settings for survivors of stroke using the COPM showed that participant satisfaction with goal achievement was independent of setting and consistent with the results of performance measured by IADL and health outcome scales (Law, Wishart, & Guyatt, 2000). A study by Simmons and colleagues found that using the COPM in combination with the FIM enhanced accuracy in prediction of outcomes for rehabilitative services for people in adult physical disabilities settings (Simmons, Crepeau, & White, 2000). These and several other studies have demonstrated that the COPM correlates well with other measures of ADL outcome, motivates active participation and adherence to rehabilitation regimens, and improves client satisfaction with services for a variety of diagnostic groups and ages (Carpenter, Baker, & Tyldesley, 2001; Gilbertson & Langhorne, 2000; Law et al., 1997; Ripat, Etcheverry, Cooper, & Tate, 2001; Wressle, Eeg-Olofsson, Marcusson, & Henriksson, 2002). The COPM appears to provide useful and important information regarding ADL and IADL performance from the perspective of the recipient of care.

Measures of ADL/IADL for Children

Assessment tools specifically designed to measure functionality in ADL and IADL in children include the Functional Independence Measure for Children (WEEFIM™) and the Pediatric Evaluation of Disability Inventory (PEDI).

WeeFIM™

In 1987, the FIM was adapted to provide a reliable and valid functional assessment tool that would be useful for children. The resulting tool, the WeeFIM, was designed to measure functional ability in a developmental context (System, 1990). The scale has 18 items. Each item is considered in relation to chronological age, developmental norms, and realistic expectations for children from 6 months to 7 years of age. The WeeFIM uses the same 7-point ordinal scale as the FIM to assess level of function. The WeeFIM is intended to give clinicians a view of the child's actual daily performance in six areas, including self-care, mobility, locomotion, sphincter control, communication, and social cognition.

Studies of the WeeFIM have shown a strong correlation between the scale scores and age, with the subscale scores involving gross and fine motor skill demonstrating the highest correlations (Ottenbacher et al., 1999). Data have shown that tasks on the WeeFIM demonstrate a developmental sequence, with an observed positive relationship between the complexity of the task and the age at which children achieve independence in its performance (Braun & Granger, 1991). Repeated evaluations of the scale and comparisons of personal and telephone interview ratings have demonstrated that the scale has good stability and equivalence reliability (Ottenbacher, Taylor, et al., 1996).

Validity studies of the WeeFIM have been encouraging. The score correlates well with other developmental tests, including the Vineland Adaptive Behaviors Scales and the Battelle Developmental Inventory Screening Test (Azaula et al., 2000). Studies have shown that the WeeFIM demonstrates acceptable validity in tracking the developmental status of children without disabilities across cultures as well as that of children with a host of conditions, ranging from preterm infants and children with various syndromes at birth to children who experience brain or spinal injury after birth (Christiansen, 2004b).

Pediatric Assessment of Disability Inventory (PEDI)

The PEDI is a comprehensive assessment that samples key functional capabilities and performance in children from the ages of 6 months to 7 years 6 months (Haley, Coster, Ludlow, Haltiwanger, & Andrellos, 1992). The scale was developed to measure functional deficits and developmental delays and to monitor progress in children having a variety of disabling conditions. Professionals may administer the PEDI through structured interviews or by parental reports (Haley et al., 1992).

The PEDI measures capability and performance in the areas of self-care, mobility, and social function. Capability is determined by identifying the functional skills for which a child has demonstrated mastery, with scores reflected on the instrument's Functional Skills Scales. Two other subscales are provided. The Caregiver Assistance scale measures the extent of help provided to the child during typical daily situations, and the Modifications scale measures environmental modifications and equipment that the child routinely uses in daily activities. The PEDI includes 197 items that measure functional skills and 20 items that measure caregiver assistance and environmental modifications (Table 3.1).

During development of the PEDI, content validity was determined through use of a multidisciplinary panel of experts (Haley et al., 1992). Items were derived from a wide array of functional performance and development scales. Normative data were collected from 412 children and families from the Northeastern United States, with a sample stratified to represent national population demographics. A detailed manual with scale development data, administration instructions, and scoring is available, as are published scoring forms and software.

The PEDI's six domain scores enable the tester to develop a profile of the client's relative strengths

Table 3.1. Performance Items in the Pediatric Evaluation of Disability Inventory

Functional Skills Content (197 Items)

Self-Care	Mobility	Social Function
Fasteners	Ability to negotiate outdoor surfaces	Community function
Hairbrushing	Bed mobility/transfers	Complexity of expressive communication
Handwashing	Car transfers	Comprehension of sentence complexity
Management of bladder	Chair/wheelchair transfers	Comprehension of word meanings
Management of bowel	Distance traveled and speed indoors	Functional use of expressive
Nose care	Distance traveled and speed outdoors	communication
Pants	Going down stairs	Household chores
Pullover/front-opening	Going up stairs	Peer interactions
garments	Method of indoor locomotion	Problem resolution
Shoes/socks	Method of outdoor locomotion	Self-protection
Toileting tasks	Pulls or carries objects	Self-information
Toothbrushing	Toilet transfers	Social interactive play
Types of food textures	Tub transfers	Time orientation
Use of drinking containers	Bed mobility/transfers	Functional comprehension
Use of utensils	Car transfers	Functional expression
Washing body and face	Chair/toilet transfers	Joint problem solving
Bathing	Indoor locomotion	Play with peers
Bladder management	Outdoor locomotion	Safety
Bowel management	Stairs	
Dressing lower body	Tub transfers	
Dressing upper body		
Eating		
Grooming		
Toileting		

Note. Adapted from "Functional Evaluation and Management of Self-Care and Other Activities of Daily Living," by C. H. Christiansen, in *Rehabilitation Medicine: Principles and Practice* (4th ed.), by J. Delisa et al. (Eds.), 2004, Philadelphia: Lippincott Williams & Wilkins. Copyright © 2004 by Lippincott, Williams & Wilkins. Adapted with permission.

and weaknesses in functional skills and caregiver assistance. No composite summary score is provided; the rationale is that doing so would obscure meaningful differences in functional performance within specific domains. Scaled scores can be computed to provide an indication of where a child performs relative to the maximum possible. The average time for administration is 45 min to 60 min.

The PEDI's psychometric properties are reported in the administration manual. Reliability (internal consistency) for the six scale scores was excellent. Initial data collected on the normative sample reflected an expected progression of functional skills according to age. Initial concurrent validity was established through comparison of scores on the PEDI with scores on the Battelle Developmental Inventory Screening Test and the WeeFIM. These correlations were generally high for self-care and mobility but were lower for social function. Early studies of the PEDI's ability to detect change yielded mixed results. One clinical sample of children with mild to moderate traumatic injuries demonstrated positive changes on the PEDI in all domains. Another clinical sample involving children with multiple significant disabilities showed positive change after eight

months only on the mobility scale. Some scores for this group decreased, indicating that the children were falling behind their peers in age-expected functional levels. Ludlow and Haley (1996) studied the influence of setting (context) on rating of mobility activities and found that parents in the home setting tend to use stricter criteria in their ratings than did rehabilitation professionals in the school setting, although both can be trained to attain a satisfactory level of consistency.

Several clinical studies have used the PEDI with children having conditions that affected their developmental status. The PEDI also has been used to measure outcomes following targeted medical and surgical interventions. Ketelaar and colleagues (Ketelaar, Vermeer, & Helders, 1998) studied the properties of 17 scales assessing the functional motor abilities of children with cerebral palsy and concluded that the PEDI was one of only two measures that demonstrated both acceptable psychometric properties and the capability to document changes in function over time.

Reports from several studies regarding the suitability of using the PEDI with other cultural groups have led to specific recommendations for item modifications when the scale is used outside the United States. The PEDI can be described as an instrument that is useful for measuring basic and extended functional ADL status and changes in children with disabilities from 6 months to 7 years 6 months of age.

Measures of IADL (EADL)

IADL are defined as activities that are oriented toward interacting with the environment; often are complex; and generally are optional in nature, meaning that they may be delegated to another person (AOTA, 2002). Wade (1992) has suggested that these types of ADL be described as Extended Activities of Daily Living, or EADL. Other terms in use for similar scale items are Social ADL and Advanced ADL (Chong, 1995). Several scales focus specifically on IADL (EADL) performance, including the Assessment of Motor and Process Skills (AMPS), the Nottingham Extended Activities of Daily Living Index (NEADL), and the Frenchay Activities Index, (FAI).

Assessment of Motor and Process Skills (AMPS)

The AMPS is an observational evaluation system that simultaneously examines a client's ability to perform IADL and the underlying motor and process capacities necessary for their successful performance (Fisher, 1994). The AMPS requires a clinician to observe a person performing IADL as he or she would normally perform them. The client selects 2 or 3 familiar tasks from among more than 50 possible tasks described in the AMPS manual. After the client performs the tasks, the clinician rates the person's performance in two skill areas: IADL motor and IADL process (Table 3.2).

The AMPS defines *motor skills* as observable actions that are supported by underlying abilities, including postural control, mobility, coordination, and strength. In the AMPS, motor-skill items represent an observable taxonomy of actions that are taken to move the body and objects during actual performance of a task. In comparison, *process skills* include actions that demonstrate the organization and execution of a series of actions over time to complete a specified task. Thus, process skills may be related to a person's underlying attention, conceptual, organizational, and adaptive capabilities. Items in the AMPS address 16 motor skills and 20 process skills, which together represent a universal taxonomy of actions observable during the performance of any task (see Table 3.2).

During each task performed for the assessment, the person is rated on a 4-point scale. Each point has

Table 3.2. Skills Measured Through Task Performance Using the Assessment of Motor and Process Skills

Motor Skills		
Paces	Inquires	Searches/Locates
Attends	Initiates	Gathers
Chooses	Continues	Organizes
Uses	Sequences	Restores
Handles	Terminates	Navigates
Heeds		

Process Skills		
Stabilizes	Coordinates	Lifts
Aligns	Manipulates	Calibrates
Positions	Flows	Grips
Walks	Moves	Paces
Reaches	Transports	Endures
Bends		

Process Skills—Adaptation	
Notices/Responds	Adjusts
Accommodates	Benefits

a specific label. A score of 1 is *deficit*; 2 is *ineffective*; 3 is *questionable*; and 4 is *competent*. The raw ordinal scores are analyzed using a probability model known as many-faceted Rasch analysis. This approach rests on a mathematical model of likelihood that the person will receive a given score on each of the motor- and process-skill items.

The AMPS motor and process scales represent continua of increasing IADL motor- or process-skill ability, and the person's estimated position on the AMPS motor and process scales, expressed in "logits," represents his or her IADL motor- and process-skill ability (Fisher, 1993). The Rasch analysis produces an estimated "person ability," which is plotted on a linear scale. Person ability is defined by the easiness and simplicity of each skill item and adjusted for the rater who scored the task performance (Kinnman, Andersson, Wetterquist, Kinnman, & Andersson, 2000; McNuty & Fisher, 2000).

Because the AMPS adjusts the person ability measures for task simplicity, a therapist can use them to predict whether a client will have the motor and process skills necessary to perform tasks that are more difficult than those demonstrated in the assessment. Additionally, because the AMPS includes 50 possible IADL tasks and each person is observed performing only 2 or 3, many possible alternative task combinations exist. Regardless of how many different tasks the individual performs, however, the ability measure is always adjusted to account for the ease and simplicity of those particular tasks. Therefore, direct comparisons can be made, even among people who performed completely different tasks.

Several investigations have been reported that use the AMPS to assess people with a variety of conditions, including psychiatric, orthopedic, and neurological disorders (Mercier, Audet, Hebert, Rochette, & Dubois, 2001); cognitive disorders (Nygard, Bernspang, Fisher, & Winblad, 1994; Darragh, Sample, & Fisher, 1998); and developmental disabilities (McNulty & Fisher, 2000). A school-based version of the AMPS is now available. The tool's ability to analyze the separate contributions of motor and process variables has provided knowledge about the specific variables that contribute to task limitations in various conditions. Validity studies have suggested that the AMPS can help predict home safety (McNulty & Fisher, 2000) and measure improvements following intervention for multiple sclerosis (Kinnman et al., 2000) and stroke (Tham, Ginsburg, Fisher, & Tegner, 2001). The AMPS also has demonstrated consistency across different cultural groups (Fisher & Duran, 2000; Fisher, Liu, Velozo, & Pan, 1992). These studies have also established the reliability and validity of the AMPS.

Nottingham Extended Activity of Daily Living Scale (NEADL)

The NEADL was developed by Nouri and Lincoln (1987) and is widely used throughout Europe and in other countries. This self-report index organizes 22 items into four sections: mobility, kitchen tasks, domestic tasks, and leisure activities (Table 3.3). Scoring uses a 4-item set of discrete categories that range from *not done at all* to *done alone easily*. Unfortunately, no guidelines currently exist for assigning scores. Because of the range of EADL tasks reported, the scale has intuitive appeal as an outcome measure of rehabilitation and social participation.

The accumulating literature on the use of the NEADL is beginning to demonstrate that it is suitable for evaluating EADL function in the community. Although most reported studies involve participants who had received rehabilitation following stroke (Lincoln, Gladman, Berman, Noad, & Challen, 2000; Rodgers et al., 1997; Walker, Gladman, Lincoln, Siemonsma, & Whiteley, 2000), the measure has been used with other diagnostic groups, such as people with pulmonary problems (Bestall et al., 1999; Dyer, Singh, Stockley, Sinclair, & Hill, 2002; Garrod, Bestall, Paul, Wedzicha, & Jones, 2000; Yohannes, Roomi, Winn, & Connolly, 2000), elderly people in the community (Burch, Longbottom, McKay, Borland, & Prevost, 2000; Weatherall, 2000), and patients with hip replace-

ment (Harwood & Ebrahim, 2000). For the patients with hip replacement, Harwood and Ebrahim compared the responsiveness of the NEADL with two other measures. In that study, the NEADL was viewed as less sensitive to change in function than the SF-36 or the London Handicap Scale in measuring activity and social participation for patients with hip replacement. Despite this limitation, the scale has shown evidence of acceptable scalability, concurrent validity, and construct validity. In a study of survivors of stroke in Taiwan, Hsueh and colleagues found that with minor modification to two items, the NEADL had satisfactory scalability and reproducibility and correlated with age and scores on the Barthel Index (Hsueh et al., 2000). The scale also has been useful as a measure of the effectiveness of rehabilitation strategies, such as ADL training (Walker, Drummond, & Lincoln, 1996).

Frenchay Activities Index (FAI)

The Frenchay Activities Index was developed initially for use in clinical social work for survivors of stroke and has emerged as a frequently used measure of EADL (Buck, Jacoby, Massey, & Ford, 2000; Holbrook & Skilbeck, 1983). The FAI consists of 15 items divided into two sections. The first section addresses activities performed within the 3 months preceding completion of the scale and includes standard mobility, household maintenance, and meal preparation items. The second section addresses activities performed within the 6 months preceding completion of the scale and includes work, leisure, travel, and household or car maintenance items. Items are scored on a 4-point scale that ranges from 0 to 3 according to well-defined guidelines. The index is designed as a mailed questionnaire to be completed by self-report.

Turnbull et al. (2000) studied 1,280 people to construct preliminary norms and to determine evidence of reliability and validity. They concluded that the FAI is reliable and shows good evidence of validity with an elderly population, but would benefit from adding items relating to sports, physical exercise, and caring for children. Adding such items would enhance the FAI's usefulness in assessing a broader segment of the population. Green and colleagues studied the test–retest reliability of the FAI and other scales of stroke outcome. They found that the FAI had only moderate reliability and had higher random error when stroke survivors were measured twice within a 1-week interval (Green, Forster, & Young, 2001).

Although most of the studies using the FAI have been related to outcomes following stroke (Dennis, O'Rourke, Slattery, Staniforth, & Warlow, 1997;

Table 3.3. Nottingham Extended Activities of Daily Living Index

Questions	Answers			
	Not At All	**With Help**	**Alone With Difficulty**	**Alone Easily**
Mobility—Do you:				
Walk around outside?				
Climb stairs?				
Get in and out of the car?				
Walk over uneven ground?				
Cross roads?				
Travel on public transport?				
Kitchen tasks—Do you:				
Manage to feed yourself?				
Manage to make yourself a hot drink?				
Take hot drinks from one room to another?				
Do the washing up?				
Make yourself a hot snack?				
Domestic tasks—Do you:				
Manage your own money when you are out?				
Wash small items of clothing?				
Do your own shopping?				
Do a full clothes wash?				
Leisure activities—Do you:				
Read newspapers or books?				
Use the telephone?				
Go out socially?				
Manage your own garden?				
Drive a car?				

Note. Based on Nouri, F., & Lincoln, N. (1987). An extended activities of daily living scale for survivors of stroke. *Clinical Rehabilitation, 1,* 301–305.

Kwakkel, Kollen, & Wagenaar, 2002; Sveen, Bautz-Holter, Sodring, Wyller, & Laake, 1999; Young, Bogle, & Forster, 2001), the index also has been used for other populations, including those with complex disabilities (Haig, Nagy, Lebreck, & Stein, 1995), patients with venous leg ulcers (Walters, Morrell, & Dixon, 1999), and caregivers (Mant, Carter, Wade, & Winner, 2000). The scale also has been translated for and used to study rehabilitation outcomes in Japan (Hachisuka et al., 1999), China (Hsieh & Hsueh, 1999), Denmark (Pedersen, Jorgensen, Nakayama, Raaschou, & Olsen, 1997), and Spain (Carod-Artal, Egido, Gonzalez, & de Seijas, 2000).

One study showed that the FAI has excellent interrater reliability (Piercy, Carter, Mant, & Wade, 2000). However, Schuling and others suggested that the instrument's reliability could be improved by deleting two items and creating two subscale scores, one for domestic activities and the other for outdoor activities (Schuling, Dehaan, Limburg, & Groenier, 1993). Studies using the FAI and measures of BADL, particularly the Barthel Index, demonstrated that the scales measure different factors and may be useful in combination (Hsieh & Hsueh, 1999).

Measures of Leisure Activity

Historically, developments in leisure theory and measurement have occurred largely outside the field of occupational therapy, principally in leisure science, therapeutic recreation, and related fields. Measures in these fields have concerned themselves with leisure awareness or knowledge, leisure attitudes and interests, skills, leisure satisfaction, and participation. Three notable measures of leisure activity are the Leisure Satisfaction Questionnaire, the Leisure Competence Measure, and the Leisure Diagnostic Battery (LDB).

Leisure Satisfaction Questionnaire

Developed by Beard and Ragheb in 1980, the Leisure Satisfaction Questionnaire consists of 51 items scored on a 5-point scale (Beard & Ragheb, 1980). The self-report instrument provides information on six aspects of leisure engagement, including psychological, educational, social, relaxation, physiological, and aesthetic domains. It requires approximately 30 min to complete.

Many experts in leisure studies have validated the content validity of the Leisure Satisfaction Questionnaire Reliability estimates for this tool range from .82 to .86 (Beard & Ragheb, 1980). Unfortunately, few studies have been done to test the validity of this scale. One study, reported by Kanters

(1995), failed to support a hypothesis that increased leisure satisfaction would be associated with reduced stress. Lloyd and Auld (2002) found that leisure satisfaction, as measured by the Leisure Satisfaction Questionnaire, was the best predictor of quality of life in a sample of people studied. Pearson (1998) showed that leisure satisfaction and job satisfaction were positive and significant predictors of psychological health in a sample of employed people.

Leisure Competence Measure

The Leisure Competence Measure was developed in 1997 by Kloseck and Crilly (Kloseck & Crilly, 1997). The scale is designed as a measure of adult leisure functioning and as an instrument to document change in leisure functioning over time. Kloseck and Crilly selected items based on leisure science theory using information provided by 25 content experts. Items in the scale are organized into nine categories—leisure awareness, leisure attitude, leisure skills, cultural behaviors, social behaviors, interpersonal skills, community integration, social contact, and community participation—with each item rated on a 7-point Likert scale. The rater assigns points to each item based on observation, the client's record, an interview, and reports from other people who are aware of the client's behaviors.

The Leisure Competence Measure can be administered in about 1 hr, with additional time required for scoring. No normative data are available, but reliability estimates for internal consistency and stability over time are above .90. The scale has been reported as sensitive to changes in leisure participation over time (Strain, Grabusic, Searle, & Dunn, 2002), and construct validity studies have shown that it correlates significantly with mental state, life satisfaction, and depression (Searle, Mahon, & Iso-Ahola, 1995). The Leisure Competence Measure also has shown sensitivity to measuring change following leisure education (Searle, Mahon, Iso-Ahola, & Sdrolias, 1998).

Leisure Diagnostic Battery (LDB)

The LDB was developed in 1986 as a self-report tool to determine a person's perceptions of his or her leisure competence. This scale can be used with adolescents and with adults of all ages. Version A of the LDB is designed for adolescents. It includes 95 items related to competence, control, needs, depth, and playfulness; 24 items related to perceived barriers to leisure participation; and 28 items related to knowledge of leisure activities. Items are rated on a 3-point scale on which subjects are asked to determine whether a statement about leisure sounds like them, sounds a little like them, or does not sound like them. A 25-item short form of the LDB also is available for either version of the battery. Administration of the long-form LDB requires approximately 40 min, and administration of the short-form LDB requires approximately 15 min. An administration manual is available, and an automated scoring and report-writing system is available on the Internet for use with desktop computers.

Several studies have validated the LDB, including a study that confirmed by factor analysis the independence of the battery's separate scales (J. Dunn, 1987; Ellis & Witt, 1986). The scale has been shown to have internal consistency, with alpha coefficients of .83 to .94 for the long form and .89 to .94 for the short form (Chang & Card, 1994). Correlational studies have validated the LDB with other measures of leisure, including knowledge of leisure activities and barriers. Scores on the battery are sensitive to change on the basis of clients' participation in recreation programs.

Measures of Children's Play Activity

Instruments specifically designed to measure play activity in children include the Preschool Play Scale—Revised (PPS–R) and the Test of Playfulness (TOP).

Preschool Play Scale–Revised (PPS–R)

In 1974, Knox developed the Play Scale, a structured observational scale that could be used to determine a child's developmental play age and provide a profile of the play behaviors of children (Knox, 1974). The original scale measured four dimensions: space management, material management, imitation, and participation. Revised by Bledsoe and Shepherd in 1982, the scale was renamed the Preschool Play Scale, or PPS (Bledsoe & Shepherd, 1982). Study of the revised scale's reliability and validity suggested that it provided consistent and valid information on childhood play (Harrison & Kielhofner, 1986). Harrison and Kielhofner recommended that the PPS be revised to include a dimension that measured the degree of a child's engagement in play. Other studies showed that the PPS could not measure differences in play between age groups or in children with conditions affecting their development (Bledsoe & Shepherd, 1982; Morrison, Bundy, & Fisher, 1991).

In 1997, Knox further revised the PPS and renamed it the Preschool Play Scale—Revised (PPS–R; Knox, 1997). Changes included revisions to the definitions of the dimensions and the renaming of the imitation dimension. The PPS–R now focuses on the child's capacity to play and is suitable for use with children from birth to 6 years of age. The scale is designed to function both as a diagnostic tool and as an outcome measure to determine the effectiveness of intervention. The PPS–R remains an observational assessment of four play dimensions, which are now defined as space management, material management, imitation, and participation. While observing the child at play in familiar environments (both outside and indoors), the examiner scores the child's behaviors on items associated with each dimension. Dimension scores are determined by averaging the item scores, and a total score is determined by averaging the scores on individual dimensions. The PPS–R requires about 1 hr to administer.

Early reliability data had shown that the first version of the scale had good interrater reliability. (Bledsoe & Shepherd, 1982). Because the PPS has evolved on the basis of thorough reviews of the literature, its content validity can be described as good. Studies also have shown that the PPS correlates significantly with measures of social play development and chronological age (Knox, 1997).

Test of Playfulness (TOP)

In 1997, Bundy developed the TOP to measure four elements of playfulness in children: intrinsic motivation, internal control, freedom from some constraints of reality, and the ability to give and read cues (Bundy, 1997). The scale applies for all children, from infants through adolescence. TOP data have been collected on children from 3 months to 15 years of age.

Administration of the scale involves observing a child during 15 to 20 min of free play in an environment familiar to the child. The TOP consists of 24 items, with each item rated on a 4-point scale to reflect the extent of play, intensity, or skill.

Rasch analysis revealed evidence that 100% of the raters scored the TOP reliably, and data for 88% of the children with disabilities conformed to the pattern of playfulness typical of most of the children represented in the test's normative data set. Four TOP items accounted for most of the unexpected ratings. The TOP has been found to be significantly correlated with its companion instrument, the Test of Environmental Supportiveness (Bronson & Bundy, 2001). In another study, children diagnosed with attention deficit hyperactivity disorder (ADHD) were found to have lower mean scores on the TOP than were children without ADHD. A study by Harkness and Bundy (2001) showed no significant differences between comparison groups of children with and without disabilities and also demonstrated acceptable reliability for administration. The TOP is unavailable commercially.

It is easy to administer, however, and interpretation of the scale serves as a useful guide to intervention.

Measures of School and Work Performance

Tools for measuring school- and work-related occupational performance include the School Function Assessment (SFA), the VALPAR Component Work Samples (VALPAR), the Career Ability Placement Survey (CAPS), and the Employee Aptitude Survey (EAS). Note that these tests measure functional performance of cognitive and motor skills necessary for productive engagement in activities necessary for school or work.

School Function Assessment (SFA)

The SFA measures the functional skills children must have to perform necessary education-related and social tasks in elementary school. The scale was designed to facilitate collaborative program planning for children with disabilities. Published in 1998, this new test is early in its development, so information is limited regarding its reliability and validity.

Scores on the SFA are derived from observations of a child's performance in the school setting using 26 scales. Each scale is scored using either a 4- or 6-point rating. The SFA can be administered in two ways: Items may be completed in a team setting or a leader may collect the scores from school professionals who have observed the performance of the child and completed the scale in the academic setting.

Items for the SFA were selected from a review of the literature that identified those tasks that were related to successful school performance. The items for the scale were developed through an iterative statistical process that involved a broad sample of children with and without disabilities from across the United States and Puerto Rico. Development studies of the scale showed that it has excellent reliability (Coster, Deeney, Haltiwanger, & Haley, 1998). The developers report that the SFA has excellent predictive validity and is capable of discriminating between students who are at risk and those who are more likely to succeed in the academic environment. The scales with the lowest reliability are those associated with task support (Coster, 1998).

VALPAR

The VALPAR consists of 23 simulated work sample performance tests that are designed to assess the ability of an individual to successfully engage in various work-related tasks. Each sample task has been standardized and can be evaluated according to job requirements identified by the U.S. Department of Labor (DOL) taxonomy. The VALPAR is suitable for use by adolescents and adults. Completion of each work component requires from 10 min to 30 min.

The VALPAR compares client scores to two main types of criterion-referenced standards: the U.S. Department of Labor's work-related factor system as described in the *Revised Handbook for Analyzing Jobs* (DOL, 1991) and the Methods-Time Measurement (MTM) standards. MTM standards may be used in two ways. They may be interpreted directly, or they may be used to help determine, whether the client has demonstrated the DOL factors at the levels needed to succeed in specific jobs and occupations. VALPAR Component Work Samples 1, 2, 4, 8, 9, and 10 can be modified for use by people with blindness and visual impairments using a "B-Kit" available from the publisher.

The VALPAR has an examiner's manual with detailed instructions. Stability for the VALPAR is reported as good to excellent for Work Samples 14 through 16, using test–retest correlations. Criterion validity as reported in the manual is good for most samples. Table 3.4 includes a list of the work samples and a description of the abilities measured by each test.

Career Ability Placement Survey (CAPS)

The CAPS is a timed and standardized paper-and-pencil test battery consisting of eight subtests. The test battery measures a person's abilities in the conceptual skills required for entry-level performance in the majority of jobs found in 14 occupational clusters listed in the *Dictionary of Occupational Titles* maintained by the DOL (Knapp, Knapp, & Knapp-Lee, 1992). The subtests measure abilities in mechanical reasoning, spatial relations, verbal reasoning, numerical ability, language usage, word knowledge, perceptual speed and accuracy, and manual speed and dexterity. The CAPS is suitable for administration to clients who are in junior high school or older. It requires approximately 50 min to administer and score. Examiners can score the CAPS subtests manually or use machine scoring. The subtests also can be self-scored by the client or examinee. The CAPS is part of the COPSystem (Career Occupational Preference System), a battery of work ability, interest, and value tests that is widely used in Canada.

Extensive research on the CAPS has demonstrated strong evidence of reliability and validity. Internal consistency, stability, and interrater coefficients have been reported as satisfactory to excellent

Table 3.4. VALPAR

Ability	Description
Small tools (mechanical)	Measures the ability to make precise finger and hand movements and to work with small tools in tight or awkward spaces. The work sample simulates light work and makes the following physical demands on the client: reaching, handling, fingering, feeling, near acuity, depth perception, and accommodation. Significant motor coordination, finger dexterity, and manual dexterity are called for to perform the work sample satisfactorily.
Size discrimination	Measures the ability to perform work tasks involving size discrimination, manual dexterity, and finger dexterity. The work sample simulates light work and makes the following physical demands on the client: reaching, fingering, feeling, near acuity, depth perception, and accommodation. Significant motor coordination and manual dexterity are called for to perform the work sample at a competitive level.
Numerical sorting	Assesses the ability to perform work tasks involving sorting, categorizing, filing by number arrangement, and using numbers and numerical series. The work sample simulates light work and makes the following demands: reaching, fingering, near acuity, depth perception, and accommodation.
Upper-extremity range of motion	Assesses upper-extremity range of motion and work tolerance in the upper body, including shoulders, arms, elbows, wrists, hands, and fingers. The work sample simulates light work and makes the following physical demands on the client: reaching, fingering, feeling, near acuity, depth perception, accommodation, and color vision.
Clerical comprehension and aptitude	Measures a variety of clerical work skills, including those required in mail sorting, filing, telephone answering, typing, and bookkeeping. The work sample simulates sedentary and light work and makes the following physical demands on the client: reaching, handling, fingering, hearing, near acuity, depth perception, and accommodation.
Independent problem solving	Measures the ability to pay attention to detail and to compare and discern differences among variously colored geometric designs. The work sample simulates sedentary work and makes the following physical demands on the client: reaching, handling, near acuity, accommodation, and color vision.
Multilevel sorting	Measures the ability to make rapid sorting decisions involving several levels of visual discrimination of color, numbers, letters, and combinations of these. The work sample simulates light work and involves repetitive finger grasping and reaching. The work sample makes the following physical demands on the client: reaching, fingering, near acuity, depth perception, accommodation, color vision, and field of vision.
Simulated assembly	Assesses the ability to perform repetitive assembly work requiring manipulation and bilateral use of the upper extremities. The work sample simulates light work and makes the following physical demands on the client: reaching, handling, fingering, feeling, near acuity, depth perception, accommodation, and field of vision.
Whole body range of motion	Assesses whole-body range of motion, agility, and stamina through gross body movements of the trunk, arms, hands, legs, and fingers. The effects of kneeling, bending, stooping, repeated crouching, and overhead reaching on various work-related physical skills are assessed. The work sample simulates light work and makes the following physical demands on the client: stooping, crouching, reaching, handling, fingering, feeling, near visual acuity, depth perception, and other visual abilities.
Tri-level measurement	Measures work skills related to inspection and measurement tasks, ranging from simple to very precise. The work sample simulates light work and makes the following physical demands on the client: reaching, handling, fingering, feeling, near acuity, depth perception, and accommodation.
Eye–hand–foot coordination	Measures the ability to move the eyes, hands, and feet in coordination. The work sample simulates light work and makes the following physical demands on the client: reaching, handling, fingering, near acuity, depth perception, and field of vision.

Continued

Table 3.4. *Continued*

Ability	Description
Soldering and inspection (electronic)	Measures the ability to use small tools and to make precise hand and finger movements in close coordination with the eyes. The work sample exercises call for skills similar to those required in occupations involving fabricating, processing, or repairing materials and examining and measuring for the purpose of grading and sorting and other industrial production work. This work sample simulates sedentary work and makes the following physical demands on the client: reaching, handling, fingering, near acuity, depth perception, and accommodation.
Integrated peer performance	Measures a client's instruction-following ability, hand and finger dexterity, and color discrimination skills. Special emphasis is placed on each client's ability to interact effectively with both peers and supervisors and his or her ability to work as a team member.
Electrical circuitry and print reading	Measures work skills related to understanding and working with electrical circuits. The client uses a variety of tools to test for circuit continuity and repair circuits. He or she must also read electrical schematic prints and install wires, diodes, and resistors. The work sample simulates sedentary work and makes the following physical demands on the client: reaching, handling, fingering, feeling, near acuity, depth perception, accommodation, and color vision.
Drafting	Measures work skills required in occupations involving drafting. The work sample may be used to assess both current levels of achievement and potential for achievement in drafting skills. This work sample simulates sedentary work and makes the following physical demands on the client: reaching, handling, fingering, near acuity, depth perception, and visual accommodation. There are six scored exercises in this sample that range from simple measuring tasks to relatively complex drafting and blueprint reading.
Prevocational readiness	Is divided into four subtests: Developmental Assessment, Workshop Evaluation, Interpersonal/Social Skills, and Money Handling Skills. Each of the subtests requires little or no reliance on language or reading skills. A client can respond by pointing, gesturing, talking, or using sign language.
CUBE (conceptual understanding through blind evaluation)	Measures various skills and abilities that are used to compensate for loss of vision by persons with visual impairment and blindness. Assessed skills are relevant to both daily living and vocational situations. These skills include spatial aptitude and motor coordination, problem-solving skills, and tactile and auditory perceptual abilities. The work sample establishes baseline measures that may be compared with scores after orientation and mobility training and rehabilitation teaching to gauge progress toward established client goals. Subtests include Tactual Perception, Mobility and Discrimination Skills, Space Organization and Memory, Assembly and Packaging, and Audile Perception.
Dynamic physical capacities	Measures the physical capacities associated with simulating the work of a shipping and receiving clerk. The work sample assesses strength levels ranging from sedentary to very heavy and makes the following physical demands, among others: reaching, handling, near acuity, climbing, balancing, stooping, crouching, and visual accommodation.
Physical capacities and mobility screening evaluation	Provides objective scores on a variety of strength measures. The work sample exercises also permit the evaluator to make pass–fail judgments on a number of dimensions of mobility. The work sample is divided into two parts. Part 1, Dynamic Strength, consists of six exercises: Lifting, Continuous Lifting, Two-Handed Grip, Palm Press, Horizontal Press, and Vertical Press. Part 2, Mobility Evaluation, has 15 exercises that require the client to balance on each leg, walk forward, walk backward, walk from heel to toe, walk on toe, walk on heel, squat, climb, kneel, crawl, stoop, and crouch.
Mechanical assembly alignment and hammering	Measures work skills that require proper selection, placement, and use of a variety of hand tools according to instructions and routine. The tasks involve assembling articles, fastening them together with bolts and washers, driving objects into grooves, and moderately precise, light hammering. The work sample simulates light and sedentary work and makes the following physical demands on the client: reaching, handling, fingering, near acuity, and depth perception.

Continued

Table 3.4. *Continued*

Ability	Description
Mechanical reasoning and machine tending	Measures work skills involving machine tending, positioning, and guiding items into a machine or under a needle; and assembling and disassembling various materials using hand tools. The work sample simulates sedentary work and makes the following physical demands on the client: reaching, handling, fingering, feeling, near acuity, depth perception, and accommodation.
Fine finger dexterity	Measures the ability to perform work tasks that require a high level of finger dexterity. The work sample simulates sedentary work and makes the following physical demands on the client: reaching, handling, fingering, feeling, near acuity, depth perception, and visual accommodation.
Independent perceptual screening–spatial aptitude	Measures the ability to envision geometric forms and to comprehend two-dimensional representations of three-dimensional objects. The work sample simulates sedentary work and makes the following physical demands on the client: reaching, handling, fingering, feeling, near acuity, and accommodation.

(Knapp, Knapp, & Michael, 1977). Validity has been demonstrated through studies of the association of CAPS test scores with scores of clients on comparable tests, such as the EAS, General Aptitude Test Battery, and others (Katz, Beers, Geckle, & Goldstein, 1989; Knapp, Knapp, Strand, & Michael, 1978; Knapp-Lee, 1995). Factor analysis of the CAPS has identified three primary factors, including Verbal Comprehension, Perceptual Skill, and Response Speed (Knapp et al., 1992).

Employer Aptitude Survey (EAS)

The EAS is a battery of ten standardized and timed multiple-choice subtests designed to measure the cognitive, perceptual, and psychomotor abilities required for successful job performance in a wide variety of occupations. Each of the EAS tests can be used either individually or as part of a battery. The 10 subtests measure verbal comprehension, numerical ability, visual pursuit, visual speed and accuracy, space visualization, numerical reasoning, verbal reasoning, verbal fluency, manual speed and accuracy, and symbolic reasoning (Ruch & Stang, 1994). The EAS is suitable for use with clients who are 12 years of age or older. Each subtest requires approximately 5 min to 10 min to administer.

The EAS has shown satisfactory reliability (Ruch & Stang, 1994). Content-related evidence of validity for the EAS was gathered during the test construction process by representatively sampling defined content domains. Test developers first identified 10 abilities as important for a wide variety of jobs, then selected item types that had been shown to tap the ability well. Criterion-related evidence of validity for the EAS has been gathered for more than 40 years (Table 3.5). Summaries of 725 validity coefficients from 160 studies appear in the technical man-

ual for the survey (Grimsley, Ruch, Ruch, Warren, & Ford, 1983). The EAS has been found to be statistically predictive of both training success and job performance. Construct validity evidence for the EAS, provided by factor analyses and correlations with other measures of identified constructs, shows that common, general mental abilities are associated with certain job categories (Table 3.5). Factor analysis has identified eight primary factors across the eight subtests. Percentile norms are available for close to 100 occupational and educational classifications based on more than 200,000 test scores. Computer-based, Web-based, and paper-and-pencil versions of the tests are available.

Measures of the Performance Environment

All human activities take place within an environmental context. For assessments conducted outside a rehabilitation center, hospital, or skilled care facility, it is appropriate and relevant to determine the safety and adequacy of the setting and the extent to which the environment supports the performance of activities and occupations in the home or workplace. Any one instrument will face challenges in measuring the many environmental factors that can influence engagement and performance in occupations. Cooper, Letts, and colleagues have suggested that because occupational engagement represents a transaction between an individual and the environment in which the occupation takes place, the best measures incorporate the dynamic nature of that transaction—what they refer to as the interface between the individual, the nature of an occupation, and the environment (Cooper, Letts, Rigby, Stewart, & Strong, 2001).

Table 3.5. Summary of Correlation Coefficients for Studies of the Employment Aptitude Survey and Criterion Variables

Performance Dimensions	Occupational Grouping									
	Professional, Managerial, and Supervisory		Clerical		Light Industry, Production, Mechanical		Technical		All Jobs	
	Job Performance	Training Success	Job Performance	Training Success	Job Performance	Training Success	Job Performance	Training Success	Job Performance	Training Success
Verbal comprehension	.53	.42	.38	—	.35	.63	.17	.45	.35	.53
Numerical ability	.55	.60	.46	—	.38	.69	.53	.76	.41	.66
Visual pursuit	—	.27	—	—	.35	—	—	.41	.37	.39
Visual speed and accuracy	—	.28	.46	—	.32	.31	.31	.40	.39	.37
Space visualization	—	.34	.50	—	.38	.48	.38	.47	.38	.45
Numerical reasoning	.53	.31	.29	—	—	.31	.52	.61	.10	.51
Verbal reasoning	.53	.29	.46	—	.13	—	.33	.48	.33	.47
Word fluency	—	.40	—	—	—	—	—	.22	.47	.41
Manual speed and accuracy	—	.27	.27	—	.29	—	—	.30	.22	.34
Symbolic reasoning	—	.48	—	—	—	—	.57	.53	.44	.59

Scales that measure the performance environment include two major categories of tools. The Safety Assessment of Function and the Environment for Rehabilitation (SAFER) Tool, the Home Occupation Environment Assessment (HOEA), and the revised Home Observation for Measurement of the Environment (HOME) examine factors in the home. The Work Environment Scale (WES) focuses on the work environment. The Environmental Independence Interaction Scale (EIIS) measures factors that relate to independent performance for people receiving rehabilitation services.

Safety Assessment of Function and the Environment for Rehabilitation (SAFER) Tool

The SAFER Tool was designed to identify risk factors in the living setting that can result in injury and to permit recommendations regarding safety (Letts & Marshall, 1995; Oliver, Blathwayt, Brackley, & Tamaki, 1993). The SAFER Tool uses 97 items grouped into 14 domains: living situation, mobility, kitchen, fire hazards, eating, household, dressing, grooming, bathroom, medication, communication, wandering, memory aids, and general. The SAFER Tool was developed by occupational therapists in the province of Ontario, Canada, to address the need for

an "acceptable, standardized instrument focusing on safety and function within the home environment" (Letts & Marshall, 1995, p. 53; Oliver et al., 1993).

Items to be assessed within the client's living environment are listed adjacent to three columns, which are labeled "Addressed," "Not Applicable," and "Problem." The evaluator checks off the correct columns as he or she makes observations about the relevant items. Items that are not relevant for given settings (e.g., elevators in a single-story home) are marked "Not applicable."

An interesting attribute of the SAFER Tool is the choice of items that reflect a transactional relationship between the individual and the home environment. The items were selected systematically by a panel of clinicians and seniors, and some items were discarded after analysis of content and construct validity. The item-selection process also provided a basis for developing guidelines to assist clinicians in using the tool. These guidelines have been organized in the form of questions to consider when completing an environmental assessment.

The SAFER Tool is a descriptive environmental assessment that demonstrates acceptable reliability and validity in measuring a person's ability to function safely within a home environment. A recent study of the SAFER Tool demonstrated that environments with greater safety risk correlated with cognitive impairment, suggesting that a relationship exists between level of independence and safety (Letts, Scott, Burtney, Marshall, & McKean, 1998).

Home Occupation Environment Assessment (HOEA)

The HOEA is an assessment tool developed specifically for use with clients with dementia (Baum, Edwards, Bradford, & Lane, 1995). Through items that address specific behavioral and environmental factors, the HOEA assesses the client's ability to live safely in a given environment. Items on the scale were developed on the basis of expert opinion and then factor analyzed to determine which item clusters correlated with high risk. The therapist uses a checklist to indicate whether a given item has been assessed and to assign a score. The HOEA uses a 4-point scale: no problem observed, requires monitoring, requires attention, or high risk situation.

Behavioral items include impaired judgment, disheveled appearance, possible abuse or neglect, depressed mood, difficulties with finance, difficulties with managing medications, awareness of surroundings, understands questions, slurred speech, slow response, difficult to understand, hearing problem, smell, and vision. Environmental item categories include accessibility within the home, sanitation, food storage, and general safety issues. The HOEA is a new scale, so it has not yet been validated or studied extensively. Research continues, but further study is needed with this instrument aimed at people with cognitive deficits.

Home Observation for Measure of Environment (HOME)

The HOME is a standardized screening instrument designed to identify attributes of the home environment that contribute to cognitive, social, and emotional development in children. The scale is used to evaluate the environments of children from birth through 13 years of age. Three versions of the scale are available: one for infants (birth to 3 years old); a second for preschoolers (3 years old to 6 years old); and a third, middle childhood version, for children from 6 years old to 13 years old. The scale requires active assistance from a second professional or a caregiver who can be a service provider and takes about 2 hr to complete. The infant version has 45 items, the preschool version has 55 items, and the middle childhood version has 59 items.

The scale is scored nominally (plus or minus for each item) and measures abilities, activities, environmental factors, and life habits. The factors addressed in the scale include social skills and behaviors; physical attributes of the home environment (lighting, safety, size, location, equipment, technology, appliances, tools, and toys); social aspects of the environment (stimulation, social support, communication, and family organization); and interpersonal relations (family, relatives, friends, community life, and use of services).

The reliability of the HOME as an assessment tool is good. Studies also support the validity of this scale. Studies have examined the content of the scales, and factor and item analysis have supported the underlying structure. Studies also have supported the construct and criterion validity of the scale.

Work Environment Scale (WES)

The Work Environment Scale was designed to allow individuals to evaluate productivity, assess employee satisfaction, and clarify employee work expectations to ensure a healthy work environment (Moos, 1993, 1994). The WES consists of 90 items organized as 10 subscales of 9 items each. A 40-item short form of the WES also is available. The subscales assess the following work environment factors: involvement, coworker cohesion, supervisory support, autonomy, task orientation, work pressure, clarity, managerial control, innovation, and physical comfort. The WES is designed for completion by adult workers but can be completed by service providers as well. The WES can be completed through a structured interview or in a naturalistic context by observing the work setting. The scale takes approximately 30 min to complete. Scoring is complex, so examiner training is recommended.

The WES can be administered to individuals or groups. The manual provides normative data and information on clinical, consulting, and program evaluation uses. It also has updated and expanded research information. Normative data for the WES have been collected from more than 8,000 workers in a variety of work settings (Moos, 1981). The user's guide assists with the interpretation of results and provides scale assessment information. The WES comes in a self-score format with an interpretative report form that can be used to explain results.

Reliability of the WES is considered to be excellent. (Abraham & Foley, 1984; Moos, 1981). Studies have demonstrated that the WES has good content, construct, and criterion-related validity (Moos, 1994; Moos & Moos, 1998).

Environment Independencce Interaction Scale (EIIS)

The EIIS was developed to measure contextual factors that are significantly related to independent performance among people receiving rehabilitation services (Teel, Dunn, Jackson, & Duncan, 1997). The EIIS identifies four domains as contextual factors: physical factors (including nonhuman aspects, such as objects and devices that enhance or inhibit performance); social factors (including the availability and actions of significant people in the client's environment); cultural factors (including customs, beliefs, and expectations); and temporal factors (including timing of interventions and time available for practicing skills).

The content of the EIIS was developed in concert with the construction of a conceptual model known as the Ecology of Human Performance (EHP). The EIIS and EHP were based on an extensive review of the literature that identified environmental factors related to rehabilitation success (W. W. Dunn, Brown, & McCuigan, 1994). Different groups of caregivers were used to test the original version of the scale, including family members of people receiving rehabilitation at home, clients receiving care in facilities, and professionals providing care in facilities.

The EIIS consists of 20 items; 5 items rate factors in each of the physical and social environment areas, 6 items rate the cultural environment, and 4 items assess temporal factors. Using a 5-point Likert scale with values representing ranges between *not at all* to *a great deal*, informants express their opinions regarding attitudes, care practices, and features of the home- or facility-based rehabilitation program in which the client of interest is receiving care.

Reliability has been reported as good to excellent (Teel et al., 1997).

Studies of the scale's validity have been limited. Content validity can be judged as excellent based on the manner in which items were chosen. Evidence of construct and criterion validity is being gathered. The score provided by the EIIS is intended to show the extent to which a rehabilitation environment supports or interferes with a client's independence (Teel et al., 1997).

Measures of Social Participation

The final area appropriate for use in developing an occupational profile is social participation. Few well-established scales address this domain in the context of activities. Five potentially suitable scales are the Activity Card Sort (ACS), the Assessment of Communication and Interaction Skills (ACIS), the Interview Schedule for Social Interaction (ISSI), the Reintegration to Normal Living Index (RNL), and the Community Integration Questionnaire (CIQ). Other scales noted in the literature may be suitable for assessment in this domain. The scales presented here are intended to be representative of the larger domain of available instruments.

Activity Card Sort (ACS)

The ACS is a tool for making a broad assessment of life activity. Developed by Baum (1993), it was designed to determine an individual's level of participation in instrumental, leisure, and social activities. The scale's Q-Sort methodology can be used with clients or people familiar with the client's life activities (Figure 3.4). Although it was originally designed for the assessment of people with cognitive deficits, the ACS can be used with adult populations with or without conditions that limit function (Baum, 1993).

Q-Sort methodology uses cards that are sorted into categories by the client or proxy (a person completing the assessment on behalf of the client). The Activity Card Sort uses 80 cards with photographs of activities that are sorted into five categories (never done, not done as an older adult, do now, do less, and given up). The categories can be modified according to the questions of interest to the evaluator.

Three versions of the ACS have been developed: a healthy adults version, an institutional version, and a recovering client version. The versions differ with respect to the categories used for sorting the cards. For example, the institutional version sorts the activity cards into two groups (done prior to illness and not done). This approach allows the therapist to identify premorbid activity data that is useful for planning intervention.

Administration of the ACS takes approximately 20 min. If the provider wishes to interview the client about details associated with sorting results, the interview will lengthen the time needed for administration. Because the ACS is a method for gathering data rather than a scale, it is flexible and can be adjusted to work with various client groups and cultures by adding or substituting cards depicting group-appropriate photographs of activities.

The second edition of the ACS added 7 new activities to the original list of 73, bringing the total to 80. In an unpublished study of survivors of stroke, Edwards showed that the percentage of activities regained since suffering the stroke was a better predictor of a client's quality of life than traditional measures of function. N. Katz and colleagues (N. Katz, Karpin, Lak, Furman, & Hartman-Maier, 2003) re-

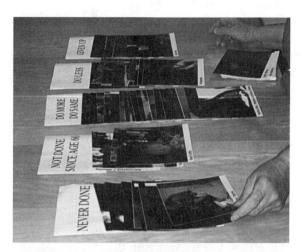

Figure 3.3. The Activity Card Sort consists of a set of labeled cards with photographs of common household and leisure tasks. The client, using a Q-Sort method, places the cards into defined categories depicting current functional status. Photo by M. C. Baum.

ported on a reliability and validity study of a version of the ACS that had been modified for use in Israel. Their version used 88 cards and reported good internal consistency values using Cronbach's alpha for instrumental activities of daily living and social cultural activities. Lower coefficients were found for activities described as low and high physical leisure activities. A comparison of participant groups on total retained activity level and individual activity areas showed a significant group effect on all comparisons, adding to the evidence that the ACS can be a valid method for distinguishing among groups according to their engagement in and perception of activities (N. Katz et al., 2003).

Assessment of Communication and Interaction Skills (ACIS)

The Assessment of Communication and Interaction Skills (ACIS) is an observational rating scale that measures a client's social interaction abilities (Forsyth, Lai, & Kielhofner, 2001; Simon, 1989). Based on the conceptual framework of the model of human occupation, the ACIS is intended to capture characteristics of social interaction during participation in ordinary everyday activities. The current version of the scale reflects several revisions designed to allow the scale to precisely use behavioral criteria to identify the demonstration of skills used in social interaction.

The ACIS consists of 22 observational skill items grouped into three domains: physicality, information exchange, and relations. The clinician rates each skill item after observing the client in a social situation using a 4-point rating scale. The scoring of

individual items permits the identification of strengths and weaknesses useful for social skills intervention. Items are scored after observation in four types of situations: an unstructured situation, a parallel task group, a cooperative group situation, and a dyadic (one-to-one) situation.

Studies with earlier versions of the ACIS resulted in refinement of the skill item definitions. One study that used Rasch analysis found evidence of construct validity, but shortcomings in the scale's ability to distinguish among clients with known social deficits (Salamy, 1993). A more recent study using 52 trained raters established the construct validity of the scale through comparison of the calibrated and ranked statistics using Rasch analysis (Forsyth et al., 2001). In this study, the scale was able to discriminate among clients with different diagnostic profiles, demonstrated unidimensionality, and demonstrated satisfactory interrater reliability. The ACIS has not yet been well researched and therefore must be viewed as an emerging but promising measure of skill in social participation.

Interview Schedule for Social Interaction (ISSI)

The Interview Schedule for Social Interaction is a well-validated structured interview. It consists of 52 items that provide scores in four areas: availability of attachments or close relationships, adequacy of attachments, availability of social interaction or more distant relationships, and adequacy of social interaction (Henderson, Duncan-Jones, Byrne, & Scott, 1980). Varying response formats are available. On average, the interview requires about 45 min to administer (Henderson, 1980).

The ISSI has satisfactory internal consistency, and factor analysis has confirmed the validity of the four subscales as measuring distinct facets of social interaction (Duncan-Jones, 1981a, 1981b).

Studies have shown evidence of construct validity in the ISSI. ISSI scores are associated with marital status and age and correlate significantly in expected directions with measures of neuroticism, depression, and extraversion (Morris, Robinson, Raphael, & Bishop, 1991; Thomas, Garry, Goodwin, & Goodwin, 1985). The scale does not seem to be influenced by social desirability response tendency, or the tendency of subjects to change their natural responses based on their perceptions that it will reflect a more favorable view of themselves. Norms are available for defined populations (Henderson, Byrne, & Duncan-Jones, 1981). The scale has been well accepted by clinicians and seems suitable for measuring behaviors related to social interaction and clients' tendencies and resources that would affect social participation.

Reintegration to Normal Living Scale (RNL)

The Reintegration to Normal Living Scale is a 15-item measure developed with input from health care consumers, family members, and clinicians concerning the factors that explain community reintegration following functional disruption related to injury or illness (Wood-Dauphinee, Opzoomer, Williams, Marchand, & Spitzer, 1988). The RNL typically is used with rehabilitation clients who have experienced sudden onset disability (Wood-Dauphinee & Willliams, 1987).

Items consist of statements to which the client provides a response using a visual analogue scale anchored with the statements "Fully describes my situation" or "Does not describe my situation." Scoring is based on the placement of marks on the analogue scale. Scores are converted to percentages.

The RNL requires approximately 10 min to complete. It can be administered through interview or completed by the client. Reliability for the measure is excellent (Wood-Dauphinee & Willliams, 1987). Factor analysis supports a one-factor solution that explains 49% of the variation in client scores. Content validity of the RNL seems excellent based on the iterative three-stage process used in the scale's development. The scale also has evidenced criterion and construct validity, with scores on the RNL correlating significantly with work and disease status but not with living situation. The RNL also correlates with measures of quality of life and affect.

Community Integration Questionnaire (CIQ)

The Community Integration Questionnaire was developed to measure social disadvantage as an aspect of outcome following rehabilitation following brain injury (Willer, Rosenthal, Kreutzer, Gordon, & Rempel, 1993). Although the scale was developed for a specific population (people who had sustained brain injuries), it has been used more broadly. The CIQ consists of 15 items contained in three subscales pertaining to home integration, social integration, and engagement in productive activities. Items are scored with a 3-point response option that varies with each subscale. The CIQ can be administered in approximately 10 min, either as a telephone interview or directly with clients.

Reliability for the CIQ is satisfactory, using measures of internal consistency and stability (Willer, Linn, & Allen, 1992).

Content for the CIQ was derived from the literature and a panel of consumers, rehabilitation professionals, and researchers (Willer et al., 1993). Scores on the CIQ have correlated significantly with other measures of community integration, and the scale is able to discriminate between client groups who are able bodied and those who are disabled (Willer, Allen, Liss, & Zicht, 1991).

Summary

The process of developing a client's occupational profile involves using observations and instruments from several domains. Useful instruments have been developed for measuring functional skills in the areas of ADL, IADL, leisure, play, school, and work. Additional instruments are available for measuring the performance environment and social participation. Table 3.6 presents a summary of the characteristics of these assessment instruments.

Effective assessment of occupational performance is essential to planning and modifying intervention strategies and making informed recommendations about safe and satisfying performance options for clients. The choice of an instrument for assessing a client will depend on the characteristics of the setting, the characteristics of the client, and the purpose of the assessment. No one "gold standard" for occupational assessment ideally suits every purpose. Ultimately, the choice of assessment tools must be geared toward the development of a useful occupational profile.

A great need exists for more reports of how well existing scales perform in varied settings and with different populations. Are the instruments sensitive to change? Do they predict future occupational performance at home or in the natural living environment? Can existing interview and self-report instruments be modified to include observations of performance in addition to reported performance? Studies also are needed that support the development and validation of existing scales. The use of ad hoc or "homemade" evaluations is no longer acceptable. Occupational therapists have extensive expertise in the assessment of function and in interventions that help adapt tasks, tools, and environments so that occupations can be pursued. Therefore, occupational therapists should be at the forefront of the development of performance-based assessments related to the important need to engage in activities and participate in the social world.

Acknowledgment

Catherine Backman, PhD, OT(C), made important contributions to earlier versions of this chapter. The author is indebted to her for her past and continuing support.

Table 3.6. Summary of Characteristics of Instruments Reviewed

Instrument	Area(s) Measured	Reliability	Validity	Measurement Method(s)
Activity Card Sort (ACS)	IADL/leisure/social	Internal consistency = .61–.82	Evidence of content and criterion validity	Q-sort
Assessment of Communication and Interaction Skills (ACIS)	Social interaction skills (physicality, information exchange, and relations)	*r* = .96	Evidence of content, criterion, and construct validity (few studies)	Observation of performance
Assessment of Motor and Process Skills (AMPS)	IADL/education tasks	95% interrater reliability using Rasch analysis	Validity testing ongoing; concurrent validity established	Observation of performance
Barthel Index (BI)	Basic ADL (extended version measures additional functional items)	Stability = .89 Interrater = .95	Criterion = .89 Detects change in parallel with Katz	Interview Observation Chart review
Canadian Occupational Performance Measure (COPM)	ADL/IADL/leisure	Stability = .63–.84 ICC = .90 and above	Evidence of content and criterion validity	Interview
Career Ability Placement Survey (CAPS)	Work-related conceptual skills and perceptual/manual speed and dexterity	Split-half = .70–.95 Test–retest = Interrater =	Evidence of content, concurrent, criterion, and construct validity	Written performance test
Community Integration Questionnaire (CIQ)	Social participation (engagement in productive activities in the home and community)	Internal consistency = .76 Test–retest = .90	Evidence of content, concurrent, and criterion validity	Interview
Employee Aptitude Survey (EAS)	Work-related cognitive, perceptual, and psychomotor abilities	Alternate forms = .76–.91 Test–retest = .75	Evidence of content, concurrent, criterion, and construct validity	Written performance test
Environmental Independence Interaction Scale (EIIS)	Living context (physical, social, and temporal factors that influence independence)	Internal consistency = .92–.96; individual areas have alpha coefficients of .68–.90	Evidence of content validity, but other validity studies are under way	Report based on observation
Frenchay Activities Index (FAI)	IADL/work/leisure/social	Kappa = .60 Interrater = .93	Evidence of concurrent, construct, and criterion validity	Report/interview (mailed version)
Functional Independence Measure (FIM)	ADL/IADL	Interrater = .95 Test–retest = .95 Equivalence = .92 Subttests = .78–.95	Large number of studies showing concurrent, predictive, and construct validity	Interview Telephone report Direct observation
Functional Independence Measure for Children (WeeFIM)	ADL/social cognition	Interrater = .98 Stability = .83–.99 ICC = .95 total score ICC = .73–.99 for subscales	Scores predict amount of caregiver assistance needed; correlates with measures of developmental status; has criterion validity	Interview Observation

Continued

Table 3.6. *Continued*

Instrument	Area(s) Measured	Reliability	Validity	Measurement Method(s)
Home Observation for Measurement of the Environment (HOME)	Performance context (home); attributes that influence cognitive, social, and emotional development of children	Internal consistency = .89 or greater Interrater ≥ .90 Stability = .64	Evidence of content, criterion, and construct validity	Interview/survey
Home Occupation Environment Assessment (HOEA)	Performance context (home)	Interrater = .95	Content through expert opinion; factor analysis	Observation
Interview Schedule for Social Interaction (ISSI)	Social interaction	Internal consistency = .67–.81 Test–retest = .75–.79	Evidence of content, concurrent, criterion, and construct validity	Interview
Katz Index of Independence in ADL	Basic ADL	Scalability = .74–.88 Interrater =	Criterion = discharge score; predicts need for personal assistance	Observation
Leisure Competence Measure	Leisure behaviors	Internal consistency and stability > .90	Evidence of content, concurrent, and criterion validity	Report Interview/survey
Leisure Diagnostic Battery (LDB)	Leisure knowledge, needs, and attitudes	Internal consistency = .83–.94 for long version and .89–.94 for short form	Evidence of concurrent, criterion, and construct validity (including confirmatory factory analysis)	Interview/survey
Leisure Satisfaction Questionnaire	Leisure satisfaction	Internal consistency = .82–.86	Evidence of content and predictive validity	Interview/survey
Nottingham Extended Activities of Daily Living Scale (NEADL)	IADL/leisure	Internal consistency = .72–.94 Interrater reliability = .81–.90	Evidence of construct and concurrent validity	Report
Pediatric Evaluation of Disability Index (PEDI)	ADL/cognition	Interrater reliability = .96–.99 Internal consistency = .95–.99	Expert panel content: scores correlate with age and with WeeFIM and Battelle Scores (.62–.97)	Interview Observation
Performance Assessment of Self Care Skills (PASS)	ADL/IADL	Interrater agreement = 96–99% Internal consistency and test–retest > .80	Evidence of content, concurrent, criterion, and construct validity	Observation
Preschool Play Scale (Revised) (PPS–R)	Play behaviors (underlying capacity to play)	Interrater = .88–.99 Test–retest = .91–.97	Evidence of content, concurrent, and criterion validity	Report/survey
Reintegration to Normal Living Index (RNL)	Activity participation following rehabilitation	Internal consistency = .90–.95	Evidence of content, criterion, and construct validity	Interview/ self-report
Safety Assessment of Function and the Environment for Rehabilitation (SAFER) Tool	Features (safety) of living context	Interrater = .80 Internal consistency = .83	Evidence of content and concurrent validity	Observation

Continued

Table 3.6. *Continued*

Instrument	Area(s) Measured	Reliability	Validity	Measurement Method(s)
School Functional Assessment (SFA)	Learning and social skills	Internal consistency = .92–.98 ICC = .80–.99	Evidence of concurrent and criterion validity	Observation
Test of Playfulness (TOP)	Play behaviors	Interrater ≥ .90	Evidence of concurrent, construct, and criterion validity	Observation
VALPAR Component Work Samples	Work performance	Stability = .70–.99	Evidence of criterion validity for all samples	Observation of performance
Work Environment Scale (WES)	Work context (productivity, satisfaction, expectations)	Internal consistency ≥ .69–.86 Test–retest = .69–.83 Stability = .51–.63	Evidence of content, construct, and criterion validity	Interview/survey

Note. ADL = activities of daily living; IADL = instrumental activities of daily living; ICC = intraclass correlation coefficient.

Study Questions

1. What is an analysis of occupational performance?
2. Distinguish between the properties of reliability and validity in determining the merits of a particular assessment instrument.
3. Define the term *occupational profile*. What sources of information can the occupational therapist use in compiling an occupational profile?
4. What are the major differences between scales that measure ADL skills and scales that measure IADL skills?
5. Identify two instruments for each of the following categories of occupational performance: ADL, IADL, leisure, play, education, work, and social participation.
6. What client factors does the Assessment of Motor and Process Skills measure?
7. When assessing a performance context, what types of information should be sought that will assist in the analysis of occupational performance?

References

Abraham, I., & Foley, T. (1984). The Work Environment Scale and the Ward Atmosphere Scale (short forms): Psychometric data. *Perceptual and Motor Skills, 58*(1), 319–322.

American Occupational Therapy Association. (2002). Occupational therapy practice framework: Domain and process. *American Journal of Occupational Therapy, 56,* 609–639.

Azaula, M., Msall, M., Buck, G., Tremont, M., Wilczenski, F., & Rogers, B. (2000). Measuring functional status and family support in older school-aged children with cerebral palsy: Comparison of three instruments. *Archives of Physical Medicine and Rehabilitation, 81*(3), 307–311.

Baum, C. M. (1993). *The effects of occupation on behaviors of persons with senile dementia of the Alzheimer's type and their carers.* Washington University, St. Louis, MO.

Baum, C. M. (1995). The contribution of occupation to function in persons with Alzheimer's disease. *Journal of Occupational Science: Australia, 2,* 59–67.

Baum, C., Edwards, D. F., Bradford, T., & Lane, R. (1995). *Home Occupation-Environment Assessment.* St. Louis, MO: Washington University, Occupational Therapy Program.

Beard, J., & Ragheb, M. (1980). The Leisure Satisfaction Questionnaire. *Journal of Leisure Research, 12*(1), 20–32.

Bent, N., Jones, A., Molloy, I., Chamberlain, M., & Tennant, A. (2001). Factors determining participation in young adults with a physical disability: A pilot study. *Clinical Rehabilitation, 15,* 552–561.

Bestall, J. C., Paul, E. A., Garrod, R., Garnham, R., Jones, P. W., & Wedzicha, J. A. (1999). Usefulness of the Medical Research Council (MRC) dyspnoea scale as a measure of disability in patients with chronic obstructive pulmonary disease. *Thorax, 54,* 581–586.

Bledsoe, N., & Shepherd, J. (1982). A study of the reliability and validity of a preschool play scale. *American Journal of Occupational Therapy, 36,* 783–788.

Bodiam, C. (1999). The use of the Canadian Occupational Performance Measure for the assessment of outcome on a neurorehabilitation unit. *British Journal of Occupational Therapy, 2*(3), 123–126.

Braun, S., & Granger, C. (1991). A practical approach to functional assessment in pediatrics. *Occupational Therapy Practice, 2,* 46–51.

Bronson, M., & Bundy, A. C. (2001). A correlational study of a test of playfulness and a test of environmental supportiveness for play. *OTJR: Occupation, Participation and Health, 21*(4), 242–259.

Brorsson, B., & Asberg, K. (1984). Katz index of independence in ADL: Reliability and validity in short-term care. *Scandinavian Journal of Rehabilitation Medicine, 16,* 125–132.

Buck, D., Jacoby, A., Massey, A., & Ford, G. S. (2000). Evaluation of measures used to assess quality of life after stroke. *Stroke, 31,* 2004–2010.

Bundy, A. C. (1997). Play and playfulness: What to look for. In L. Parham & L. Fazio (Eds.), *Play in occupational therapy for children* (pp. 52–66). St. Louis, MO: Mosby.

Burch, S., Longbottom, J., McKay, M., Borland, C., & Prevost, T. (2000). The Huntingdon Day Hospital Trial: Secondary outcome measures. *Clinical Rehabilitation, 14,* 447–453.

Carod-Artal, J., Egido, J. A., Gonzalez, J. L., & de Seijas, E. V. (2000). Quality of life among stroke survivors evaluated 1 year after stroke: Experience of a stroke unit. *Stroke, 31,* 2995–3000.

Carpenter, L., Baker, G., & Tyldesley, B. (2001). The use of the Canadian Occupational Performance Measure as an outcome of a pain management program. *Canadian Journal of Occupational Therapy, 68*(1), 16–22.

Chang, Y., & Card, J. (1994). The reliability of the Leisure Diagnostic Battery Short Form Version AB in assessing healthy, older individuals: A preliminary study. *Therapeutic Recreation Journal, 28,* 163–167.

Chesworth, C., Duffy, R., Hodnett, J., & Knight, A. (2002). Measuring clinical effectiveness in mental health: Is the Canadian Occupational Performance an appropriate measure? *British Journal of Occupational Therapy, 65*(1), 30–34.

Chong, D. S. (1995). Measurement of instrumental activities of daily living in stroke. *Stroke, 26,* 1119–1122.

Christiansen, C. H. (2004). Functional evaluation and management of self care and other activities of daily living. In J. DeLisa & B. Gans (Eds.), *Rehabilitation medicine: Principles and practice.* Philadelphia: Lippincott Williams & Wilkins.

Cooper, B., Letts, L., Rigby, P., Stewart, D., & Strong, S. (2001). Measuring environmental factors. In M. Law, C. Baum, & W. Dunn (Eds.), *Measuring occupational performance: Supporting best practice in occupational therapy* (pp. 229–256). Thorofare, NJ: Slack.

Coster, W. (1998). Occupation centered assessment of children. *American Journal of Occupational Therapy, 52,* 337–344.

Coster, W., Deeney, T., Haltiwanger, J., & Haley. S. (1998). *Manual for the School Function Assessment.* San Antonio, TX: Psychological Corporation.

Darragh, A. R., Sample, P. L., & Fisher, A. G. (1998). Environmental effect on functional task performance in adults with acquired brain injuries: Use of the Assessment of Motor and Process Skills. *Archives of Physical Medicine and Rehabilitation, 79,* 418–423.

DeJong, G., Branch, L., & Corcoran, P. (1996). Independent living outcomes in spinal cord injury: Multivariate analyses. *Archives of Physical Medicine and Rehabilitation, 77,* 883–888.

Dennis, M., O'Rourke, S., Slattery, J., Staniforth, T., & Warlow, C. (1997). Evaluation of a stroke family care worker: Results of a randomized controlled trial. *British Medical Journal, 314,* 1071–1076.

Duncan-Jones, P. (1981a). The structure of social relationships: Analysis of a survey instrument. Part 1. *Social Psychiatry, 16,* 55–61.

Duncan-Jones, P. (1981b). The structure of social relationships: Analysis of a survey instrument. Part 2. *Social Psychiatry, 16,* 143–149.

Dunn, J. (1987). *Generalizability of the Leisure Diagnostic Battery.* Unpublished doctoral dissertation, University of Illinois, Champaign.

Dunn, W. W., Brown, C., & McCuigan, A. (1994). The ecology of human performance: A framework for considering the effect of context. *American Journal of Occupational Therapy, 48,* 595–607.

Dyer, C., Singh, S., Stockley, R., Sinclair, A., & Hill, S. (2002). The incremental shuttle walking test in elderly people with chronic airflow limitation. *Thorax, 57,* 34–38.

Edwards, D. A. (1995). Unpublished raw data.

Ellis, G. D., & Witt, P. A. (1986). The Leisure Diagnostic Battery: Past, present and future. *Therapeutic Recreation Journal, 19,* 31–47.

Ellul, J., Watkins, C., & Barer, D. (1998). Estimating total Barthel scores from just three items: The European Stroke Database "minimum dataset" for assessing functional status at discharge from hospital. *Age and Ageing, 27*(2), 115–122.

Finlayson, M., Havens, B., Holm, M., & Van Denend, T. (2003). Integrating a performance-based observation measure of functional status into a population-based longitudinal study of aging. *Canadian Journal on Aging, 22*(2), 185–195.

Fisher, A. (1993). The assessment of IADL motor skill: An application of the many-faceted Rasch analysis. *American Journal of Occupational Therapy, 47,* 319–329.

Fisher, A. (1994). *Assessment of Motor and Process Skills (research edition 7.0).* Fort Collins: Colorado State University.

Fisher, A., & Duran, L. (2000). ADL performance of black Americans and white Americans on the Assessment of Motor and Process Skills. *American Journal of Occupational Therapy, 54,* 607–613.

Fisher, A., Liu, Y., Velozo, C., & Pan, A. (1992). Cross-cultural assessment of process skills. *American Journal of Occupational Therapy, 46,* 876–885.

Forsyth, K., Lai, J., & Kielhofner, G. (2001). The Assessment of Communication and Interaction Skills (ACIS): A measurement profile. *British Journal of Occupational Therapy, 62*(2), 69–74.

Garrod, R., Bestall, J. C., Paul, E. A., Wedzicha, J. A., & Jones, P. W. (2000). Development and validation of a standardized measure of activity of daily living in patients with severe COPD: The London Chest Activity of Daily Living Scale (LCADL). *Respiratory Medicine, 94,* 589–596.

Gilbertson, L., & Langhorne, P. (2000). Home-based occupational therapy: Stroke patients' satisfaction with occupational performance and service provision. *British Journal of Occupational Therapy, 63*(10), 464–468.

Gompertz, P., Pound, P., & Ebrahim, S. (1994). A postal version of the Barthel Index. *Clinical Rehabilitation, 8*(3), 233–239.

Granger, C., Deutsch, A., & Linn, R. (1998). Rasch analysis of the Functional Independence Measure FIM™

Mastery Test. *Archives of Physical Medicine and Rehabilitation, 79,* 52–57.

Granger, C., Hamilton, B., Gresham, G., & Kramer, A. (1989). The stroke rehabilitation outcome study: Part II. Relative merits of the total Barthel Index score and a four-item sub score in predicting patient outcomes. *Archives of Physical Medicine and Rehabilitation, 70,* 100–103.

Green, J., Forster, A., & Young, J. D. R. (2001). A test-retest reliability study of the Barthel Index, the Rivermead Mobility Index, the Nottingham Extended Activities of Daily Living Scale and the Frenchay Activities Index in survivors of stroke. *Disability and Rehabilitation, 23,* 670–676.

Grimsley, G., Ruch, F. L., Ruch, W., Warren, N. D., & Ford, J. S. (1983). *Employee Aptitude Survey technical manual.* Glendale, CA: Psychological Services.

Guttman, L. E. (1950). The basis for scalogram analysis. In S. Stouffer, L. Guttman, E. Suchman, P. Lazarsfield, S. Star, & J. Clausen (Eds.), *Measurement and prediction* (pp. 60–90). Princeton, NJ: Princeton University Press.

Hachisuka, K., Saeki, S., Tsutsui, Y., Chisaka, H., Ogata, H., Iwata, N., et al. (1999). Gender-related differences in scores of the Barthel Index and Frenchay Activities Index in randomly sampled elderly persons living at home in Japan. *Journal of Clinical Epidemiology, 52,* 1089–1094.

Haig, A., Nagy, A., Lebreck, D., & Stein, G. (1995). Outpatient planning for persons with physical disabilities: A randomized prospective trial of physiatrist alone versus a multidisciplinary team. *Archives of Physical Medicine and Rehabilitation, 76,* 341–348.

Haley, S., Coster, W., Ludlow, L., Haltiwanger, J., & Andrellos, P. (1992). *Pediatric Evaluation of Disability Inventory: Development, standardization and administration manual.* Boston: PEDI Research Group.

Hall, K., Mann, N., High, W., Wright, J., Kreutzer, J., & Wood, D. (1996). Functional measures after traumatic brain injury: Ceiling effects of FIM, FIM+FAM, DRS, and CIQ. *Journal of Head Trauma Rehabilitation, 11*(5), 27–39.

Hamilton, B., Granger, C., Sherwin, F., Zielezny, M., & Tashman, M. (1987). A uniform national data system for medical rehabilitation. In M. Fuhrer (Ed.), *Rehabilitation outcomes: Analysis and measurement* (pp. 137–147). Baltimore: Brookes.

Harkness, L., & Bundy, A. C. (2001). The test of playfulness and children with physical disabilities. *OTJR: Occupation, Participation and Health, 21*(2), 73–89.

Harrison, H., & Kielhofner, G. (1986). Examining reliability and validity of the Preschool Play Scale with handicapped children. *American Journal of Occupational Therapy, 40,* 167–173.

Harwood, R. H., & Ebrahim, S. (2000). A comparison of the responsiveness of the Nottingham Extended Activities of Daily Living Scale, London Handicap Scale and SF-36. *Disability and Rehabilitation, 22,* 786–793.

Henderson, S. (1980). A development in social psychiatry: The systematic study of social bonds. *Journal of Nervous and Mental Diseases, 168,* 63–69.

Henderson, S., Byrne, D., & Duncan-Jones, P. (1981). *Neurosis and the social environment.* New York: Academic Press.

Henderson, S., Duncan-Jones, P., Byrne, D., & Scott, R. (1980). Measuring social relationships: The Interview Schedule for Social Interaction. *Psychological Medicine, 10,* 723–734.

Hertanu, J., Demopoulos, J., Yang, W., Calhoun, W., & Fenigstein, H. (1984). Stroke rehabilitation: Correlation and prognostic value of computerized tomography and sequential functional assessments. *Archives of Physical Medicine and Rehabilitation, 65,* 505–508.

Hoenig, H., Hoff, J., McIntyre, L., & Branch, L. (2001). The Self-Reported Functional Measure: Predictive validity for health utilization in multiple sclerosis and spinal cord injury. *Archives of Physical Medicine and Rehabilitation, 82,* 613–618.

Holbrook, M., & Skilbeck, C. (1983). An activities index for use with stroke. *Age & Ageing, 12,* 166–170.

Holm, M. B., & Rogers, J. C. (1999). Functional assessment: Performance assessment of self-care skills. In B. Hemphill-Pearson (Ed.), *Assessments in occupational therapy mental health: An integrative approach* (pp. 113–124). Thorofare, NJ: Slack.

Hsieh, C., & Hsueh, I. (1999). A cross validation of the comprehensive assessment of activities of daily living after stroke. *Scandinavian Journal of Rehabilitation Medicine, 31*(2), 83–88.

Hsueh, I. P., Huang, S. L., Chen, M. H., Jush, S. D., & Hsieh, C. L. (2000). Evaluation of survivors of stroke with the extended activities of daily living scale in Taiwan. *Disability and Rehabilitation, 22,* 495–500.

Kanters, M. (1995, October). *Leisure satisfaction, stress and health.* Unpublished paper presented at the Leisure Research Symposium, San Antonio, TX.

Karamehmetoglu, S., Karacan, I., Elbasi, N., Demirel, G., Koyuncu, H., & Dosoglu, M. (1997). The Functional Independence Measure in spinal cord injured patients: Comparison of questioning with observational rating. *Spinal Cord, 35*(1), 22–25.

Katz, L., Beers, S., Geckle, M., & Goldstein, G. (1989). The clinical use of the Career Ability Placement Survey versus the GATB for persons having psychiatric disabilities. *Journal of Applied Rehabilitation Counseling, 20*(1), 13–19.

Katz, N., Karpin, H., Lak, A., Furman, T., & Hartman-Maeir, A. (2003). Participation in occupational performance: Reliability and validity of the Activity Card Sort. *OTJR: Occupation, Participation and Health, 23*(1), 10–17.

Katz, S., Downs, T., Cash, H., & Grotz, R. (1970). Progress in development of an Index of ADL. *Gerontologist, 10,* 20–30.

Katz, S., Ford, A. B., Moskowitz, M., Jackson, B. A., & Jaffe, M. W. (1963). Studies of illness in the aged. The index of ADL: A standardized measure of biological and psychosocial function. *Journal of the American Medical Association, 185,* 914–919.

Ketelaar, M., Vermeer, A., & Helders, P. (1998). Functional motor abilities of children with cerebral palsy: A systematic literature review of assessment measures. *Clinical Rehabilitation, 12*(5), 369–380.

Kinnman, J., Andersson, U., Wetterqvist, L., Kinnman, Y., & Andersson, U. (2000). Cooling suit for multiple sclerosis: Functional improvement in daily living? *Scandinavian Journal of Rehabilitation Medicine, 32*(1), 20–24.

Kloseck, M., & Crilly, R. (1997). *Leisure Competence Measure: Adult Version.* London, Ontario, Canada: Data System.

Knapp, L., Knapp, R., & Knapp-Lee, L. (1992). *Career Ability Placement Survey technical manual*. San Diego, CA: EdITS.

Knapp, L., Knapp, R., & Michael, W. (1977). Stability and concurrent validity of the Career Ability Placement Survey (CAPS) against the DAP and GATB. *Educational and Psychological Measurement, 37*, 1081–1085.

Knapp, L., Knapp, R., Strand, L. I., & Michael, W. (1978). Comparative validity of the Career Ability Placement Survey and the GATB for predicting high school course marks. *Educational and Psychological Measurement, 38*, 1053–1056.

Knapp-Lee, L. (1995). Use of the COP system in career assessment. *Journal of Career Assessment, 3*, 411–428.

Knox, S. (1974). A play scale. In Reilly, M (Ed.), *Play as exploratory learning* (pp. 247–266). Beverly Hills, CA: Sage.

Knox, S. (1997). Development and current use of the Knox Preschool Play Scale. In L. D. Parham & L. S. Fazio (Eds.), *Play in occupational therapy for children* (pp. 35–51). St. Louis, MO: Mosby.

Kwakkel, G., Kollen, B., & Wagenaar, R. (2002). Long term effects of intensity of upper and lower limb training after stroke: A randomized trial. *Journal of Neurology, Neurosurgery, and Psychiatry, 72*, 473–479.

Law, M., Baptiste, S., McColl, M., Opzoomer, A., Polatajko, H., & Pollock, N. (1990). The Canadian Occupational Performance Measure: An outcome measure for occupational therapy. *Canadian Journal of Occupational Therapy, 57*(2), 82–87.

Law, M., Polotajko, H., Pollock, N., McColl, M., Carswell, A., & Baptiste, S. (1994). Pilot testing of the Canadian Occupational Performance Measure: Clinical and measurement issues. *Canadian Journal of Occupational Therapy, 61*(4), 191–197.

Law, M., Russell, D., Pollock, N., Rosenbaum, P., Walter, S., & King, G. (1997). A comparison of intensive neurodevelopmental therapy plus casting and a regular occupational therapy program for children with cerebral palsy. *Developmental Medicine and Child Neurology, 39*, 664–670.

Law, M., Wishart, L., & Guyatt, G. (2000). The use of a simulated environment (Easy Street) to retrain independent living skills in elderly persons: A randomized controlled trial. *Journal of Gerontology (Medical Sciences), 55*, M578–M584.

Letts, L., & Marshall, L. (1995). Evaluating the validity and consistency of the SAFER tool. *Physical and Occupational Therapy in Geriatrics, 13*, 49–66.

Letts, L., Scott, S., Burtney, J., Marshall, L., & McKean, M. (1998). The reliability and validity of the Safety Assessment of Function and the Environment for Rehabilitation (SAFER) tool. *British Journal of Occupational Therapy, 61*, 127–132.

Lincoln, N. B., Gladman, J. R. F., Berman, P., Noad, R. F., & Challen, K. (2000). Functional recovery of community survivors of stroke. *Disability and Rehabilitation, 22*(3), 135–139.

Lloyd, K., & Auld, C. (2002). The role of leisure in determining quality of life: Issues of content and measurement. *Social Indicators Research, 57*(1), 43–71.

Ludlow, L., & Haley, S. (1996). Effect of context in rating of mobility activities in children with disabilities: An assessment using the pediatric evaluation of disability inventory. *Education and Psychological Measurement, 56*(1), 122–129.

Mahoney, F., & Barthel, D. (1965). Functional evaluation: The Barthel Index. *Maryland State Medical Journal, 14*, 56–61.

Mant, J., Carter, J., Wade, D. T., & Winner, S. (2000). Family support for stroke: A randomized controlled trial. *Lancet, 356*, 808–813.

McDowell, I., & Newell, C. (1996). *Measuring health: A guide to rating scales and questionnaires*. New York: Oxford University Press.

McNulty, M., & Fisher, A. (2000). Validity of using the Assessment of Motor and Process Skills to estimate overall home safety in persons with psychiatric conditions. *American Journal of Occupational Therapy, 55*, 649–655.

Mercier, L., Audet, T., Hebert, R., Rochette, A., & Dubois, M. F. (2001). Impact of motor, cognitive, and perceptual disorders on ability to perform activities of daily living after stroke. *Stroke, 32*, 2602–2608.

Moos, R. (1981). *A social climate scale: Work environmental scale manual*. Palo Alto, CA: Consulting Psychologists Press.

Moos, R. (1993). *Work Environment Scale: An annotated bibliography*. Palo Alto, CA: Stanford University Medical Center.

Moos, R. (1994). Work as human context. In M. Pallack & R. Perloff (Eds.), *Psychology and work: Productivity, change and employment* (Vol. 5, pp. 9–52). Washington, DC: American Psychological Association.

Moos, R., & Moos, B. (1998). The staff workplace and the quality and outcome of substance abuse treatment. *Journal of Studies on Alcohol, 59*, 43–51.

Morris, P. L. P., Robinson, R. G., Raphael, B., & Bishop, D. P. (1991). The relationship between the perception of social support and post-stroke depression in hospitalized patients. *Psychiatry, 54*, 306–316.

Morrison, C., Bundy, A., & Fisher, A. G. (1991). The contribution of motor skills and playfulness to play performance of preschool aged children. *American Journal of Occupational Therapy, 45*, 687–694.

Nouri, F., & Lincoln, N. (1987). An extended activities of daily living scale for survivors of stroke. *Clinical Rehabilitation, 1*, 301–305.

Nygard, L., Bernspang, B., Fisher, A., & Winblad, B. (1994). Comparing motor and process ability of persons with suspected dementia in home and clinical settings. *American Journal of Occupational Therapy, 48*, 689–696.

Oliver, R., Blathwayt, J., Brackley, C., & Tamaki, T. (1993). Development of the Safety Assessment of Function and Environment for Rehabilitation (SAFER) tool. *Canadian Journal of Occupational Therapy, 60*, 78–82.

Ottenbacher, K., Hsu, Y., Granger, C., & Fiedler, R. (1996). The reliability of the Functional Independence Measure: A quantitative review. *Archives of Physical Medicine and Rehabilitation, 77*, 1226–1232.

Ottenbacher, K., Msall, M., Lyon, N., Duffy, L., Granger C. V., & Braun, S. (1997). Interrater agreement and stability of the functional independence measure for children (WeeFIM™): Use in children with developmental disabilities. *Archives of Physical Medicine and Rehabilitation, 78*, 1309–1315.

Ottenbacher, K., Msall, M., Lyon, N., Duffy, L., Granger, C., & Braun, S. (1999). Measuring developmental and functional status in children with disabilities. *Developmental Medicine and Child Neurology, 41*(3), 186–194.

Ottenbacher, K., Taylor, E., Msall, M., Braun, S., Lane, S., Granger, C., et al. (1996). The stability and equivalence reliability of the functional independence measure for children (WeeFIM)®. *Developmental Medicine and Child Neurology, 38*, 907–916.

Pearson, Q. (1998). Job satisfaction, leisure satisfaction, and psychological health. *Career Development Quarterly, 46*, 416–426.

Pedersen, P. M., Jorgensen, H. S., Nakayama, H., Raaschou, H. O., & Olsen, T. S. (1997). Comprehensive assessment of activities of daily living in stroke: The Copenhagen Stroke Study. *Archives of Physical Medicine and Rehabilitation, 78,*161–165.

Piercy, M., Carter, J., Mant, J., & Wade, D. T. (2000). Interrater reliability of the Frenchay Activities Index in patients with stroke and their carers. *Clinical Rehabilitation, 14*, 433–440.

Pollock, N. (1993). Client-centered assessment. *American Journal of Occupational Therapy, 47*, 298–301.

Prosiegel, M., Boettger, S., Give, T., Koenig, N., Marolf, M., Vaney, C., et al. (1996). The Extended Barthel Index: A new scale for the assessment of disability in neurological patients. *Neurorehabilitation, 1*, 7–13.

Ripat, J., Etcheverry, E., Cooper, J., & Tate, R. (2001). A comparison of the Canadian Occupational Performance Measure and the Health Assessment Questionnaire. *Canadian Journal of Occupational Therapy, 68*(4), 247–253.

Rodgers, H., Soutter, J., Kaiser, W., Pearson, P., Dobson, R., Skilbeck, C., et al. (1997). Early supported hospital discharge following acute stroke: Pilot study results. *Clinical Rehabilitation, 11*, 280–287.

Rogers, J. C., & Holm, M. (1994). *Performance assessment of self care skills (PASS)*. Pittsburgh, PA: University of Pittsburgh.

Rogers, J. C., & Holm, M. B. (2000). Daily-living skills and habits of older women with depression. *Occupational Therapy Journal of Research, 20*, 68s–85s.

Rogers, J. C., Holm, M., Beach, S., Schulz, R., Cipriani, J., Fox, A., et al. (2003). Concordance of four methods of disability assessment using performance in the home as the criterion method. *Arthritis and Rheumatism, 49*, 640–647.

Rogers, J. C., Holm, M., Beach, S., Schulz, R., & Starz, T. (2001). Task independence, safety, and adequacy among nondisabled and osteoarthritis: Disabled older women. *Arthritis and Rheumatism, 45*, 410–418.

Rogers, J. C., Holm, M., Goldstein, G., McCue, M., & Nussbaum, P. (1994). Stability and change in functional assessment of patients with geropsychiatric disorders. *American Journal of Occupational Therapy, 48*, 914–918.

Ruch, W., & Stang, S. (1994). *Employee Aptitude Survey examiner's manual* (2nd ed.). Glendale, CA: Psychological Services.

Salamy, M. (1993). *Construct validity of the assessment for communication and interaction skills*. Unpublished master's thesis, University of Illinois, Chicago.

Samsa, G., Hoenig, H., & Branch, L. (2001). Relationship between self-reported disability and caregiver hours. *Archives of Physical Medicine and Rehabilitation, 80*, 674–684.

Schuling, J., Dehaan, R., Limburg, M., & Groenier, K. (1993). The Frenchay Activities Index: Assessment of functional status in survivors of stroke. *Stroke, 24*, 1173–1177.

Searle, M., Mahon, M., & Iso-Ahola, S. (1995). Enhancing a sense of independence and psychological well-being among the elderly: A field experiment. *Journal of Leisure Research, 27*(2), 107–124.

Searle, M., Mahon, M., Iso-Ahola, S., & Sdrolias, H. (1998). Examining the long term effects of leisure education on a sense of independence and psychological well-being among the elderly. *Journal of Leisure Research, 30*(3), 331–340.

Sewell, L., & Singh, S. (2001). The Canadian Occupational Performance Measure: Is it a reliable measure in clients with chronic obstructive pulmonary disease? *British Journal of Occupational Therapy, 64*(6), 305–310.

Simmons, D., Crepeau, E., & White, B. (2000). The predictive power of narrative data in occupational therapy evaluation. *American Journal of Occupational Therapy, 54*, 471–476.

Simon, S. (1989). *The development of an assessment for communication and interaction skills*. Unpublished master's thesis, University of Illinois, Chicago.

Strain, L., Grabusic, C., Searle, M., & Dunn, N. (2002). Continuing and ceasing leisure activities in later life: A longitudinal study. *Gerontologist, 42*(2), 217–223.

Sveen, U., Bautz-Holter, E., Sodring, K. M., Wyller, T. B., & Laake, K. (1999). Association between impairments, self-care ability and social activities 1 year after stroke. *Disability and Rehabilitation, 21*(8), 372–377.

System, U. D. (1990). *Guide for the use of the pediatric functional independence measure*. Buffalo: Research Foundation—State University of New York.

Teel, C., Dunn, W. W., Jackson, S., & Duncan, P. (1997). The role of the environment in fostering independence: Conceptual and methodological issues in developing an instrument. *Topics in Stroke Rehabilitation, 4*(1), 28–40.

Tham, K., Ginsburg, E., Fisher, A. G., & Tegner, R. (2001). Training to improve awareness of disabilities in clients with unilateral neglect. *American Journal of Occupational Therapy, 55*, 46–54.

Thomas, P. D., Garry, P. J., Goodwin, J. M., & Goodwin, J. S. (1985). Social bonds in a healthy elderly sample: Characteristics and associated variables. *Social Science and Medicine, 20*, 365–369.

Trombly, C., Radomski, M., & Davis, E. (1998). Achievement of self-identified goals by adults with traumatic brain injury: Phase I. *American Journal of Occupational Therapy, 52*, 810–818.

Turnbull, J., Kersten, P., Habib, M., McLellan, D., Mullee, M., & George, S. (2000). Validation of the Frenchay Activities Index in a general population aged 16 and over. *Archives of Physical Medicine and Rehabilitation, 81*, 1034–1038.

U.S. Department of Labor. (1991). *Revised handbook for analyzing jobs*. Washington, DC: U.S. Government Printing Office.

Wade, D. (1992). *Measurement in neurological rehabilitation*. Oxford, England: Oxford University Press.

Walker, M. F., Drummond, A. E. R., & Lincoln, N. B. (1996). Evaluation of dressing practice for survivors of stroke after discharge from hospital: A crossover design study. *Clinical Rehabilitation, 10*(1), 23–31.

Walker, M., Gladman, J., Lincoln, N., Siemonsma, P., & Whiteley, T. L. (2000). Occupational therapy for survivors of stroke not admitted to hospital: A randomized controlled trial. *Lancet, 354*, 278–280.

Walters, S., Morrell, C., & Dixon, S. (1999). Measuring health-related quality of life in patients with venous leg ulcers. *Quality of Life Research, 8,* 327–336.

Weatherall, M. (2000). A randomized controlled trial of the Geriatric Depression Scale in an inpatient ward for older adults. *Clinical Rehabilitation, 14*(2), 186– 191.

Willer, B., Allen, K., Liss, M., & Zicht, M. (1991). Problems and coping strategies of individuals with traumatic brain injury and their spouses. *Archives of Physical Medicine and Rehabilitation, 72,* 460–464.

Willer, B., Linn, R., & Allen, K. (1992). Community integration and barriers to integration for individuals with brain injury. In M. Finlayson & S. Garner (Eds.), *Brain injury rehabilitation: Clinical considerations* (pp. 355–375). Baltimore: Williams & Wilkins.

Willer, B., Rosenthal, M., Kreutzer, J., Gordon, W., & Rempel, R. (1993). Assessment of community integration following rehabilitation for traumatic brain injury. *Journal of Head Trauma Rehabilitation, 8,* 75–87.

Wood-Dauphinee, S., Opzoomer, A., Williams, J., Marchand, B., & Spitzer, W. (1988). Assessment of global function: The Reintegration to Normal Living Index. *Archives of Physical Medicine and Rehabilitation, 69,* 583–590.

Wood-Dauphinee, S., & Willliams, J. (1987). Reintegration to normal living as proxy to quality of life. *Journal of Chronic Diseases, 40,* 491–499.

Wressle, E., Eeg-Olofsson, A., Marcusson, J., & Henriksson, C. (2002). Improved client participation in the rehabilitation process using a client-centered goal formulation structure. *Journal of Rehabilitation Medicine, 34*(1), 5–11.

Wylie, C., & White, B. (1964). A measure of disability. *Archives of Environmental Health, 8,* 834–839.

Yohannes, A. M., Roomi, J., Winn, S., & Connolly, M. J. (2000). The Manchester Respiratory Activities of Daily Living questionnaire: Development, reliability, validity, and responsiveness to pulmonary rehabilitation. *Journal of the American Geriatrics Society, 48,* 1496–1500.

Young, J., Bogle, S., & Forster, A. (2001). Determinants of social outcome measured by the Frenchay Activities Index at one year after stroke onset. *Cerebrovascular Diseases, 12*(2), 114–120.

Chapter 4

Planning Intervention

PENELOPE A. MOYERS, EdD, OTR, FAOTA

CHARLES H. CHRISTIANSEN, EdD, OTR, OT(C), FAOTA

KEY TERMS

health promotion

ICF

intervention plan

modification

occupational performance
  problem statement

prevention

remediation

OBJECTIVES

Upon completion of this chapter, the reader will be able to

- Appreciate the difference between independence and interdependence;

- Understand that intervention planning requires critical reasoning;

- List the elements of an intervention plan;

- Understand the difference between intervention approaches and types of intervention;

- Identify and understand the distinctions among the various intervention approaches of remediation/restoration/establishment, maintain, modify, prevent, and promote;

- Appreciate the need for client and caregiver collaboration throughout the intervention planning process;

- Write appropriate intervention goals, including all the necessary elements;

- Delineate the criteria for selecting outcome measures; and

- Understand the importance of theory and use of evidence-based information in selecting intervention approaches and types of intervention.

This chapter describes the client-centered and evidence-based occupational therapy processes that support efficient and effective intervention planning. The *Occupational Therapy Practice Framework: Domain and Process* (American Occupational Therapy Association [AOTA], 2002), hereafter referred to as the *Framework*, provides the terminology that guides intervention planning. The World Health Organization's (2001) *International Classification of Functioning, Disability, and Health* (ICF) prompts the occupational therapist to focus intervention planning on the client's need to engage in activity and to participate in various contexts (see Table 4.1). In this chapter, the occupational areas of activities of daily living (ADL) and instrumental activities of daily living (IADL) are highlighted in the discussion about intervention planning.

Prerequisite to Planning

In working with clients, the goal of occupational therapy is to focus on the occupations and activities that the clients have determined they need and want to do (Pierce, 1998). Good intervention planning depends on the occupational therapist's having worked through the occupational therapy process of *evaluation,* which involves completing an occupational profile and in-depth analyses of the occupational performances that the client or the client's caregivers have indicated are important for improved performance (AOTA, 2002). The occupational profile enables the occupational therapist to understand the "client's occupational history and experiences, patterns of daily living, interests, values, and needs" (AOTA, 2002, p. 614). An occupational profile also helps the occupational therapist

determine the client's current concerns about performing these important daily life activities.

During the process of occupational performance analysis, the occupational therapist observes the client's current performance in one or more occupations and activities of concern in a variety of situations. The occupational therapist notes how the interaction among the person, the activity, and the environment influences occupational performance (Baum & Law, 1997). The ultimate purpose of the analysis is to determine whether the client can engage in occupations in a way that supports participation in his or her usual living environments, or *contexts* (AOTA, 2002, p. 611). During the analysis, the occupational therapist notes the way in which the selected activities, when performed in specific environments, make demands on the client's body functions and structures, performance skills, and current habits and routines. Ultimately, the occupational therapist highlights assets and barriers to performance within social roles.

Identifying Occupational Performance Problems

On the basis of the evaluation and the reason for the referral to occupational therapy, the occupational therapist formulates an occupational performance problem statement that succinctly describes the occupational status of a person and identifies the problems amenable to intervention. The occupational performance problem statement involves several elements (Table 4.2). It is imperative to work with the client and caregivers to prioritize the occupations and activities so that the intervention is properly focused (Matheson, 1998). This list of pri-

Table 4.1. World Health Organization *International Classification of Functioning, Disability, and Health* **(2001)**

Parts	Components (Definition)	Positive Aspect	Negative Aspect
Functioning and Disability	Body functions and structures (Physiology and anatomy)	Functional and structural integrity	Impairment
	Activities and participation (Task execution and involvement)	Activities and participation	Activity limitation or participation restriction
Contextual Factors	Environmental factors (Physical, social, attitudinal environments)	Facilitators	Barriers
	Personal factors (Attributes)	Not applicable	Not applicable

Table 4.2. Elements of the Occupational Performance Problem Statement

1. Intervention focus or the prioritized occupations and activities, performance skills (motor, process, communication/interaction), or habits and routines needing development to support participation in social roles within context(s).

2. Underlying factors contributing to the performance problem:
   • Client factors
     – Body functions
     – Body structures
   • Activity demands
     – Objects used and their properties
     – Space and social demands
     – Sequencing and timing
     – Required actions/body functions/body structures.

3. Impact of contexts on performance in terms of barriers and supports and in terms of standards or criteria for measuring performance. Contexts include
   • Cultural
   • Physical
   • Social
   • Personal
   • Spiritual
   • Temporal
   • Virtual.

orities is perhaps the most significant aspect of the occupational performance problem statement because it is heavily influenced by the social roles that the client values.

For example, the client may demonstrate problems in many ADL areas but prefers to concentrate first on feeding and functional mobility, even though dressing and bathing also are problems. The client might indicate that he or she wants to be able to go out to eat with family members because this social interaction would provide the motivation needed to keep working on other problem areas later. The client might therefore initially need total assistance with dressing and bathing in order to focus on the two prioritized activities necessary for social participation as a family member.

Given the prioritized list of activities targeted for improvement, the occupational therapist must delineate the performance skills and patterns inherent in performance, the underlying factors contributing to the performance problem, and the ways in which the context influences performance. Issues of skill and habit, along with underlying factors, often may be anticipated in light of the medical or diagnostic information available from the physician. Consider the following information pertinent to people who have experienced a cerebrovascular accident (CVA),

or stroke. A CVA in the brain's right hemisphere causes a left hemiplegia. After a stroke, clients are sometimes depressed, and depression can influence motivation to engage in intervention activities. The person also may have specific perceptual problems and problem-solving limitations. CVAs may occur in people with other medical problems, such as obesity, hypertension, and macular degeneration. These medical problems are examples of diagnostic factors that influence decisions relevant to planning an intervention for someone who has suffered a stroke.

Using the *Framework* (AOTA, 2002) as a guide, the evaluation helps the occupational therapist determine whether the client has problems with motor, process, or communication and interaction skills and whether the skills are environmentally dependent, are nonexistent, have atrophied, or have become impaired because of the medical condition (Holm, Rogers, & Stone, 2003). The performance problem statement also indicates the performance pattern issues that might interfere with occupational performance, such as the presence of environmentally dependent habits, underdeveloped or obligatory habits, ineffectual habits, or inappropriate habits (Holm, Rogers, & Stone, 2003).

The underlying factors influencing occupational performance include client factors (which involve a range of body function and body structure impairments) and activity demands. The body function impairments most often amenable to occupational therapy interventions include mental or cognitive functions, sensory disorders and pain, neuromusculoskeletal and movement-related dysfunction, cardiovascular and respiratory disorders, and skin problems that require special adaptive precautions or procedures (AOTA, 2002). The occupational therapist analyzes the prioritized list of occupations and activities in order to understand the way in which the objects used, the space and social demands, the sequencing and timing, and required actions make demands on the client's present level of body functioning or state of the body structures. This analysis of activity demands helps to prioritize the impairments of body function that need intervention and to indicate how each activity may need modification.

Finally, the occupational therapist analyzes the context in which performance needs to occur in terms of the way in which that context supports or inhibits performance. Understanding context helps the occupational therapist identify the context modifications needed and delineate how performance outcomes may be judged. According to the *Framework* (AOTA, 2002), cultural, physical, social, personal, spiritual, temporal, and virtual contexts could need modification or could provide information regarding expectations for performance. For instance, the physical environment could be modified for a person with a CVA so as to facilitate wheelchair access (e.g., by building ramps into the home, replacing carpeting with wood or linoleum flooring, and widening doors). The personal context, such as age, gender, and socioeconomic and educational status, helps the therapist understand performance expectations and priorities, social roles, and resources needed.

Formulation of the occupational performance problem statement is a complex process involving critical reasoning. Experienced occupational therapists are able to use their previous client intervention experiences to help them analyze the information available to them and discern patterns, enabling them to quickly develop tentative hypotheses about the most important occupational performance problems and their underlying factors (Robertson, 1996).

Thus, identification of occupational performance problems results from a client-centered approach to problem identification; from careful attention to medical and occupational therapy profile information; from observation data and assessment results that confirm hypotheses about the relationships among underlying factors, occupational performance, and contexts; and from the occupational therapist's previous experiences with similar client situations.

Intervention Process

According to the *Framework* (AOTA, 2002), the intervention process is divided into three parts: creating the intervention plan, implementing intervention, and intervention review. This chapter focuses on only the first part of the intervention process or the intervention plan (Table 4.3). The principles of client-centered care dictate that intervention planning be a collaborative process among the client,

Table 4.3. Intervention Plan Components

Intervention Goals	Definitions
• Time frame	Days, weeks, or months
• Underlying factors	Client factors
• Activity method change	Steps, techniques, procedures, equipment, context modification
• Focus of intervention	Occupational area, performance skills, performance patterns
• Measurement parameter	Independence/assistance levels, safety, quality/adequacy
Intervention Approaches	**Match Intervention Focus**
• Remediation/ Restoration/ Establishment	Impairments
	Performance skills and patterns
	Habilitation of skills and patterns
• Maintain	Protection of current performance
• Modify	Activities, contexts, caregivers
• Prevent	Risk reduction
• Promote	Lifestyle change
Types of Intervention	**Definitions**
• Therapeutic use of self	Planned use of personality, insights, perceptions, and judgments
• Therapeutic use of occupations and activities	Occupation-based activities in client's own context; purposeful activities occur in therapeutically designed context; preparatory methods prepare for occupational performance
• Consultation process	Therapist not directly responsible for intervention
• Education process	Imparting knowledge and information
Mechanisms of Service Delivery	**Definitions**
• Frequency	Number times per week
• Duration	Total number of visits or total time period
• Personnel involved	Occupational therapist, occupational therapy assistant, caregivers
• Location of intervention	Clinical sites, occupational performance contexts, community settings
Referrals and Recommendations	**Examples**
• Referrals	Expert occupational therapists, other health care professionals
• Recommendations	Community resources
Outcome Measures	**Examples**
	Performance, client satisfaction, role competence, adaptation, health and wellness, prevention, quality of life

the caregiver, and the occupational therapist (Law & Mills, 1998). Occupational therapy assistants may contribute to the planning process within their competency and under supervision, but responsibility for the final development of the plan is within the scope of only the occupational therapist's practice (AOTA, 2000). The content of the intervention plan is based on the results of the occupational profile and analyses and on the occupational performance problem statement. The plan is formulated to guide intervention so that either the occupational performance of specific activities in a variety of contexts improves or the risk for activity limitations and participation restrictions diminishes. The intervention plan normally includes objective and measurable goals that are accomplishable within a given time frame, the occupational therapy intervention approach and types of intervention, the mechanism of service delivery, the discharge plan, chosen outcome measures, and recommendations or referrals to others as needed (AOTA, 2002).

Intervention Goals

Goals should reflect the client's priorities for improvement in occupational performance (Matheson, 1998). Box 4.1 illustrates how the occupational therapist works with Irene to verbalize her goals for therapy (see Chapter 3). Goals focus the intervention on occupational areas, performance skills, and performance patterns. Intervention goals are client centered when they are written in collaboration with the client and caregivers in order to achieve significant changes in social participation. Goals may be divided into long- and short-term goals: The long-

term goal reflects the outcome expected by the time of discontinuation of therapy, and the short-term goals consist of the various steps needed to reach the final outcome. When the intervention time period is of short duration, however, the occupational therapist may not need to separate goals in this manner.

Whatever the type, goals must indicate the change in underlying factors that will lead to an improvement in occupational performance, and they must delineate the time frame in which goal achievement is expected. Goals also indicate any change in context and activity method that will support performance. For example, a measurable goal might be written in the following manner:

> Within four weeks [time frame], client will demonstrate the upper extremity strength and endurance [underlying factors] to use assistive devices and a modified task procedure [activity method change or context modification] to dress [occupational area or focus of intervention] independently within 30 min [measurement parameters of independence level and societal standard].

Note that the method or parameter for measuring achievement of goals may vary among institutions and therapists (Table 4.3). Goals may be written in terms of the level of independence the person can be expected to achieve (Box 4.2) or in terms of the level of assistance needed in the performance of the valued occupations and activities (Table 4.4). Another measure of change could be in the client's ability to perform the occupations and activities in a safe manner. The quality or adequacy of performance may improve (Holm, Rogers, & James, 2003): Parameters such as levels of difficulty, pain, fatigue

---

Box 4.1. Goal Setting for Irene

[See evaluation results from Chapter 3]

Irene is lonely and unhappy about her life and wants to go back to doing things she enjoys. She feels worthless and guilty about the burden she is placing on her daughter but does not know how to get out of it. She knows she cannot drive unless her vision improves, so she will need to readjust how she does things. Her fatigue makes it difficult for her to even want to try. The therapist helped her focus on actions by asking her to identify goals she would like to achieve within the next 2 months.

Irene's goal areas are as follows:
- Complete bathing and dressing tasks daily in a timely manner without fatigue

- Prepare a light meal daily without fatigue
- Complete one housekeeping task each day without fatigue
- Resume walking for pleasure at least twice per week
- Attend a church group meeting or social activity at least once per week
- Spend time reading or enjoying a leisure activity instead of sleeping excessively.

The therapist then uses these prioritized goal areas to create specific, measurable goals for tracking Irene's progress.

Box 4.2. Independence or Interdependence?

What does independence mean? Certainly, it means more than simply doing something on your own. A person can be considered independent while performing tasks that require the use of adapted devices or environments or while overseeing others to meet various needs. In truth, few people in the modern world can claim that they are entirely self-reliant. Most of us depend on others extensively as we manage the affairs of our daily lives. The dependence is practical—we depend on those who transport goods to the market; on those who manufacture and sell goods; and on those who work in service occupations, such as police officers, hairstylists, butchers, mechanics, bus drivers, and employees of public utilities.

We also depend on other people for emotional support and behavioral models and expectations that guide and influence our behavior. Our understanding of the events in our daily lives is derived from shared interpretations of the world around us. Therefore, it can be said that we are dependent on others for providing the structure that gives us our sense that the reality of daily life has stability and continuity. We are not independent, but interdependent.

Many people have argued that making independence a principal goal in occupational therapy is a misleading and a potentially damaging concept. Instead, adopting a recovery model that recognizes and values *interdependence* will improve therapy and more accurately reflect the realities of our social existence. A focus on interdependence can provide a broader, more socially appropriate set of options for the therapist in planning intervention than can an emphasis on independence. The primary objective may thus involve helping the client learn how to take advantage of the view that we are all interdependent by nature, thereby defining performance outcome success as effectively creating and managing this web of interdependence.

and dyspnea, and satisfaction may change; duration may increase; societal standards may be achieved; fewer resources may be used or existing resources may be used more effectively; or aberrant performance behaviors may be extinguished.

Intervention Approaches

In collaboration with the client and caregivers, the occupational therapist selects the therapy approaches best suited for the focus of intervention, the client's values and capacity for learning, the prognosis for the impairments, the time available for intervention, the probable discharge environment, and the expected client follow-through with recommendations (Holm, Rogers, & James, 2003). According to the *Framework* (AOTA, 2002), the main intervention approaches are remediation, restoration, or establishment (habilitation); modification; maintenance; prevention; and health promotion. These categories are summarized below. Throughout the following discussion, refer to Table 4.5 to see how the occupational therapist may address Irene's goals through the use of a combination of approaches.

Table 4.4. Levels of Performance Assistance and Levels of Independence

Assistance Level (Independence Level)	Definition
Total assistance (dependent)	The need for 100% physical and cognitive assistance to perform functional activities
Maximum assistance (25% independent)	The need for 75% physical and cognitive assistance to perform functional activities
Moderate assistance (50% independent)	The need for 50% physical and cognitive assistance to perform functional activities
Minimum assistance (75% independent)	The need for 25% physical and cognitive assistance to perform functional activities
Standby assistance	The need for supervision to perform new activity procedures without error and with anticipation of the need for using appropriate safety precautions
Independent status (100% independent)	No physical or cognitive assistance is required to safely perform functional activities

Table 4.5. One Example of an Intervention Approach for Each of Irene's Goals

Goal	Remediation	Modification	Maintenance	Prevention	Health Promotion
			Intervention Approaches		
Complete bathing and dressing tasks daily in a timely manner without fatigue	Use or complete a strengthening program to improve grip for ease in bathing and dressing	Bathe and dress at a time with higher energy or before bed	Irene and her daughter will learn energy conservation principles and remediation techniques	Use nonskid flooring on the tub and make sure grab bars are positioned properly and secured	Recall the importance of bathing and proper dressing as fundamental to social interactions and sense of well-being
Prepare a light meal daily without fatigue	Complete a strengthening program to improve arm strength for ease in meal preparation	Sit to cook (use a stool) and use energy-saving devices (e.g., electric mixer)	Use daily planners and organizational strategies for meal planning	Irene's daughter arranges supplies to eliminate need for risky reaching or bending	Irene's daughter finds healthy foods and snacks that come in convenient sizes and packaging
Complete one housekeeping task each day without fatigue	Build endurance through an exercise program	Modify routines and habits to incorporate energy conservation principles (e.g., spread the task throughout the day)	Irene's daughter organizes cleaning supplies and equipment to be easily accessible	Rest before getting tired	Use a method of prioritizing activities such that energy is saved for the most valued activities
Resume walking for pleasure at least twice per week	Develop a progressive walking schedule that gradually builds endurance	Bring an adapted cane that opens to a stool for needed rests	Interpret and implement a written walking program	Use comfortable clothing and sturdy walking shoes	Join or create a peer group of walkers for support and socialization, and walk in stimulating places such as a mall or sports center
Attend a church group meeting or social activity at least once per week	Complete memory and cognitive retraining	Irene's daughter arranges rides from the group members	Irene's daughter develops a car pool list and has Irene swap rides for other services such as bringing treats	Plan day to allow rest before attending the group	Learn about the importance of meaningful activity to health and quality of life
Spend time reading or enjoying a leisure activity instead of sleeping excessively	Complete visual exercises, including eye patching	Use books on tape, magnifiers, or both when vision is poor	Irene's daughter has supplies readily available for games and crafts that interest her	Understand precautions related to her weak grip and sensory changes	Participate in a book club or activity group for social and mental stimulation

Remediation/Restoration/Establishment

Remediation approaches focus on impairments in body functions and body structures, such as range of motion and strength; therefore, these approaches attempt to influence biological, physiological, or neurological processes. Restoration approaches are used to reestablish the client's performance skills and healthy habits and routines. If skills and habits have never been learned, then establishing the necessary motor, process, and communication and interaction skills is necessary, as is organizing those skills into new habit patterns and routines. Typically, ADL improvements take place over extended periods and involve the careful structuring of tasks, frequent monitoring to identify problems, and feedback to correct performance errors.

Modification

Modification also may be termed *compensation* or *adaptation*. Regardless of word choice, the objective is to identify new ways to accomplish the required task using remaining performance capabilities. Often, the context can be modified to enable successful performance. Thus, modification approaches may focus on modifying the activity, the context, or both. Many strategies can be used to modify an activity and the context in which it is performed to enable one to satisfactorily meet ADL goals. First, the client can be taught to perform the activity within his or her capabilities. Doing so often involves a change in task method, such as putting on pants while seated instead of standing. Second, the context can be modified to permit accomplishment of the task despite limitations in ability or skill, such as installing grab bars in the shower stall. Third, systems or devices can be designed or acquired to enable performance despite limited cognition, strength, or sensory ability, such as using a transfer board to enable car-to-wheelchair transfer. Another modification approach involves having an agent or a caregiver assist with the portions of the task that overly tax the client's current capabilities, such as the caregiver's carrying the client's lunch tray from the cafeteria line to the table. Each category of modification approaches is described in more detail in the sections that follow.

Use of Adaptive Systems and Devices

Occupational therapy practitioners often use the broad term *assistive technology* to refer to the systems and devices designed to help clients compensate for lost or diminished functions. Devices range from those described as *low technology*, such as special utensils with built-up handles and shoelaces that can be tied with one hand, to *high-technology* devices, which include remote-control devices that activate appliances and speech synthesizers that store and speak words and sentences. Clients may need equipment at one phase of their intervention, but not once remediation or habilitation approaches have improved capacity in body function and body structure. The prescription of adaptive systems and devices should be made carefully after fully understanding the client's capabilities, the client's psychological reaction to the equipment, the equipment's impact on performance safety, the client's financial limitations, the context in which the equipment is to be used, the ease in which the equipment can be incorporated into habit patterns and routines, and the fluctuations in the client's energy and time availability.

Environmental Modifications

Environmental modifications can vary from rearranging furniture to major alterations in the design of rooms or dwellings. Common examples include widening doorways, building ramps, and converting family rooms into bedrooms because of the lack of wheelchair access to bedrooms located on a second story of the house. Within bathrooms, the addition of grab bars, special toilet seats, and other safety equipment can dramatically improve ADL completion.

In the United States, the Americans With Disabilities Act (ADA) and efforts by advocacy groups and people in the universal design movement have made apparent the need to design environments so that access is available without the need for special accommodations. The ADA, however, has been instrumental in promoting the modification of environments created prior to the emphasis on universal access. Without universal access, people with impairments may experience activity limitations and participation restrictions. Unfortunately, people with disabilities often encounter bureaucratic obstacles that preclude timely completion of necessary environmental modifications.

Use of Caregivers

Another strategy available to clients involves training family members and other caregivers, such as paid personal care attendants, to assist in the performance of various ADL. To help the caregivers be effective, the occupational therapist needs to determine the activities for which assistance is required as well as the level of assistance that is needed. For some activities, the client may need total assistance, whereas with other activities, the client might need only stand-by assistance. The level of assistance needed might vary according to the time of day, fatigue or pain level, or the context of the performance. Changes in health status or activity priorities also might lead to the need for different levels of assistance. Because therapy time frames probably limit the involvement of the occupational therapist in determining all the assistance needs and how they might vary, it is important to help the client gain a realistic and thorough understanding of his or her strengths and limitations related to ADL and IADL.

Maintenance

Maintenance involves strategies designed to ensure that the client does not lose current levels of functioning, to ensure that the improvements in occupational performance remain once therapy is withdrawn, or to slow the anticipated loss of functioning associated with a progressive condition such as Alzheimer's disease. Maintenance could involve training caregivers to ensure that clients follow therapeutic recommendations, training the client to use exercise routines or splinting schedules, and incorporating planned therapy "booster" sessions to briefly retrain the client because of gradual degradation of performance skills and patterns.

Prevention

Prevention as a primary category of intervention promotes safety and prevents health problems. The occupational therapist seeks to identify risk factors before an accident occurs to improve safety and reduce the risk of injury, hospitalization, chronic disability, and death. ADL and IADL not only support social participation but also promote nutrition and hygiene; in certain cases, they prevent specific health problems (e.g., taking medication to control diabetes, HIV, or epilepsy). Thus, by enabling the client to complete ADL, prevention is taking place. The occupational therapist must always emphasize safety in the performance of tasks. For people with visual difficulties, sensory deficits, balance disorders, or other conditions that place them at risk for personal injury, attention must be paid to object placement, environmental design (lighting and nonslip surfaces), location of safety apparatus (e.g., grab bars), and use of safe task methods.

Health Promotion

The final intervention approach involves health promotion. Because the time and energy available for occupational performance may be limited, teaching clients how to manage and conserve their resources is an important part of helping them successfully adapt to their impairments and activity limitations. For instance, the client may prefer to have a personal care assistant do most of his or her hygiene and dressing activities in order to conserve energy for more enjoyable activities, such as cooking or shopping. Moreover, by learning how to structure one's daily routine, unnecessary stress and its physical consequences can be avoided. Health promotion also involves strategies to improve the client's sense of life satisfaction and well-being. Lifestyles that include goal-directed occupations that reflect competence, that are viewed as less stressful, and that permit meaning and the adequate expression of personal identity are likely to result in greater levels of life satisfaction (Christiansen, Backman, Little, & Nguyen, 1999).

Choosing Specific Types of Intervention

Once approaches are chosen, the occupational therapist, in collaboration with the client and caregivers, selects the types of interventions within the major approaches described previously that are effective in leading to the desired changes in occupational performance. Intervention types include therapeutic use of self (i.e., planned use of personality, insights, perceptions, and judgments), therapeutic use of occupations and activities, consultation, and education (AOTA, 2002). When using therapeutic occupations, the therapist most likely will use a combination of occupation-based activity (i.e., meaningful activities within the client's own context), purposeful activity (i.e., goal-directed activities within a therapeutic context), and preparatory methods (e.g., sensory input, physical agent modalities, splinting, and exercise).

Table 4.6 illustrates a sample intervention plan designed for a person with a CVA. Occupational therapists also work with clients with substance use disorders. Types of intervention can be delineated for clients with mental illness, as well as for those with physical impairments. For instance, a remediation or restoration approach may be needed if the focus of intervention is on changing the client's addictive substance use pattern. The therapist may use an education process that helps the client identify his or her addictive habit patterns and create healthy replacement patterns (Moyers & Stoffel, 2001). During this education process, the therapist may adopt a therapeutic use of self that is accepting of the client's responsibility for leading the change process and that is motivating to facilitate the client's belief in the likelihood of success (Miller & Rollnick, 2002). In addition, a prevention approach

Table 4.6. Sample Occupational Therapy Intervention Plan

Problem Statement	Goals	Approaches	Types of Intervention
Medical • Right cerebrovascular accident • Depression *Performance* • Unable to initiate complete dressing or bathing tasks without verbal cues and physical assistance *Underlying factors* • Mental functions • Sensory functions • Neuromusculoskeletal	• Within 4 weeks, client will demonstrate the upper-extremity strength and endurance to use assistive devices and a modified task procedure to dress independently within 30 minutes • Within 4 weeks, client will demonstrate the motor planning to shower independently using adaptive equipment	• Education of clients and caregivers • Restoration of motor skill and habit patterns and routines • Remediation of strength and endurance • Use of adaptive equipment, context modifications, and safe practices • Modification of activity demands • Remediation of motor planning • Modification of physical context • Prevention of safety error	• Consultation with caregivers about physical context modifications for home bathroom • Use of neuromotor techniques to facilitate normal tone, strength, and range of motion • Use of purposeful activity and occupation-based activity to restore skills and habits and to remediate motor planning

that focuses on development of coping skills may be required so that the client does not relapse back into the "full-blown" addictive pattern of behavior (Stoffel, 1992). Intervention could include an education process to learn the coping skills along with engagement in both occupation-based and purposeful activity (in which coping skills have to be used during the activity performance; Stoffel & Moyers, 2001). In addition, the therapist may need to take a modification approach to the client's social context so that the client spends less time with those who use substances and more time with people who can model effective recovery habits, routines, and skills (Moyers, 1997). This modification could be achieved by using the occupation-based activity of attending Alcoholics Anonymous (AA) social events and activities, which incorporate an education process whereby AA support groups teach the client about a recovery lifestyle.

Formulating a Successful Plan of Care: Theory- and Evidence-Based Intervention

To achieve the desired outcomes of occupational therapy intervention, the therapist not only relies on client and caregiver collaboration but also is aware of the way in which current theories and evidence support the approaches and interventions recommended to the client. With the focus of intervention on occupational areas, performance skills, and performance patterns, the occupational therapist must use practice models and theories that address successful changes not only in underlying factors but also in current occupational performance

(Baum & Baptiste, 2002). The use of multiple practice models may be necessary because some models may address only underlying factors and some may address only occupational performance. Some theories and practice models are specific to certain approaches or intervention types, such as learning theories that guide the use of education as a type of intervention.

The occupational therapist should use theory to guide intervention planning; in addition, he or she must critically appraise the latest research that demonstrates the efficacy and effectiveness of the approaches and types of intervention. The therapist also should analyze the outcomes he or she typically achieves when using a specific approach and intervention. In the absence of research, the occupational therapist needs to be knowledgeable of the latest expert opinions and theoretical developments supporting these approaches and types of interventions.

Mechanisms of Service Delivery

Once the intervention approach and intervention types are selected, the occupational therapist determines the mechanisms of service delivery. Several people may provide the intervention, including the occupational therapist and the occupational therapy assistant. The practitioners may train the client to implement home programs or train the caregivers to assist in the intervention process. The location of intervention is an important consideration, one that may vary to include clinical sites, such as a hospital room, clinic, or agency; key occupation contexts, such as the home, work sites, or schools; or various community settings, such as where the client shops, eats in restaurants, or goes to church. The frequency of intervention and the duration of therapy needed to achieve the therapy goals are determined on the basis of the therapist's experience with other clients, outcomes data, research studies, expert opinion, and client preference.

Discharge Plans

Another important aspect of an effective intervention plan is the incorporation of plans consistent with the context of the environment to which the client is discharged. For instance, the client may prefer to return home and live independently and want to develop an intervention plan that is based on that assumption. After the occupational therapist conducts a realistic evaluation and develops an understanding of the client's prognosis, however, it may be apparent that such a discharge assumption is inappropriate. For example, it could require either the training of caregivers in the home or a clinical environment providing more intensive therapy before discharge to home.

The context often dictates the intervention priorities and approaches, particularly when the therapist decides to emphasize modification over remediation. If a client is home alone during a major part of the day, the more immediate need might be to ensure that he or she can access prepared meals or light snacks; the remediation of range of motion, strength, and coordination needed to use the oven can come later. Being alone may require adaptation of kitchen habits to improve the safety of meal preparation, such as using the microwave instead of the stove. In this way, the client can still cook when alone, even though body functions have not improved adequately for oven operation.

Referral

A successful plan includes recommendations for referral to other occupational therapists who possess specific kinds of expertise (e.g., splinting, therapy for eating and swallowing, hand therapy). Referral also may be needed to other professionals, such as physical therapists, physicians, psychologists, social workers, dieticians, or speech and language pathologists. The occupational therapist can recommend involvement in specific support groups, fitness centers, or other types of activity groups or clubs to support engagement in enjoyable and healthy activities. The therapist informs the client of community resources, such as parks, museums, universities, volunteer opportunities, and funding sources, to additionally support engagement in occupation.

Outcome Measures

The occupational therapist, the client, and the caregivers will not know whether therapy is successful unless the therapist selects outcome measures to indicate progress. Typically, a variety of outcome measures are needed, depending on the outcomes described in the intervention goals. Outcome measures will need to be selected according to the instruments that best measure occupational performance, client satisfaction, role competence, adaptation, health and wellness, prevention, and quality of life (AOTA, 2002). To select the best outcome measure, the occupational therapist must ensure that the instrument focuses on the construct that is most affected by the intervention plan and the intervention process, is least affected by outside influences, is relevant for the client's age or other personal characteristics, and is easily interpreted (Finch, Brooks, Stratford, & Mayo, 2002).

In measuring occupational performance, the occupational therapist should select the outcome instrument according to the occupational area of interest and the specific activities involved, such as using an ADL instrument that emphasizes dressing, bathing, toileting, feeding, and personal device use (Dittmar, 1997). The occupational performance instrument must be sensitive to measuring improvement. When a performance deficit is not present but the need to prevent problems in daily life occupations exists, the instrument should be able to measure enhancements (AOTA, 2002). Role competence requires selection of an instrument that measures performance against a specific criterion or standard. Instruments that measure adaptation will provide outcome data about changes in how the client responds to an occupational challenge, such as ability to use relapse-specific coping skills to avoid using addictive substances.

Client satisfaction involves measurement of the client's perception and affective response to the occupational therapy process (AOTA, 2002; Elliott-Burke & Pothast, 1998; Simon & Patrick, 1998). Health-related quality-of-life outcome measures might be useful in measuring various aspects of health and wellness, prevention, and life satisfaction. Quality-of-life measures assess various domains such as physical, emotional, cognitive, and social role functioning and perceptions of health and well-being (Finch et al., 2002; Wan, Counte, & Cella, 1998). Such measures can be generic in that they can be used with a broad population, or they can be disease specific (e.g., arthritis; Stanton, Gresham, & Dittmar, 1997). Often, disease-specific quality-of-life measures enable the person to compare him- or herself with others possessing similar health conditions.

Summary

The mainstay of occupational therapy practice consists of strategies that enable people to engage in daily occupations. Intervention planning is a process that bridges evaluation and intervention and requires a careful, analytical process of critical reasoning.

The evaluation phase includes an occupational profile and the analysis of occupational performance derived from interviews, the client's medical and occupational history, observations, and results from specific assessment instruments. Next, the occupational therapist generates a performance problem statement that indicates the client's occupational performance status and occupational performance problem priorities; it also lists the underlying factors contributing to the performance problem. The occupational performance problem statement is the basis for intervention planning. It is part of a plan of care that delineates measurable goals to indicate the outcomes expected by the end of therapy.

Given the focus of the intervention, occupational therapists work with the client to select the most appropriate mixture of intervention approaches and types of intervention. This process is based on a critical appraisal of the evidence regarding intervention effectiveness and on the therapist's up-to-date knowledge of relevant theories and practice models. A successful intervention plan uses the appropriate mechanisms of service delivery and reflects understanding of the discharge context. The plan includes recommendations regarding the use of community resources and referrals to appropriate professionals. Outcome measures are selected that will best demonstrate to the client whether occupational performance has been improved or enhanced; whether changes have occurred in role competence, ability to adapt to occupational challenges, and health-related quality of life; and whether the client is satisfied with the occupational therapy process.

Study Questions

1. What are the elements of an occupational therapy performance problem statement?
2. What measurement parameters are useful in writing measurable goals?
3. Write some measurable intervention goals that include all the necessary aspects.
4. What is the difference between intervention approach and type of intervention? Give examples of each.
5. Compare and contrast remediation, restoration, and establishment.
6. Describe the aspects of a successful intervention plan.
7. How does the occupational therapist know which outcome measure to select?

References

American Occupational Therapy Association. (2000). Standards of practice for occupational therapy. *American Journal of Occupational Therapy, 52,* 866–869.

American Occupational Therapy Association. (2002). Occupational therapy practice framework: Domain and process. *American Journal of Occupational Therapy, 56,* 609–639.

Baum, C. M., & Baptiste, S. (2002). Reframing occupational therapy practice. In M. Law, C. M. Baum, & S. Baptiste (Eds.), *Occupation-based practice: Fostering performance and participation* (pp. 3–16). Thorofare, NJ: Slack.

Baum, C. M., & Law, M. (1997). Occupational therapy practice: Focusing on occupational performance. *American Journal of Occupational Therapy, 51,* 277–288.

Christiansen, C., Backman, C., Little, B. R., & Nguyen, A. (1999). Occupations and well-being: A study of personal projects. *American Journal of Occupational Therapy, 53,* 91–100.

Dittmar, S. S. (1997). Selection and administration of functional assessment and rehabilitation outcome measures. In S. S. Dittmar & G. E. Gresham (Eds.), *Functional assessment and outcome measures for the rehabilitation health professional* (pp. 11–15). Gaithersburg, MD: Aspen.

Elliott-Burke, T. L., & Pothast, L. (1998). Measuring patient satisfaction in an outpatient orthopedic setting, part 1: Key drivers and results. In E. A. Dobrzykowski (Ed.), *Essential readings in rehabilitation outcomes measurement* (pp. 71–77). Gaithersburg, MD: Aspen.

Finch, E., Brooks, D., Stratford, P. W., & Mayo, N. E. (2002). *Physical rehabilitation outcome measures: A guide to enhanced clinical decision making* (2nd ed.). Toronto: Canadian Physiotherapy Association.

Holm, M. B., Rogers, J. C., & James, A. B. (2003). Interventions for activities of daily living. In E. B. Crepeau, E. S. Cohn, & B. A. Boyt Schell (Eds.), *Willard & Spackman's occupational therapy* (10th ed., pp. 491–533). Philadelphia: Lippincott Williams & Wilkins.

Holm, M. B., Rogers, J. C., & Stone, R. G. (2003). Person–task–environment interventions: A decision-making guide. In E. B. Crepeau, E. S. Cohn, & B. A. Boyt Schell (Eds.), *Willard & Spackman's occupational therapy* (10th ed., pp. 460–490). Philadelphia: Lippincott Williams & Wilkins.

Law, M., & Mills, J. (1998). Client-centered occupational therapy. In M. Law (Ed.), *Client-centered occupational therapy* (pp. 1–18). Thorofare, NJ: Slack.

Matheson, L. (1998). Engaging the person in the process: Planning together for occupational therapy intervention. In M. Law (Ed.), *Client-centered occupational therapy* (pp. 107–122). Thorofare, NJ: Slack.

Miller, W. R., & Rollnick, S. (2002). *Motivational interviewing: Preparing people to change addictive behavior* (2nd ed.). New York: Guilford.

Moyers, P. A. (1997). Occupational meanings and spirituality: The quest for sobriety. *American Journal of Occupational Therapy, 51,* 207–214.

Moyers, P. A., & Stoffel, V. C. (2001). Community-based approaches for substance use disorders. In M. Scaffa (Ed.), *Occupational therapy in community-based practice settings* (pp. 318–342). Philadelphia: F. A. Davis.

Pierce, D. (1998). What is the source of occupation's treatment power? *American Journal of Occupational Therapy, 52,* 490–491.

Robertson, L. J. (1996). Clinical reasoning, part 2: Novice/expert differences. *British Journal of Occupational Therapy, 59,* 212–216.

Simon, S. S., & Patrick, A. (1998). Understanding and assessing consumer satisfaction in rehabilitation. In E. A. Dobrzykowski (Ed.), *Essential readings in rehabilitation outcomes measurement* (pp. 104–116). Gaithersburg, MD: Aspen.

Stanton, M. P., Gresham, G. E., & Dittmar, S. S. (1997). Relationship among measures of disease, general health, and functional status. In S. S. Dittmar & G.E. Gresham (Eds.), *Functional assessment and outcome measures for the rehabilitation health professional* (pp. 31–36). Gaithersburg, MD: Aspen.

Stoffel, V. C. (1992). The Americans With Disabilities Act of 1990 as applied to an adult with alcohol dependence. *American Journal of Occupational Therapy, 46,* 640–644.

Stoffel, V. C., & Moyers, P. A. (2001). *AOTA evidence-based practice project: Treatment effectiveness as applied to substance use disorders in adolescents and adults.* Unpublished manuscript.

Wan, G. J., Counte, M. A., & Cella, D. F. (1998). A framework for organizing health related quality of life research. In E. A. Dobrzykowski (Ed.), *Essential readings in rehabilitation outcomes measurement* (pp. 16–21). Gaithersburg, MD: Aspen.

World Health Organization. (2001). *International classification of functioning, disability and health.* Geneva, Switzerland: Author.

Chapter 5

Methods for Promoting Basic and Instrumental Activities of Daily Living

LAURA K. VOGTLE, PHD, OTR/L, ATP

MARTHA E. SNELL, PHD

KEY TERMS

acquisition

age appropriate

antecedent events

baseline data

consequences

fluency

generalization

graduated guidance

maintenance

partial participation

participation

probe data

response prompts

stages of learning

stimulus prompts

system of least prompts

time delay

training data

OBJECTIVES

Upon completion of this chapter, the reader will be able to

• Discuss the need for age-appropriate, client-centered occupations for clients;

• Describe the stages of learning and relate them to age-appropriate and occupationally relevant goals;

• Discuss how task analysis is used in teaching self-care skills;

• Describe the different components of teaching strategies, including the use of prompts and feedback and different kinds of antecedents and consequences for teaching self-care skills;

• Understand the need for systematic evaluation of teaching strategies used with clients; and

• Understand the importance of careful documentation and graphing of baseline and training data for measuring change and supporting reimbursement requests.

Regardless of what occupations are being taught to whom, some general principles and methods of good instruction should be used during intervention. When the person receiving intervention has cognitive limitations, teaching should reflect additional guidelines, and the occupational therapist should consider supplementary methods. The purpose of this chapter is to describe some of the principles and methods for occupational therapists to use when working with people who have cognitive limitations. The chapter is organized into four sections: (1) initial planning of goals and intervention, (2) direct assessment of occupational performance on chosen goals, (3) teaching strategies to be used during intervention, and (4) intervention review.

Initial Planning of Intervention

Guiding Principles for Selecting Appropriate Intervention

The occupational therapist should select interventions that

- Are suited to the client's chronological age;
- Are outcomes needed by that person now and later in life;
- Are valued by the client, his or her family and peers, or both;
- Are likely to be achieved with or without task modifications;
- Can be integrated into daily routines and become useful habits;
- Can be supported by the contexts within which the client functions;
- Will meaningfully contribute to the client's independence; and
- May improve the client's positive self-image.

Perhaps the most important aspect of occupational therapy intervention is the selection of appropriate occupational outcomes. Although it is possible to devise strategies to develop just about any occupational skill, if inappropriate long-term goals are the focus of therapy, both the client's and the therapist's time are wasted. For example, when modifications such as shoes that use hook-and-loop fasteners or elastic laces are available and preferred by the client, teaching him or her to tie shoes can be an inappropriate goal. Therapists should consider several principles when selecting therapy goals for occupational performance areas:

- Occupations chosen for intervention need to consider the client's chronological age.

- Selected goals should be useful to the client in current and future life contexts.
- Goals should be those that the client, the family, or both deem important.
- Goals should enable the person to achieve occupations carried out by the typical population, such as basic and instrumental activities of daily living (ADL), leisure, work, play, and social participation.
- Even if partial participation, rather than independent occupational performance, is the goal, objectives that are realistic for the client and suited to his or her life should be selected.

When providing services for people with cognitive impairments, therapists often choose to target narrow aspects of performance, such as motor or process skills, using activities appropriate for people younger than the client. This approach violates the first principle cited above. Sometimes the occupation or outcome targeted is valid (i.e., is meaningful and age appropriate), but the activities, materials, or methods used during the intervention are not. For example, teenagers with apraxia may be asked to toss bean bags into a wooden frog's mouth to improve eye–hand coordination so that the teenager can participate in computer games with friends. This kind of intervention is not occupation based and could be construed as culturally, socially, or temporally demeaning. Incorporating the computer game itself as the intervention, rather than focusing on the motor skills needed to perform the occupation, is more likely to be meaningful and build the performance needed to incorporate the occupation into routines later in life.

The remaining principles address other aspects of occupations and participation: Goals or activities selected for intervention should be those that are meaningful to the client, that are commonly performed in familiar contexts and that, if not learned, will need to be carried out by someone else. Client-centered occupational goals are more likely to be integrated into daily routines, are not forgotten through disuse, and promote less dependence on others. Evidence suggests that goals written by families and clients promote "ownership" of the goals and are more likely to result in long-term success (Mackey & McQueen, 1998). Such outcomes have purpose in daily contexts and thus are valued by others. Learning to perform occupations that are valued by people in the client's social and cultural environments improves the way the client is viewed by others and by him- or herself (Guidetti & Soderback, 2001; Kellegrew & Allen, 1996). Selecting goals that have little value or purpose to the client means that the occupations will not be used once they are learned.

Some clients have significant impairments in performance skills that make it more feasible to learn to perform part of an activity than to attempt the entire task. This practice, known as *partial participation,* was identified some years ago and was reviewed recently (Baumgart et al., 1982; Ferguson & Baumgart, 1991). It includes the following elements:

1. Receiving help from others on difficult steps (Bosner & Belifore, 2001)
2. Changing the order of the steps of the activity
3. Changing the rules of the activity
4. Adding assistive technology.

Careful selection of activities that incorporate partial participation is important so that the skills learned will fit into the client's and caregiver's various contexts and thus become part of the daily routine. It is important for the occupational therapist to review intervention progress periodically, however, because the client may be able to learn more steps of the activity and thus require modifications in occupational performance, habits, and routines (Ferguson & Baumgart, 1991).

Occupations important to the client and family often involve part of a daily schedule or routine and thus may include instrumental activities of daily living (IADL). Brown, Evans, Weed, and Owen (1987) described two types of related skills that can help occupational therapy practitioners build a core ADL task to become part of a larger routine or role. *Extension skills* include the ability to initiate a routine, prepare for the activity, monitor the speed and quality (i.e., tempo) of the activity, solve problems, and terminate the activity or clean up when done. *Enrichment skills* involve expressive communication (through nonsymbolic or symbolic means), social behavior, and making choices (Table 5.1).

Practitioners working in a team setting need to avoid "dividing up" the client into parts that reflect each team member's professional territory. Pooling talents only strengthens teaching. Depending on the context, a variety of people (e.g., staff, peers, family members) may contribute to teaching an ADL. Therapists tend to pay closer attention to teaching the motor and cognitive learning requirements involved than families do; however, everyone who assists in teaching or supervising task or activity performance should be alert to the variety of

extension and expansion skills that are embedded within personal ADL.

Ecological Inventories

How does one determine which occupations are important to a particular person? The most important source of this information is the client and family. If the client is at all able to give information through interview or direct assessment, he or she must contribute to the initial assessment. Skill checklists, such as ADL inventories, are often used to assess current abilities and identify goals. They can be particularly valuable for clients who are unable to contribute to interviews. Although ADL checklists can help determine whether a person has the obvious prerequisite skills, they also may lead practitioners to focus on skills that are not needed or are less needed than others. Sometimes the sequencing nature of a checklist causes clinicians to regard tasks appearing earlier on the list as prerequisites to later skills, when they may not be. This is particularly true for early childhood assessments, such as the Denver II (Frankenburg, Dodds, Archer, Shapiro, & Bresnick, 1992). To avoid this problem and develop a more comprehensive picture of the client in his or her routine environments, therapists can use other indirect methods, such as interviewing people in the following categories:

- Those who know most about the individual's current performance needs, such as parents and family members, past teachers, peers, and practitioners
- Those who would be familiar with upcoming participation needs, such as the next teacher or practitioner, peers, job coaches, and so forth.

Some examples of indirect methods of functional assessment are the Canadian Occupational Performance Measure (Law, Baptiste, Carswell, Polatajko, & Pollack, 1998), the Pediatric Evaluation of Disability Inventory (Haley, Ludlow, & Coster, 1993), the Klein–Bell Activities of Daily Living Scale (Law & Usher, 1988), the Functional Independence Measure (Hamilton, Laughlin, Fiedler, & Granger, 1994), and the Functional Independence Measure for Children (McCabe & Granger, 1990). Comparable assessments exist in special education and are called *ecological inventories* and *environmental assessments* (Brown & Snell, 2000; Ford et al., 1989; Giangreco, Cloninger, & Iverson, 1993). Using these kinds of tools, occupational therapists can assess references for goals through direct interview or by ob-

Table 5.1. Activity Analysis Illustrating the Sensory-Motor Task Component Model Used for Treatment Planning

Activity Step	Activity Component	Sensory Component	Motor Component	Grasp Component
Inspects nails to see if they are dirty or jagged	Initiation of task	Vision, light touch	Finger extension, wrist extension, forearm supination and pronation	N/A
Finds and selects materials	Preparation for task	Vision, light touch, pressure discrimination	Finger flexion/extension, wrist extension, elbow flexion and extension, possible shoulder action	Radial digital grasp, lateral tip pinch, pad to pad pinch
Cleans and trims nails	Core steps of task	Vision, pain, light touch, pressure discrimination	MP and IP flexion/ extension/abduction for all digits, including the thumb, wrist flexion/ extension, ulnar/radial deviation, isolated finger control	Lateral tip pinch, pad to pad pinch, possible gross grasp
Checks nails for cleanliness and neatness	Quality monitoring	Vision	MP and IP flexion/wrist extension, possible shoulder action	N/A
Grooms nails within an acceptable amount of time	Tempo monitoring	Rapid motor response to sensory input	Use of feedforward and feedback mechanisms to ensure motor efficiency, finger flexion and extension, possible shoulder action	Rapid change of grasp patterns as required by the task
Resolves problems that arise (such as locating materials)	Problem solving	Variable	Variable	Variable
Puts trimming supplies away	Termination of task	Vision, light touch, pressure discrimination	Finger flexion/extension, wrist extension, elbow flexion and extension, possible shoulder action	Radial digital grasp, lateral tip pinch, pad to pad pinch
Communicates about any aspect of nail grooming (such as length of nails, hangnail)	Communication	Variable	Variable	N/A
Makes choices within task (such as to polish or not)	Choice making	Variable	Variable	Variable
Performs routine at appropriate time and location	Social aspect of task	Variable	Variable	Variable

Note. MP = metacarpophalangeal joints; IP = interphalangeal joints.

Source. Adapted from "Making Functional Skills Function: A Component Model," by F. Brown, I. M. Evans, K. Weed, and V. Owen, 1987, *Journal of the Association for Persons with Severe Handicaps, 12*, p. 122. Copyright © 1987 by the Association for Persons with Severe Handicaps. Adapted by permission.

servation, and they can ask "informants," who know the client or who know settings the client will use in the future, questions such as the following:

- What skills do you think are important for _____ to learn?
- What skills are required of _____ that he or she does not know or that others must perform regularly?
- Are there some skills critical to _____'s safety and health that he or she might learn partially or totally?
- What skills are expected of _____'s peers in the same activities and places?
- Could _____ learn to assist with this skill (partial participation) or to perform the skill with adaptations? Without adaptations?

Therapists also can ask clients a variety of questions (or may observe them with input from the people who know them to deduce the answers), such as the following:

- What occupations do you want to learn?
- What part of this occupation is hard for you? Is easy for you?

Therapists may examine program entry requirements or visit programs, desired places of employment, or future residences to consider creative accommodation and to understand what occupations are needed for the client to participate. Once complete information is obtained, therapists work with the client, family, and client's team to set priorities. They consider assessment information from all team members at this time. The skills that seem most needed and functional for the client typically become intervention objectives (sometimes called *habilitation targets*).

Stages of Learning

Learning may be viewed as occurring in stages or phases, from initial instruction, or *acquisition,* to expanded instruction, or *generalized skills* (Snell & Brown, 2000). During acquisition, clients receive assistance and feedback (i.e., reinforcement and error correction) to help them progress to the stage of self-regulated, developed occupations. *Prompting* (also called *scaffolding*), is the term for the verbal and nonverbal assistance provided to the client to help them move from initial learning to mastery of a skill (Wang, Bernas, & Eberhard, 2001). The type and frequency of prompting depends on the client's cognitive and motor abilities, the contexts in which he or she functions, and his or her personal preferences. Most clinicians agree that such assistance should be provided initially to decrease frustration with new or difficult tasks and to facilitate success. As the client's competence increases, prompting is reduced.

Figure 5.1 illustrates the relationship among the following four stages of learning (Snell & Brown, 2000):

1. *Acquisition* is the initial learning of an activity. In this stage, clients may not be able to perform the target skill at all or may perform with limited competence. Performance accuracy ranges from 0 to 60%.
2. *Maintenance* involves routinely using a skill and improving its accuracy under fairly stable and familiar conditions. At this stage, clients perform the target skill with limited competence but do not initiate the task during the typical daily routine. Performance accuracy is roughly 60% or better.
3. *Fluency* or *proficiency* involves improving the accuracy, quality, and speed of performance.

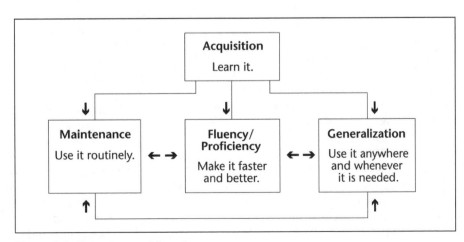

Figure 5.1. Four stages of learning.

At this stage, clients perform the activity with limited competence in that they may be too slow, careless, or inattentive to detail. Accuracy is roughly 60% or better.

4. *Generalization* refers to performance under changing conditions (e.g., location, materials, time, task variation). At this stage, clients perform the activity with limited competence in that they fail to initiate or are unable to complete the task when the performance context changes in some way. Performance accuracy is roughly 60% or better.

Given these brief descriptions, it is clear that intervention approaches and criteria should vary somewhat to match the different stages of learning. When therapy personnel view learning in these four stages, they are more likely to

- Adjust their intervention methods as they shift their focus from one stage to another;
- Avoid overemphasizing new activities; and
- Broaden their focus so that maintenance, fluency, and skill generalization are valued equally to acquisition of new activities.

Strategies to promote engagement in targeted occupations can focus concurrently on maintenance, fluency, and generalization if practitioners are clear about their goals, if instruction is not too complex, and if task performance data are kept to evaluate whether learning is occurring. The following case may help clarify this process.

Following a head injury, 13-year-old April wanted to learn to put her shoes, socks, and ankle-foot-orthoses (AFOs) on fast enough that she could put them on every day before school rather than have her parents do it for her. The project was undertaken in June with hopes for proficiency in the activity by early September. The final goal of 10 to 15 min for putting on the items was determined with input from the parents.

In the acquisition phase, the therapist worked with April on accuracy: getting shoes and socks on over her heels and putting on the AFOs correctly. Once April achieved successful performance on these difficult steps about two-thirds of the time, the focus shifted to maintenance, or performance of the activity in her daily routine. Her parents agreed that she could perform the activity by herself on weekends, and they would simply check whether the items were on correctly when she was finished and document her performance speed.

April then began to work on independent maintenance of her skills. Her parents agreed to purchase shoes that use hook-and-loop fasteners to eliminate lacing and tying, which could improve her speed from her initial time of 40 min. Throughout the summer, April worked hard and used a clock to time herself. Her efforts to use the shoes and her daily monitoring of performance time represent a focus on fluency learning.

By mid-July, April was able to get the AFOs on tight enough that her family no longer worried about blisters. Her time was reduced to 25 min—good, but still short of her goal. April and her parents made several additional task improvements that were aimed at improving fluency even more. First, April would get up early enough to put on her shoes before her parents left for work. With this arrangement, she usually managed to get up 4 or 5 days per week to work on speed. Second, the therapist made improvements in the AFO's hook-and-loop fasteners, which made the task easier. By the start of school, April was able to get all items on in 15 min and was willing to get up early enough to put them on by herself each day. Once back in school, April asked to work on generalizing the skill from home to the physical context of school. By the end of October, she was able to change her shoes for physical education in 10 min without help.

Maintenance and generalization are promoted even during acquisition, when therapists select activities that are functional, needed, or valued by others, because those activities will be routinely required in multiple contexts. When the occupational therapist selects activities suited to the client's age, the client may be more inclined to develop the habit of using them. Peers, family members, and practitioners will be more likely to encourage activities seen as typical in a specified context, as they would occupations or behaviors typical of a younger person.

When clients' skills are not fluent, other people are not likely to incorporate those skills into routines. Consider the following scenarios:

- A fifth-grade boy writes so slowly that his parents always do his assigned homework.
- Caregivers for a 30-year-old woman with cerebral palsy living in a group home often feed her because the client makes a mess when feeding herself.

- A young woman knows how to make up beds but cannot be hired for motel housekeeping because she drapes sheets and blankets unevenly and does not smooth out the wrinkles.

The examples describe fluency and generalization problems; unless the intervention process addresses them, instruction will not result in occupational performance that others value. Stated another way, activities that cannot be performed at a reasonable speed, with required accuracy and quality, and regardless of changes in activity demands and context will not be valued by the people in the client's social context.

During the acquisition stage, practitioners can incorporate elements into the intervention plan that will promote generalization into multiple physical or social contexts, as in the following examples:

- Provide intervention in natural or as close to natural contexts as possible.
- Use "real," not simulated, materials that are appropriate to the task (e.g., real shoes to teach dressing and shoe tying; real clothes to teach dressing and buttoning, not button boards or dolls, although larger clothes may be used during early instruction).
- Use multiple teaching examples (e.g., staff members, peers, physical and social contexts, and materials).
- Select teaching examples carefully, starting with those that best reflect the range of variation (e.g., for upper-body dressing, a turtleneck, tank top, and T-shirt are typically taught first because they best reflect the range of variations in collar, sleeve length, fit, and fabric from a group of eight pullover shirts; Day & Horner, 1986). The strategy of teaching the general case first teaches clients a generalized skill that is durable across commonly expected changes in contextual and activity demand requirements.

Goals must specify the occupation; the desired outcome, or *criterion,* for performance; and the context in which the behavior or skill will be performed. The conditions for successful occupational performance involve temporal and physical context, the presence or absence of others, the activity demands involved, and any assistance or adaptations needed. A general rule to follow is to let the client's or family's reality dictate the conditions for learning. If the client shows little or no learning under natural conditions, then the conditions or activity demands may be simplified. For example, the therapist could provide fewer variations in material,

location, times, and practitioners, or less noise and distraction. Eventually, however, the client must learn to perform the activity in typical contexts, or the occupation will not become part of his or her habits, routines, or roles. For example, McInerney and McInerney (1992) identified the goal of riding the bus to the mall as an outcome for 29 adults with developmental disabilities and first used simulated, then community contexts to successfully reach their criterion for performance.

The occupational therapist collaborates with other team members to rewrite selected teaching goals as instructional objectives. The following example illustrates the objective April's team wrote for the skill of putting on shoes and socks:

> *Target objective:* April will be able to put on her shoes, socks, and AFOs in 10 min each morning at home before school without assistance from her parents.

- *Behavior:* Putting on shoes that use hook-and-loop fasteners, socks, and AFOs
- *Performance criterion:* 10 min
- *Conditions or context:* Sitting on the floor in her bedroom
- *When:* Each morning before school
- *Where:* At home
- *Who is present:* No one
- *Materials:* Shoes, socks, and AFOs
- *Assistance:* None
- *Modifications:* Hook-and-loop fasteners.

Direct Evaluation of Skills

We have referred to assessment and data collection as an "evil necessity." We use that label for several reasons:

- Clients seldom learn during evaluation, so it seems like wasted time.
- Many therapists find assessment or data collection tedious and time consuming, especially when time with clients is restricted by reimbursement requirements or caseload size.
- Many therapists are inexperienced in evaluating the evaluation data gathered and applying it to the intervention, thus they cannot justify the effort it takes.

Collecting performance data is necessary because it provides objective information relevant to the performance of the target goal and enables the therapist to determine whether a therapy intervention has succeeded. When data indicate minimal or slower progress than expected, the therapy approach or conditions can be changed. Likewise, if the data indicate that the goal has been met, then instruction can be directed toward a different stage of learning for the same occupation or toward other occupations, as shown in the following example:

> Ron, an adolescent with a spinal cord injury, has learned to perform several wheelchair push-ups every 15 min; his consistency over an 8-hr day is 60%. On the basis of these data, his therapist might direct therapy toward improved consistency of performance while shifting the focus of intervention toward several new goals. Those goals might include promoting his routine and spontaneous use of the skill in all the situations in which training has occurred (i.e., maintenance) and extending the expectation for routine performance of push-ups to the home or school setting (i.e., generalization).

Assessment Data

Many kinds of data are pertinent to therapy intervention. The following section specifically discusses two kinds of data, client performance data and data collected from observation during both intervention and natural settings or conditions.

Observational Data

This discussion primarily addresses *client performance data:* data that measure some aspect of occupational performance relevant to the goals set by the therapist, client, and family. Such data are collected mainly through direct observation of the client during performance of the activity, but valuable data can be collected *after* the skill has been performed, as seen in the following three examples:

Measure the *permanent products* resulting from the performance (e.g., estimating the spillage on the table and floor after he finishes eating).

> *Socially validate* the client's performance by (1) seeking the opinions of peers or caregivers on the performance of a skill they regularly see (e.g., "Is the client eating neatly enough?") or (2) comparing the client's performance with that of peers for the same skill (How fast and how neatly do the client's peers eat?).

Test and Training Data

Observational data on occupational performance may be collected under two conditions. *Training data* reflect student performance during training or treatment sessions (e.g., when assistance, corrective feedback, and reinforcement are provided according to the therapy plan). *Test data* (also called *probe data*) reflect performance during nontraining conditions, such as daily routines when little or no assistance or feedback is available other than that naturally occurring in the environment (also referred to as *criterion conditions*). Test data often show lower performance than do training data. Both training and test data can be useful to practitioners.

Discrete and Chained Target Behaviors

Target behaviors can be thought of as being either *discrete* (i.e., distinct behaviors that stand alone) or *chained* (i.e., involving a sequence of discrete behaviors). Therapists target many types of discrete behaviors, such as lip closure, steps taken during walking, ability to grasp during household chores, and time required to dress. Discrete behavior targets typically are defined in specific terms so they can be observed and then counted during a fixed period of time or over a set number of opportunities, as illustrated in the following example:

> The therapist defines grasping behaviors during the occupation of play for Muriel, a 5-year-old with cerebral palsy. Grasp is the "correct response," and failure to grasp is the "incorrect response." The therapist then identifies daily activities during which grasping occurs and can be measured, and he or she defines the length of the observation period. The therapist could calculate Muriel's *rate of performance* (in this case, the number of successful and unsuccessful grasping behaviors Muriel makes during 10 min of toy-and-block play with peers in kindergarten), but because this outcome might be highly variable because of changing activity demands during play, a better measurement procedure might be (1) to count her successful and unsuccessful attempts at grasp during the first 10 opportunities during playtime and (2) divide the number of successful and unsuccessful grasps by the total number of opportunities (i.e., 10). Focusing on the first opportunities to grasp rather than a length of time allows the therapist to observe an activity in which grasp is used, which may not happen in some play activities.

Chained behaviors are those involving a sequence of behaviors or skills that constitute an activity or are needed to complete the activity. Behavior sequences often are identified as steps in a task or activity analysis of the skill. Examples include dressing tasks; standing and transfer tasks; some vocational skills; and most grooming, housekeeping, and cooking tasks. Activity analyses frequently serve as the guide for intervention and evaluation because they list the behaviors and the sequence involved in performing activities targeted for intervention.

Activity Analysis

Activity analysis can be defined as the process of breaking down routines into discrete components. Another commonly used term for this process found in the literature is *task analysis*. Often the occupations that therapists identify for intervention are divided into steps according to the occupational profile (see Chapter 3; Watson & Wilson, 2003). Commercially available activity analyses may seem to be time-savers; however, they fail to individualize the activity to the client's important contexts, individual factors, performance skills, and activity demands. Rather, to develop a good activity analysis, several steps are important:

1. Spend time observing the client and others performing the activity.
2. Develop the best approaches for completing the activity.
3. Ask others' opinions about the activity performance (including the person who will learn it and family members who will support it).
4. Field-test the activity analysis and revise it as necessary.

5. To promote generalization across contexts, develop an activity analysis that is relatively generic or suits a number of situations in which the client will need to perform the activity.

The activity analysis in Figure 5.2 divides eating, drinking, and wiping with a napkin into response steps and identifies the relevant stimuli (i.e., *discriminative stimuli*) for each response. Such stimuli are sensory feedback in the activity that cue the resulting response. In contrast, the approach illustrated in Table 5.1 focuses on component or performance skills involved in the skill or activity—it analyzes the sensory, motor, and grasp components in addition to the behavior chain or core steps involved in the skill or activity. What the activity analysis methods have in common is their delineation of sequenced, observable behaviors that lead to the accomplishment of a given activity. The kind of activity analysis used will depend on the needs of the client, the user of the analysis (i.e., therapist, teacher, or parent), and the therapeutic goals.

The following guidelines are valuable in developing an activity analysis:

1. Use steps of fairly even "size."
2. Be sure each step is observable and results in a visible change in behavior.

Behavior	Discriminative Stimuli	Response
Spoon	"Eat"	Grasp spoon
	Spoon in hand	Scoop food
	Food in spoon	Raise spoon to lips
	Spoon touching lips	Open mouth
	Mouth open	Put spoon in mouth
	Food in mouth	Remove spoon
	Spoon out of mouth	Lower spoon
	Spoon on table	Release grasp
Cup	"Drink"	Grasp cup
	Cup in hand	Raise cup to lips
	Cup touches lips	Tilt cup to mouth
	Liquid in mouth	Close mouth and drink
	Liquid swallowed	Lower cup to table
	Cup on table	Release grasp
Napkin	"Wipe"	Grasp napkin
	Napkin in hand	Raise hand to face
	Napkin touching face	Wipe face
	Face wiped	Lower napkin
	Napkin on table	Release grasp

Note. From "Using Constant Time Delay to Teach Self-Feeding to Young Students With Severe/Profound Handicaps: Evidence of Limited Effectiveness," by B. C. Collins, D. L. Gast, M.Wolery, A. Holcombe, and J. Letherby, 1991, *Journal of Developmental and Physical Difficulties, 3,* p. 163. Copyright © 1991 by Plenum Publishing. Reprinted by permission.

Figure 5.2. Task analysis for teaching spoon, cup, and napkin use.

3. Order the steps in a logical sequence, but indicate when the sequence is optional.

4. Distinguish any steps requiring another person's assistance and the parts of the activity performed by people other than the student or client.

5. Write the specific steps in second-person singular (so that they can be used as verbal prompts).

6. Use language meaningful to the student or client with whom it will be used, and place in parentheses any additional information that may be difficult for the client to understand but is needed for the observer (e.g., "using a pincer grasp").

7. Place the steps on an activity analysis data sheet, which allows the user to record step-by-step data over a number of days (see Figure 5.3; Snell & Brown, 2000).

Conducting Assessments With Activity Analyses

Once a good activity analysis is prepared, the therapist uses it as a guide for observing and measuring the client's performance and for teaching the activity. The therapist asks the client to perform the activity. Each step in the activity analysis is then observed and scored as correct or incorrect.

Chris is a 3 1/2-year-old boy who attends a preschool five mornings per week. His therapy is integrated into daily activities in order to address performance skill needs and improve the likelihood that he will generalize his learning to the daily routine. Before being taught this activity, Chris waited for help to sit down and stand up from a chair because his balance was unsteady, and he sometimes fell when not assisted. His therapists and teachers planned to use a total task approach to develop his ability to both sit in and stand up from a chair so that whenever training and practice occurred, each step would be performed in order and with the needed assistance provided. His teachers used the task analysis to guide their observation of his performance on each step. (Figure 5.3)

Two methods of observation can be used during assessment:

1. *Single-opportunity activity analysis assessment:* The client is asked to perform the activity. Testing stops after the first error, and all remaining steps are scored as errors. Errors include performing the wrong step, making a mistake on a step, taking too long (if time is important), or not performing.

Name: Chris
Instructor: Maura
Instructional Cue: "Find your chair"
Program: Sitting
Method: Least to Most/4-sec latency

Objective: Given a natural opportunity or a request to sit in a preschool cube chair for an activity and a response latency of 4 second, Chris will perform correctly on at least 88% (7 of 8 steps) of the task analysis without assistance for three consecutive training opportunities and one probe.

	Date Baseline*					Date Training																		Probe
	2/27*	3/4*	3/5*	3/6*	3/7*	3/18	3/19	3/20	3/21	3/22	3/25	4/8	4/11	4/12	4/16	4/17	4/18	4/22	4/23	4/26	4/29	4/30	5/1	5/2*
1. Face cube chair	—	—	—	—	—	P	P	P	P	P	V	+	+	+	+	+	+	+	+	+	+	+	+	+
2. Bend forward	—	—	—	—	—	P	P	P	P	P	V	+	+	+	+	+	+	+	+	+	+	+	+	+
3. Grip arm handles	—	—	—	—	—	G	+	G	G	G	V	+	+	+	+	+	+	V	+	+	+	+	+	+
4. Shift right arm to left arm handle	—	—	—	—	—	P	P	P	P	P	P	+	+	+	+	+	G	+	+	+	+	+	+	+
5. Twist trunk and hips	—	—	—	—	—	P	P	P	+	+	V	+	+	V	V	+	+	+	+	+	+	+	+	+
6. Lower bottom to chair	—	—	—	—	+	+	+	+	+	+	+	+	+	+	+	+	+	+	+	+	+	+	+	+
7. Reposition hands and feet	+	—	+	+	+	+	+	+	+	+	+	+	+	+	+	+	+	+	+	P	+	+	+	+
8. Push bottom to back of chair using feet and hands	+	+	+	+	+	+	+	+	+	+	+	+	+	+	+	+	+	+	+	P	+	+	+	+
	25	13	25	25	38	58	50	38	50	50	38	100	100	88	88	100	88	88	100	75	100	100	100	100*

Key:

Baseline*	Training
(+) independent	(+) independent
(—) error	(V) verbal prompt
	(G) gestural prompt
	(P) physical prompt

Figure 5.3. Task analysis data sheet for Chris's objective of sitting down in a chair.

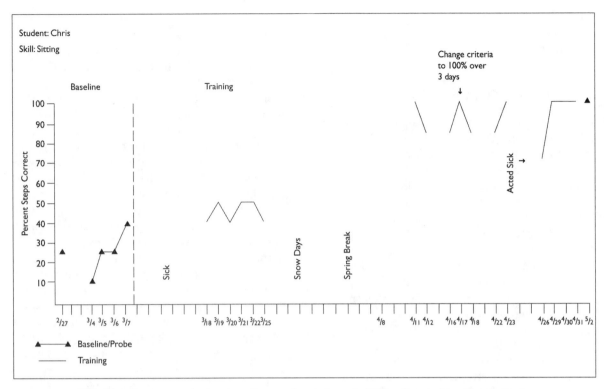

Figure 5.4. Chris's performance during baseline and training of sitting. Created by Maura Burke. Used with permission.

2. *Multiple-opportunity activity analysis assessment:* The client is asked to perform the activity, and each step is observed. Whenever an error occurs it is recorded, and the evaluator positions the student for the next step. Positioning for testing a step is done without comment or instruction because this is a testing, not teaching, context.

Chris's teacher and therapist decided to use a multiple-opportunity activity analytic assessment approach so they could observe his performance on all steps during each test. His baseline performance over 5 days of assessment was collected and graphed (Figures 5.3 and 5.4). He consistently missed the first five steps but was successful on the last three, although his performance was inconsistent and slightly improved over the 5 days. His baseline performance seems to indicate that Chris did not know how to perform the activity, so selecting the task as a goal was appropriate. His parents and teacher also identified independent sitting and standing as skills needed for many daily activities at home and at school.

When enrichment goals (i.e., communication, choice making, and social goals) are addressed at the same time as core skills, they can simply be placed on the activity analysis sheet. For example, if the therapist wants to give the client a choice about which chair to sit in or about verbalizing his or her success (e.g., Chris sometimes says "Sit!" when he is successful), those choice-making and communication goals can go directly into the activity sequence. Enrichment behaviors that are not readily predictable can simply be listed at the end of the activity analysis, with a frequency count entered for each observation. Therapists who must keep a record of significant problem behaviors that occur (e.g., having tantrums, falling down, or legs giving out) can add them to the end of the activity steps as well.

The graph of Chris's performance data (Figure 5.4) is summarized in percentage form (i.e., the percentage of eight steps performed correctly during each observation). Because Chris is still in the acquisition stage (less than 60% correct), his team decided to include only core behaviors in the activity analysis. Extension and enrichment skills might be added later. If enrichment behaviors are added to an activity analysis, however, they should be graphed separately from the core skill steps. Any problem behaviors added to the bottom of the activity analysis also need to be analyzed separately because the intended goal is to decrease their frequency by replacing them with more appropriate behaviors. The use of data and graphing is discussed in the last section of this chapter.

Intervention Strategies

Before discussing general teaching strategies, it might be helpful to review Table 5.2, which illustrates the events that may take place before and after the targeted self-care behavior. These events, discussed next, can be incorporated into intervention strategies. Antecedent events are those that occur before the target behavior or goal; some events are intentionally arranged and are called *controlling antecedents,* whereas other antecedents may not be under the practitioner's control and are called *relevant antecedent stimuli,* as in the following example:

> Just prior to his lessons on spoon, cup, and napkin use at lunch, Sam, who has autism, is hungry. Hunger serves as a powerful internal antecedent stimulus. The school bell ringing at lunchtime and classmates rushing to their lockers to get packed lunches also are stimuli that establish that it is lunchtime. Once the children are seated in the lunchroom, more specific stimuli are present, such as the therapist's request to Sam ("Let's eat") and the task-discriminative stimuli (S^D) created by performing each response in the chain of taking a spoonful of food.

As shown in Table 5.2, performance of each response creates an antecedent discriminative stimulus relevant to the next response in the chain.

To teach Sam the three targeted mealtime skills, his therapists decided to use physical prompts such as hand-over-hand assists and planned antecedent events; they used only as much hand-over-hand assistance as was needed to get Sam to demonstrate each behavior in the three targeted chains. The physical prompt worked for Sam: The physical assistance prompts controlled his behavior. The discriminative stimuli that resulted from performing each step of the task, however, did not yet control the responses that they preceded. When the therapist placed the spoon in Sam's hand, he seemed to know he needed to scoop some food, but he did not yet respond in a way that got food on the spoon. One major goal of instruction was to fade out the controlling antecedents that were provided by teachers or practitioners (e.g., requests to eat and physical prompts). At the same time, Sam was taught to attend to the relevant antecedent stimuli (e.g., food on his plate with a spoon, napkin, and filled glass beside it; spoon in hand; food on spoon; and spoon touching lips).

Table 5.2 includes *consequences,* or the events (either planned or unplanned) that may be used following a target response to reinforce desired behavior. During treatment sessions, consequences may include any of the following examples:

- Comments or information given about the accuracy or success of the response (e.g., "that's right")
- Feedback about an error (e.g., "Remember to hold the bottom of the zipper" while pointing to the end of the zipper)
- Reinforcement (e.g., approval, praise, pat on the back, activity choice, tangibles)
- Correction (e.g., modeling the missed step and giving the client an opportunity to perform it with help)

Table 5.2. Possible Antecedent and Consequence Events That May Precede and Follow the Target Response

Antecedent Events		Response	Consequences
New Stimuli "To Be Learned"	**Controlling Stimuli or Prompts**		
Teacher's request	*Response Prompts:*	*Correct response*	*Confirmation*
Task materials	Verbal instructions		
	Pictorial prompts	*Approximation*	*Reinforcement:*
Time of day	Gestures or pointing		Self-reinforcement
		Incorrect response:	Praise and approval
Location	Modeling	Error	Choice
		No response	Preferred activity
People present	Physical assistance (partial or full)	Inappropriate behavior	Tangible reinforcer
Internal stimuli			
	Stimulus Prompts:		*Error feedback:*
	Color coding		Pause for self-correction
	Stimulus fading		Ignore and no S^{R+}
			correction

Note. S^{R+} indicates no positive reinforcement.

- Extinction (e.g., ignoring errors and withholding comments when performance is not "up to par")
- Punishing consequences (e.g., withholding reinforcement, giving sharp criticism, requiring excessive practice following an error, or time out).

Much of the early special education research on self-care instruction of people with developmental disabilities involved punishing consequences or intensive teaching practices (e.g., excessively lengthy training sessions; Farlow & Snell, 2000). Now, however, punishing consequences are regarded as unethical and socially invalid practices. For most people, punishment does not contribute to creating good learning conditions for the following reasons:

- The therapist is put into a position of "me against you" control, emphasizing the negative aspects of a therapeutic relationship, which may hinder the practitioner's effectiveness as a clinician.
- Punitive methods often are socially invalid or unacceptable to professionals, peers, or care providers and may violate the client's basic rights.
- When a problem behavior exists that is not serious, it is best to ignore it, redirect the client, and focus on teaching needed skills or alternative replacement skills. If the problem behavior harms the client, others, or task materials, a careful study of the situation (i.e., a functional assessment) is indicated and a behavior support plan may be required.

Problem behavior is beyond the scope of this chapter; the reader should consult any of a variety of useful references on problem behavior for more information (e.g., Carr et al., 1994; Janney & Snell, 2000; O'Neill et al., 1997).

Artificial and Natural Prompts and Feedback

Antecedent events and consequences can be naturally occurring or intentionally arranged by a therapist. They also can either help or hinder learning. As clients advance into different stages of learning for specific occupations, artificial antecedent events and consequences should be faded out, leaving only the consequences that are natural, as illustrated in Table 5.2; the latter are the stimuli or activity demands that clients must deal with in everyday living. The intervention task becomes one of directing clients to attend to cues in the environment that assist them in performing activities. In many cases, the occupational therapist should emphasize natural cues as prompts from the beginning of learning, as in the following examples:

Sam, who has autism, is learning to use a spoon and napkin and will benefit from having his teachers call attention to his peers, who sit nearby and can remind him to wipe his face clean.

Rose, an older woman who has recently had a stroke, is relearning many of the daily living skills she once performed with ease. The therapist's verbal, gestural, and physical assists will be helpful, as will the confirmations about her performance and the help with her errors. Rose must learn to pay attention to the visual and tactile cues from the left side of her body and the cues of material placement. Doing so will permit her to self-regulate and recognize whether her body is moving as it should be while she is dressing or helping her daughter with meal preparation (e.g., patting lettuce dry and putting salad in a bowl). In place of the therapist's consequences, the comments and reactions of others that naturally occur will become the corrective and reinforcing consequences.

For many youth and adults, the natural antecedent of peer modeling and the consequence of peer approval provide important means by which they can judge their own performances (Farmer-Dougan, 1994; Kellegrew & Allen, 1996). Other studies have incorporated a process called *peer mediation* to successfully deliver interventions using peer modeling, natural cues and prompts, and feedback in natural environments (Odom et al., 2003; Robertson, Green, Alper, Schloss, & Kohler, 2003).

Antecedents: Instructional Cues

An instructional cue can be a request to perform a target skill or goal (e.g., "Get your lunch" or "Find your chair"), or it may consist of other stimuli that alert the client to perform the activity without a request:

Sam follows his peers to the cafeteria line; their actions of lining up, getting a tray, taking a spoon and fork, moving down the line, and so on, cue him to begin the activity of moving through the line to get his lunch.

One common error of therapists and teachers is the tendency to say too much. When the instructional cue is a request, it should be stated just once, and in a way the client understands. Instructional cues should not be questions ("Do you want to tie your shoes?") unless the client is being given an option to do the task. To make cues understandable, the therapist must be familiar with the client's level of comprehension. Spoken instructional cues may be accompanied by gestures, if symbolic communication is less meaningful, or by signs, pictures, or symbols, if the client uses those kinds of cues to augment or replace verbal communication. When the client does not make the desired response, assistance or prompts should be given to encourage his or her performance, rather than just repeating the cue.

The best conditions for teaching most people involve embedding instruction within the activity or routine, thus providing many natural cues for the client (e.g., location, activity materials, time of day, others performing a similar activity, and the need for the activity to be completed).

> For Chris, who is learning to sit and stand by himself during preschool activities, the natural cues include his peers getting cube chairs, the teacher calling for circle time, and others taking a seat. Chris's performance after several weeks of training was good enough for his therapist to replace the instructional cue "Find your chair" with directing his attention to natural cues. Whenever Chris fails to perform the first activity step, the teacher and therapist use one of three kinds of prompts (verbal, gestural, or physical) given in order of increasing assistance, and only as needed.

Antecedents: Prompts

Prompts fall into two general categories: *response prompts* and *stimulus prompts* (see Table 5.2). The discussion in this section focuses on response prompts because they are more versatile than stimulus prompts for self-care activities and require less effort to use.

Stimulus prompts (also called *stimulus modification procedures;* Wolery, Ault, & Doyle, 1992) require a gradual change from easy to hard (e.g., teaching a person to write her name by fading, when the level of prompts are decreased from more assistance to less assistance, the stimulus prompts from tracing letters to thickly dotted letters, to thinly dotted letters, to, finally, no dotted guidelines). Response prompts, however, encompass various types of therapist assistance that are directed toward encouraging the client's response. In order of increasing assistance, response prompts include the following types of prompt:

- Specific verbal instructions (e.g., "Open the shampoo")
- Pictorial or two-dimensional prompts, such as showing the client photos of activity steps (see Lancioni & O'Reilly, 2001; Mirenda,

MacGregor, & Kelly-Keough, 2002, for a review of the effectiveness of picture cues and others)
- Gestures, such as pointing to needed materials or gesturing toward children's seats when it is time to begin class
- Models or demonstrations of the target response
- Physical assistance, either partial (e.g., nudging a client's hand toward the toothpaste) or full (e.g., using hand-over-hand assistance to get the client to pick up the toothpaste; Wolery et al., 1992).

Prompts can be given individually (e.g., a verbal request to pick up the soap in a handwashing task), in combinations (e.g., a verbal request plus pointing to the soap), or as part of a planned hierarchy of prompts given one at a time, as needed.

Latency

To allow clients to initiate prompted performance on the activity step, a therapist often provides a short *latency* (i.e., period of time) before prompting a client to initiate the activity step without help as well as after prompting a client. The latency may be as short as 2 to 3 sec or as long as 15 sec but it needs to be determined on an individualized basis, according the client's natural response latency on known activities (i.e., how long it takes the client to initiate a fairly familiar task step). Response latency will be slower when performance skills are impaired, as when muscle tone is atypical, movement is less volitional, or vision is limited. Piazza, Anderson, and Fisher (1993) described an example of the successful use of prompts followed by latency when teaching girls with Rett syndrome to feed themselves.

Selection of Prompts

Prompts must be selected to fit the client, situation, and activity. For example, some clients with cerebral palsy or other neurological conditions may understand the activity and the order of its steps, but they need to learn to organize and use smaller ranges of movement. For these clients, sensory prompts such as deep pressure on an extremity may be far more effective than verbal or model prompts:

> In a three-step task analysis of standing up from sitting written for Chris, the therapist provides support at the knees after Chris scoots to the edge of the chair and then positions his hands on the arm rests. At this point, Chris can push up to stand.
>
> Some prompts depend on the client's already having certain performance skills; if he

or she does not have those skills, the prompt is not a *controlling stimulus* for a given response: Rose's therapist made some activity-step photos to prompt her completion of daily living tasks, but because Rose has limited vision and does not readily associate pictured items with three-dimensional items, the photos will not prompt the required response. Her therapist will need to select another prompt that works for Rose or enlarge the photos and teach her to associate them with objects first.

Some kinds of assistance may be permanently added to the activity when clients cannot master certain steps independently. This approach is known as *permanent assistance* or *partial participation*. It may involve prolonged personal assistance, including various therapy techniques, such as cues to initiate motion or assist in movement; support at a point of control (e.g., hips, elbow); or even performance of entire steps.

> The occupational therapist applies a tactile cue at the forearm and wrist whenever working with John on dressing skills. This permanent prompt is continued (rather than faded out) because it cues John to move his arm forward to initiate donning a shirt. In the same dressing activity, the therapist completes several difficult nontarget steps (she places the shirt over John's head and holds one sleeve out), but she teaches the remaining activity steps.

Fading

A client who does not know the steps to a particular activity can be prompted in many ways. But because all prompts must be faded out for the client to achieve complete independence, prompts must be added to instruction with care. Unneeded or excessive assistance will only increase dependence on the therapist or caregiver. Therapists can simply apply prompts singly or in combination without an organized approach for eliminating them; however, prompts need to be faded eventually, and abrupt fading may result in performance setbacks for many clients with developmental disabilities. The sections that follow describe five effective prompting procedures in order of increasing intrusiveness and difficulty: observation learning (i.e., *modeling*), time delay, simultaneous prompting, system of least prompts, and graduated guidance. All but modeling incorporate fading strategies.

Modeling. Several studies support the use of *modeling*, that is, learning by watching someone else perform a target activity partially or fully. This ordinary approach to teaching or intervention has been referred to as *observation learning* (Wolery et al., 1992) and *passive observation* (Biederman, Fairhall, Raven, & Davey, 1998) and has been effective with a wide range of clients for many functional tasks. Some occupational therapists refer to this type of learning as a *see-then-do* method. Because modeling is a fairly nonintrusive, natural approach that has a good success record, it is a good choice before other, more complex prompting methods are used.

To learn through modeling, the client requires focused attention, memory, and the ability to imitate. When clients are missing some of these skills, the approach can be simplified and coupled with reinforcement for improved attending or imitating. Model prompts may be repeated, exaggerated, or given partially, and they may be paired with other prompts such as gesturing or partial physical prompts. Researchers, however, have shown that uncomplicated modeling of entire activities also can be effective. For example, passive observation of the whole activity without verbal prompting was more successful in teaching a range of dressing, eating, and grooming activities to school-age clients who had Down syndrome than was hand-over-hand guidance with verbal prompts across activity steps (Biederman et al., 1998).

Wolery et al. (1992) have repeatedly demonstrated the success of observational learning in small groups of students with the same targeted activities. Instruction was directed to one student for all or half of an activity while one or two other students watched; instruction then moved to another student while others observed. Even when no praise was provided for observing, students learned activities they had observed being taught to peers but were never directly taught to them. With observational learning, students may be praised (or prompted, if necessary) for attending to the model because they must see the model before they can learn by this method!

Simultaneous Prompting. Simultaneous prompting involves providing teaching trials and testing trials during daily ADL routines. Prompts are not gradually faded; they are simply present during teaching trials and absent during testing trials. This method has been applied more often to academic tasks than to teaching ADL occupations (Sewell, Collins, Hemmeter, & Schuster, 1998), but it is simple to use and has research support, as noted in Sewall et al., so it is included here. To use simultaneous prompting, the therapist gives the controlling prompt (the one that is known) at the same time that the target stimulus (the one that is not known) is being taught. In the following example, physical prompts are the controlling stimuli, and the target stimulus is putting on a pullover:

> Lynn, who is almost 3 years old and developmentally delayed, chooses dress-up play and selects a green pullover shirt from the clothing box. The therapist points to it, saying, "Put on your shirt." At the command, the therapist immediately places her hands over Lynn's arms and physically guides her through each step in the task until the shirt is on. The therapist explains in simple language what is happening as each step is performed and delivers praise after each activity step as long as Lynn allows her guidance. When finished, the therapist offers Lynn an activity-based choice while holding up materials: "Do you want to cook something, or should we sweep?"

During intermittent testing trials, the therapist simply withholds prompts or physical assistance, gives 5 sec for the client to initiate the activity step and 25 sec to complete a step, and offers praise when the step is completed. Errors and failures to respond are ignored, but the therapist performs the activity step and repeats the specific direction, giving the client an opportunity to perform each activity step in sequence. Criterion is reached when the client performs the activity completely during several consecutive testing trials:

> After Lynn could complete all dressing steps during three testing trials in a row, her team regarded her performance as meeting criterion, and the skill became one to maintain and generalize to her home environment.

Time Delay. Another approach for giving and fading assistance is to pause or add a delay period before giving a prompt. During delay periods, the client may either wait for assistance or try the response on his or her own. If the learner tries, the response may be correct or incorrect.

> Sam is learning some basic eating skills (see Figure 5.2). His therapists decide that a physical prompt is best for him and plan to fade the prompt using time delay. They start teaching each skill using a no-delay period (0 sec) between the discriminative stimulus (S^D) and the prompt, so Sam receives physical prompts continually through each spoon, napkin, and cup cycle for several meals. Then his therapist inserts a 4-sec pause between each S^D and the prompt, allowing Sam time to attempt the response without help. For some steps in the

tasks, Sam waits for assistance (prompted correct responses); for others, he completes the steps (independent responses). On a few steps, he tries on his own and makes errors, and the therapist immediately repeats that step with help. Because Sam can eat faster when he tries on his own rather than wait out the delay for help, time delay seems to motivate him to initiate without help; however, because help is forthcoming at the end of a delay period, an uncertain client could simply wait.

Therapists using time delay more often adopt a simple constant delay approach (e.g., no delay followed by delays of 4 sec). They also may use progressive delay trials, in which a delay is gradually increased from 0 to 6 or 8 sec or longer, depending on the client's natural response latency (Schuster & Griffen, 1990; Snell & Brown, 2000). Time delay has been found effective across many academic tasks as well as IADL and ADL (Collins, Gast, Wolery, Holcombe, & Leatherby, 1991; Hughes, Schuster, & Nelson, 1993; Wolery, Ault, Gast, Doyle, & Griffen, 1991). Progressive time delay is more complicated than constant delay, and applying either time delay approach to a chained activity such as eating or dressing is more complicated than applying it to a discrete response (e.g., lip closure or grasping) or repeated responses (e.g., stepping). Balancing the effectiveness of a teaching approach with staff requirements is something teams must consider in their choice of prompting methods. The principle of parsimony—to seek the simplest effective method—is one that teams should heed as they make their choices (Etzel & LeBlanc, 1979).

When using either delay approach, the therapist needs to select a single prompt (e.g., modeling) or a combined prompt (e.g., verbal plus physical cues), rather than a hierarchy of prompts, and should plan how and when to increase the delay. The best guide is to increase the delay only after a period of several sessions or trials of successful waiting responses (i.e., the client does not make an error but allows him- or herself to be prompted) or correct responses (i.e., the client makes the response during the delay without help). If the client makes errors before the prompt, the delay might be shortened for several trials. If the client makes an error after the prompt, the prompt may not work for that person. If this pattern happens repeatedly, another prompt should be considered. The delay should not increase following errors; instead, the therapist should determine what type of error has occurred and address it accordingly. These decisions rely on the team's thinking about the task, the client, and the client's performance.

System of Least Prompts.

Chris, the preschooler learning to sit in and stand up from a chair, did not readily perform the steps in these activities. His therapist plans to use a prompting procedure and discusses the options with his team. Because Chris can follow some verbal–gestural directions and often imitates models, they choose a prompting procedure with a "built-in" means for fading: a system of least prompts.

A system of least intrusive prompts, also called *least prompts* for short, involves selecting a hierarchy of prompts that "work" both for the client and the activity. These prompts are used one at a time, starting with less assistance and moving to more assistance. Therapists select a latency period, and the student initiates the response with no help or with no additional help:

Because of cerebral palsy, Chris has high tone and a movement disorder, which slow his response time. In consultation with Chris's preschool teachers, his therapist decides to use a slightly long latency of 5 sec. Thus, his therapist will pause for 5 sec following her instructional cue, before giving any assistance, to let him initiate the first step in the target task. If he begins to make an error, she will interrupt the error with the least intrusive level of assistance. She will pause for the 5-sec latency after giving any type of assistance or prompt to allow him to initiate the step with a certain amount of assistance.

Typically, three levels of prompt are used:

1. *Verbal instructions:* The therapist provides simple statements for each activity step.
2. *Verbal instructions plus a model or gesture:* Depending on the step, the therapist will point to the materials needed; for other activities, a brief demonstration of all or part of the movement required may be used.
3. *Verbal instructions plus physical assistance:* The therapist provides only as much guidance as is needed, placing a hand on the person's hand, wrist, forearm, or elbow or at control points such as the knees, shoulders, waist, or hips.

With Chris, the therapist decides to use only two levels of prompts (verbal plus gesture and verbal plus physical assistance) but starts with the least intrusive prompt and proceeds to more intrusive prompts if Chris cannot complete a particular step of the task or if he makes an error and needs more help. For each step of the task, the therapist initially waits for Chris's initiation during the latency before giving any help. If he does not initiate or makes an error, the therapist offers a verbal prompt plus a pointing gesture and waits. If he does not initiate the step within 4 sec, does not complete the response, or makes an error, the therapist moves to the most intrusive prompt and physically helps him complete the step.

A least prompts system is adaptable to many activities and clients; it has been demonstrated to be effective for people with mental retardation and other disabilities across many ADL (Snell, 1997). One downside to this system is that it is initially a bit complex for therapists to learn. It uses artificial instructor prompts rather than natural ones, and it can appear to be quite intrusive to clients. Examples include physically helping a client move through the step of opening the toothpaste or grasping a box of cereal in the grocery store. A least prompts system that uses modeling and physical prompts is better during acquisition, whereas more subtle prompts are better used during subsequent learning stages. Examples of subtle prompts include an initial nod to encourage a hesitant client to keep going, followed by a nonspecific verbal prompt of "What's next?" which is followed, finally, by gestures toward relevant stimuli (e.g., materials needed or part of the body to move), if needed.

Client factors need to be considered when choosing prompts. Some people are tactilely defensive and do not like to be touched; others cannot use certain prompts because of their skill limitations (not everyone can imitate a model prompt or follow verbal instructions). Therefore, the occupational therapist needs to select prompts that work with a particular client or select prompts that can be learned after being associated with meaningful prompts. Least prompts systems require that at least two levels of prompts be selected, that they be arranged in a hierarchy from least to most intrusive, and that prompts be preceded by a latency period. In some cases, the later (more intrusive) prompts in the hierarchy might be more consistently effective than the earlier (less intrusive) prompts. This situation is satisfactory as long as all the selected prompts are at least partially effective with a client. Given these basic characteristics, the least prompts system can be adapted to suit many different clients and activities (Kellegrew, 1998).

Prompt systems, especially least prompts and time delay, offer several advantages: They have a built-in plan for fading out assistance, they result in fewer errors than most teaching methods, and they have a research basis of demonstrated effectiveness. When therapists rely only on consequences to teach new skills, students may become discouraged by their errors and fail to make progress. The combined use of antecedent–prompt strategies with planned consequences is the best teaching approach.

Graduated Guidance. Therapists using graduated guidance apply more intrusive physical prompts first, then fade them out. Several variations of graduated guidance have been applied when teaching ADL skills to people with disabilities. In the hand-to-shoulder approach, therapists initially provide full hand-over-hand guidance throughout the activity, but they give only the amount of assistance that is needed for the client to complete the activity. This requirement—"to give only as much help as is needed"—means that therapists must become highly sensitive to the pressure cues clients give back as they are being assisted. If the client's hands move in the desired direction during a dressing task, the therapist tries to "back off" and give less guidance; but if the client stops forward movement before he or she should, the therapist provides the movement. The general order of fading assistance is from the client's hands upward to the shoulder. Ultimately, physical assistance is eliminated entirely. This approach has been used to teach eating behaviors (Denny et. al., 2000) and dressing skills (McKelvey, Sisson, Van Hasselt, & Hersen, 1992).

One difficulty with graduated guidance is deciding when to reduce assistance. The best approach is to try reducing assistance periodically while encouraging the student or client to perform with less assistance. The client's own movements are the best guides to where less assistance is needed. Another approach is to use a brief waiting period before physically assisting each step (or some steps) in the activity, thereby giving the client opportunities to initiate each step before being prompted. This approach enables the therapist to eliminate prompts if the client then performs the step. Watching the client perform without any help (e.g., when testing performance) also can help determine which steps may need less assistance.

A second graduated guidance approach involves using three different levels of physical assistance, again ranging from more assistance to less assistance during training:

1. Full hand-over-hand assist
2. Two-finger assist
3. "Shadowing" the person's hand from about 1 to 2 in.

This approach has been used to teach dressing skills (McKelvey et al., 1992; Reese & Snell, 1991) and self-care skills (Farlow & Snell, 2000). In both graduated guidance approaches, if the client resists the prompted movement, the therapist may maintain contact with the client but simply wait until no resistance is felt before continuing to assist. When the therapist has successfully reduced assistance, he or she should praise the client's increased effort. When the client seems to require additional assistance, it can be provided. Graduated guidance allows the client to "get the feel" of the movement required by a skill and gradually take more responsibility for making the movement without the therapist's guidance. This method does not work for people who are tactilely defensive, do not like to be guided, or choose to move very quickly; nor will it work for those who become dependent on physical assistance. Unnaturally intensive training and punitive correction methods often have been coupled with graduated guidance; those strategies are not recommended. Graduated guidance may be appropriate when it is suited to the client and if less intrusive prompting methods have not been successful.

Consequences

Table 5.2 shows some of the consequences that adults and peers can offer to a client to reinforce a target response. The following practices for using positive consequences are recommended for most clients.

Reinforcement Schedule

During acquisition, reinforcement following correct and approximate responses (even when the client is prompted) facilitates learning. Reinforcement should occur more frequently during acquisition than during subsequent stages of learning, but it should be "thinned" to an intermittent frequency so the student learns to perform without constant reinforcement from others. If reinforcement schedules are not reduced over time, students may fail to use the skill under natural conditions, when little reinforcement is forthcoming.

Appropriateness for Client

Reinforcing consequences should suit the learning situation and the client's chronological age, preferences, level of understanding. Some clients find simple confirmation reinforcing ("That's right"), whereas others benefit more from task-specific praise ("Good job sweeping in the corner"). For some students, a choice of preferred activities can be provided at the end of a relatively long activity during the acquisition stage. Letting the client have a choice about the reinforcing consequence is always better than trying to anticipate what he or she might find enjoyable.

Natural Reinforcers

During late stages of learning, it is good to teach the client to self-monitor his or her performance by asking and answering, "How well did I do this time?" It also is helpful to teach clients to look to natural forms of self-reinforcement: In the examples used elsewhere in this chapter, Sam may be permitted to eat a preferred finger food after a session of teaching spoon use, April may choose the preferred activities whenever she reaches her time goals for putting on her shoes and AFOs, or Chris may participate in the next activity once seated in a circle at preschool (Koegel, Koegel, & Carter, 1999). The therapist reinforces good behavior by rewarding the client for doing a good job with an activity the client enjoys.

Consequences also are part of prompt systems. For least prompts and graduated guidance and for single prompts (with time delay or simply with a fixed latency), praise is the typical consequence for completing a step. Only if concrete reinforcers are needed should they be added, and they, too, should be appropriate to the client. During acquisition, praise can be given following the completion of every step, whether or not the step was prompted. As learning progresses, the reinforcing consequences need to be decreased; praise and other reinforcing consequences therefore are reserved for progress on difficult steps and are not given for steps completed with the most intrusive prompts.

Consequences Following Errors

When clients or patients make errors, the therapist can respond in many different ways. The stage of learning and the type of error made will influence the consequence, as will many of the client's characteristics (e.g., age, disabilities, and skills). Consider Chris, the preschooler who is learning to sit down and stand up:

> Before Chris has learned sitting and standing to about 60% accuracy, the therapist will need to correct any errors (e.g., pointing to the chair arms and saying, "Grab the chair right here") by showing Chris how to respond.

Corrections typically involve giving assistance following mistakes. Some prompt systems provide clear ways to respond to errors. For example, in a least prompts approach the therapist interrupts any

mistakes with the next prompt in the hierarchy. If the incorrect response is simply a failure to respond, however, then the next prompt in the hierarchy is given following the latency. In graduated guidance, the therapist also responds to errors by giving more (typically physical) assistance.

> If Linda, who is learning to brush her teeth, fails to remove the cap before squeezing the tube of toothpaste, the therapist may move her guiding hand away from Linda's elbow (a point of less assistance) to the wrist or hand (both points of greater assistance) and ask her to repeat the missed step. Once Linda has learned more of the toothbrushing activity, the therapist might ask her, "What's next?" (a nonspecific verbal prompt) when Linda hesitates on a step she has done before without help. Alternatively, the therapist may simply wait longer, giving Linda time to correct herself.

Both approaches encourage client self-correction and independence, something that is especially desirable during the later stages of learning. Clients in advanced stages of learning a skill may simply check with the therapist when they have completed the activity; if it has not been done adequately, the therapist might withhold approval or ask the client to try again. As we have noted earlier, the use of punitive consequences for errors is inappropriate.

Review of Progress and Intervention

This section describes procedures for reviewing outcomes of therapeutic intervention. Therapists may not always have the opportunity to follow up on specific process recommendations. For example, return visits to occupational therapy may not be approved by reimbursement agencies, and in early intervention and school system settings, therapists commonly treat children once a week for short periods. Under such circumstances, opportunities for review of intervention outcomes may be restricted by time constraints or may not be possible at all. These unfortunate situations are realities in the current practice environment. Therapists should take time to read the following sections and consider ways to modify the review methods to suit individual settings and needs. For instance, when the therapist is not routinely present in a classroom setting, the teacher or aide may be able to collect information. Some families are good at collecting detailed information as well.

Client testing and training performance data may be used in a number of ways. Test data help teachers and therapists with the following tasks:

1. Deciding what learning areas to target, depending on the client's *baseline data* (i.e., performance before instruction begins)
2. Judging progress once training has begun by monitoring the client's progress using criterion or test conditions (also known as *probing*, or collecting *probe performance data*); whenever possible, it is best to use test data collected in the context in which the goal behavior is used because doing so provides a realistic picture of learning
3. Deciding on environmental changes, such as hospital discharge or transition to another unit or service.

Baseline and Test Data

Baseline data should be collected over at least two sessions, or until they seem fairly stable—that is, not varying by 40% or more in either direction (Farlow & Snell, 1994). If only one assessment is possible, therapists might ask family members, the client, or others who are familiar with the client's performance how well the client currently performs the activity and use that information to estimate whether performance is stable. When these data are representative of the client's performance, then instruction can begin with baseline performance serving as a benchmark: a guide for judging progress made during training.

> Chris's baseline performance was measured over a week and indicated some improvement. Test data involved repeating the test observation after teaching had begun (Figure 5.4).

Many of us have found that test observations need not be taken more than once every 5 training days (when training or therapy is daily) unless progress is poor. Even then, training data, rather than test data, are more useful when analyzing the reasons for lack of progress (see Farlow & Snell, 1994). Both baseline and test data typically are recorded using symbols for correct and incorrect responses (see Figure 5.3). Test data may be summarized as the percentage correct (i.e., the number of correct responses divided by the total number of opportunities). It is useful to record the data on the same graph as the training data but to use different symbols to distinguish between them (see Figures 5.3 and 5.4). Moreover, the ungraphed, step-by-step, task analysis data should be saved and dated because it is a record of which steps were correct and

which were missed. Chris's trial-by-trial data are shown in Figure 5.3, and his percentage correct performance is graphed in Figure 5.4.

Training Data

Training data are collected during the intervention session. Typically, clients perform a given activity better during training than during test conditions. This phenomenon can be painfully obvious to therapists who treat in one-on-one intervention sessions, then find that task performance plummets in contexts such as the classroom or home! When recording training data, use symbols for correct responses and for the types and amounts of assistance the client needs to complete the behavior or step in the activity. If several prompts are possible, different symbols may indicate which prompt obtained the response (e.g., V for verbal, G for gestural, M for model, or P for physical assistance). Thus, steps in the three activities in Figure 5.2 (spoon, cup, and napkin use) could be either rated "correct" or noted with a P to indicate that a physical prompt was given (see Figure 5.3).

If parents, caregivers, teachers, or spouses will be collecting data, remember to take time to teach them how to record correctly. Training data provide the therapist with objective information about how the client responds to the therapy program and can be used to support requests from reimbursement sources for further sessions. Like test data, training data should be preserved in an ungraphed form (so the information on individual steps is not lost) as well as graphed using the percentage correct or the number of steps correct. Note that in Figure 5.3, Chris's baseline and test data are indicated with an asterisk.

Using Data

Besides simply scanning graphs for trends in progress and for variability, teachers and therapists can examine "raw" or ungraphed (step-by-step) data for specific error patterns or problem areas that provide clues to needed changes if progress is poor. Dated anecdotal records about student behavior, interfering circumstances, and illnesses also will help resolve why progress may be inadequate. These kinds of data are particularly helpful in clients with complex problems, such as sensory disturbances.

> Chris's data indicate steady progress on the first five steps of the task during March and April. On April 26 he required some physical assistance on steps he usually got correct, and the teacher noted on the graph that he did

not appear to feel well that day. Because his performance was soon back to its higher level, the teachers made no changes in the program (see Figure 5.3).

Farlow and Snell (1994) provided a detailed method for using data effectively; Brown and Snell (2000) also provided some guidelines for this approach. Ottenbacher's (1986) book *Evaluating Clinical Change: Strategies for Occupational and Physical Therapists* gives similar information. Several steps are involved in analyzing data to improve treatment programming:

1. *Collect data relevant to the treatment goals.* Collect training data whenever the client is seen—several times a week is optimal, but that is unusual in most therapy settings. Collect test data in other settings periodically, or have others involved in the client's life do so.

2. *Preserve step-by-step data and graph data.* Indicate on the graph the dates and types of data: baseline, intervention, test, and training. In addition, note (and date) any relevant anecdotal comments pertinent to the performance data. Use graphs that show all attendance dates so that absences, vacations, and other missed days are clear (see Figure 5.4). Connect data that are from continuous periods of time.

3. *Determine trend if possible.* If the data seem to be reliable and representative of the client's performance, determine the trend after graphing 6 to 8 data points. The trend will be ascending, flat, or descending. If the data are not representative (e.g., the client has been sick) or not reliable (e.g., for three of the data points, the aide "recalled" the performance instead of recording the data during the performance), examine the trend after more data have been collected.

Chris's initial flat progress in March was followed after spring break by perfect performance during training. This higher-than-criterion performance caused the therapist and teacher to increase the criterion to 100% (Figure 5.4).

3a. *Ascending trends:* If the trend is ascending, continue the program unless the intervention goal has been met, in which case the goal needs to be changed.

3b. *Flat or descending trends:* If the trend is flat or descending, work with the client, the client's team, or both, depending on the

setting, to determine the possible reason(s) for the lack of progress.

In determining the reasons for lack of progress, the therapist should consider the following questions:

- Is there a cyclical variability? Are some days or sessions worse because of a weekend, the occupational therapist or occupational therapy assistant, a prescribed medication, or other changing factors?
- Are test data better than training data? If so, what are the differences between the two situations?
- Does the client have difficulty with the same step(s) across sessions?
- What is the pattern of errors? Is it a specific step? Are the errors setting-, time-, or staff-specific? Are they a result of the client's not attempting the activity or performing incorrectly? Is the client reinforced to continue performing the activity incorrectly after making errors?

In addition, the therapist should conduct the following tasks:

- Make comparisons. Compare the client's performance on other activities and behaviors with the declining performance. Are the errors similar? Does the target behavior interact with other behaviors? Are problem behaviors increasing? Does the program prevent access to other interactions and activities?
- Develop a possible explanation. Working with the client or client's team, develop a feasible explanation for the lack of progress.
- Plan program improvements. As a team, decide on programmatic changes that will address the possible reasons for the behavior. If more than one explanation is developed, determine which ones should dictate program change, perhaps by making more observations.

Consider the example of Millie:

Millie is an adolescent who is working on improving her use of a power wheelchair at school. Millie's lack of progress in driving seems cyclical or related to sessions that isolate her from peers, but she is improving during training sessions held during physical education class with peers and at lunch time in the cafeteria. Anecdotal records state that Millie often refuses to try driving during the sessions in which no progress is being made and has cried several times. Two possible explanations are as follows:

1. When there is progress, Millie's trainers are doing something more effective than what her trainers are doing at other times.
2. Millie enjoys instruction in the context of her peers—perhaps it's the cheering they sometimes give her when she tries harder at driving.

The first explanation was ruled out after team members realized that instructors during physical education and lunch were rotated and not specific to those times. Millie's team then decided to focus on the second explanation. They asked Millie whether she might prefer to have a peer volunteer help during the times that peers had not been present. When Millie indicated she would like this, they recruited volunteers and included them in all training sessions in which little progress was occurring. Data collected after this change indicated that her progress showed ascending trends in all sessions.

In current practice settings, reimbursement sources usually require ongoing evaluation. Therapists gather and examine student performance data to address the program evaluation steps described in the previous paragraph. Relevant data include test and training data, which should be supplemented with anecdotal notes about the client's performance and social validation of the progress attained. To validate clients' progress socially, therapists can use the following approaches:

1. Query clients themselves, their peers or family members, and teachers and therapists to obtain subjective opinions about progress.
2. Compare clients' performance with that of their peers.

Evaluation is never simple, but it need not be overly complex to provide information pertinent to the effectiveness of a therapy program. The evaluation process should be *ongoing,* if possible, and not applied at the conclusion of a program or a school year. In ongoing evaluation, the data are continually analyzed to clarify the reasons for the progress (or lack of progress) and to design the needed program changes. The data are then used to monitor whether program changes actually lead to performance improvements.

Summary

The goal of most occupational therapy intervention strategies is to provide intervention to clients in ways that promote learning and encourage their occupational performance during daily routines and in their usual physical and social environments. Therapists therefore need to target goals that will be meaningful to individual clients; to use methods that are relatively uncomplicated, are effective, and respect the client; and to review clients' progress on an ongoing basis.

Study Questions

1. Discuss the rationale for setting goals that are appropriate to chronological age.
2. How does a person who can do only part of an activity initially become independent in that activity over time?
3. How do the stages of learning fit into occupational therapy goal setting?
4. Why are multiple sources of data important in planning self-care treatment? Name several such sources.
5. Discuss the consideration an occupational therapist should give to antecedent events and consequences used in treatment. Why are they important?
6. What is the difference between baseline and training data? How can an occupational therapist, who may see a patient only once a week, collect training data?
7. What influence can graphed information have on setting occupational therapy goals and treatment?

References

Baumgart, D., Brown, L., Pumpian, I., Nisbet, J., Ford, A., Sweet, M., et al. (1982). Principle of partial participation and individualized adaptations in educational programs for severely handicapped students. *Journal of the Association for the Severely Handicapped, 7,* 17–27.

Biederman, G. B., Fairhall, J. L., Raven, K. A., & Davey, V. A. (1998). Verbal prompting, hand-over-hand instruction, and passive observation in teaching children with developmental disabilities. *Exceptional Children, 64,* 503–511.

Brown, F., Evans, I., Weed, K., & Owen, V. (1987). Delineating functional competencies: A component model. *Journal of the Association for Persons with Severe Handicaps, 12,* 117–124.

Brown, F., & Snell, M. E. (2000). Meaningful assessment. In M. E. Snell & F. Brown (Eds.), *Instruction of students with severe disabilities* (5th ed., pp. 67–114). Upper Saddle River, NJ: Merrill/Prentice Hall.

Carr, E. G., Levin, L., McConnachie, G., Carlson, J. I., Kemp, D. C., & Smith, C. E. (1994). *Communication-based intervention for problem behavior. A user's guide for producing positive change.* Baltimore: Brookes.

Collins, B. C., Gast, D. L., Wolery, M., Holcombe, A., & Leatherby, J. (1991). Using constant time delay to teach self-feeding to young students with severe/profound handicaps: Evidence of limited effectiveness.

Journal of Developmental and Physical Disabilities, 3, 157–179.

Day, H. H., & Horner, R. H. (1986). Response variation and the generalization of a dressing skill: Comparison of single instance and general case instruction. *Applied Research in Mental Retardation, 7,* 189–202.

Denny, M., Marchand-Martella, N., Martella, R. C., Reilly, J. R., Reilly, J. F., & Cleanthous, C. C. (2000). Using parent-delivered graduated guidance to teach functional living skills to a child with cri du chat syndrome. *Education and Treatment of Children, 23,* 441–454.

Etzel, B. C., & LeBlanc, J. M. (1979). The simplest treatment alternative: Appropriate instructional control and errorless learning procedures for the difficult-to-teach child. *Journal of Autism and Developmental Disorders, 9,* 361–382.

Farlow, L. J., & Snell, M. E. (1994). *Making the most of student performance data* (Research to Practice Series). Washington, DC: American Association on Mental Retardation.

Farlow, L. J., & Snell, M. E. (2000). Teaching self care skills. In M. E. Snell & F. Brown (Eds.), *Instruction of students with severe disabilities* (5th ed., pp. 331–380). Upper Saddle River, NJ: Merrill/Prentice Hall.

Farmer-Dougan, V. (1994). Increasing requests by adults with developmental disabilities using incidental teaching by peers. *Journal of Applied Behavior Analysis, 27,* 533–544.

Ferguson, D. L., & Baumgart, D. (1991). Partial participation revisited. *Journal of the Association for Persons with Severe Handicaps, 16,* 218–227.

Ford, A., Schnorr, R., Meyer, L., Davern, L., Black, J., & Dempsey, P. (1989). *The Syracuse community-referenced curriculum guide for students with moderate and severe disabilities.* Baltimore: Brookes.

Frankenburg, W. K., Dodds, J., Archer, P., Shapiro, H., & Bresnick, B. (1992). The Denver II: A major revision and re-standardization of the Denver Developmental Screening Test. *Pediatrics, 89*(1), 91–96.

Giangreco, M. F., Cloninger, C. J., & Iverson, V. S. (1993). *C.O.A.C.H.: Choosing options and accommodations for children.* Baltimore: Brookes.

Guidetti, S., & Soderback, I. (2001). Description of self-care training in occupational therapy: Case studies of five Kenyan children with cerebral palsy. *Occupational Therapy International, 8*(1), 34–48.

Haley, S. M., Ludlow, L. H., & Coster, W. J. (1993). Pediatric Evaluation of Disability Inventory: Clinical interpretation of summary scores using Rasch rating scale methodology. *Physical Medicine and Rehabilitation Clinics of North America, 4,* 529–540.

Hamilton, B. L., Laughlin, J. A., Fiedler, R. C., & Granger, C. V. (1994). Interrater reliability of the 7-level Functional Independence Measure (FIM). *Scandinavian Journal of Rehabilitation Medicine, 26,* 115–116.

Hughes, M. W., Schuster, J. W., & Nelson, C. M. (1993). The acquisition of independent dressing skills by students with multiple disabilities. *Journal of Developmental and Physical Disabilities, 5,* 233–295.

Janney, R. E., & Snell, M. E. (2000). *Teacher's guide to inclusive practices: Behavioral support.* Baltimore: Brookes.

Kellegrew, D. H. (1998). Creating opportunities for occupation: An intervention to promote the self-care independence of young children with special needs. *American Journal of Occupational Therapy, 52,* 457–465.

Kellegrew, D. H., & Allen, D. (1996). Occupational therapy in full-inclusion classrooms: A case study from the Moorpark Model. *American Journal of Occupational Therapy, 50,* 718–724.

Lancioni, G. E., & O'Reilly, M. F. (2001). Self-management of instruction cues for occupation: Review of studies with people with severe and profound disabilities. *Research in Developmental Disabilities, 22,* 41–65.

Law, M., Baptiste, S., Carswell, A., Polatajko, H., & Pollock, N. (1998). *Canadian Occupational Performance Measure* (3rd ed.). Ottawa: Canadian Association of Occupational Therapists Publications ACE.

Law, M., & Usher, P. (1988). Validation of the Klein-Bell Activities of Daily Living Scale for Children. *Canadian Journal of Occupational Therapy, 55,* 63–68.

Mackey, S., & McQueen, J. (1998). Exploring the association between integrated therapy and inclusive education. *British Journal of Special Education, 25*(1), 22–27.

McCabe, M. A., & Granger, C. V. (1990). Content validity of a pediatric Functional Independence Measure. *Applied Nursing Research, 3*(3), 120–122.

McInerney, C. A., & McInerney, M. (1992). A mobility skills training program for adults with developmental disabilities. *American Journal of Occupational Therapy, 46,* 233–239.

McKelvey, J., Sisson, L. A., Van Hasselt, V. B., & Hersen, M. (1992). An approach to teaching self-dressing to a child with dual sensory impairment. *Teaching Exceptional Children, 25,* 12–15.

Mirenda, P., MacGregor, T., & Kelly-Keogh, S. (2002). Teaching communication skills for behavioral support in the context of family life. In J. M. Lucyshyn, G. Dunlap, & R. W. Albin (Eds.), *Families and positive behavior support: Addressing problem behaviors in family contexts* (pp. 185–207). Baltimore: Brookes.

Odom, S., Brown, W. H., Frey, T., Karasu, N., Smith-Canter, L., & Strain, P. (2003). Evidence-based practices for young children with autism: Contributions for single-subject design research. *Focus on Autism and Other Developmental Disabilities, 18*(3), 166–176.

O'Neill, R. E., Horner, R. H., Albin, R. W., Sprague, J. R., Storey, K., & Newton, J. S. (1997). *Functional assessment and program development for problem behavior.* Pacific Grove, CA: Brooks/Cole.

Ottenbacher, K. J. (1986). *Evaluating clinical change. Strategies for occupational and physical therapists.* Baltimore: Williams & Wilkins.

Piazza, C. C., Anderson, C., & Fisher, W. (1993). Teaching self-feeding skills to patients with Rett syndrome. *Developmental Medicine and Child Neurology, 35,* 991–996.

Reese, G. M., & Snell, M. E. (1991). Putting on and removing coats and jackets: The acquisition and maintenance of skills by children with severe multiple disabilities. *Education and Training in Mental Retardation, 26,* 398–410.

Robertson, J., Green, K., Alper, S., Schloss, P., & Kohler, F. (2003). Using a peer-mediated intervention to facilitate children's participation in inclusive child daycare activities. *Education and Treatment of Children, 26*(2), 182–197.

Schuster, J. W., & Griffen, A. K. (1990). Using time delay with task analyses. *Teaching Exceptional Children, 22*(4), 49–53.

Sewell, T. J., Collins, B. C., Hemmeter, M. L., & Schuster, J. W. (1998). Using simultaneous prompting within an activity-based format to teach dressing skills to preschoolers with developmental delays. *Journal of Early Intervention, 21,* 132–145.

Snell, M. E. (1997). Teaching children and young adults with mental retardation in school programs: Current research. *Behaviour Change, 14,* 73–105.

Snell, M. E., & Brown, F. (2000). Measurement, analysis, and evaluation. In M. E. Snell & F. Brown (Eds.), *Instruction of students with severe disabilities* (5th ed., pp. 173–206). Upper Saddle River, NJ: Merrill/Prentice Hall.

Wang, X., Bernas, R., & Eberhard, P. (2001, April). *Children's early literacy environment in Chinese and American Indian families.* Paper presented at the biennial meeting of the Society for Research in Child Development, Minneapolis, MN.

Watson, D. E., & Wilson, S. E. (2003). *Task analysis: An individual and population approach* (2nd ed.). Bethesda, MD: American Occupational Therapy Association.

Wolery, M., Ault, M. J., & Doyle, P. M. (1992). *Teaching students with moderate to severe disabilities.* White Plains, NY: Longman.

Wolery, M., Ault, M. J., Gast, D. L., Doyle, P. M., & Griffen, A. K. (1991). Teaching chained tasks in dyads: Acquisition of target and observational behaviors. *Journal of Special Education, 25,* 198–220.

Chapter 6

Adaptive Strategies for Children With Developmental Disabilities

Karin J. Barnes, PhD, OTR

Jane Case-Smith, EdD, OT/L, FAOTA

KEY TERMS

adaptive equipment

augmentative and alternative communication

cerebral palsy

developmental disabilities

functional mobility

positioning

postural stability

powered mobility

sensory defensiveness (hypersensitivity)

OBJECTIVES

Upon completion of this chapter, the reader will be able to

- Discuss school, home, and play environments of children and provide examples of occupational therapy processes designed to support engagement within these contexts for children with developmental disabilities;
- Describe the developmental sequences of feeding, dressing, bathing, toileting, communication, and mobility skills;
- Explain those performance skills, client factors, and contextual concerns that influence the achievement of eating, dressing, bathing, toileting, communication, and mobility skills of children;
- Describe intervention strategies to improve mealtime skills of children with impairments in motor, sensory-processing, and behavioral skills;
- Illustrate intervention strategies to improve dressing skills of children with motor, sensory-processing, and cognitive impairments;
- Explain intervention strategies to improve bathing skills in children with motor, sensory, and cognitive impairments;
- Explain intervention strategies to improve toileting skills of children with motor impairments;
- Describe the selection of and interventions to promote the use of augmentative and alternative communication systems; and
- Describe the types and selection of mobility devices and interventions to promote independence in the mobility for children with motor impairments.

Addressing the occupations (activities of daily living [ADL], instrumental activities of daily living [IADL], education, play, and social participation) of children with disabilities requires knowledge of how performance skills and patterns develop within childhood contexts. The child's skills and limitations must be viewed in the personal, social, and cultural context of the family and in the physical context of the home, school, and play areas. Children learn these occupations as a part of everyday family and community life. Thus, the intervention processes designed to improve children's meaningful engagement in occupations require an understanding of the transactions among the child, the occupation or activity, and these contexts (American Occupational Therapy Association [AOTA], 2002).

Infants and children have unique contexts and activity demands that influence their occupations and activities. For example, a childhood occupation of playing in the sandbox at the playground requires responding to the other children in the box (social context), playing with the sand (physical context), and taking turns driving the toy truck through the sand (social and space demands and sequencing the activity). The contexts and activity demands also influence the occupational therapy process with children with disabilities. For example, when an occupational therapist provides intervention for a boy with autism who wishes to play in a sandbox at the playground, the therapist must take into account the child's difficulty in coping with the tactile sensory environment of the sand; his difficulty comprehending the concepts involved in sharing, taking turns, and social space; and the unpredictable auditory stimuli of the playground.

For many children with disabilities, engagement in occupation cannot be taken for granted. As a case in point, in the United States more than 6.5 million children with disabilities were served by the public schools and early childhood intervention systems in the 2000–2001 school year (U.S. Department of Education, 2002). In school, children learn to play and socialize with peers of various levels of ability and to interact with educators, including occupational therapists. The development of their occupations may be impeded unless attention is given to the factors that influence them. Occupational therapists can provide interventions to support the child, family, and other professionals, so that the child can develop and participate in meaningful occupations.

This chapter discusses the occupational therapy process for children with disabilities. The *Occupa-tional Therapy Practice Framework: Domain and Process* (AOTA, 2002) provides a basis for understanding how specific occupations of children with disabilities are viewed in the occupational therapy process. The chapter covers school, home, and play contexts and the occupations of eating, dressing, bathing, toileting, communication, and functional mobility; it also identifies intervention principles, which are based on analysis of the child and his or her contexts. Several case studies illustrate the principles.

School Contexts

Schools have classrooms, halls, gyms, cafeterias, libraries, playgrounds, buses, and principal's offices and a host of different people, including teachers, students, bus drivers, and parents. These settings and people influence children's learning and shape their developing occupations and activities. Schools are the places in which children learn academic, athletic, vocational, social, and community skills. Participation within the school context has long been considered an important right for children with disabilities in the United States, as first written into law in 1975 and has been reaffirmed legislatively and by professional groups since then (AOTA, 1999; U.S. Department of Education, 2002).

The physical context of a school setting can play a major role in school occupation success for a child with a disability. For example, a youth who has cerebral palsy and uses a wheelchair may not be able to complete a vocational assembly task if he or she becomes too tired wheeling back and forth among different workstations spaced several feet apart. The occupational therapist can evaluate how school environments influence the school occupations of specific students with disabilities. Hanft and Place (1996) listed several environmental factors that should be noted in all relevant school settings:

- Room arrangement
- Traffic patterns
- Sensory environments (auditory, visual, tactile, kinesthetic, and movement).

The elements of the sensory environment may be evaluated informally or formally to determine their impact on student occupations. Sensory Profile (Dunn, 1999), an assessment tool, evaluates a child's ability to process sensory information in the environment; this information can be useful for the school occupational therapist and may be especially important for children who have sensory-processing impairments, such as autism or fragile X syndrome (Roley, Blanche, & Schaaf, 2001).

Additionally, the occupational therapist should evaluate the impact of architectural structures of the school environment on clients' occupations, including the following elements (Barnes, 1991):

- Distances between schoolrooms
- Hallway accessibility
- Lighting and flooring
- Types of stairs, elevators, and ramps
- Doorway and entrance accessibility (weight and width of door, threshold height)
- Bathroom facilities
- Playground surface and accessibility of playground equipment
- Cafeteria access
- Work surfaces
- Equipment, including chairs, tables, blackboards, computers, and closets.

The School Function Assessment is a comprehensive assessment of the child's skills within the school's physical context, including the activity demands (Coster, Deeney, Haltiwanger, & Haley, 1998). This assessment tool is designed to assist occupational therapists in evaluating an elementary school student's participation in various school-related activity settings; support needs; and performance of specific, school-related functional activities (Coster et al., 1998). The School Setting Interview (Hoffman, Hemmingsson, & Kielhofner, 1999) is another occupational therapy instrument designed to assess student–environment fit and to identify accommodation needs for students with disabilities in schools. For example, this instrument can help determine whether limited reach and poor balance prevent a student with spastic diplegia from participating in an art class occupation. The occupational therapist can adjust the angle and width of the table to compensate for reaching limitations and provide a chair with lateral support for balance. The student can then concentrate on his or her artistic endeavors instead of physical abilities.

The cultural and social contexts of a student's school environment influence performance. In determining occupational needs of a student with a disability, the occupational therapist must take into account the social and cultural contexts of the student. Students usually wish to perform occupations that meet the social expectations of other students. Peer support is critical for social and academic inclusion of students with disabilities (Thousand, Villa, & Nevin, 1994). Evaluation and intervention strategies must include these cultural and social contexts. The Occupational Therapy Psychosocial Assessment of Learning (Townsend et al., 1999) assesses psychosocial skills and the match between the student and the environment.

Home Contexts

Addressing the needs that support the engagement in occupation of children with disabilities requires that the occupational therapist recognize the child as a part of his or her primary environment, the home. The physical, cultural, and personal contexts of the home and the family are vitally important and must be taken into account throughout the occupational therapy process. These contextual issues profoundly affect the development of the child's occupations and can determine the success of an occupational therapy intervention.

A vast range of home contexts influence children's everyday performance. Homes can be small apartments, large houses, or mobile homes, located in rural, suburban, or urban areas. Families vary in size, familiar relationships, ages of members, ethnicity, and socioeconomic status. These differences affect the importance placed on the attainment of childhood occupations. For example, in many Far Eastern cultures, the mother feeds children until 5 or 6 years of age because it is an important demonstration of the mother's affection. Teaching a child from a family within this culture to eat independently at 2 or 3 years of age would be inappropriate because it would interfere with this act of motherly love (Chan, 1998). Other mealtime rituals differ among ethnic groups and according to the family's values. For example, some families do not have established mealtimes, whereas others reserve the family's evening meal as the most important time of the day. Table 6.1 provides examples of family variables that highly influence a child's developmental skills.

Play Contexts

Play, an important childhood occupation, is affected by the context in which it occurs. This vital childhood occupation can be compromised when a child does not have the physical, social, or cultural support needed to nurture it (Law, 2002). For example, when the parents of a child with spina bifida are busy taking care of the health maintenance of their child, play development may be impeded because the parents do not have enough time to devote to playing with their child. The physical context of the home affects a child's play as well. Children who use walking devices may have difficulty engaging in play activities when small or crowded home environments prevent the play movements.

Table 6.1. Family Variables That Influence a Child's Developmental Skills

Variable	Influence on Development
Culture	Does the family value independence? What foods are accepted? What clothing is appropriate? Is assistive technology accepted? What family traditions and rituals must be respected in designing intervention?
Time	Are family members able to extend the time required in care of the child? When in the family's daily routine can self-care skills be practiced?
Commitment	Are the parents committed to the effort needed to promote independence? Can family members apply the self-care interventions with consistency and regularity?
Communication	Do family members communicate daily problems and successes with each other?
Adaptability and flexibility	Can family roles adapt to changes in routines? Can family members share caregiving responsibilities?

Access to playgrounds in the community and at school affects play. Children with disabilities may not have as many opportunities to play in playgrounds at school and in other community settings. Limited access to and use of playgrounds can decrease social interactions, development of motor skills, exploration of the environment, and the development of personal achievement (Frost, 1992). Occupational therapists may evaluate the contextual aspects of play of children with disabilities in order to provide interventions designed to encourage playground use. The following design elements can increase physical accessibility to playground equipment (Holmstrand, 2003):

- Elevated sandboxes so children in wheelchairs can roll up to them
- Overhead bars and rings that have been lowered so children in wheelchairs can reach them
- Bridges wide enough for wheelchairs and children who use crutches
- Swings with adequate trunk support
- Easy-to-reach manipulatives and activities, such as tic-tac-toe, on panels and tables.

Accessibility guidelines for play areas, playgrounds, and play equipment have been developed by the U.S. Architectural and Transportation Barriers Compliance Board (2001) and may be found at http://www.access-board.gov/play/guide/intro.htm.

The occupational therapist can determine intervention strategies that help the student meet his or her individual home, school, and play goals by determining the relationship of environmental con-

texts to the child's abilities. The occupational therapist evaluates the contextual factors that impede the student's occupations and, in collaboration with parents and educators, applies strategies to improve performance. Interventions that target contextual factors involve maintenance, modification, and prevention strategies as outlined in the AOTA *Framework* (2002; see Table 6.2 for examples). Intervention to improve contextual factors may be used in conjunction with interventions focused on performance skill and patterns, activity demands, and client factors.

Eating and Self-Feeding

Development of Eating and Self-Feeding

Full-term infants are born with the ability to consume nutrition, thereby sustaining life and growth. They first accomplish eating using rooting (to find the nipple) and sucking (to express liquid from the nipple). The gag reflex and automatic cough are also present (to prevent aspiration of liquids), ensuring that the ingested liquid moves through the correct passageway to the stomach. These early reflexes are integrated at 2 to 3 months of age; infants develop rhythmic sucking movements at that point. From sucking, the development of more advanced eating proceeds quite rapidly so that by 2 years of age, children are proficient in drinking, chewing, and biting. Typical development of eating is presented in Table 6.3.

Not all children follow a typical sequence of development of self-feeding, but it is helpful to

Table 6.2. Examples of Occupational Therapy Contextual Interventions for the Child's School, Home, and Play Areas

Intervention Approaches	Contextual Examples
Create the context to support the child's occupation.	*School:* Strategically place a child with an attention deficit within the classroom to optimize visual perception and learning. *Home:* Arrange bedroom to reduce sensory distractions and provide a calming environment for an adolescent with fragile X syndrome. *Play Area:* Create play area that allows a child in a wheelchair easy access.
Maintain the child's occupation by providing contextual support.	*School:* Maintain handwriting skills by providing visual reminders of letter formation in the front of the classroom. *Home:* Maintain acquired social awareness and skills of a child with conduct disorder by placing behavioral reminder signs in the dining and TV rooms. *Play Area:* Maintain acquired play skills of a child with athetosis by removal of potentially hazardous equipment in the gymnasium.
Modify the context to allow the child's occupation.	*School:* Change circle time from a floor activity to a chair-sitting activity for all students so that a student in a wheelchair will be at the same height as the other students. *Home:* Remove a bathroom wall so that a child in a wheelchair has easier access to the toilet and bathtub. *Play Area:* Provide additional space between the backyard play equipment for easier access of children using walking devices.
Prevent problems for the child's occupational performance by addressing contextual issues.	*School:* Prevent social ridicule of a student who sits on a ball seat to improve self-regulation, by allowing all students the opportunity to use the special seat at other times. *Home:* Prevent parental back injuries by removal of architectural barriers at the house entrance, for a youth in a wheelchair. *Play Area:* Prevent overstimulation and possible socially unaccepted behavior of a child with autism by allowing only small groups of children in the play area.

Note: The italic terms used in the intervention approaches column are from "Occupational Therapy Practice Framework: Domain and Process," by American Occupational Therapy Association, 2002, *American Journal of Occupational Therapy, 56,* pp. 609–639. Used with permission.

identify the usual sequence (without focusing on age) in order to provide general guidelines for the expected order in which skills develop. Infants practice self-feeding for many months before they accomplish independence at mealtime. Bringing the hand to the mouth is one of the first motor behaviors that an infant demonstrates, and he or she may hold a bottle by 6 months. Finger-feeding a cracker or soft cookie is generally accomplished by 8 months.

By 7 to 8 months of age, an infant usually can sit in a high chair with the family at the dinner table. While observing the other family members, he or she engages in food play or finger-feeding. An infant may play with a spoon by banging it on the high chair tray. Dried cereal or small bits of soft foods provide entertainment and multiple opportunities to practice pincer grasp and finger skills. The selection of finger foods should match the child's oral motor skills. Nuts, hard candy, popcorn, grapes, and hot dogs cut width-wise are not recommended, because they can totally occlude

the airway if aspirated. Soft foods that dissolve in the mouth or require minimal chewing and cannot block the airway are appropriate for first finger-feeding.

To develop independent spoon-feeding, an infant must understand the use of a tool and must have control of midrange elbow, forearm, and wrist movements, including supination and pronation. Spoon-feeding often develops between 15 and 18 months of age. At this time, shoulder and wrist stability are adequate for holding the spoon to scoop the food and bring it to the mouth with minimal spillage. The child holds the spoon in a pronated gross grasp and brings the spoon to the mouth using exaggerated shoulder and elbow movements.

By age 24 months, the child uses a supinated grasp of the spoon, holding it in the radial fingers. The subtle movements at the wrist and forearm needed to obtain the food and efficiently enter the spoon into the mouth also emerge at this age. With this increased control, the child may begin to use a

Table 6.3. Typical Development of Oral Eating

Age	Eating Skill	Type of Food and Utensil
Neonate	Oral reflexes of rooting and sucking; sucking is strong and rhythmic	Breast or bottle
1 month	Sucking: rhythmic back-and-forth tongue movement with jaw opening and closing	Breast or bottle
4 months	Strong sucking: tongue moves up and down, good lip seal	Breast or bottle
6 months	Efficient sucking, good jaw stability and lip seal	Breast or bottle, may introduce the cup, may begin pureed foods
9 months	Long sequence of continuous sucking; jaw stability improves on cup; uses a munching pattern with pureed foods; beginning of diagonal jaw movements; lateral tongue movements	Pureed and soft foods, bottle or breast, cup
12 months	Rotary chewing movements; active upper lip in removing food; licking present	Soft foods, some table foods, bottle or breast, cup
18 months	Well-coordinated rotary chewing; controlled and sustained biting; mobile tongue, including tongue elevation	Table foods, soft meat
24 months	Well-graded and sustained bite; circular rotary jaw movements; tongue reaches lips and all gum surfaces; good lip closure; good jaw stabilization on cup	Most meats and soft vegetables, cup without lid

fork and to eat foods that are more difficult to handle (e.g., peas, corn, rice, and cold cereal).

Between 6 and 12 months of age the child learns cup drinking, initially with a cup that has a lid and a spout. Some children can best manage a cup with handles; others prefer a small plastic cup without handles. A child tends to spill from a cup until 24 months of age, when jaw stability and hand control increase (Case-Smith & Humphry, 2001; Morris & Klein, 2000).

Performance Variables That Influence Eating and Self-Feeding

Problems With Motor Skills

Eating requires coordination, strength, and energy. The child must use a versatile sequence of oral movements in which tongue, cheek, jaw, and lip movements are coordinated. Children with significant motor problems (e.g., cerebral palsy or trisomy 21 syndrome) often have difficulty coordinating the sequence of oral movements necessary for successful feeding. Children with cerebral palsy and trisomy 21 syndrome frequently exhibit low muscle tone (i.e., *hypotonia*) in the face, neck, and trunk, which results in instability of the head and trunk.

This postural instability may cause poor postural alignment; the child may fall into trunk and cervical flexion unless properly positioned. The child also may demonstrate hyperextension of the neck, thereby placing him or her at risk for aspiration due to improper alignment of the pharynx.

The jaw of a child with low muscle tone often moves in wide excursions, completely open or closed, without controlled midrange movement. The graded jaw mobility and stability needed for chewing and cup drinking are lacking. The child's mouth is often open, which makes swallowing difficult and may result in drooling.

In a child with hypotonia, the tongue may be inactive and move primarily with movement of the lower jaw. The tongue may exhibit primitive extension and retraction (i.e., the tongue extends beyond the lips and is held in the back of the mouth) rather than move up and down or side to side. Extreme movements of the jaw and tongue can disrupt coordination of the suck-swallow-breathe pattern. The extreme movement of the tongue may relate to poor neck and jaw stability, because the tongue does not have a sufficient base of stability for controlled movement. Hypotonia also may involve the lips, rendering them relatively inactive. As a result, the child's ability to seal the lips on the bottle's nipple, the cup's rim, or the spoon is inadequate and results in food loss or air intake. Hypotonic cheeks create difficulty in maintaining food on the chewing surfaces of the teeth or gathered together in the tongue's center for swallow.

Alternatively, a child can demonstrate excess muscle tone (i.e., *hypertonicity* or *spasticity*) or fluctuating muscle tone in the face and oral area. A child with spasticity may exhibit tonic oral reflexes or abnormal motor patterns that disrupt the rhythm and sequence of eating and put the child at risk for aspiration. Table 6.4 lists some of the functional problems associated with developmental disabilities.

Sensitivity to Touch

The sensory systems also contribute to development of feeding skills. A child with touch defensiveness of the face and oral areas demonstrates aversion to touch on or in the mouth and to textured foods inside the mouth. Such children may spit, choke, or gag when food is placed in the mouth, particularly if the food's texture is unfamiliar. For the child with hypersensitivity to touch, feeding is associated with genuine discomfort. Introduction of new textures usually results in aversive responses in any young infant. When the child has hypersensitivity to oral touch, however, these responses continue well beyond the

time usually required of children to develop tolerance. Hypersensitivity to oral touch can limit the child's amount of nutritional intake and the variety of foods that are accepted. It also can result in negative or oppositional behaviors at mealtime. For example, children with autism may experience this discomfort and have no method of communicating their dislike other than through negative or disruptive behaviors (Klein & Delaney, 1994).

Problems in Interaction Skills

Feeding difficulties are often accompanied by interaction and communication problems. The child may not engage in feeding and may disengage by refusing to eat, throwing food, spitting food, or crying. These behaviors inevitably create stress for the family members and disrupt an important family routine, and they also can limit essential nutritional intake. Parents often misunderstand the child's negative responses, and they become anxious about the child's limited nutritional intake and negative behaviors. The parents' increased attention can be rewarding to the child, leading him or her to repeat the disruptive behaviors to gain the parents' attention and emotional response. Mealtime scenarios of the child refusing to participate in eating can become routine if appropriate interventions are not implemented.

Table 6.4. Problems in Eating and Self-Feeding Associated With Developmental Disabilities

Condition	Associated Feeding Problems
Cerebral palsy	Primitive sucking and chewing Hyper- or hypotonia Difficulty sequencing suck, swallow, and breathe Difficulty coordinating lip, tongue, and jaw mobility Postural instability
Sensory-processing dysfunction	Poor tolerance of tactile input Limited chewing and biting skills Oral motor-planning problems Sensory defensiveness
Autism or pervasive developmental disorder	Sensory defensiveness Poor tolerance of specific tastes Difficulty in communicating about feeding Fetishes about feeding (i.e., only eats certain foods)
Respiratory or cardiac problems	Poor endurance Difficulty coordinating between swallowing and breathing Purposely limits intake to limit workload of eating and digestion
Severe sensorimotor disabilities	Poor stability and mobility of oral structures Limited control of chewing and drinking Swallowing problems and risk of aspiration Nutritionally at risk because of oral motor and communication problems
Failure to thrive	Negative interactions between feeder/caregiver and child Behavioral problems associated with meals

Interaction problems are prevalent during feeding for several reasons. First, for the child with severe limitations in motor control, eating may be the only opportunity to exercise control over the social environment. No one can force the child to eat, and refusal to eat almost always causes a reaction in the caregiver or feeder, allowing the child to feel some control over his or her environment. Second, the child quickly becomes aware that the parent is concerned and anxious about the refusal to eat. Generating this emotional response reinforces the behavior. The child quickly learns that negative behaviors at mealtime draw increased attention.

Contextual Variables That Influence Eating and Self-Feeding

Social Context

Eating and feeding almost always involve interaction with others. Initially, feeding is an intimate experience between mother and child (Humphry, 1991; Humphry & Rourk, 1991). The give-and-take and communication between parent and child during eating contribute to building their relationship. Early in development, the parent establishes an eating rhythm, making sustained eye contact, holding and patting the child, and initiating first communications (for example, when the infant signals hunger and satiation). Therefore, this is an initial time for responsive give-and-take between parent and child (Kelly & Barnard, 2000).

When the child makes an attempt to interact but receives no response, he or she may become passive and no longer initiate communication. In infants with failure to thrive, the parent may not respond to the infant's signals or may not read the infant's cues.

A medical problem associated with interactional problems during feeding is congenital heart disease (CHD). Infants with CHD often refuse to eat, and parents report that feeding their infants is difficult and anxiety-producing (Clemente, Baines, Shinebourne, & Stein, 2001), particularly when the infants become breathless and fatigued during the process. Parents of children with CHD and other significant health problems frequently worry about feeding safety and the adequacy of nutritional intake. They often report that feeding their children with medical problems becomes a task characterized as stressful rather than pleasurable.

The family structure affects the child's development of eating skills (Case-Smith & Humphry, 2001). In single-parent families or when one parent is frequently away from home, feeding responsibili-

---

Box 6.1. Failure to Thrive

Failure to thrive (FTT) is the abnormal retardation of growth and development of an infant resulting from conditions that interfere with normal metabolism, appetite, and activity. The resulting prolonged nutritional deficiency may cause permanent, irreversible retardation of physical, mental, and social development.

FTT can be caused by a multitude of birth defects and genetic problems that leave babies unable to suck or swallow or to process the food they have eaten. It also has been linked to psychosocial causes, such as severe maternal deprivation. Many infants with feeding problems are exquisitely sensitive to their environment. They may not sleep well and respond poorly to changes in their schedules. They startle easily at bright lights and noises, and they never cry or fuss because they are hungry. Many FTT children have exceptionally sensitive oral reflexes that cause them to reject or gag on pureed or solid foods.

Because FTT is such an elusive medical problem that can strike children from any social or ethnic background, many families struggle for months before they get adequate medical guidance. Parents who feel their child is not thriving and have not been informed of medical or developmental problems should ask their physician or occupational therapist for a referral to a pediatric gastroenterologist, a nutritionist, or both. Getting help early is important because retardation in growth and mental development at a young age is generally irreversible.

---

ties may fall onto one person. This responsibility can be overwhelming if a child must be fed four to five meals per day, each requiring an hour. One mother explained,

> I am the only one who can feed him. The staff at the child care center try to feed him, but they worry when he chokes and they do not know how to hold him and place the spoon so that he can swallow. He is starving when he comes home from child care, so I feed him a small meal then and dinner later. Since his birth 4 years ago, I have fed him almost every meal.

Although parents often bottle-feed infants on their laps and, later, face-to-face in the high chair, preschool children generally participate in family mealtime by sitting with other family members at the dinner table. Family mealtimes can help a child build skills, because he or she now has multiple role models and is usually highly motivated to become a full participant in the meal. This social environment can reinforce the child's efforts to eat, but it can also compound his or her frustrations about eating, resulting in disruptive, acting-out behaviors.

Most families establish a routine that allows the child to participate in the family mealtime, thereby maintaining the social benefits of family gatherings and promoting the child's mealtime skills. If the child requires supportive seating, the wheelchair can be placed near the table. When specific handling techniques are required, the child may be fed before the mealtime and be allowed to play with food on the tray while the other family members eat. Establishing eating as a social event is an important goal for every child, even when oral motor skills are limited.

Cultural Context

Cultural background highly influences the eating routine, the amounts and types of food given to the child, how the child is served, and how much independence is valued. In certain cultures, large amounts of food are served, which can be overwhelming to a young child who struggles to eat. Although every culture has certain foods that are easier to masticate (e.g., rice, curry, cornmeal, and yogurt), some cultures have standard food items that consist of fatty meats or foods that are difficult to chew.

Cultural context can affect feeding practices of families that have continued through generations. Schulze, Harwood, and Schoelmerich (2001) compared the feeding practices of Anglo-American and Puerto Rican–American mothers whose infants were 12 months of age. Anglo mothers encouraged their infants to self-feed, whereas Puerto Rican mothers spoon-fed or bottle-fed their infants. Only 1 in 28 Puerto Rican infants self-fed, but 26 of 32 Anglo infants self-fed. Anglo mothers reported that they expected their infants to self-feed earlier and expressed the importance of autonomy. Puerto Rican mothers placed more emphasis on maintaining close interpersonal relationships with their children.

Physical Context

The home and child care environments may promote or inhibit the development of eating and feeding skills. Sensory aspects of the environment, such as noise levels, amount of visual stimuli, and lighting, can interfere with a child's ability to eat. Thus, quiet, nonstimulating, and calming environments can allow the child to concentrate and perform at optimal levels. Music can promote a level of arousal that is optimal for eating (e.g., calming music that has one beat per second can promote sucking; Morris & Klein, 2000).

The physical arrangement of the home can promote or discourage development of feeding skills. Tables and chairs should be modified to meet the needs of children with disabilities. A comfortable and adaptable arrangement for feeding is needed, particularly when a child requires physical support and adapted equipment for success in feeding.

Evaluation of Eating

Evaluation of feeding and other ADL skills generally has four components. The first component is the *chart, file, or report review.* Information about medications that the child takes, developmental course, prognosis, and systemic or metabolic problems is essential before making recommendations about feeding.

The second evaluation component is the *interview of the parent or caregiver.* The perspective of the parent is critical for establishing the concerns and priorities. The caregiver's description of feeding the child and the child's ability to eat (covering the complete 24-hour daily cycle) enables the occupational therapist to understand the problem from an insider's perspective. The therapist asks questions such as those in Table 6.5 to begin to make goals and plans with the family.

The third and fourth evaluation components involve observation of the child. After gaining extensive information about what the child eats and how he or she is fed, the occupational therapist *watches the child eat.* The parent is asked to feed the child foods that he or she typically eats at home. The goal is to demonstrate feeding as it typically occurs. The occupational therapist observes parent–child interaction, documents oral motor skills, notes swallowing problems, and analyzes behaviors. This information provides an understanding of the context for feeding at home. The activity demands of eating are particularly high and must be considered in developing intervention strategies. The parent and child establish a pace and rhythm. The parent must attend to the child's ability to chew and swallow, his or her hunger level, and interest in the activity. The child needs to follow the pace of the parent and, in the case of self-feeding, establish an appropriate pace for feeding and feeding sequence.

Finally, the therapist *observes and analyzes the child's oral motor skills and sensory function.* In this focused assessment, the therapist may try specific handling techniques (described later in the discus-

Table 6.5. Occupational Therapist's Interview With Caregiver Regarding Child's Feeding

Requested Information	Probes
Describe feeding of your child.	Who feeds him/her? How does your child respond to feeding?
Describe your child's feeding problems.	Does he/she have difficulty sucking, drinking, biting, or chewing? Does your child cough or choke?
How much help does your child need with feeding?	What are ways that you help your child eat?
How do you know when your child is hungry?	What are different behaviors that indicate your child is hungry?
How do you know when your child has had enough?	When and why do you think your child stops eating? (Endurance can be an issue.)
When and how often is your child fed?	How long does a meal take?
Describe your child's diet.	Include fomula, milk, and all foods.
Describe where your child is fed.	In highchair, on lap, at table, or in wheelchair. Describe child's position.
What equipment is used in feeding?	Describe bottles, nipples, spoon, and adapted equipment.
Describe your child's response to feeding.	When does he/she most enjoy feeding?
How does your child react to new foods, foods with different textures or tastes?	Does his/her response vary according to the time or day? According to the place?
Describe the environment during feeding.	Who is present? What is the actvity/noise level?
What recommendations have been given to you regarding feeding?	How have these recommendations worked?

sion of interventions) to determine their potential use in promoting the child's feeding skills. Different textures are given to the child to assess his or her sensory tolerance. A variety of food textures (e.g., viscous and chewy, crunchy, and mixed) are used to assess the child's sensory tolerance, sensory preferences, and range of oral motor skills.

When self-feeding is evaluated, the child is placed in supportive seating and observed using fingers, utensils, cups, and straws to eat and drink. Use of a variety of foods is also important for evaluation of self-feeding. The parents are interviewed as to how, where, and what the child eats at home. The therapist must respect cultural differences in how food is eaten, including use of a bottle well beyond the first year and use of utensils that are culturally specific.

Consultation with the physician and nutritionist is important to designing intervention, particularly when the child is diagnosed with failure to thrive, is on medications, or has a history of metabolic problems. Modifications to the child's feeding methods or diet should not be made without frequent communication with the other health care professionals who are caring for the child. In all feed-

ing interventions, the nutritional status of the child is of highest priority and cannot be compromised, particularly in children with related health concerns.

Interventions for Eating Problems

The following sections describe interventions for eating problems of children with primary motor dysfunction, sensory function problems, and interaction and communication problems.

Primary Motor Dysfunction

Intervention for primary motor dysfunction falls into two categories: positioning and direct intervention. ***Positioning.*** During eating, postural alignment and stability must be adequate to support oral motor control. Full external support is required when postural stability is low. For example, a high-back chair with lateral supports and straps may be recommended for a child with severe cerebral palsy. The goal of any positioning device is to provide the level of head and trunk support that will allow the child to demonstrate the highest level of oral motor control (Logemann, 1997).

For a child who has not developed head control, slightly reclining the chair while maintaining

90° of hip flexion can assist the child with head control and facilitate oral movements for feeding. A slightly reclined position (30°) also enables the child to use gravity to assist in the suck-swallow sequence (Morris & Klein, 2000). Whether the chair is tilted backward or is upright, neck alignment in neutral (with head directly over shoulders) or in slight flexion is critical so that the throat structures are optimally aligned for efficient swallow. A slightly forward position of the head appears to facilitate swallowing by bringing the throat structures closer together and making closure of the trachea easier. Therefore, this position of slight flexion should be considered for children with swallowing problems (Logemann, 1997). If the child is at risk for aspiration, a videofluoroscope study can reveal the head and neck position that results in optimal swallow and alert the health care provider to further swallowing problems or dangers.

Direct Intervention. With the head well supported, the therapist's or parent's fingers, or cupped hand, can be placed under or around the child's chin to enhance jaw stability. One finger places pressure through the front of the chin to promote chin tuck, and another provides support under the jaw (see Figure 6.1). The goal of this support is to assist with jaw stability and provide support for the tongue's movement. This technique of jaw support has been shown to be effective with premature infants (Einarsson-Backes, Deitz, Price, Glass, & Hays, 1994) and with children who have cerebral palsy (Gisel, Applegate-Ferrante, Benson, & Bosma, 1995).

When spoon-feeding, downward pressure on the tongue with the bowl of the spoon or the nipple can inhibit tongue retraction or protraction and facilitate sucking. This gentle pressure, rhythmically applied with a spoon, promotes a cupped tongue and an organized suck-swallow pattern.

When the occupational therapist determines a technique to be effective, he or she recommends that the technique be implemented on a regular basis. Instruction to parents and other care providers is essential and should be reinforced with modeling, pictures, or feedback as the caregiver tries the techniques. Given the stressful requirements of a child who requires specific handling techniques, feeding techniques should be taught to multiple family members and child care providers so that this responsibility can be shared. Continual monitoring of the child's response to the eating intervention is critical to assist in problem solving and to help the caregivers adapt the techniques when needed.

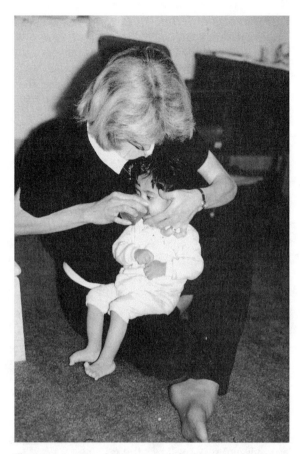

Figure 6.1. Use of jaw control during cup drinking.

Sensory Function Problems

The following sections describe interventions for eating problems of children with primary motor dysfunction, sensory function problems, and interaction and communication problems.

Modifying Sensory Aspects of Food. Altering the sensory qualities of food is another way to improve eating performance (Case-Smith & Humphry, 2001). A child's tongue movement is guided by the texture of food or drink and responds to the sensory stimulus in the mouth. Foods that are smooth and stick together can facilitate organized tongue responses. Thick, heavy, and cohesive foods (such as oatmeal or puddings) tend to facilitate an efficient suck-swallow pattern. Highly textured foods result in increased tongue movements. Foods that break apart and fill the mouth with sensory input can cause disorganized responses, coughing, or choking.

To promote mature oral movements, the occupational therapist carefully selects appropriate food textures to use in therapy sessions and to recommend to the family. The therapist selects food textures for the child according to the child's level of oral motor skill and sensory tolerance. Some guidelines for texture selection are provided in Table 6.6. A combination of strategies can be more successful than selecting any one method. Foods that are contraindicated for a child with severe oral motor problems are those that break apart into small pieces that are difficult to manage (e.g., raw carrots or crisp cookies) and those that are tough and require a grinding motion to masticate.

Strategies for Sensitivity to Touch. When a child has hypersensitivity to touch (or tactile defensiveness), the face and oral areas often are particularly sensitive. Hypersensitivity of the oral area may be a result of an extended period of nonoral feeding or a lack of appropriate oral experiences. The occupational therapist evaluates the child's sensory function through a combination of observation and parent interview. The therapist asks the parents about the range of food textures that the child tolerates and then observes the child as he or she is offered a variety of food textures. Aversive responses, choking, gagging, or expressions of discomfort all can indicate sensory-processing problems.

When the child has oral tactile hypersensitivity, multisensory experiences at times other than mealtime can decrease the child's response to touch. Oral play with rubber toys and a warm, wet washcloth can be helpful, and children generally enjoy these textures. In particular, rubber toys promote tongue and jaw movements, and use of these toys is an acceptable method of desensitizing the oral area. Brushing with a regular or NUK toothbrush helps desensitize the child's mouth (see Figure 6.2). Asking the parent to brush the child's teeth and gums twice a day may easily fit into the family's daily routine. Routines vary, however, and parents may select more playful methods of oral stimulation.

Table 6.6. Guidelines for Selection of Food Texture

Developmental Level	Recommendation
Child demonstrates a munching pattern and does not have lateral tongue movements.	Use pureed, smooth foods.
Child has poor tongue control and an inefficient suck-swallow pattern.	Avoid thin liquids and thicken liquids when possible.
Child is demonstrating beginning chewing skills.	Use soft foods that have cohesion (e.g., cheeses, chicken, well-cooked vegetables with no skins). Graham crackers, butter cookies, and some cereals are good foods for chewing because they dissolve quickly once inside the mouth, presenting less risk of choking.
Child maintains a munching or sucking pattern for an extended period of time.	A food grinder is an excellent method for varying the texture of food and allowing the child to eat a variety of foods despite low-level oral motor skills.
Child demonstrates beginning chewing skills but tends to mash foods between the tongue and upper palate.	Grainy breads and crackers are better than soft white breads or white crackers, which tend to stick to the upper palate.
Child demonstrates some lateral movement of the tongue.	Add foods with texture (e.g., peas, beans) to smooth and cohesive foods (e.g., mashed potatoes). Thicker foods tend to stay in the mouth longer and increase the work of the tongue, and they are easier to control. Peanut butter is an example of a food that is generally too thick when consumed by itself.
Child needs additional muscle tone and strength for effective biting and chewing.	Some foods can increase muscle tone for improved chewing. Viscous foods such as fruit rollups promote rotary chewing and graded jaw movements. Some dried fruits (e.g., apricots, apples) can be used to increase chewing. Tough or fibrous meats are contraindicated in children without basic chewing skills.
Child with beginning chewing skills has not yet developed controlled bite.	The therapist should hold a long piece of vegetable or meat between the side teeth to promote graded biting. Strips of cheese or lunch meat can be used. Soft cookies and crackers placed to the side can also promote controlled biting. Pretzels and apple slices require more jaw strength and can be tried as a next step in biting skill.

Case Study 6.1. Trevor: A Child With Oral Motor Dysfunction

History

Trevor had a history of neonatal asphyxia. Initially, he was extremely hypotonic and moved little. He was given liquids through an oral-gastric tube, but his oral sucking was adequate for oral feeding by 3 weeks of age. During bottle-feeding, he was positioned upright with head well supported, jaw support was applied, and a soft preemie nipple was used. This method was slow, but his growth was adequate with nutritional supplements.

Current Feeding Problem

Trevor was bottle-fed until 10 months, when his mother expressed interest in attempting pureed foods. At this point several problems had to be overcome:

- He exhibited a pattern of spastic quadriparesis.
- He demonstrated extreme hypersensitivity because he had not experienced texture in his mouth.
- When textures were attempted, he spit them out and turned his head.
- His head and trunk control remained poor.
- He required full support to sit.

When a spoon was introduced, Trevor demonstrated wide jaw excursions: His mouth opened to its full range and then clamped shut on the spoon in a tonic bite. His tongue moved in extension-retraction and was not effective in taking the food from the spoon. Lateral tongue movement was poorly controlled. He gagged easily if the spoon was placed in the center of his tongue. His suck-swallow was disorganized, and he often coughed when given small amounts of food.

Intervention

Positioning. Trevor required full head and trunk support for feeding. A feeder chair was used because it provided complete support, had a strapping system, and helped maintain a position of 90° hip flexion. He tended to arch in all positions; therefore, additional support was provided at the anterior upper trunk to maintain his alignment. Backward pressure on the front of his chest helped maintain a position of chin tuck, which is important for efficient suck-swallow. Although the strapping helped with his postural alignment, he attempted to arch and hyperextend his head. A small pad was placed behind his head to prevent hyperextension and to promote chin tuck. The feeding chair was placed at a 60° angle so that gravity assisted his oral movements and swallow. This angle also prevented food loss from his mouth.

Handling. To decrease his sensory defensiveness before feeding, his mother gently stroked the area around his mouth and his lips with a warm washcloth. She also stroked his gums and rubbed his tongue. Trevor liked this input and would frequently bite the washcloth and smile.

During feeding the mother was instructed to use jaw control. She placed her hand around his jaw with her third finger under his mandible, her index finger along his cheek, and her thumb on his front mandible to reinforce his chin tuck. Her hand prevented his wide jaw movement and gave support to his tongue to move the food back in his mouth for swallowing. She placed the spoon in the center of his tongue and pressed down gently to facilitate a suck-swallow response. Smooth pureed foods were used; textured food was avoided until his suck-swallow became more reliable.

Family Variables. The mother generally fed Trevor. She frequently asked the therapist if she was applying the techniques correctly. The therapist reassured her often that her gentle touches and careful attention to his responses were important to the success of the feeding efforts. She was always responsive to his cues and waited patiently for his responses. Although her hesitancy established a comfortable pace for Trevor, the time required for a meal was not realistic in the family's busy daily schedule. The practitioner encouraged her to place slightly more food on the spoon and to establish a somewhat quicker pace. This was possible after Trevor's initial hypersensitivity was reduced. The therapist reassured the mother that Trevor would indicate if the amount or pace exceeded his capability. With practice she became more comfortable and feeding became more efficient.

The therapist discussed with the mother who else could be trained to feed Trevor and who might give her respite from this responsibility. She identified her mother as someone else who could help and was the best candidate for learning the techniques.

These methods worked fairly well; however, Trevor could take in only small amounts of food on the spoon, and his suck-swallow response was slow and inefficient, thereby requiring several attempts. He required 15 minutes to eat a bowl of pureed food. This level of oral feeding was acceptable because his primary nutritional source was formula from the bottle. The mother's goal in the following 6 months was to increase the amount of food he could take by mouth and to increase the textures that were acceptable to him. The grandmother attended the following therapy sessions and learned how to position and handle Trevor for feeding. One day each week, she helped care for Trevor, giving his mother a day of respite.

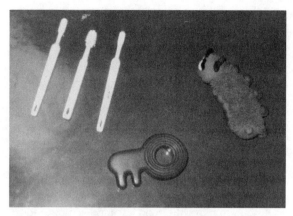

Figure 6.2. A Nuk® toothbrush set and rubber toys. These items help desensitize the mouth, and children often enjoy chewing them.

The time just before mealtime is an optimal time to desensitize the oral area to improve acceptance and tolerance of the meal. The amount and type of sensory input must depend on the child's responses to touch. In children with severe tactile hypersensitivity, the therapist should begin with application of deep pressure around and in the mouth, stroking with the finger inside a nipple or a washcloth. Taste experiences can be added by dipping the washcloth or nipple in juice or strained fruits. Toothbrushing, with extra input to the gums and sides of the tongue, also can help prepare the child for feeding. If the parent or therapist establishes the same routine for desensitization each time (e.g., begins around the mouth and then rubs along the gum line) the child generally demonstrates more tolerance of the stimulation.

Guidelines for introducing food textures to children with sensory-processing problems are presented in Table 6.7. Among the most difficult textures to tolerate are small, discrete bits of food, such as small pieces of meat, corn, or raisins. With some children, incorporating textured food into smooth food substances, such as pudding or applesauce, may make the texture tolerable. Other children, however, expel any discrete bit of food from the mouth.

Understanding the basis of the child's oral hypersensitivity is important when planning an intervention program. Oral hypersensitivity that relates to a neurological impairment is often among the most difficult to overcome. When sensory intolerance appears related to lack of oral sensory experience, as in a child who is fed with a gastrostomy tube, the hypersensitivity may be easier to overcome. This child generally improves rapidly when given graded sensory experiences. Although the guidelines in Table 6.7 apply to many children, every child is unique and has individual preferences for oral sensory experience, food textures, and tastes.

Interaction and Communication Problems

Interaction problems during feeding are not easily solved. Often interaction problems reflect long-standing concerns. Negative feeding interactions can indicate the child's frustration and distress related to hunger or discomfort when eating. These negative interactions also may reflect habits and routines that the child has adopted because he or she has been rewarded with attention when practicing negative behaviors. The following guidelines for occupational therapists can help improve children's behaviors during mealtime and snacks.

- Perform a functional analysis of the problem. What initiates the negative behaviors? Often the behavior is a form of communication. What is the child attempting to communicate by his or her behaviors?
- When the source of the disruptive behaviors is identified, discuss with the parent or caregiver how that situation can be avoided or how it can be modified so that the disruptive behavior is not needed.
- Help the parent or caregiver read the child's cues. Problems often occur when a child's gestures and speech are difficult to understand and cues are subtle. Help the parent or caregiver increase sensitivity to the child's gestures or facial expressions that indicate discomfort, satiation, or dislike of a food.
- Recommend that the feeders give the child choices during feeding so that he or she participates in the meal. Giving the child simple choices at mealtime can promote the child's feeling of control. The child can select which food to eat or indicate when a bite is desired. The child should direct the pace and sequence of the meal (e.g., choosing a drink over solid food, or meat instead of a vegetable).
- Explain to the family that a child who struggles to eat or has oral hypersensitivity needs consistent praise and positive feedback. Positive interaction between the child and parent or other family members can be as important as the amount of nutritional intake. Each influences the other.
- Teach the family to use behavioral management techniques when behaviors become highly disruptive to the family mealtime. A

Table 6.7. Food Texture Progression

Recommendations	Examples	Nutritional Value	Precautions
1. To facilitate sucking and swallowing, use pureed or soft foods.	Gelatin	High sugar Limited protein value	Avoid gelatin with fruit pieces.
	Pureed meats and vegetables	Good variety of vitamins and protein	Avoid using baby foods for extended periods.
	Pudding or custard	High carbohydrates; milk provides calcium and protein	Tapioca pudding can be very offensive to hyper-sensitive children and may provide extra stimulus to hyposensitive children.
	Applesauce	Low calorie; high fluid content	
2. To facilitate sucking and swallowing, use a heavy food that easily forms a bolus and gives proprioceptive input.	Mashed potatoes (excellent consistency for providing proprioceptive input)	High carbohydrate; adding margarine provides calories; adding powdered milk adds protein and calcium	Mixing firm bits of food with mashed potatoes may not be tolerated by sensitive children; incon-sistency in texture may cause choking.
	Oatmeal	High carbohydrate; milk adds calcium and protein	
3. Liquids may need to be thickened to improve and facilitate swallowing.	Liquids may be thickened with yogurt, wheat germ, gelatin, cereal, carrageen	Yogurt: protein and calcium Wheat germ: carbohydrates and fiber Gelatin: see above Cereal: carbohydrates, vitamins (depends on the type of cereal)	Avoid high carbohydrates to thicken liquids; when food pools in the back of mouth, alternate with thinner liquids; avoid cornstarch.
4. To promote chewing initially, use chewy or gummy foods that hold together to make a bolus.	Bananas; cheese; progress to chicken, lunch meat, marshmallows, soft vegetables, crackers, dried fruit, apples, zwieback toast, graham crackers	Fruits: carbohydrates and vitamins Cheese: protein and calcium Meat: protein Vegetables: vitamins and complex carbohydrates	Avoid foods and meats that break apart; avoid vegetables with skins unless well cooked.
5. To promote chewing when jaw is more stable but movement is primitive, use crispy or harder solids.	Crackers, graham crackers, dried fruit	Crackers: complex carbohydrates Graham crackers: complex carbohydrates and fiber Dried fruit: high-calorie carbohydrates	If you use carrots or beef jerky, avoid allowing child to bite off pieces. Use of tough meat may increase abnormal postures.
6. To desensitize the mouth, grade the texture of the food; use a blender, if possible, to make small variations in texture.	Begin with pureed, then progress to soft foods, then lumpy or solid.	Different nutrients can be provided in a variety of textures.	Do not begin with lumpy foods—a hypersensitive child will be intolerant of these. When blending foods, avoid mixing all foods together.
Use a variety of tastes, textures, and temperatures.	Be creative, given the above guidelines.	Variety should improve the nutritional balance.	Consult nutritionist and occupational or speech therapist for advice.

regimen can be established that defines limits to the child's behavior and specific consequences when the child exceeds the limits. When the discipline technique is consistently applied, the child learns which behaviors are allowed and which are not. "Time out" or elimination of something desired can be effective consequences of disruptive behaviors (Hall & Hall, 1998).

Interventions for Self-Feeding Problems Related to Motor Function

When children have motor function limitations that interfere with self-feeding, a variety of therapeutic interventions may be needed to increase their skills. The following sections describe positioning, handling, and adaptive equipment.

Positioning

Correct alignment and adequate support for the trunk and head are essential for eye–hand coordination in self-feeding and eventual independence in this occupation. The midrange movement of the hand and arm through space requires either well-developed trunk stability or sufficient external support to keep the trunk aligned and stable. The child must feel secure and relaxed during self-feeding in order to use the strength, control, and endurance needed to eat an entire meal. Correct positioning (i.e., the chin tucked, shoulders depressed and slightly forward, and the pelvis in neutral alignment) allows the child to use both hands at midline and in midspace for spoon-to-mouth eating and cup drinking. This position can be maintained in a wheelchair or feeder chair with adequate pelvic, hip, and lateral trunk supports. When the child tends to retract his or her shoulders, padded humeral "wings" attached to the back of the chair can help maintain the child's arms in a forward, shoulder-protracted position. The wings help maintain a scapular position that allows for neutral shoulder rotation and forearm supination (Danella & Vogtle, 1992).

When the shoulder is unstable, an external support to the upper arm or elbow can help the child control a hand-to-mouth pattern. The child can stabilize his or her arm on a small bolster placed under the arm. The bolster separates the child's elbow from the trunk, thereby maintaining a position of some shoulder abduction. Then, stabilizing the elbow on a tray or table, the child scoops food and reaches his or her mouth with minimal movement of the shoulder and elbow. The bolster, in combination with the tray surface, serves as a lever that helps the child effectively engage in hand-to-mouth motion.

Simply raising the tray or table surface can also help the child whose hand-to-mouth pattern is unstable. With the child bearing weight on his or her elbows, raising the height of the wheelchair tray promotes upright sitting and humeral abduction (Morris & Klein, 2000). This postural help can improve hand-to-mouth control, as the child stabilizes the elbows on the tray and then uses simple elbow flexion and extension to feed. An elevated, well-fitting tray can enable the child with motor problems to gain the postural control needed to self-feed independently when given easily managed foods (Figure 6.3).

Handling

For the child with athetoid cerebral palsy and limited control of arms in space, handling during feeding should emphasize postural stability and proximal support of the arms (Boehme, 1988). An aide, parent, therapist, or therapist assistant can provide the shoulder depression and protraction and scapular stability during self-feeding. Support and guidance of the upper arm may be needed to establish a smooth hand-to-mouth pattern. This support should help the child stabilize his or her arm in space rather than move it through the range, allowing the child to be an active participant in the feeding process. The therapist therefore should provide the least amount of support needed to allow the child to self-feed successfully, and this support should be able to be reduced with practice.

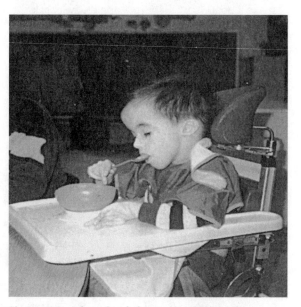

Figure 6.3. A boy feeds himself, with his elbow resting on an elevated tray.

To provide subtle guidance of the spoon to mouth, the occupational therapist can hold the spoon handle in between his or her own extended index and third fingers. The therapist slips these fingers holding the handle into the child's palm and places his or her thumb on the dorsum of the child's hand. Using a gross grasp, the child holds onto the therapist's fingers that align the spoon handle, and the therapist then facilitates a self-feeding pattern by subtly guiding the hand-to-mouth pattern. This strategy is particularly successful with a child who has developed a basic hand-to-mouth pattern but spills frequently. The therapist's or parent's fingers inside the child's hand support the small movements of hand and wrist needed to place the spoon in the mouth and to reduce spillage.

The physical and social context for implementing these strategies should be considered. Feeding strategies can limit face-to-face communication, and the positions required to use these strategies can make implementation during family mealtime difficult (e.g., the feeder may have to sit beside rather than in front of the child). The techniques can be most appropriately implemented during snack time at school or at home. When providing these techniques, the caregiver should work to decrease the amount of physical assistance, so that the child continually makes small gains in independence during the meal.

Adaptive Equipment

Adaptive equipment for feeding is readily available and often is helpful in enabling independence in self-feeding. Parents have frequently remarked that adapted utensils, plates, and cups help increase the child's ability to self-feed and decrease spillage and frustration. Helpful feeding equipment includes built-up handles; plates with high, curved rims and nonskid pads; and cups with handles and lids (Scherzer & Tscharnuter, 1991; Figure 6.4). Morris and Klein (2000) provided numerous examples of utensils, cups, and bowls that enable a child to self-feed successfully.

Characteristics of spoons that assist the child in self-feeding are enlarged handles, flat spoon bowls, and angled handles. Cups with lids reduce spillage. Lids without spouts may be helpful when the child exhibits suckling (in and out) tongue movement. Straws can promote the child's ability to suck and can allow the child to drink without lifting the cup from the table surface. More sophisticated adaptive equipment, such as an electric feeder, may enable a child to self-feed without using his or her arms; however, the cost and difficulty in setup should be a consideration in the purchase of such devices. Criteria for selecting adaptive equipment to improve the child's independence in self-feeding include safety, durability, ease of cleaning and use, and developmental appropriateness.

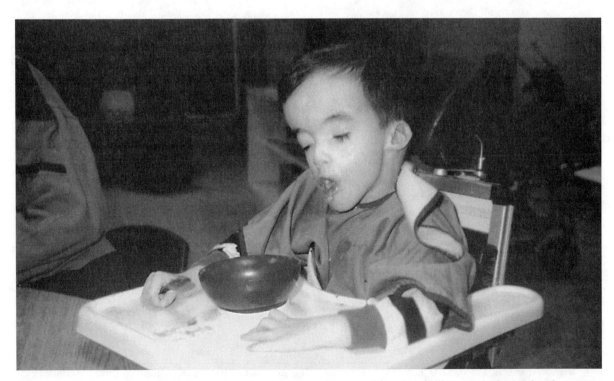

Figure 6.4. A bowl with a high rim and suction cup at its base enables the child to eat independently.

Dressing

Development of Dressing Skills

Dressing proficiencies in children typically develop over a 4- to 5-year period within the first 6 years of life. The emergence of these capabilities depends on the child's interest and self-initiative and the value that family members place on dressing independence.

The child first begins to participate in dressing at about 12 months of age, when he or she holds out an arm or leg to allow the parent to put the garment over the body part or when the child decides to remove shoes or pants on his or her own. It is not until 5 or 6 years of age that the child can accomplish the most difficult fasteners. The child will use the rest of the childhood years to refine dressing skills and develop clothing preferences in accordance with cultural and social contexts. Table 6.8 provides some guidelines to the sequence and typical ages that specific dressing skills are accomplished.

Performance Variables That Influence Dressing

Problems in Motor Skills

Dressing requires basic and complex motor skills. Balance, postural stability, and flexibility are needed to reach one's feet, head, and other body parts. Strength is needed to fit tight clothing over body parts and pull on shoes. Dexterity and eye–hand coordination are needed to close and open fastenings, button, and tie. For children with motor problems, dressing may be difficult. Poor postural control and abnormal movement patterns interfere with dressing development and routines. Problems in dexterity and two-hand coordination may interfere with ability to fasten and properly arrange clothing.

Problems in Sensory and Mental Functions

A child must be able to tolerate and accept the feel of clothing next to his or her skin. Most children tolerate touch, but some children do not tolerate certain textures. Infants' clothing is typically soft,

Table 6.8. Sequence of Typical Development of Dressing

Age (in years)	Self-Dressing Skills	Age (in years)	Self-Dressing Skills
1	Cooperates with dressing (holds out arms and feet) Pulls off shoes, removes socks Pushes arms through sleeves and legs through pants	3½	Finds front of clothing Snaps or hooks front fastener Unzips front zipper on jacket, separating zipper Puts on mittens Buttons series of three or four buttons Unbuckles shoe or belt Dresses with supervision (help with front and back)
2	Removes unfastened coat Removes shoes if laces are untied Helps pull down pants Finds armholes in over-the-head shirt		
2½	Removes pull-down pants with elastic waist Assists in pulling on socks Puts on front-button coat, shirt Unbuttons large buttons	4	Removes pullover garment independently Buckles shoes or belt Zips jacket zipper Puts on socks correctly Puts on shoes with assistance in tying laces Laces shoes Consistently identifies the front and back of garments
3	Puts on over-the-head shirt with minimal assistance Puts on shoes without fasteners (may be on wrong foot) Puts on socks (may be with heel on top) Independent in pulling down pants Zips and unzips jacket once on track Needs assistance to remove over-the-head shirt Buttons large front buttons	4½	Puts belt in loops
		5	Ties and unties knots Dresses unsupervised
		6	Closes back zipper Ties bow knot Buttons back buttons Snaps back snaps

Note. From *Pre-Dressing Skills,* by M. D. Klein, 1988, Tucson, AZ: Therapy SkillBuilders. Copyright 1988 by Therapy SkillBuilders. Adapted with permission.

but clothing for older children can be stiff or rough. Children must learn to accept the increasing variety in clothing materials. Body awareness and body scheme are inherent in the task of dressing. A child learns to match body parts to clothing pieces and in the process learns the important perceptual concepts of front, back, right, and left. Visual perception and somatosensory information are important to recognizing clothing characteristics and how they fit the body (Shepherd, 2001).

Infants and children with problems in sensory function, such as sensitivity to touch, may not tolerate certain types of materials or clothing. They may become irritable when dressed or may resist dressing. Some children may insist on wearing only clothes of their preferred texture (e.g., a girl who insists on wearing the same dress day after day).

Children with sensory processing and perception difficulties may have inadequate body scheme, difficulty distinguishing right and left sides, visual perception problems, dyspraxia, and directionality problems, all of which can delay the development of dressing skills. Children with cognitive delays also may experience those difficulties. Tying or buckling shoes, putting legs in the correct pants legs, and lining up buttons can be difficult tasks for children with impairments in cognitive and perceptional abilities. Appropriate dressing also requires that the child be able to assess his or her appearance.

Contextual Variables That Influence Dressing

The degree to which a child participates in dressing is highly influenced by the social context of the family. Family economic status and available resources for clothing affect dressing performance. Parents' time resources determine the morning and evening routines and how much time can be devoted to dressing.

Cultural values often influence how much independence in dressing is valued. In the Anglo-American culture, independence at early ages is highly valued (Lynch & Hanson, 1998), whereas in Asian, Hispanic, and Middle Eastern cultures, interdependence may be more valued; the parents' dressing a preschool child is not only accepted but also valued as a way of demonstrating affection and caring. Mothers may expect and want to dress their children until school age (i.e., 6 years of age; Chan, 1998).

Cultural values also influence dressing traditions and the type of clothes worn. People from some Middle Eastern cultures may prefer to cover almost all body parts, including the head. Children may be required to wear multiple layers of clothing or may wear simple, one-piece clothing.

The occupational therapist must be sensitive to whether the family values the child's independence in dressing. Families who value interdependence among its members may view dressing as an opportunity for engagement with the child and not necessarily expect independence. Parents of a child with disabilities may highly value their child's physical appearance, as expressed in clothing. They may want their child to appear as normal or attractive as possible, to reduce the stigma they may experience and to increase others' acceptance. Occupational therapists should recognize and respect this need, and dressing interventions should incorporate this value into the procedures.

Interventions for Dressing

When a child with a disability is introduced to dressing interventions, the activity should take

Case Study 6.2. Megan: An Illustration of Family Values and Dressing

Megan was a beautiful 7-year-old girl who had cerebral palsy, and her mother always dressed her in the most fashionable styles. Megan's wardrobe included items such as blue denim overalls, which had multiple fasteners at the shoulder and waist, and short pants and dresses with tiny buttons in awkward positions. The outfits made it impossible for Megan to manage her clothing for independent toileting. The teaching staff members at school were frustrated because she remained dependent in dressing tasks when she could have been independent if she wore simpler, easy-to-manage clothes.

The occupational therapist suggested that Megan wear sweatshirts and sweatpants with an elastic waist to school so that she could be independent in toileting. This suggestion angered the parents because they highly valued Megan's appearance and beautifully tailored clothes. They valued how others at school perceived her appearance much more than how independently she was able to function at school. The occupational therapist provided suggestions for clothing that was both fashionable and easy to manage; however, the parents continued to primarily use clothing that created the image they held of their daughter as a beautiful, meticulously dressed child. The school-based team decided that respect for the parents' priorities was most important; therefore, throughout the school year, the teachers continued to help Megan with toileting and dressing.

place cooperatively between parents and the child. The child begins to participate more in dressing, and the parents allow the child to attempt the performance skills required to dress and undress. Occupational therapy dressing interventions for children with developmental disabilities can use preparatory methods (e.g., improvement of motor skills), purposeful activities (e.g., dressing games), actual engagement in dressing, and environmental modifications (e.g., modifications to the closet).

Improving Motor Performance Skills

When a child has difficulty dressing because of movement problems, occupational therapy intervention may include the establishment of motor skills that support the occupation of dressing. For example, a young child with poor trunk control can be dressed in a supported sitting position. The child can sit between the parent's legs to support the pelvis and lower trunk. Seated behind the child, the parent guides the child's movements as the child pushes the arms and legs through sleeves and pants legs. This activity allows the child to practice bilateral movements and develop trunk control, both of which are needed to don shirts and pants. Table 6.9 presents a motor analysis for donning a T-shirt.

To increase dressing performance, dressing practice can be integrated into therapy sessions. The therapist should work to make dressing a natural and fun part of the therapy session. For example, children can put on exercise clothing to "work out," dress up in silly clothes, or dress up to pretend to be someone else (e.g., a teacher, firefighter, farmer, or chef). Dressing interventions using therapeutic positioning should focus on the motor performance skills identified as missing or delayed. Practice on a low bench with the therapist sitting behind the child can allow for a dynamic interplay between the therapist and child during a dressing activity. When practicing at home, dressing activities in a small chair with armrests or dressing on the floor with the child's back supported against a wall may provide adequate surfaces for trunk support and postural stabilization.

Upper-body dressing interventions for children with movement disorders include enhancing postural stability and symmetry, bilateral coordination, controlled reach (including reach overhead and across midline), and use of hands in space. Interventions for lower-body dressing require, in addition, well-developed trunk control, sitting equilibrium, and leg movements. For example, to place the feet through pants legs, a child must reach forward and across the midline with the arms extended. This serial skill is quite difficult for children with cerebral palsy because it involves a combination of shoulder flexion and elbow extension with shoulder mobility, elbow stability, trunk control, and active leg movements.

Table 6.9. Motor Analysis for Donning a T-Shirt

Donning a T-Shirt	Observe
Reach for shirt	Shoulder stability in directed reach Trunk control in forward weight shift Quality of reach—smooth and directed Symmetry of bilateral reach
Grasp of shirt	Hand opening Grasping pattern and control Use of two hands together Isolated distal finger prehension
Bring T-shirt over head	Use of two hands together Ability to maintain grasp during active movement of shoulder and elbow Adequate shoulder range for bringing shirt over top of head Smooth bilateral shoulder flexion with elbow flexion Maintenance of head and trunk stability Resistive grasp and arm flexion during forceful movement of shirt opening over head
Right arm through sleeve	Ability to locate arm opening (using visual or tactile perception or both) Ability to stabilize shirt with left hand Shoulder extension with elbow flexion to position arm Shoulder abduction with elbow extension to push arm through sleeve
Left arm through sleeve	Same, location of the sleeve is usually easier May require slightly greater arm strength to push through sleeve if the T-shirt fits tightly

Adapting Techniques for Dressing

Occupational therapists have long studied the performance issues of dressing to determine the best ways to modify the sequences and required actions needed for children with disabilities ("Dressing Techniques for the Cerebral Palsied Child," 1954; Klein, 1988). Techniques have been developed to simplify the actions, steps, and sequences required during dressing. For example, children may be taught a modified way to don their coats by laying the coat on the floor upside down and pushing both hands through the sleeves, lifting the coat overhead. This technique requires over-the-head arm movement but eliminates crossing the midline and reaching behind the trunk. One-hand tying techniques can be used for children with limited bilateral hand skills. Children with limited motor-sequencing skills may learn to tie their shoes using the "bunny ear" method, which requires simple, symmetrical hand movements, rather than the complex, asymmetrical movements of the "over and around" method. Parents should give the child sufficient time to work on dressing without rushing.

Adapting Equipment for Dressing

Supportive positioning and sitting are primary methods to adapt dressing so that a child has the trunk stability to become independent in this occupation. When a child with a movement disability is unstable in sitting and lacks the balance needed to reach forward and to the sides, seating should be provided that is safely supportive to the trunk, including the pelvis and shoulders. Some children dress in their wheelchair so that they can shift their weight side to side and use the armrests for support. The child may dress in the corner of a room, so that the walls support his or her trunk in side-to-side movements (Shepherd, 2001). Other children may use stools, bolsters, and railings to provide the external support needed during dressing.

Buttonhooks, long shoehorns, long-reach zipper aids, and adapted shoe ties are examples of equipment that can increase a child's dressing independence (Klein, 1988; Shepherd, 2001). Metal rings can be placed on the zipper. A dressing stick can aid in donning socks when range of motion is limited in the shoulder or the lower extremity. These devices are inexpensive and can be quite helpful, especially when the child approaches adolescence and independence in dressing becomes more important.

Modifying Activity Demands Through Appropriate Clothing

Clothing for children with movement impairments should be easy to don and doff. Pullover garments should have easy, wide openings with necklines that can stretch. Flexible, elasticized waistbands and large sleeve openings are helpful. Garments that enable the child to dress independently are loose fitting and use stretchy (knit) fabrics, elastic waistbands, and few (or no) fastenings. Hook-and-loop fasteners can replace buttons, zippers, and shoelaces. Examples of clothing easy to don and doff are sweatshirts and pants, oversized T-shirts, and elastic-waist shorts and skirts. These types of clothing often are available in attractive styles, and many children enjoy wearing "oversized" clothing; however, occupational therapists should be sensitive to the parents' and child's preferences. Clothing selection is the family's choice and should be based on their likes and dislikes, their cultural background, and the resources available to invest in clothing.

Hook-and-loop fasteners are helpful, and the use of clothing with fasteners for children with hand skill difficulties should be avoided. For children who have difficulty identifying the front and back or the right and left sides of garments, tags can be sewn inside the garment to help with correct orientation for donning. Sometimes garments can be marked inside with permanent colors for right and left. It is best to purchase clothing for which the front and back and right and left can be easily distinguished. T-shirts and sweatshirts with designs on the front are recommended for this purpose. For children with tactile hypersensitivity, clothes should "feel good." Soft, knit fabrics are generally easier to tolerate than stiff fabrics. Children vary in their response to the texture of clothing, however; given the great variety of fabrics available, children can be allowed to feel and select their clothes before purchase.

Modifying Dressing Routines

Children with hypersensitivity to touch may benefit from preparatory routines before dressing. Joint compression or deep tactile pressure techniques may help calm or organize the child before dressing. If the parent is helping the child dress, firm touch and secure holding can help the child tolerate the tactile input of the material to his or her skin, because sensation can be overwhelming. Using a set routine in dressing (e.g., always donning the pants first and the shirt last) can help prepare and organize the child. Verbal cuing about the dressing activity also can help the child know what touch inputs to expect.

Children with figure ground problems benefit when the environment is well organized and uncluttered. The parents can place clothing so that it is sequenced in the order of donning and is oriented correctly (top to bottom, right to left).

Teaching Strategies

Children with developmental disabilities, such as motor planning or cognitive problems, can benefit from practicing dressing with feedback from parents. The steps of dressing activities can be verbally reinforced, and verbal and gestural prompts can guide the child toward the next step (Van Houton, 1998). The backward chaining method can be effective in teaching a child to dress. In backward chaining, the parent performs most of the dressing task, allowing the child to complete the final steps. Over time, the parent performs fewer of the beginning steps, allowing the child greater participation in completing the task (Klein, 1988). This approach results in successful task completion and a sense of accomplishment in dressing.

Bathing

Development of Bathing Skills

Bathing is a relaxing and pleasurable activity for most children and parents. Bath time generally includes playful interaction and learning about both one's body and hygiene. It is important that children with disabilities experience bathing as a relaxing, enjoyable experience in which they are comfortable and safe.

Children usually become interested in washing themselves by 2 years of age. At this point, a child typically has mastered postural control coupled with prehension skills, allowing water play and movement about the tub or shower. The child's participation indicates a tolerance and enjoyment of the sensory experience of bathing or showering. By 4 years of age, the child may wash and dry with supervision. Four-year-olds typically have developed the motor skills to move in and out of the tub with supervision. Complete independence in bathing cannot be expected until 8 years of age, at which time the child can independently and safely wash all body parts.

Performance Variables That Influence Bathing

Problems in Motor Skills

Postural stability and sitting balance are required for the child to sit in the bathtub because the tub is slippery and hard and the risk of injurious falls is great. These skills are quite difficult for children with movement problems, such as cerebral palsy, ataxia, or trisomy 21 syndrome. To use a washcloth or soap, the child must maintain his or her grasp during active range of the shoulder and arm while maintaining an upright posture. Reaching and adequately cleaning all body parts can be a formidable task.

Problems in Sensory Functions

Bathing and showering have intense sensory components: the temperature, tactile, auditory, visual, and proprioceptive components are different from those of the other daily occupations of children. Children with sensitivity to touch or other sensory-processing problems may have a low tolerance for bathing activities and respond negatively to the bathing experience with temper tantrums and other behavioral disruptions (Table 6.10).

Problems in Mental Functions

Bathing is a complex activity that requires the cognitive ability to understand safety issues and actions, plan and execute a series of motor tasks, use the equipment and materials of the bathtub, and appreciate the concept of hygiene. Independence in bathing, as in many other activities of living, requires adequate attention span, reasoning skills, social skills, understanding of personal welfare, and adaptive and responsible behaviors (Furuno et al., 1994). Children with mental retardation, attention

Table 6.10. Issues in Bathing by Diagnosis

Diagnosis	Potential Problems
Cerebral palsy	Sitting balance in tub Easily startled Range of motion limitation affecting reach to all body parts Reaching and washing hair Transferring in and out of tub Poor control of the soap and washcloth in hands
Spina bifida	Sitting balance Sensation in legs Motor planning Tactile defensiveness
Hypersensitivities	Aversion to bathing; may have a tantrum at bath time Does not bath thoroughly because uncomfortable
Cognitive delays	Has difficulty sequencing the bathing task Does not thoroughly complete task Limited dexterity and delayed fine motor skills

deficit disorder, autism, or other impairments of mental function may have difficulty executing bathing activities. For example, a child with mental retardation may not be able to carry out the series of tasks required to use a washcloth to clean body parts. A child with attention deficit disorder may have difficulty completing the tasks of bathing because of distractibility. Children with body scheme difficulties may not understand the parent's verbal cues about washing specific body parts, and they may ignore some body parts.

Contextual Variables That Influence Bathing

Cultural values influence how the family defines bathing, how often bathing is performed, and the importance of hygiene. In many cultures, bathing once a week is the norm, and daily bathing is considered excessive. Parents may continue sponge-bathing outside a bathtub for the first 3 to 4 years of the child's life. Often parents have rituals about bathing (e.g., regularity of hair washing) that are highly ingrained. Sensitive questioning about traditions or habits related to bathing allows the therapist to understand this routine and offer the most helpful recommendations for improving the child's performance of this activity.

Interventions for Bathing

Improving Motor Performance Skills

Bath time may be a time in which the parents encourage the child with a movement disability to practice and develop desirable motor skills. The child can practice both the stability and mobility needed in washing him- or herself. Obviously, close parental supervision is necessary to prevent falls or other injuries. Through a motor analysis of the bathing tasks by the occupational therapist, specific motor skills can be targeted to become a focus of bathing activities. The movements that limit bathing independence often involve reaching to the feet, back, and head. Bathing intervention activities that improve reach to various body parts are directed toward improving range of motion, strength, and postural stability as the means to support participation in bath activities.

Children with cerebral palsy frequently have difficulty with bathing components such as reaching their feet, top of head, and back due to tight muscle groups and postural instability. Interventions outside bath time may be used to target motor skills to improve bathing activities. Activities to increase range of motion at the hips, legs, and arms can be implemented. Postural stability with scapular stability and mobility are emphasized in interven-

tion activities. The child should be given opportunities to practice activities similar to the activities of bathing, such as grasping an object while moving the upper arm through internal and external rotation. These movements may help the child develop the active range and arm–hand control needed to manage a washcloth. Other intervention activities may be designed to improve the motor skills of bathing for washing the back and head and for getting out of the bathtub and drying off.

In addition to the development of the child's motor skills, the occupational therapist will address the issue of safe movement in and out of the tub or shower. These methods must keep in mind the physical safety of the parents as well as the child. The occupational therapist can recommend methods for lifting the child into the tub and achieving secure sitting stability once in the tub. For example, a small child with cerebral palsy should be held symmetrically in slight trunk and neck flexion while being moved in and out of the tub. This method of securely holding reduces the possibility of the child exhibiting a startle response and falling backward or to the side.

Adapting Equipment for Bathing

The average bathroom environment contains many physical barriers for children with disabilities and their parents. An occupational therapist can assist the family in developing ways to eliminate barriers or accommodate them with the use of adaptive equipment or modified arrangements.

When the family has the financial means, structural changes may be made to the bathtub or shower to allow easy and safe access. Such modifications include changes in the showerheads or faucets, replacement of traditional showers or tubs with wheelchair roll-in showers or tubs with non-skid surfaces, and installation of permanent grab bars and rails. These costly changes should be made with consultation from plumbers, architects, and/or contractors.

A variety of adaptations to assist in bathing can be made without structural modifications. Nonskid bath mats or rubber appliqués may be placed on the tub bottom and sides to prevent slips and aid in transfers.

A variety of commercially available bath chairs can be used to support the child during bathing and transfers to and from the tub. Hammock chairs made of plastic netting stretched over PVC piping support the child's head and trunk in a semireclined position. The hammock chairs, which are commercially available or can be fabricated, offer the child stability and safety and raise the position of the child in the tub to ease the bathing task for the parent. Commercially available bathtub rings allow children with head control but poor sitting balance an increased sense of security in the tub because they securely hold the lower trunk upright (Shepherd, 2001). Tub benches, which extend outside the tub, allow for sliding into the tub to eliminate lifts and positioning by the parents. Wheeled shower chairs may be used to move an older child into an accessible shower stall.

Handheld showerhead extensions can be attached to the bathtub faucets, enabling the bather to direct water to different body parts without body movement and shifts in posture. For the child with limitations in balance and motor control, a handheld shower helps the child or parent easily reach all body parts and rinse without submersion in the water (e.g., for the child in a tub chair). Parents may find that use of simple household equipment, such as sponges with handles, bath mitts, liquid soaps, and pitchers for rinsing, can decrease movement and reaching as they bathe their children. Additional options for adapted bathing equipment are available as the child grows to adult size and are described in detail elsewhere in this book.

Modifying Bathing Routines

When sensory function problems, such as tactile defensiveness or auditory hypersensitivity, are present, the occupational therapist first helps the parent understand that the child's aversive response to bathing is a sensory-processing problem. When the child's negative behaviors are understood as an aversive response, parents can more readily adopt a positive, confident approach using verbal cuing, reassurance, and changes to the sensory environment.

For a child with tactile defensiveness, parents can apply deep pressure techniques before the bath to improve tolerance to tactile input. The therapist may recommend that the washcloth and towel be used with deep pressure in rhythmic, organized strokes to increase acceptance of the bathing procedures. The extremities and back should be washed before the stomach and face. After bathing, the child can be wrapped tightly in a towel and held snugly in the parent's lap. This procedure can be followed by deep rubbing of arms and legs using lotion or oils. Drying and applying lotions after bathing are natural and enjoyable methods of helping the child adjust to stimuli perceived as unpleasant and develop more tolerance of bathing. Children with auditory processing problems, as frequently seen in children with autism, may best respond to bathing if they

enter the bathroom after the noise of the water filling the tub is over and bathroom fans are turned off.

Toilet Hygiene

Development of Toilet Hygiene

The developmental process toward independence in toilet activities is initiated once the child demonstrates recognition that he or she has had bladder or bowel elimination, usually at 12 to 15 months of age (Rogers & D'Eugenio, 1991). This recognition may be expressed, through verbalization or gesture, as displeasure about wet or soiled diapers. Gradually, the child becomes increasingly aware of the processes of elimination. He or she begins to show interest in the toileting of other family members and begins to associate the toilet with elimination.

Toilet training begins by teaching the child to recognize when he or she needs to eliminate and to go to the toilet to do so. Success comes over time by rewarding approximations and with the use of much prompting by the parents. The length of time to train a child from diapers to the use of a toilet varies greatly from child to child and from family to family. Most children have developed bladder and bowel control during day and night, with occasional accidents, by 4 or 5 years of age (Brown et. al., 1991). The manner in which parents and other caregivers train this occupation varies considerably, depending on the methods and the age at which the process starts.

Performance Variables That Influence Toilet Hygiene

Problems in Motor Skills

Independent toileting requires numerous motor skills that vary by gender, by the type of clothing worn, and by the facility used. The child has to be able to accomplish a series of varied motor activities. He or she has to have the balancing skills to sit safely on the toilet, shift weight to wipe, and move on and off the toilet. The child must have the active range of motion for reaching for toilet tissue, wiping the perineal area, and flushing the toilet. Prehensile skills are needed to grasp toilet tissue, wipe, and flush. Additionally, the child requires motor skills to unfasten, remove, and refasten clothing and underwear.

Children with motor-skill difficulties may have problems with the task of toileting as a result of difficulty with any of the performance skills listed above. For example, a child with trisomy 21 syndrome may have difficulty with fastening clothing, grasping toilet tissue, and wiping as a result of low muscle tone, poor bilateral coordination, and immature grasping patterns. A child with hypertonic cerebral palsy may have difficulty balancing on the toilet, wiping, and handling clothing because of spasticity in the hips, lack of trunk stability, and poor hand skills. Boys who have motor-skill difficulties and who wish to stand in front of the toilet to urinate may not be able to stand, balance, unfasten pants, and direct urine into the toilet.

Problems in Mental Functions

Numerous steps are involved in toileting, and they are completed in a specific order to ensure elimination success. Children with mental retardation or other cognitive disabilities may have difficulty remembering the steps and their order, or they may have limited focus and concentration to perform all steps in a timely manner. They may not recognize the need to eliminate until the need is urgent and convenient opportunities have passed.

Contextual Variables That Influence Toilet Hygiene

Toileting is a personal and private activity; families have differing opinions about its development and the way it is accomplished. Difficulty in bowel and bladder control can affect the child's self-esteem and body image (Erickson & McPhee, 1998). Cultural and social norms surrounding toileting and sexuality should be considered by occupational therapists working with the families of children with disabilities so that toileting interventions will be contextually appropriate for the child and the family.

Interventions for Toilet Hygiene

Improving Motor Performance Skills

Activities to improve the underlying motor-skill problems associated with toileting problems may be an important focus in occupational therapy interventions. Through a carefully developed occupational profile and intervention plan, the occupational therapist can help develop activities to improve motor skills. For example, if a child with trisomy 21 syndrome has difficulty with fastening clothing during toileting, this can be practiced at times other than toileting. Later, as the child improves this skill, it may be used in actual toileting. For a child with trunk balance instability, intervention may target this performance skill so that it may be incorporated when toileting.

The motor steps of toileting may be modified to help a child successfully accomplish toileting. Children with trunk weakness can sit backward on the toilet seat, using the toilet tank as a support for the arms and trunk as the child eliminates. Children who have balancing problems may grasp and hold toilet tissue before sitting on the toilet, thereby reducing the need to reach while sitting on the toilet seat.

An important component of toileting intervention is communication of the handling and transferring steps to the parents and other caregivers. The occupational therapist can show the parents the best techniques for clothes handling, transferring at the toilet, and cleaning the perineal area. The therapist can instruct the parents in ways to accommodate for poor balance and stability and compensate for limited range of motion and prehension skills during toileting. For example, a child with spastic diplegia may require parental assistance to pull down underwear and transfer safely to the toilet seat. An occupational therapist can show the parents the best way to hold the child's arms so that he or she can assist in pulling down underwear and how to hold on to the child's hips during transferring to ensure safety and comfort.

Using Adaptive Equipment for Toileting

Toileting should be accomplished with ease and with as little frustration as possible. The use of adaptive equipment can help achieve this goal for many children with disabilities in their home and school environments.

Equipment for Sitting and Standing Stability. When a child's sitting balance is inadequate to use a toilet safely, external assistance can be considered. After the child is on the toilet, a table may be placed in front of the toilet; the child rests his or her arms on the table to provide balance while eliminating. Balancing during elimination, transferring on and off the toilet, and handling of clothing can be aided by the use of rails or bars installed to the sides and back of the toilet. These rails or bars, which should be installed by a carpenter to ensure durability and safety, allow the child to hold on as he or she uses the toilet. Adaptive toilet seating that provides a back, sides, and armrests can be placed over the toilet. Toilet seat adaptation to make the seat smaller can help provide sitting stability. If the child has poor head control, the seat back can include head wings for lateral stability of the child's head. Toilet seat adaptations should be securely installed so that the movement on and off the toilet will not cause equipment slippage.

Small children should have adequate foot support when sitting on toilets. Foot support helps the child feel secure and can help relax tight muscles in the legs and hips, thereby aiding in elimination and cleaning. Foot rests or raised flooring surfaces around the toilet may be built or purchased; they must be safely secured to prevent tripping. The use of smaller and lower toilets, particularly in school settings, can provide foot support.

Equipment for Reaching Difficulties. The occupational therapist and caregivers may consider using equipment to compensate for reaching problems in toilet tissue and wiping. Reachers may be used to obtain tissue and wipe the perineum. The tissue dispenser can be moved to a location within the child's reach. Additionally, the use of disposable wipes that clean better than toilet tissue can be considered.

The occupational therapist, parents, and other caregivers must weigh several considerations in the use of toileting adaptive equipment, including safety, speed in use, durability, ease in cleaning, flexibility, and costs. Occupational therapists usually have access to numerous rehabilitation catalogs containing adaptive toileting equipment; such catalogs can be used to compare and evaluate the best

equipment for the needs of the child. If the equipment is for the child's school environment, its use by other children must be taken into account.

Functional Communication

Communication skills are essential to living in social groups. Communication begins with the eye contact between the parent and the neonate and develops throughout childhood. Milestones in oral and gestural communication are presented in Table 6.11. The variables that contribute to written and oral communication are complex and multifaceted. Augmentative and alternative communication (AAC) systems are available to increase a person's conversational skills or to improve graphic communication skills. When an AAC system is considered for a child, the occupational therapist is one member of the professional team that will assist in selecting, positioning for, training in, and using the system.

Table 6.11. Milestones in the Development of Communication

Age	Communication Skills	Age	Communication Skills
3 months	Quiets to voice Looks at person who is talking Reacts to tone of voice Smiles to person who is talking	18 months	Imitates environment sounds during play Retrieves objects on verbal request Uses inflection Greets familiar people with an appropriate vocalization
6 months	Repeats sounds that are imitated by a caregiver Imitates inflection Turns head when name is called Stops activity when name is called Begins to listen Requests a toy with a gesture	21 months	Identifies at least four animals Identifies 15 or more pictures of common objects Uses inflection patterns Experiments with two-word utterances
9 months	Imitates familiar two-syllable words (baba, dada) Makes gestures for "up" and "bye-bye" Responds to "no" Uses eye gaze during communication	24 months	Imitates three-syllable words Follows three-part commands Uses greetings and farewells appropriately Says "no" Uses words in play Uses words to describe remote events Uses words to request action Answers simple questions with a verbal response
12 months	Imitates two-syllable words (different sounds) Identifies three objects Responds to "give me" Takes turns		
15 months	Imitates new two-syllable words Follows simple commands Identifies most common objects when they are named Appropriately indicates "yes" or "no" in response to questions Identifies two body parts Uses words to express wants		

Note: From *The Carolina Curriculum for Infants and Toddlers With Special Needs, Third Edition,* by N. M. Johnson-Martin, S. M. Attermeier, and B. J. Hacker, 2004, Baltimore: Paul H. Brookes Publishing Company. Adapted with permission.

Performance Variables That Influence Use of AAC Systems

Augmentative and alternative communication systems are most often considered for children with moderate to severe cerebral palsy, when oral motor delays interfere with speech production. When a child has a relatively high cognitive level and severe motor problems, simple communication by gesture is inadequate and a communication method that simulates speech becomes a priority. When evaluating whether or not an AAC system is an appropriate intervention, it is important to assess motor skills (i.e., posture, mobility, and manipulation) and client factor skills (i.e., cognition). Assessment of motor and cognition skills will help the professional team decide which device will work, how the child will access it, and what level of complexity is appropriate. In addition, assessment of the cultural, social, personal, and physical contexts is essential because contextual supports and accommodations are critical to effective use of AAC systems.

Motor Skills

To access AAC systems, the client needs to be in a position that optimizes his or her ability to control the device for the length of a communication interaction. If the trunk or head is unstable, external support is critical. In evaluating the child's posture and motor skills, the occupational therapist should ask the following questions:

- Is the child's head stable and in a position that allows complete viewing of the keyboard? Is the head sufficiently stable that he or she can control eye movements to scan the keys or track the cursor?
- Are the trunk and shoulders sufficiently stable for controlled arm movement and adequate active range of arms?
- Is trunk control adequate to maintain a midline position during arm and hand movements?
- Is trunk stability sufficient that the child can maintain upright posture through a communication exchange?
- How will the child control the device (i.e., hands, head, or eyes)?

Cognitive Functions

Cognition is highly related to the client's communication interests and needs. Operation of an AAC device can require only basic skills, or it can require highly sophisticated skills. The basic skills needed to operate ACC devices successfully include alertness,

attention span, vigilance, understanding of cause and effect, ability to express preferences, ability to make choices, understanding of object or pictorial permanence, and understanding of symbolic representation.

Cognitive skills that directly relate to AAC choice include understanding symbols, categorization, sequencing, matching, and sorting (Cook & Hussey, 2002). Memory is important: The child must remember the meaning of the symbols on the keyboard, and many of the new devices require multiple steps to enter into the system and select a correct page for the topic of conversation. When an encoded or symbol system is used (and most AAC systems involve encoding) the child must remember what each symbol represents and how combinations of symbols mean different words.

Evaluation of cognition and language should include receptive and expressive language, level of problem solving, and memory; the emphasis is on the child's ability to understand and remember symbols. Children with severe cognitive disabilities who have extreme limitation in the abilities listed above may still be able to benefit from a simple AAC device (e.g., some devices have only 14 word choices). Systems appropriate for these children are those that enable the child to communicate basic needs and make simple decisions (McNaughton & Light, 1989).

Visual Functions

AAC devices require adequate visual acuity and perceptual skills. In addition, the client must be able to scan and track to follow the sequence of letters or symbols on the device. If the client has difficulty with visual scanning, the number and placement of keys must be considered. Increasing the size of the keys, increasing the contrast between the key and the background, and increasing the spacing between the keys can accommodate problems in visual acuity. Various foreground–background combinations can be tried to improve the contrast. The issues of greatest concern in visual perception are spatial relationships, form recognition and constancy, and figure ground discrimination (Cook & Hussey, 2002). Each area of visual perception has specific implications for the layout of keys and the system's configuration.

Contextual Variables That Influence Use of AAC Systems

Family Considerations

The family members' interest in and enthusiasm about technology determines whether an AAC device will work for the child. When a family is comfortable with using technology, a sophisticated device can be considered. Families who seem perplexed by technology or avoid technology as much as possible should use a simple AAC device or method. All devices require training, problem solving when they do not work, and tolerance for learning new programs and systems. All require patience to operate, and most involve some programming to update the device and to meet the child's needs appropriately.

Families that are disorganized may have difficulty maintaining the device in accessible places and keeping up with needed changes in vocabulary and required maintenance. Most often, the barriers to using augmentative communication are barriers of knowledge, because most families are unfamiliar with the equipment and need to learn how to operate it and to problem solve when the device malfunctions.

Home and School Environments

Aspects of the environment that are important to consider when evaluating for augmentative communication include how the device will be transported and how the child will be assured of consistent access to the device. If the child is mobile, a method for transporting the device is needed. The device always needs to be handled with care (e.g., it should not have liquids spilled on it). Often it is placed on the wheelchair tray; however, if the child is ambulatory, carrying the device is not always a viable option. A system for carrying the device may include placement in a book bag or hanging it on a wheeled walker. The environments in which the child will use the device may include the playground and the cafeteria, and provisions for use across environments must be made.

Social Contexts

Other children initially respond with interest to the novelty of an AAC device. After the children have become acclimated to its presence, however, they may grow impatient with the delays required to deliver a communication message using the device. Human communication occurs rapidly, at about 150 to 175 words per minute, depending on the language. A child with a disability may only produce 10 to 12 words per minute using an AAC device; the rate may be 3 to 5 words per minute for children using scanning (Cook & Hussey, 2002). Great patience is required to maintain a conversation with someone who is speaking at a rate of 3 to 12 words per minute. A conversation partner may finish sentences for the child or speak for the child without waiting for the child to initiate the communication. Users of AAC devices often adopt adaptive strategies that they implement as they are communicating with the device, including hand signals, verbalizations, or eye movements. In conversations with a user of an AAC device, the communication partner must attend to these strategies in addition to the device's synthesized speech (Bruno & Dribbon, 1998).

Interventions for Functional Communication

Designing and Selecting an AAC System

The professional team that helps a family select an AAC system must make the following decisions:

- What type of system will adequately meet the child's current communication needs?
- What system will be capable of growing with the child to meet future communication goals?
- How will the child access the system? Which selection method is most appropriate, and what type of control interface is needed?
- What skills need to be supported or developed for the child to use the system successfully?
- What are the training needs of the family, caregivers, and teachers?

A range of devices is available, but the most sophisticated device is not always the best choice. Nonelectric devices, such as picture boards and books, may be most appropriate for a new user (Musselwhite & St. Louis, 1988). In general, the advantages of nonelectric devices are that they are low cost, easily transported, easily changed and adapted, and nonthreatening and comfortable for communication partners to use (e.g., the child may use a head pointer, mouth stick, or hand to select pictures). Some disadvantages of nonelectric systems are that they do not provide an audible or visible message (e.g., on screen) and they are limited in ability to adapt to the child's expanding vocabulary.

A variety of electronic devices are available to meet the growing needs of children who have limited speech. The advantage of the current technology is that it is versatile and flexible; therefore, it is meant to grow with the child. Typically, newer devices are easier to program and reprogram, enabling the parent or teacher to regularly update the vocabulary and messages available to the child. In deciding which device to use and how to introduce it to the child, several features need to be considered:

- How will the child access the device (i.e., direct selection or scanning)?
- What vocabulary is needed? What prestored messages should be used? How much versatility in vocabulary is needed?

- What type of output does the device provide? Is the speech synthesized or digitized? Is written output provided?
- How portable is the device? Can the device be easily transported? Can it be used on a wheelchair or on other surfaces?
- Does the device include environmental controls (e.g., can it be used to operate the television or radio)? (Beukelman & Mirenda, 1998).

Children can access electronic communication devices using direct selection or scanning. In direct selection, a user points directly to the key or symbol. The child targets his or her choice and then selects it by pointing or pressing. Although hands are most often used, the head can be used with a head pointer. If the child appears to have skills to use a direct-selection device but those skills are not very strong, adaptations may be made to improve accuracy and endurance. Increasing the child's postural support, adjusting the height or angle of the device, or using a variety of tools for access (e.g., a head stick or hand stick) may enable the child to use this method successfully.

In scanning, the child is presented with a display that is sequentially scanned by a cursor or light. The child selects a symbol or key by hitting a switch or clicking the mouse when the cursor or light reaches it. Various scanning methods are available, depending on the number of symbols that the child requires for everyday communication. In item-by-item scanning, the cursor moves to all possible symbol choices one at a time. Item-by-item methods are simple but slow; therefore, this method is not feasible when many choices are available. To increase the rate of selection, row–column scanning methods can be used. In row–column scanning, the rows are lighted sequentially, and the child selects the row with the desired item in it. Then the cursor scans the columns sequentially and the child selects the item when the cursor reaches it. Most new devices make available both direct selection and scanning, giving the family and child options regarding access.

Although scanning can be accomplished with minimal motor skill, it requires controlled visual-tracking skills, attention skills, and an understanding of sequencing (Cook & Hussey, 2002). Scanning requires more time than direct selection, but it gives the user more options for access. In designing the system, a range of control interface or switches can be used to make selections; the goal is to provide optimal accuracy and speed. The following features should be considered in selecting a switch for a child:

- Type and size of activating surface
- Force and pressure required to activate the switch
- Range of motion required
- Alternatives in positioning the device
- Sensory feedback provided by the switch.

Examples of switches that can be used with AAC systems are sip and puff, joystick, and proximity switches (for more information, go to www.ablenetinc.com or www.tashinc.com). Figure 6.5 shows a dual-press switch. Innovations in scanning allow the child to make selections using wireless infrared pointing systems that can be attached

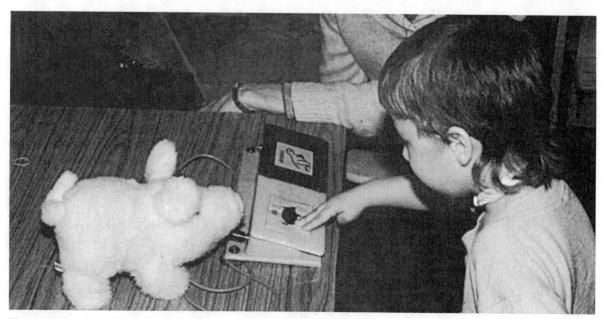

Figure 6.5. A dual switch can be introduced to facilitate decision making and turn taking.

to the head. Switch selection should be based on what the child can use reliably with a minimal effort for long periods of time.

Positioning the Device and the Child

Once a device has been selected, the occupational therapist offers recommendations as to how the device can be accessed throughout the day (Figure 6.6). If the child spends much of the day in a wheelchair that has a tray, it may be appropriate to mount the device and switch, if needed, on the tray or wheelchair. The mounting of the device can determine whether the child is able to use it efficiently or independently. The mounting can include hardware such as clamps or flexible mounting systems (e.g., gooseneck arms with clamps). The device should be mounted so that the child has adequate range of motion, strength, visual field, and motor control to operate it. Most powered wheelchairs allow for a mount that holds an AAC device that can easily be adjusted and positioned for optimal viewing and access. Mounting the device at an angle is usually ideal for viewing and for hand control. The child's wheelchair must be considered at the time of ordering an AAC device so that an integrated system can be developed that considers device interface with environmental control units, the wheelchair, and computers.

Positioning should consider the child's optimal posture for head, arm, and hand control as well as issues related to endurance and effort. An optimal seating position offers maximum postural stability and alignment. In most cases, the feet should be flat, the hips should flexed at 90°, and the trunk should be in good alignment. Correct posture can be maintained with straps, trays, and footrests.

Enhancing the Child's Performance With the Device

To help the child generalize communication skills, it is important that he or she consistently use the AAC device in home, school, and community environments. By extension, use of the device in a range of contexts is needed for skill development. The AAC device can be modified to match the skill levels of the user, and a variety of access methods should be explored when first attempting use.

A primary concern in establishing an AAC system is the accuracy of arm movement for selecting the keys. Accuracy requires both eye–hand coordination (hitting the correct key) and timing (particularly when a scanning method is used and the child must hit a switch when the cursor signals the correct letter). It is also important to evaluate speed of movement to determine the most efficient method of communication. If the child's movements are de-

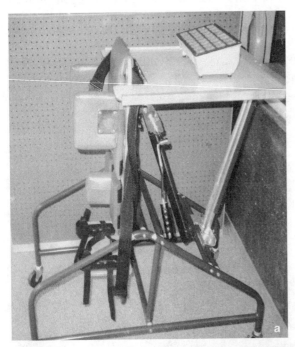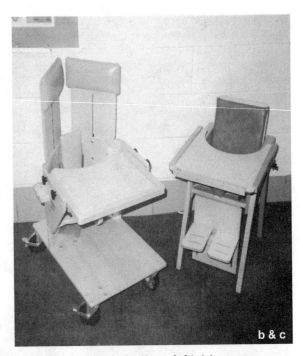

Figure 6.6. Options for positioning when using an augmentative device include (from left) (a) a prone stander, (b) a corner chair, and (c) a Rifton child's chair.

layed, then methods of selecting individual letters to spell words become impractical for producing conversational speech.

Generally, the child's arm and hand control the device and determine the type and size of keyboard that can be used. When hand movements are poorly controlled, the keys can be enlarged or a key guard can be used with the device. When hand strength is weak, a membrane keyboard can enable the child to select items using minimal pressure. Various keyboard designs can accommodate limited range of arm movement or excessive arm movement.

If the point of access is the head or eyes, the range, speed, and accuracy of head and eye movements must be evaluated. Generally, methods of access using the head and eyes require visual scanning. Therefore, timing and accuracy are critical to establishing the most practical method of communication. Sometimes a hand or head pointer device can improve accuracy; a key guard may be helpful for children who have difficulty with control or hand stability.

Integrating the AAC System Into the Home and Classroom

An AAC device becomes fully integrated into the child's daily life when it is accepted in all environments and understood by all communication partners. Because communication needs are constant, the device should always be in close proximity to the child. Extended downtime and repair time are unacceptable to the child and his or her communication partners. Therefore, good-quality devices should be obtained.

One important focus of the occupational therapist's intervention is to help integrate use of the device into the child's daily life (Figure 6.7). All the child's communication partners need to support the child's use of the system. The occupational therapist helps parents, teachers, and aides learn to operate and program the device. All communication partners should be able to solve problems so that they can prevent device failure and periods of disuse. The occupational therapist can provide initial instruction and ongoing consultation so that all caregivers and teachers understand the child's skill level, how the device operates, the child's working vocabulary, and the optimal setup for using the device. By assessing use of the device in a variety of environments, the professional team can solve problems related to device setup and environmental barriers and determine how the people present in each environment can promote efficient use of the device. Daily caregivers play a critical

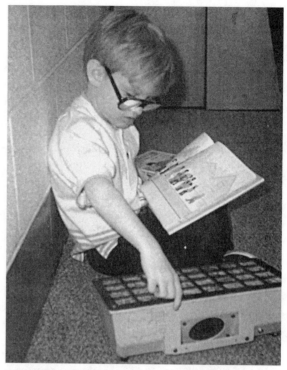

Figure 6.7. The Introtalker® communication device uses direct selection (the child touches the appropriate cell, and the device emits a word or phrase). *Note.* **For more information, contact Prentki-Romich, Wooster, OH 44691.**

role in ensuring that the child has immediate access to the device and that assistance is provided as needed.

Because even the most proficient user produces communication that is slower than normal speech, the partners must adapt the pace and rhythm to that of a natural turn-taking interaction. Patience and attentiveness beyond that required in normal conversation are necessary. It may be tempting to speak for the child rather than allow him or her to use the device. Knowing the child's vocabulary and communication skills allows the therapist and teacher to provide an optimal amount of assistance and support without communicating for the child.

As much as possible, the child's skills should be developed in natural communication experiences with peers or family members. It is important that the communication experiences are meaningful and that ongoing efforts are made to create a vocabulary and a system that enable the child to communicate at a level that matches his or her cognitive skills. The case study of Amy illustrates one type of outcome that can be realized when augmentative communication is successfully implemented.

Case Study 6.3. Amy's First AAC System

Amy was 4 years old when an AAC device was considered. She had multiple disabilities, including total blindness, cerebral palsy, and cognitive delays. She was fed with a gastrostomy tube and used only three or four sounds to indicate pleasure or displeasure. She did not sustain interaction with any of the preschool staff. She rolled from place to place, primarily away from those who attempted to hold her, as she had extreme hypersensitivity to touch. She had no opportunities for decision making, although she became highly resistant when handled or when held in a sitting position. She had approximately six signs that she used with family members, "love," "mom," "dad," "sis," "bye-bye," and "no." Her parents were highly supportive of and motivated for her to communicate with them and with her peers.

After an evaluation by an augmentative communication team, an Introtalker® with four programmed messages was introduced. The keys were identified by different textures that she was known to tolerate: corduroy, a coin, and velvet. Amy quickly became consistent in locating the message keys. Because she lacked sitting balance and had poor tolerance for being in her wheelchair, the Introtalker® was placed on the floor and she rolled to it, accessing it in a side-lying position. She had greater control in her left arm and hand and was able to locate the keys quickly by systematically touching the device with that hand. Within a month of receiving the device, she began to request it with grunts. Her use of the messages was appropriate to the situation. Within several months, the device was adapted to include 12 spaces covered with 12 different textures. She indicated "want," "down," "stop," "want music," "want mom," "want up," "love," and "want sis." The classroom staff was so excited that they could now communicate with Amy that they made every opportunity for her to use her device. After 2 years of almost no communication, Amy was able to indicate what she wanted and to make simple choices in play and daily activities.

Amy became a different child with her new communication ability, and she was more willing to participate in other classroom activities. She maintained a more positive affect and began to seek interaction. She began to laugh and giggle in the classroom and to participate more in circle and group time. The communication device was always by her side, as she learned to roll holding onto the device, and her peers became interested in using it with her. By the time Amy entered school, she was using her device with more than 30 messages programmed on different overlays.

Functional Mobility

Development of Functional Mobility

Children become mobile at an early age. Purposeful rolling often begins at 6–7 months of age, and crawling or pivoting on the abdomen begins by 7 months. Mobility milestones of the first 5 years are listed in Table 6.12. With these first forms of mobility, a child learns about the environment and begins to understand the sensory qualities of the environment as well as perceptual concepts such as depth, direction, space, and body scheme (Deitz, Swinth & White, 2002). As children become mobile, they learn about the properties of space and develop rules about exploring their environments. Studies have demonstrated that the development of mobility is related to the development of cognitive and social skills (Butler, 1997). Specific goals that can be achieved through mobility include spatial awareness, increased speed and distance, perception of directionality, and greater participation in activities

Table 6.12. Typical Development of Mobility

Age	Mobility Milestone
3–4 months	Rolls accidentally
6–7 months	Rolls in both directions Rolls sequentially and segmentally
7 months	Crawls forward on belly
8–9 months	Creeps on hands and knees Cruises sideways
11 months	Walks with one hand held Cruises in either direction
15 months	Walks independently, stopping and starting Creeps up stairs
18 months	Walks independently, seldom falls Runs stiffly Walks up stairs while holding on Walks down stairs while holding on
24 months	Runs well Walks up stairs without support Jumps down from step

(Chiulli, Corradi-Scalise, & Donatelli-Schultheiss, 1988). The development of independent mobility seems to provide the child with a sense of mastery over the environment that is critical to self-esteem and self-image.

Performance Variables That Influence Mobility

Motor Skills

Children who have motor disabilities often require devices to achieve independent mobility. Wheelchair mobility should be considered for children with limitations in strength (e.g., muscular dystrophy or myotonia), paralysis (e.g., myelomeningocele), or poor motor control (e.g., cerebral palsy). A child with limited lower-extremity strength or control and adequate upper-extremity strength and control may be a candidate for a self-propelled chair. When a child lacks postural and arm control, a transport chair, stroller, or powered mobility device should be considered.

In all types of wheelchairs, seating for optimal postural alignment and control is critical. Seating components (e.g., adapted cushions, lateral and head supports, strapping) ensure that the child is comfortable, is in good alignment for seeing the environment and functioning within it, and has an even distribution of weight. Children with severe or multiple disabilities or limited strength almost always need seating components that assist with postural stabilization and alignment. Appropriate seating generally allows for optimal control of arms and eyes as well as good respiration and skin integrity (Stoller, 1998).

Cognitive and Visual Functions

If children are to move purposefully and safely through their environments with mobility devices, they must be able to think and reason. In particular, powered mobility requires that a child can follow instructions, understand indirect cause and effect, comprehend directions involving location (i.e., directionality), and show judgment (Currie, Hardwick, & Marburger, 1998). Therefore, a certain level of cognition (e.g., capacity between 18 months and 2 years) is needed before use of a mobility device can be considered. When children are provided with powered mobility and become independent in mobility, they show increased self-initiated movement (Deitz, Swinth, & White, 2002), and they may make gains in cognition and demonstrate increased motivation to explore and interact with the environment.

Candidates for self-propelled or powered mobility devices also must have sufficient visual acuity to direct the chair. Visual acuity and perceptual dysfunctions may significantly limit a child's ability to control and direct a wheelchair and may eliminate powered mobility as an option.

Contextual Variables That Influence Mobility

A family's cultural values influence its acceptance of a mobility device. In families that greatly value independence, the idea of a self-propelled or powered wheelchair is enthusiastically accepted. Families that value interdependence may consider a wheelchair unnecessary and a disruption to their family's interaction. These families may choose to carry the child or assist the child in walking.

Family members may be concerned about the appearance of the child in a wheelchair. The wheelchair conveys the message that the child has a disability and may carry a stigma. To deemphasize the child's motor disability and nonambulatory status, parents may opt to use a stroller for a number of years.

Accessibility of the child's environments is important to successful wheelchair use. Parents are initially unprepared for their child's use of a wheelchair, so the home may lack accessibility. All the child's environments need to be assessed for accessibility to ensure success in using wheeled mobility. Transport of the wheelchair needs to be considered, because it may be a large or heavy piece of equipment.

Interventions for Functional Mobility

Although the wheelchair is the most common solution to mobility limitation, a range of devices should be considered for children. Play toys on wheels (e.g., carts or scooter boards) and strollers may be the child's first transportation devices (Swinth, 1997). Powered mobility is an option when a child is unable to propel a wheelchair manually, or it can be an appropriate choice for an additional chair when a child must independently propel long distances, as in changing classrooms in middle or high school.

Choosing the type of mobility device that best matches the child's skills and needs is a team and family decision (Currie et al., 1998). As described above, the critical variables include the child's motor skills; the child's visual perception; the child's cognition; the family's values, resources, and concerns; and the child's environments. These variables are discussed below as they relate to the following mobility devices: strollers and transport chairs, self-propelled wheelchairs, and powered chairs (including scooters).

Strollers and Transport Chairs

Child Considerations. The first mobility device of the young child is usually a stroller, because it is lightweight and practical for community travel. Strollers with firm seats and backs that can be adjusted to different angles provide greater postural support and are appropriate for young children with trunk instability. Large, sturdy strollers offer a convenient means of transportation. If the child has poor trunk and head control, a seat insert can fit into the stroller to provide additional external support. Commercial seat inserts offer secure strapping systems, footrests, and lateral supports. When the child reaches the age and size at which a stroller is no longer appropriate or no longer offers adequate support, another mobility device must be considered. If the child is unable to self-propel, a transport chair is recommended (see Figure 6.8.) Transport chairs can be customized to fit the needs of the child by selecting a variety of features that assist in maintaining postural stability and alignment. The options available include head and trunk supports, wedged or contoured seats, various strapping systems, and lap trays. Complete modular systems with replaceable and adjustable components can be modified to assist the child. These features allow for correct trunk and pelvic alignment and for postural stability (Bergen, 1990; Cook & Hussey, 2002). The entire seat tilts from upright to various reclining angles, offering the child a variety of functional positions. The upright position is selected for most fine-motor and school activities. The semireclined position may be appropriate for daily activities and can be used intermittently throughout the day to provide the child with rest in a relaxed position. All parts of the chair can be adjusted to improve the fit and to increase the child's function.

Family and Environmental Considerations. Parents may prefer strollers because a child in a stroller appears "normal" and does not carry the stigma of a child in a wheelchair. A stroller is also less expensive and more lightweight than a transport wheelchair. If the stroller provides security and good positioning, it can be a temporary option for the family before purchasing a wheelchair.

A stroller collapses easily and can be transported in a car, making it ideal for shopping, public events, or appointments away from home. The stiff structure of the stroller base does not allow for a smooth and comfortable ride over rough terrain,

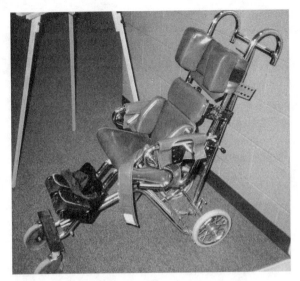

Figure 6.8. A transport chair can tilt at its base.

however. Rough terrain also may damage its structure and wheelbase. The stroller is most appropriate for use outdoors on smooth surfaces. Most strollers do not support trays and are usually fixed in a semireclined position, thus limiting their functional use in the classroom or home.

Although transport chairs are much more expensive than strollers, they are more durable and versatile, and they can grow with the child. These chairs and their special features allow for good fit and positioning of the child's posture. They also offer the child security and stability during mealtime and classroom activities, freeing the parents and teachers from the need to provide postural support.

Modern transport chairs are lighter than the earlier models, but they remain fairly heavy; this weight may present a problem for a parent who has physical limitations. Transport chairs fit children well and provide optimal postural support, so older children can stay in them for extended periods of time. This feature may be helpful during social and meal times, especially if the tilting feature is used to help the child shift his or her weight on the buttocks.

Transport chairs can be placed in most cars' front seats by collapsing the wheelbase; however, they do not always fit into compact cars. They also are difficult to lift into SUVs and vans. The family should evaluate how well the chair fits into the family automobile before purchase.

Transport chairs are versatile in that they serve as functional chairs within the home and classroom. They are usually sturdy and provide a smooth ride over uneven terrain. The tilting feature offers the child an optimal view of the room. Because of the slanting base of four small wheels, however, transport chairs require more space in the classroom and are more difficult to maneuver than small wheelchairs. Although transport chairs do not easily fit at a table, they may be ordered with a tray. Large trays with bordering rims make ideal surfaces for play, but they are sometimes awkward in small spaces.

Self-Propelled Wheelchairs

Child Considerations. The variety of manual (self-propelled) wheelchairs has increased dramatically in recent years. A manual wheelchair is an option for children who have the arm strength, control, and endurance for self-propulsion and who have the cognitive, perceptual, and visual skills to direct a chair within their environment. Most manual wheelchairs are lightweight and easily handled and transported. Small chairs that are low to the ground match the need of young children to be at the height of their peers. Small wheelchairs may not have the maneuverability of large chairs, but they are most appropriate for the classroom environments of young children.

Regular-size wheelchairs offer a choice of seat and back sizes and shapes and should be ordered to fit the child with projected growth considered. Manual sport or ultralight wheelchairs are about half the weight of a standard chair (Cook & Hussey, 2002). The amount of support the chair provides can be adjusted by adding or eliminating lateral supports, trays, and strapping. Footrests, a firm back and seat, and armrests are standard items and are available with different features and functions. Armrests can be adjusted to change the height of a lap tray for various activities. For example, the tray may be raised during self-feeding to support the hand-to-mouth movement and then lowered when the child is engaged in arts and crafts. Most manufacturers also offer a variety of back and seat designs and dimensions. Companies specializing in designing and fabricating contour seating and wheelchair equipment may also customize seating. Ultralight chairs do not have as many seating options.

Family and Environmental Considerations. Self-propelled wheelchairs, as with transport chairs and strollers, come in various weights, but they are typically lightweight and are easily collapsed and lifted into a car. Cost is a consideration, particularly when evaluating the purchase of optional features. Appearance of the chair is important, and chairs are available in a range of colors and styles. The space available in the home, community locations, child care center, and school is a factor in wheelchair choice.

Powered Chairs

Child Considerations. Children who do not have the upper-extremity strength or control necessary to propel a chair but have the cognitive, problem-solving, and perceptual skills to plan and direct chair movement from one location to another generally are candidates for powered mobility. Advancements in technology allow children with severe physical disabilities to use this option (Wright-Ott & Egilson, 2001).

Powered mobility devices also can be appropriate for children who can walk or propel a chair short distances but who have limited strength and endurance and cannot independently manage long distances. Powered mobility devices may be a choice for an older child who, on entrance to high school or college, must cover long distances daily, sometimes over rough terrain. Options for the child who would benefit from powered mobility are as follows:

- *Scooters.* Motorized scooters typically are used as additional systems for long distances by children who have adequate upper-body control to sit with minimal trunk support. Although scooters are usually considered a vehicle for community travel, they are available in a front-wheel drive, lightweight model that has enhanced maneuverability for indoor use (Wright-Ott & Egilson, 2001).
- *Standard Powered Chairs.* The child can control or drive a powered chair using a variety of input devices. Stoller (1998) listed a variety of methods to activate switches, including physical contact, muscle contraction, air pressure, light reception (i.e., infrared light switches), sound, gravitational changes (i.e., mercury switches), and magnetic fields (i.e, magnetic switches). The most typical control for a power chair is the proportional joystick. The child moves the joystick in the direction he or she wants the chair to go. The chair's speed is proportional to the amount of joystick deflection. Digital control, using a microswitch, provides the child with less control over direction and starting and stopping the chair than the proportional joystick, but speed is usually programmed into the switch system. Although switch systems offer less control, they also require less control. These switch systems include a press pad, arm slot, and individual switches (Cook & Hussey, 2002).

Switches enable the child to control the chair through sip and puff or by the head, knee, arm, foot, or other body parts using different mounting of switches. The child with fair motor control but poor strength and endurance can easily operate and direct a chair using microswitch control. When the child has poor control but forceful movement, the switch can also correct for the degree of force by responding with a programmed speed and a limited choice of directions. Accurate knowledge of vision and cognition abilities can guide the practitioner in the selection of an appropriate control interface for the chair and in training the child to use the powered mobility device.

Family and Environmental Considerations. Although powered chairs may offer the child the first and only opportunity for independent mobility, a number of variables must be considered by the family before investing in this type of device. If the powered chair is an additional mobility device for the child who already has a manual chair, the cost of an additional chair may not be covered by insurance. Because powered chairs are heavy, transporting them may require a van and a lift, even when the battery pack can be detached and lifted separately. Moreover, the home environment must be made accessible, with wide spaces to accommodate the chair's limited maneuverability. The expenses of powered mobility may be unmanageable for families and must be considered.

Some authors have advocated use of powered mobility for the young child (i.e., ages 18 to 24 months) who is immobile (Butler, 1997; Deitz et al., 2002; Trefler & Taylor, 1988). Although it may be developmentally appropriate to obtain a powered mobility device for a child before 24 months of age, the family may not yet be ready to accept the need for mobility assistance. At this early age, the family may be reluctant to accept this physical symbol of the child's disability. In addition, given the expense of the chair, the growth and development of the child should be considered when selecting the size and features. The powered chair needs ongoing maintenance and may require relatively frequent repair. The family must be willing to accept this responsibility.

Positioning and Fitting the Child to the Chair

Functional use of self-propelled wheelchairs or powered mobility devices requires correct positioning and seating. Occupational therapists and other team members evaluate the child's neuromotor, sensory, and orthopedic status to make recommendations regarding seating (Currie et al., 1998; Wright-Ott &

Egilson, 2001). The goals when recommending and selecting seating are to promote normal muscle tone while inhibiting abnormal or primitive reflexes, to prevent the development or progression of orthopedic deformities, to increase functional skills, to accommodate impaired sensation, to ensure safety, and to provide comfort. An extensive range of commercial seating systems is available (Cook & Hussey, 2002).

Taylor (1987) describes three components of evaluation for seating and positioning:

- Functional assessment of the child that includes his or her daily activities and educational goals
- Evaluation of specific positions by observing the child in different positions or on a seating simulator
- Selection of a seating system with appropriate material, size, angle, and shape.

Trunk support and pelvic alignment are critical to positioning in the chair. A child's pelvic tilt, lateral symmetry, and rotational position all must be evaluated in determining seating equipment (Currie et al., 1998). In general, the pelvis should be in neutral alignment, the back of the buttocks should be next to the chair back, and the knees should be bent at least at 90° (Stoller, 1998). Straps for the trunk can provide support and stability when the child lacks postural control. Straps that cross the chest in a *V*, *H*, or *X* design can assist with alignment, upright posture, and maintenance of posture when fatigue becomes a factor. Straps that originate on the chair back below the level of the shoulders and fit over the top of the shoulders help to effectively maintain postural alignment.

The lower extremities should be well supported, with neutral rotation at the hips and usually 90° of flexion at the hips, knees, and ankles. This positioning promotes neutral pelvic alignment and prevents posterior pelvic tilt and lower-extremity extension. Contoured seats prevent the child from scooting forward in the chair (e.g., in children with strong extensor tone).

Additional features may be added to the chair when shoulder retraction and head control are issues. Shoulder protraction wings encourage midline positioning of the upper extremities. Head supports can assist the child in maintaining his or her head at midline. When head control is poor and the head is frequently pulled into flexion, head straps or a cervical collar can be considered; however, such devices must be selected and used with care because the head may slip into an undesirable and unsafe position, thus increasing, rather than helping, poor neck alignment. A better choice may be to tilt the seating unit backward, thereby allowing gravity to assist in maintaining head alignment against the chair's back.

Functional Use of the Mobility Device in the Child's Daily Activities

Occupational therapists often focus on improving function while the child is seated in the chair (Deitz, Jaffe, Wolf, Massagli, & Anson, 1991). One primary method is to give the child a tray surface to support hand use. Trays are standard features with transport chairs and some powered chairs. Self-propelled chairs may come with desk arms to accommodate sitting at a table.

Wheelchair trays can provide a surface for eating, working on school or vocational tasks, or playing games. The tray may also provide a surface for a communication device or a computer. AAC devices usually remain with the child; therefore, mounting them on the wheelchair tray is ideal. The tray has the additional benefits of helping the child maintain an upright posture by supporting the midtrunk and maintaining the upper extremities in a functional position (Colangelo, 1999). Other performance issues to be assessed with the child in the chair are as follows:

- Can the child reach with adequate range to manage the environment (e.g., turn faucets on and off; write on the blackboard; and reach shelves, the floor, and a light switch)?
- Can the child turn the chair and maneuver it through rooms and hallways?
- Can the child propel or drive up to a table or desk and position him- or herself comfortably for tabletop activities?
- Can the child propel or drive the chair over grass, rough terrain, and other outdoor surfaces in the environment (Wolf, Massagli, Jaffe, & Deitz, 1991)?
- Can the child transfer in and out of the chair independently?
- Can the child move the chair into close proximity of classmates and peers to participate in school and play activities?
- Can the child transport a backpack and other school supplies while in the wheelchair?

The child, family, occupational therapist, and other team members can identify the limitations in the environment that require accommodation. Together, the team can help the child overcome these performance limitations. In some cases, the physical environment can be adapted. For example, table heights can be adjusted and home or school modifications can be made. The child may become independent in transferring into the chair with adapted environmental supports and modified techniques. Additionally, the social and personal contexts may be modified. For example, the teacher can modify the sequencing of group games at recess to allow the child in the wheelchair to participate. The child can be supported to play in a small group by placing a table game on the wheelchair tray with friends seated around. These contextual changes allow the child using a mobility device to meet the goals of participation in desired occupations.

Summary

Children with developmental disabilities often require assistance with their occupations, such as eating, dressing, bathing, toileting, communication, and mobility. The child's ability to achieve independence and mastery in these occupations is important to self-esteem. Autonomy also can enhance the child's interaction with family members, school educators, and peers. Occupational therapists are particularly skilled and resourceful in enhancing the child's occupations by analyzing the involved performance skills, patterns, and client factors, and by maintaining a perspective of the child's occupation as it relates to his or her culture, family, home, and school. Occupational therapists work closely with family members and other disciplines to ensure that a consistent, comprehensive approach is implemented that places the child's and family's priorities first, enables the child, and involves appropriate school and community resources. They recognize that occupational performance issues of children with developmental disabilities are often long-term and sometimes even lifelong.

This chapter has described many of the variables in the child's home and school environment that can affect performance in areas of occupation. An approach that considers the child, the family, and the environmental contexts enables the occupational therapy practitioner to offer a therapeutic approach that is based on a comprehensive, holistic understanding of the child. This understanding creates opportunities for increased mastery of the important occupations of children.

Study Questions

1. What are the environmental contexts that should be evaluated by an occupational therapist to determine their relationship to the child's success in school?

2. What are the performance skills, client factors, and contextual factors that influence eating skills of children with disabilities?

3. How can sensory-processing problems cause difficulty in dressing and bathing?

4. What interventions improve toileting for children with problems in motor skills?

5. What recommendations should the occupational therapist make for selecting an AAC device for the child with poor motor and communication skills?

6. What is the role of the occupational therapist in helping to integrate the use of an AAC device into a child's school life?

7. What variables need to be considered when recommending powered mobility to the family of a young child?

References

American Occupational Therapy Association. (1999). *Occupational therapy services for children and youth under the Individuals With Disabilities Education Act* (2nd ed.). Bethesda, MD: Author.

American Occupational Therapy Association. (2002). Occupational therapy practice framework: Domain and process. *American Journal of Occupational Therapy, 56,* 609–639.

Barnes, K. (1991). Modification of the physical environment. In C. Christiansen & C. Baum (Eds.), *Occupational therapy: Overcoming human performance deficits* (pp. 701–746). Thorofare, NJ: Slack.

Bergen, A. F. (1990). *Positioning for function: Wheelchairs and other assistive devices.* Valhalla, NY: Valhalla Rehabilitation Publications.

Beukelman, D. R., & Mirenda, P. (1998). *Augmentative and alternative communication: Management of severe communication disorders in children and adults* (2nd ed.). Baltimore: Brookes.

Boehme, R. (1988). *Improving upper body control.* Tucson, AZ: Therapy SkillBuilders.

Brown, S., D'Eugenio, D., Drews, J., Haskin, B., Lynch, E., Moersch, M., et al. (1991). *Developmental programming for infants and young children: Vol. 5. Preschool developmental profile.* Ann Arbor: University of Michigan Press.

Bruno, J., & Dribbon, M. (1998). Outcomes in AAC: Evaluating the effectiveness of a parent training program. *Augmentative and Alternative Communication, 14*(2), 59–70.

Bundy, A., Lane, S., & Murray, E. (2002). *Sensory integration theory and practice* (2nd ed.). Philadelphia: F. A. Davis.

Butler, C. (1997). Wheelchair toddlers. In J. Furumasu (Ed.), *Pediatric powered mobility: Developmental perspectives, technical issues, clinical approaches* (pp. 1–6). Arlington, VA: RESNA.

Case-Smith, J., & Humphry, R. (2001). Feeding interventions. In J. Case-Smith (Ed.), *Occupational therapy for children* (4th ed., pp. 453–488). St. Louis: Mosby.

Chan, S. (1998). Families with Asian roots. In E. Lynch & M. Hanson (Eds.), *Developing cross cultural competence* (2nd ed., pp. 251–354). Baltimore: Brookes.

Chiulli, C., Corradi-Scalise, D., & Donatelli-Schultheiss, L. (1988). Powered mobility vehicles as aids in independent locomotion for young children. *Physical Therapy, 68,* 997–999.

Clemente, C., Baines, J., Shinebourne, E., & Stein, A. (2001) Are infant behavioural feeding difficulties associated with congenital heart disease? *Child: Case, Health, and Development, 27*(1), 47–59.

Colangelo, C. A. (1999). Biomechanical frame of reference. In P. Kramer & J. Hinojosa (Eds.), *Frames of reference for pediatric occupational therapy* (2nd ed., pp. 257–322). Philadelphia: Lippincott Williams & Wilkins.

Cook, A. M., & Hussey, S. M. (2002). *Assistive technologies: Principles and practice* (2nd ed.). St. Louis: Mosby.

Coster, W., Deeney, T., Haltiwanger, J., & Haley, S. (1998). *School Function Assessment: User's manual.* San Antonio, TX: Psychological Corporation.

Currie, D., Hardwick, K., & Marburger, R. (1998). Wheelchair prescription and adaptive seating. In J. DeLisa et al. (Eds.), *Rehabilitation medicine: Principles and practice* (3rd ed., pp. 763–789). Philadelphia: Lippincott.

Danella, E., & Vogtle, L. (1992). Neurodevelopmental treatment for the young child with cerebral palsy. In J. Case-Smith & C. Pehoski (Eds.), *Development of hand skills in the child* (pp. 91–110). Rockville, MD: American Occupational Therapy Association.

Deitz, J., Jaffe, K. M., Wolf, L. S., Massagli, T. L., & Anson, D. (1991). Pediatric power wheelchairs: Evaluation of function in the home and school environments. *Assistive Technology, 3,* 24–31.

Deitz, J., Swinth, T., & White, O. (2002). Powered mobility and preschoolers with complex developmental delays. *American Journal of Occupational Therapy, 56,* 86–96.

Dressing techniques for the cerebral palsied child. (1954). *American Journal of Occupational Therapy, 8,* 8–10, 37–38.

Dunn, W. (1999). *Sensory Profile: User's manual.* San Antonio, TX: Psychological Corporation.

Einarsson-Backes, L. M., Deitz, J., Price, R., Glass, R., & Hayes, T. (1994). Effect of oral support on feeding efficiency in preterm infants. *American Journal of Occupational Therapy, 48,* 490–498.

Erickson, R., & McPhee, M. (1998). Clinical evaluation. In J. Delisa et al. (eds.) *Rehabilitation medicine: Principles and practice* (3rd ed.). Philadelphia: Lippincott.

Frost, J. (1992). *Play and playscapes.* Albany, NY: Delmar.

Furuno, S., O'Reilly, K., Hosaka, C., Inatsuka, T., Allman, T., & Zeisloft. (1994). *Hawaii Early Learning Profile, Revised.* Palo Alto, CA: VORT.

Gisel, E. G., Applegate-Ferrante, T., Benson, J., & Bosma, J. F. (1995). Effect of oral sensorimotor treatment on measures of growth, eating efficiency, and aspiration in the dysphagic child with cerebral palsy. *Developmental Medicine and Child Neurology, 37,* 528–543.

Hall, R. V., & Hall, M. (1998). *How to use time-out* (2nd ed.). Austin, TX: PRO-ED.

Hanft, B., and Place, P. (1996). *The consulting therapist.* Tucson, AZ: Therapy SkillBuilders.

Hoffman, O., Hemmingsson, H., & Kielhofner, G. (1999). *A user's manual for the School Setting Interview (SSI).* Chicago: University of Illinois.

Holmstrand, K. E. (2003). *Guidelines for safe, accessible playgrounds.* Retrieved November 30, 2003, from http://www.familyeducation.com/article/0,1120,1–1390.html.

Humphry, R. (1991). Impact of feeding problems on the parent-infant relationship. *Infants and Young Children, 3*(3), 30–38.

Humphry, R., & Rourk, M. H. (1991). When an infant has a feeding problem. *Occupational Therapy Journal of Research, 11*(2), 106–120.

Kelly, J. F., & Barnard, K. E. (2000). Assessment of parent-child interaction: Implications for early intervention. In S. Meisels & J. P. Shonkoff (Eds.). *Handbook of early intervention* (2nd ed., pp. 278–302). Cambridge, MA: Syndicate of the Press of the University of Cambridge.

Klein, M. D. (1988). *Pre-dressing skills.* Tucson, AZ: Therapy SkillBuilders.

Klein, M. D., & Delaney, T. A. (1994). *Feeding and nutrition for the child with special needs.* Tucson, AZ: Therapy SkillBuilders.

Law, M. (2002). Participation in the occupations of everyday life, 2002 Distinguished Scholar Lecture. *American Journal of Occupational Therapy, 56,* 640–649.

Logemann, J. A. (1997). *Evaluation and treatment of swallowing disorders* (2nd ed.). Austin, TX: PRO-ED.

Lynch, E., & Hanson, M. (Eds.). (1998). *Developing cross-cultural competence* (2nd ed.). Baltimore: Brookes.

McNaughton, D., & Light, J. (1989). Teaching facilitators to support the communication skills of an adult with severe cognitive disabilities: A case study. *Augmentative and Alternative Communication, 5,* 35–41.

Morris, S. E., & Klein, M. D. (2000). *Pre-feeding skills* (2nd ed.). Tucson, AZ: Therapy SkillBuilders.

Musselwhite, C., & St. Louis, K. (1988). *Communication programming for persons with severe handicaps: Vocal and augmentative strategies.* Boston: College-Hill Press.

Rogers, S., & D'Eugenio, D. (1991). *Developmental programming for infants and young children: Vol. 1. Assessment and application.* Ann Arbor: University of Michigan Press.

Roley, S. S., Blanche, E. I., & Schaaf, R. C. (2001). *Understanding the nature of sensory integration with diverse populations.* Tucson, AZ: Therapy SkillBuilders.

Scherzer, A., & Tscharnuter, I. (1991). *Early diagnosis and therapy in cerebral palsy.* New York: Marcel Dekker.

Schulze, P. A., Harwood, R. L., & Schoelmerich, A. (2001). Feeding practices and expectations among middle-class Anglo and Puerto Rican mothers of 12-month-old infants. *Journal of Cross-Cultural Psychology, 32,* 397–406.

Shepherd, J. (2001). Self-care and adaptations for independent living. In J. Case-Smith (Ed.), *Occupational therapy for children* (4th ed.). St. Louis: Mosby.

Stoller, L. (1998). *Low-tech assistive devices: A handbook for the school setting.* Framingham, MA: Therapro.

Swinth, Y. (1997). Technology for young children with disabilities. In J. Case-Smith (Ed.), *Pediatric occupational therapy and early intervention* (pp. 277–300). Andover, MA: Andover Medical Publishers.

Taylor, S. J. (1987). Evaluating the client with physical disabilities for wheelchair seating. *American Journal of Occupational Therapy, 41,* 711–716.

Thousand, J., Villa, R., & Nevin, A. (Eds.). (1994). *Creativity and collaborative learning: A practical guide to empowering students and teachers.* Baltimore: Brookes.

Townsend, S., Crey, P., Hollins, N., Helfrich, C., Blondis, M., Hoffman, A., et al. (1999). *A user's manual for Occupational Therapy Psychosocial Assessment of Learning (OT PAL).* Chicago: University of Illinois.

Trefler, E., & Taylor, S. J. (1988). Power mobility for severely physically disabled children: Evaluation and provision practices. In K. M. Jaffe (Ed.), *Childhood power mobility: Developmental, technical, and clinical perspectives* (pp. 117–126). Washington, DC: RESNA.

U.S. Architectural and Transportation Barriers Compliance Board (2001, May). *A guide to the ADA accessibility guidelines for play areas.* Retrieved November 15, 2003, from http://www.access-board.gov./play/guide/intro.htm.

U.S. Department of Education (2002). *Twenty-fourth annual report to Congress on the implementation of the Individuals With Disabilities Education Act.* Washington, DC: Author.

Van Houton, R. (1998). *How to use prompts to initiate behavior.* Austin, TX: PRO-ED.

Wolf, L. S., Massagli, T. L., Jaffe, K. M., & Deitz, J. (1991). Functional assessment of the Joncare Hi-Lo Master power wheelchair for children. *Physical and Occupational Therapy in Pediatrics, 11*(3), 57–72.

Wright-Ott, C., & Egilson, S. (2001). Mobility. In J. Case-Smith (Ed.), *Occupational therapy for children* (4th ed., pp. 609–635). St. Louis: Mosby.

Chapter 7

Adaptive Strategies for Adults With Developmental Disabilities

KRISTINE HAERTL, PHD, OTR/L

KEY TERMS

adaptive

client-centered occupation-
    based approaches

clinical approaches

compensatory

developmental disabilities

extended care network

remedial

OBJECTIVES

Upon completion of this chapter, the reader will be able to

- Describe some major challenges to occupational performance experienced by people with developmental disabilities;

- Describe major considerations in selecting theoretical approaches for evaluation and intervention in adults with developmental disabilities;

- List evaluation methods and assessment tools commonly used with people who have developmental disabilities;

- Distinguish among remedial and adaptive intervention strategies when addressing occupational performance for adults with developmental disabilities;

- Describe specific remedial and adaptive intervention strategies that occupational therapists may use to enhance the occupational performance of adults with developmental disabilities; and

- Describe the integration of the client, family, occupational therapist, extended care network, and context in providing holistic, client-centered occupational therapy for adults with developmental disabilities.

The term *developmental disabilities* often causes confusion. It may summon thoughts of mental retardation or cerebral palsy, but by definition and scope, the term also includes autism spectrum disorders, spina bifida, learning disabilities, pervasive developmental disorders, fetal alcohol syndromes, developmental sensory losses, and a host of other developmental conditions that cause physical and mental impairments. As originally used in the 1970s, the term denoted chronic neurodevelopmental conditions affecting a person's ability to function in daily life (Malone, McKinsey, Thyer, & Straka, 2000). As the terminology expanded, however, a generally accepted definition arose in Western countries centering on a developmental cognitive deficit requiring an IQ ≤ 70 and some type of functional deficit (Sonander, 2000). Within the United States, the current legal definition of developmental disabilities has broadened to include "a severe disability of an individual" that

- Is chronic;
- Is attributable to a mental or physical impairment manifested before 22 years of age;
- Results in "substantial functional limitations in three or more of the following" categories: self-care, receptive and expressive language, self-direction, learning, capacity for independent living, and economic self-sufficiency; and
- Requires interdisciplinary services (Developmental Disabilities Assistance and Bill of Rights Act, 2000).

Within this legal definition, children from birth to 9 years of age may qualify as having a developmental disability without the above functional deficits, provided they have a specific congenital or acquired condition along with a substantial developmental delay. The definition covers a wide range of conditions; therefore, clients with developmental disabilities differ greatly from one condition to another.

Occupational therapists in nearly all areas of practice will provide services to people with developmental disabilities. Clients with developmental conditions may manifest physical, psychological, intellectual, sensory–perceptual, and emotional–behavioral difficulties. Evaluation and intervention for an ambulatory client who is nonverbal, mentally retarded, and has autism will require intervention techniques that are vastly different from those involved in evaluation of and intervention with a nonambulatory, highly intelligent client who has spina bifida. Given the broad nature of develop-

mental disabilities, detailed information on evaluation and intervention techniques for every condition is beyond the scope of this chapter. Rather, this chapter presents a decision-making framework related to evaluation and intervention. It also provides general suggestions to maximize occupational performance in living skills. Information from this chapter should be considered along with the self-care strategies and techniques presented for children with developmental disabilities in Chapter 6.

Intervention Approaches

The occupational therapy literature provides a wide range of intervention approaches and frames of references for working with clients who have developmental disabilities. Occupational therapists must use effective clinical reasoning skills to choose frames of reference that are appropriate to the client. Integral to holistic practice is consideration of factors related to the client, family, context, activity, occupational therapist, team, and other concerned people (such as the conservator or guardian, group home staff, employer, and so forth), along with desired occupational performance.

Providing client-centered services to adults with developmental disabilities may prove challenging, particularly if the client has impairments that affect insight and judgment (Balboa, 2000). When working with such clients, occupational therapists should attempt to maximize client participation throughout the therapy process. Occupational therapists apply various theoretical frameworks, models, and frames of reference in working with clients who have developmental disabilities. Each approach has special considerations.

Client-Centered, Occupation-Based Approaches

In the current health care environment of shorter stays and external regulatory requirements, occupational therapists may focus too heavily on problem areas and overlook client strengths, interests, and resources. Hale (2000) found little evidence that occupational therapists routinely incorporate client strengths and resources into the specific therapy process. A comprehensive, client-centered approach to working with adults who have developmental disabilities should include an interface between the client's expressed desires (along with the priorities of the family) and the views of the client's extended care network (e.g., conservators, guardians, group home staff, and employers). Because clients with developmental conditions often have multiple, complex problems, coordinating care may prove challenging.

Client-centered approaches in occupational therapy consider the client's views and attributes along with the environmental context and occupational needs. Examples of such approaches include the Person–Environment–Occupational Performance (PEOP) Model (Christiansen & Baum, 1997), the Ecology of Human Performance Model (Dunn, Brown, & McGuigan, 1994), the Occupational Performance Process Model (Fearing, Law, & Clark, 1997), the Contemporary Task-Oriented Approach (Bass Haugen & Mathiowetz, 1995; Mathiowetz & Bass Haugen, 1994), and the Model of Human Occupation (Kielhofner, 1995). These approaches share a client-centered focus that acknowledges the roles of the client, context, and desired outcomes in occupational performance. Such a holistic approach to therapy requires a comprehensive evaluation of the client's strengths and resources (Box 7.1).

Commonly Used Theoretical Approaches

In conjunction with a holistic client-centered approach, therapists use theoretical frameworks to guide evaluation and intervention. The following provides a summary of commonly used approaches in working with developmentally disabled adult populations, along with a discussion of considerations for therapists within each approach. The examples are not meant to be inclusive of all approaches but represent examples of frameworks for practice when working with developmentally disabled clients.

Remedial vs. Adaptive Approaches

For people with developmental disabilities, therapy often focuses on remedial and adaptive strategies (Neistadt, 1990). Remedial strategies seek to improve underlying deficits. Adaptive strategies incorporate changes to the environment or to specific activities and may include the use of compensatory techniques that offset underlying deficits. Both types of strategies are used to maximize occupational performance. Occupational therapists selecting an intervention framework for an adult with developmental disabilities should

- Review the client's therapeutic history and goals,
- Assess the client's likely responses to various approaches, and
- Consider the suitability and timing of combined approaches.

An adult client with a developmental disability likely has a long history of therapeutic interventions. The occupational therapist should consult historical records pertaining to the client's responses to therapy and current occupational goals.

Clients with chronic developmental conditions will probably respond to remedial techniques differently from clients with acute conditions that require an intensive rehabilitative approach. The occupational therapist should carefully consider how and when to apply remedial approaches in conjunction with adaptive and compensatory strategies. If a client has a longstanding underlying deficit that is intrinsic to the developmental disability, prospects for remediation may be slim, and use of adaptive and compensatory strategies may be more appropriate. For example, if a client with a long history of mild mental retardation has chronic difficulties with monthly budgeting skills, it may make more sense to use adaptive strategies and external supports, such as using a financial payee with client spending privileges, rather than try to remediate the underlying cognitive and skill deficit. Such decisions are based on the client, the desired task, activity demands, and potential for remediation.

The term *age appropriate* is often used in discussions of activities with clients who have developmental disabilities. Occupational therapists must take care not to make value judgments that are based on the age appropriateness of an activity. Sociocultural and personal value systems drive concepts of age appropriateness. When selecting activities as therapeutic interventions, the therapist should consider the meaning of the activity and the functional status of the client along with a developmentally appropriate range of activities. For example, some people may assign coloring with crayons, to the developmental level of a child of elementary school age. Certainly, children in elementary school use crayons, but that does not warrant discounting coloring as an activity that may be meaningful to older clients.

John was a 42-year-old man with moderate mental retardation and obsessive qualities. The therapy team reported that he frequently engaged in self-injurious behaviors and property destruction. The team attempted to engage John in age-appropriate activities, such as involvement in sports, household maintenance, and woodworking. John rejected all of those activities; yet when his 6-year-old niece came to visit him with a coloring book and crayons, he participated in parallel process and colored for 20 consecutive min. John's occupational therapist encouraged him to explore coloring using other media to create

Box 7.1. Intervention Considerations in Adult Developmental Disability

Holistic, client-centered interventions with adults with developmental disabilities should be guided by a detailed evaluation that includes the following questions:

Client

- Who is the client, and what is his or her occupational performance profile? Occupational performance profiles summarize the client's occupational patterns, history, interests, values, and needs (American Occupational Therapy Association [AOTA], 2002).
- What is the client's status in cognitive, physical, psychological, sensory–perceptual, and social or emotional performance? What is the prognosis for improvement and change within each of these areas?
- What resources are available for the client?
- What are the client's strengths and needs? How can those strengths best be used, and how can the needs best be met?

Family

- What is the family's role in the client's life?
- How does the client view the family's role? Do conflicts exist between the client and family members?
- To what extent should the family be involved in the therapy process?
- If the client currently lives with the family, are there expectations the client will transition to another place of residence?
- Are the family's views consistent with those of the client, the interdisciplinary team, and other concerned individuals?
- What are the family's resources, strengths, and needs? How can those strengths best be used, and how can the needs best be met?

Therapist

- How best can a therapeutic relationship be developed with this client?
- Which theoretical approaches and frames of references should be used?
- What evaluation and intervention techniques are appropriate?
- What is the therapist's occupational therapy diagnosis (Rogers & Holm, 1989)? What is the client's current occupational performance status, and what are the expectations for improvement?
- Should remedial, adaptive, or compensatory strategies be used?
- How best can the therapist collaborate with the client on evaluation, realistic goal development, intervention, and discharge? For example, if a client with mild mental retardation (IQ = 65) feels strongly that he or she wants to live in an apartment and the family and team believe it would be unwise to pursue independent living, what strategies may be used to come to agreement on the therapy process?
- What are the therapist's strengths and needs? How can those strengths best be used, and how best can the needs be met?

Extended Care Network

- Who are the other important people in the client's life, and how will their relationships with the client affect the therapy process? Important people generally include group home staff; the client's conservator; and the client's guardian, friends, and employer.
- If the client will be cared for by other people (i.e., personal care attendant or group home staff), are they adequately trained, prepared, and willing to implement the therapy plan?
- What extended care network resources are available, and how best can they be used in the therapy process?
- What are the strengths and needs of the extended care network? How best can those strengths be used, and how best can the needs be met?

Environment

- What are the client's cultural, physical, social, personal, spiritual, temporal, and virtual contexts (AOTA, 2002), and how will they affect the client's occupational performance?
- What are the environmental demands for occupational performance? Are those performance outcomes reasonable? For example, will the client be required to independently make his or her own meals? If so, can the client reasonably be expected to perform the required tasks?
- Will the client's environment change? If so, what resources, adaptations, and outcomes are needed before the move? For example, will the client move to a different residence?
- What are the environmental resources, strengths, and constraints? How best can those strengths be used, and how best can the constraints be overcome? (see AOTA, 2002).

posters and designs. Although coloring was not initially identified as an appropriate activity for someone John's age, it provided meaning and satisfaction for John.

Behavioral Approaches

Occupational therapists often use behavioral approaches with people who have developmental disabilities, particularly with clients who have forms of mental retardation or conditions that result in problematic behaviors. Behavioral approaches may be used to train a person in a particular skill or to address a target behavior.

Behavioral approaches draw on the works of theorists such as Pavlov and Skinner, who focused on behavior as a process of stimulus and response (Berger, 2001). Occupational therapists facilitate desired behaviors by defining target behaviors, setting goals, and developing a plan to meet the goals through skill instruction, modeling, coaching, and behavioral reinforcement. The behavioral approach succeeds when the client generalizes learning to various environments in daily life and improves occupational performance. Examples of behavioral approaches include use of token environments, providing positive reinforcements such as extra time with staff for good behavior, and use of extinction techniques such as ignoring negative behaviors.

When using behavioral approaches with clients who are developmentally disabled, the occupational therapist must consider possible causes for any unwanted behaviors, the potential for shaping the client's behaviors, and the client's ability to generalize learning from setting to setting. To develop desired behaviors, such as learning of a new living skill, the therapist will work with the interdisciplinary team to determine the client's physical and cognitive potential as well as his or her motivation to learn the skill.

If a client has compromised cognition and difficulty with learning and generalization, the therapist must consider whether a behavioral approach will be useful. Toglia (1991) emphasized that transfer of learning occurs in degrees and that generalization occurs along a continuum. Therapists who are training clients in a specific living skill must consider not only the task but also the client's ability to transfer the skill across various contexts. People with profound cognitive deficits may not be able to generalize learning of the task, in which case the therapist should focus on a more realistic approach.

An occupational therapist must also discern whether underlying reasons are contributing to behaviors that interfere with learning a particular skill.

For example, as a therapist is teaching a client oral hygiene, the client may become self-abusive during the process of brushing his or her teeth. Before implementing a behavioral modification plan, the therapist should consider possible reasons for the self-abusive behavior other than direct opposition. Reasons may include a physical problem or sensory-processing deficit. If the client has underlying sensory defensiveness, interventions such as sensorimotor or sensory-processing techniques may effectively decrease the self-injurious behavior and help maximize function (Hanschu, 1998; Hirama, 1989; Stancliff, 1998).

Approaches Based on Sensory Processing and Sensory Integration

Sensory-based approaches assume the ability to affect the central nervous system using organized sensory input. Since the pioneering work of A. Jean Ayres (1972, 1979), similar approaches have been developed both in the United States (Oetter, Laurel, & Cool, 1991; Oetter, Richter, & Frick, 1993; Willbarger & Willbarger, 1991; Williams & Shellenberger, 1994) and abroad (Portwood, 1996). Occupational therapists long have used sensory-based approaches with clients who have developmental disabilities (Spitzer & Roley, 2001). They can be applied for many purposes, including

- Decreasing sensory defensiveness;
- Reducing negative behaviors, such as self-injurious behaviors;
- Improving underlying sensory processing and sensory integration; and
- Facilitating improved adaptive response to increase daily function.

Research has demonstrated the importance of sensory integration in performing a variety of daily occupations (Fanchiang, 1996; Kinnealey, Oliver, & Wilbarger, 1995; Spitzer & Roley, 2001). Therapists often use sensory-related approaches to improve nervous system functioning, which enhances adaptive response and improves a client's performance in areas such as dressing, toileting, and eating. For example, a therapist may initiate a brushing program before working on dressing techniques with a client who exhibits sensory defensiveness. The rationale is that the brushing program may decrease the sensory defensiveness, thereby increasing the client's ability to tolerate various textures and fabrics. Other applications may include using a weighted vest to facilitate attention to task (Fertel-Daly, Bedell, & Hinojosa, 2001) or using tactile stimulation to the gums before brushing teeth.

As developed by Ayres, classic forms of sensory integration intervention are largely client directed. Using an active therapeutic environment, occupational therapists encourage clients to naturally seek out sensory experiences. Clients with serious developmental disabilities are at increased risk for self-harm; therefore, therapists must provide maximal structure for the sensory stimulation yet offer the clients some choices in the context of treatment. The theoretical framework for the sensory integration approach assumes that the brain is plastic throughout life but that plasticity decreases with age (Bundy, Lane, & Murray, 2002).

Occupational therapists should be cautious in predicting neurological change because clients with major developmental neurological damage likely will always have some form of damage. Bundy, Lane, and Murray (2002) emphasized that Ayres's theories were not intended to explain neurological deficits in developmental disabilities such as Down syndrome and cerebral palsy, but they also emphasized that sensory-integration and sensory-processing issues may occur along with developmental disabilities. Therapists who are considering the use of sensory-processing techniques should develop a clear rationale for doing so, based on the client's diagnosis, goal areas, and evidence-based practice.

Some researchers have reported success in applying sensory-based approaches with adults (Hanschu, 1998; Reisman & Hanschu, 1992), but research has focused on pediatric populations. Continued research is needed to fully validate sensory-based treatment approaches for adults with developmental disabilities. Given the chronic nature of developmental disabilities, clients likely will need ongoing treatment or support that promotes organized sensory experiences throughout life. Willbarger (1994) emphasized the importance of an ongoing "sensory diet" to promote adaptation and optimal occupational performance. Occupational therapists may need to train clients and caregivers to implement long-term sensory diet programs at home and in the community. Therapists may adapt existing approaches, such as the ALERT Program (Williams & Shellenberger, 1994) and other psychoeducational methods, to teach clients and caregivers techniques that facilitate neurological readiness for participating in skill training and therapy.

Physical and Biomechanical Approaches

People with developmental disabilities often have accompanying physical dysfunction, particularly in disorders such as cerebral palsy and spina bifida. Oc-cupational therapists often use rehabilitative biomechanical approaches to reduce physical deficits and maximize occupational performance (J. P. Jackson & Schkade, 2001).

The biomechanical approach seeks to remediate underlying physical deficits and prevent additional problems that may affect occupational performance (J. Jackson, Gray, & Zemke, 2001). It follows a medical model of practice to a greater degree than some of the other occupation-based approaches (Pierce, 2003), and occupational therapists often use this approach with clients who have lost previous function, emphasizing rehabilitation and remediation efforts. If weakness or lack of range of motion affect the client's independence or quality of daily life, the client may benefit from biomechanical techniques, which include strength activities, stretching techniques, and exercises to increase a client's range of motion and functional mobility. Therapy should emphasize using these techniques and exercises to enhance meaningful occupational performance (J. Jackson et al., 2002). For example, rather than exercising the shoulder to increase flexion and endurance through repetitive weightlifting, similar motions may be practiced while completing a meaningful activity, such as painting a large wall mural. When planning an activity within the biomechanical approach, the therapist should consider the client's level of understanding and the perceived meaning of the activity.

Many adults with developmental disabilities have chronic physical problems that may limit the potential for remediation. Because of this, and because such clients often have multiple problems that affect their psychological, social-emotional, cognitive, and sensory systems, therapists should combine biomechanical techniques with other approaches.

Cognitive Disability Approach

The cognitive disabilities model was originally designed by Claudia Allen (1985). The model comprises six levels of cognitive function with specific skills identified in each level. The approach relies heavily on matching activities to the adult client's cognitive function and uses detailed activity analysis to provide a framework for evaluation and intervention. Allen's original applications focused on psychiatric populations, but more recently the model has been applied to other groups, such as people with various dementias (Burns, 1992). Allen and Blue's (1998) publication on how to make clinical judgments within the cognitive disabilities model further extended the model to two distinct groups:

- Clients whose cognitive function is expected to improve rapidly, such as people with head injuries and stroke, and
- Clients with long-term cognitive disabilities whose function is expected to remain static or decline, such as regressed psychiatric patients and people with dementia.

Despite Allen and Blue's (1998) investigation, research on the cognitive disability model generally has focused on populations with psychiatric and dementing conditions. Nonetheless, Harjamaki (2000) found that occupational therapists working with people with developmental disabilities reported using the Allen Assessments, particularly the Allen Cognitive Level Test (ACL), more frequently than other commonly used evaluation tools.

Therapists may find the cognitive disability approach or cognitive disability model helpful, particularly in providing a framework for understanding the client's general cognitive levels and how they relate to occupational performance. In teaching clients living skills, therapists may find particular aspects of the model useful, such as the framework for activity analysis. Earhart (1992) created a detailed analysis of activities that describes a wide variety of ADL and client abilities at each cognitive level. Such analysis may prove helpful in evaluation, intervention, and client and caregiver education.

Occupational therapists should be cautious about using the cognitive disability approach to make any long-term prognosis for a client's future capabilities. Bruce and Borg (2002) identified three limitations of the cognitive disability model:

- It tries to treat too broad a range of problems.
- It contradicts other theoretical models that assume an ability to remediate underlying problems.
- It assumes that interventions using crafts as media will generalize to home and community environments.

Given these cautions, occupational therapists should be careful to maintain a client-centered focus when deciding how and when to apply the model, although they need not discount it entirely.

Additional Cognitive Approaches

Occupational therapists also use other cognitive approaches, including Abreu's (1992, 1998) quadraphonic approach; Toglia's (1991) multicontextual approach; Toglia's (1998) dynamic interactional model of cognition; and cognitive–behavioral approaches built on the work of theorists such as Ellis, Bandura, and Meichenbaum (Bruce & Borg, 2002). Toglia's and Abreu's works often are described in terms of rehabilitation after an acquired brain injury but may provide a framework for understanding the role of cognition in occupational therapy evaluation and intervention.

Cognitive–behavioral applications seek to change behaviors through education and skill building. Using this model, therapy may include both work with the client and education of the client's family and caregivers about the client's disability, suggested techniques to be used with the client, specific home programs, and available resources.

When selecting theoretical approaches to address cognition in adults with developmental disabilities, it is important to consider the client's cognitive level and his or her ability to learn and develop some level of insight. Describing evaluation and intervention techniques used with clients who had severe disabilities and profound retardation, Kellogg (1998) identified the barriers to evaluation and intervention with such clients, including significant difficulties in communication, mobility, interaction, and daily living skills. Clients who are profoundly retarded are unlikely to respond well to traditional evaluation techniques or to efforts aimed at client education. Because many clients with developmental disabilities have mental retardation in conjunction with other disabilities, therapists selecting approaches to address cognition should consider each client's learning potential as well as priorities for therapy.

Evaluation

The *Occupational Therapy Practice Framework* (Practice Framework; American Occupational Therapy Association [AOTA], 2002) describes evaluation as a process that includes identification of occupational needs, problems, and concerns. Formal evaluation methods may be inappropriate, however, when working with people who have profound developmental disabilities. Therapists often identify occupational needs using observation, historical records, and caregiver reports. Evaluations also involve analyzing the client's strengths and any barriers to occupational performance in the client's physical, mental, psychological, social, emotional, sensory–perceptual, and cognitive performance.

Before selecting tools and methods for evaluating an adult with developmental disabilities, the occupational therapist must consider the purpose of the evaluation and the client's ability to engage in the evaluation process. Common purposes for evaluation include

- Initial identification of occupational needs and strengths;
- Identification of intervention goals;
- Monitoring of change over time;
- Monitoring of response to therapy;
- Recommendation for discharge placement;
- Recommendation for special programming, home programming, or specific interventions; and
- Determination of a client's level of functioning for court purposes (e.g., to qualify the client to receive public funds or services).

The definition of developmental disabilities includes criteria for establishing a functional deficit. Accordingly, occupational therapists sometimes are solicited to act as expert witnesses in court to evaluate the extent of a client's functional deficit. They also may perform evaluations for legal situations involving petitions for guardians or conservators, consideration of the need for a court-appointed payee or, less commonly, parental rights. Most often, they evaluate adults with developmental disabilities for purposes relating to therapy.

Assessment Tools

The *Framework* identifies two substeps of evaluation: (1) to produce a client occupational profile to identify needs and priorities and (2) to conduct an "analysis of occupational performance . . . identifying occupational performance issues" and evaluate factors that hinder performance (AOTA, 2002, p. 616). Evaluations often include formal and informal assessments. Standardized tools may not work well with clients who have extensive developmental disabilities, in part because standardized tests often require rigid testing circumstances and procedures. Many adults with developmental disabilities require adaptations to perform the test, which makes it difficult to accurately conduct the test using standardized procedures (Bachner, 1998). As a result, when standardized instruments are used, they often consist of structured interviews of caregivers or observations of clients in natural contexts.

When working with adults who have developmental disabilities, occupational therapists commonly use one or more assessment instruments (Table 7.1), including the following examples:

- AAMR Adaptive Behavior Scales (Nihira, Leland, & Lambert, 1993)
- Assessment of Motor and Process Skills (Fisher, 1997)

- Functional Independence Measure (*Guide for the Uniform Data Set for Medical Rehabilitation*, 1999)
- Scales of Independent Behavior–Revised (Bruininks, Woodcock, Weatherman, & Hill, 1996)
- Sensory Integration Inventory–Revised for Individuals With Developmental Disabilities (Reisman & Hanschu, 1992)
- Vineland Adaptive Behavior Scales–Revised (Sparrow, Balla, & Cicchetti, 1984).

Various standardized developmental assessments also can be used with adults who have developmental disabilities. However, since many such tools are normed for pediatric populations, therapists should use the tools with caution.

Typically, a caregiver or other person highly familiar with the client will complete the assessment instrument. The therapist then scores the responses, producing a standardized score along a continuum of performance. These types of instruments often benefit the intervention process, but they should be used in conjunction with additional evaluation techniques.

When selecting assessment tools to use with a client who has developmental disabilities, the therapist should take into account the client's diagnosis, the areas identified for assessment, the utility and psychometric properties of the assessment tool, and whether the tool can be used to accurately test the client. Therapists also must choose whether to adopt a holistic, top-down approach using occupation-based tools or a bottom-up approach using component-based assessments. In either situation, considerations should include specific barriers to occupational performance and whether remedial or adaptive approaches best suit the intervention.

Use of observation, history taking, checklists, and interviews of the client, family, and caregivers are crucial in the evaluation of adults with developmental disabilities. Babola (2000) presented Spencer and Sample's (1993) Performance Inventory as a possible interview and observation tool for use with clients who have developmental disabilities (Appendix 7.A). This tool identifies a client's current level of functioning and priorities of intervention in five domains: domestic and home, general community, vocational, recreational and leisure, and school.

Another tool that has been identified as useful in evaluating adults with developmental disabilities is the nonstandardized "Let's Do Lunch" assessment (Appendix 7.B). This tool provides a framework for assessing clients' strengths and difficulties when eating (Bachner, 1998). The assessment is adminis-

Table 7.1. Examples of Assessments Used in Adult Populations With Developmental Disabilities

Assessment Tool	Type	Description
AAMR Adaptive Behavior Scale–Residential and Community (Nihira, Leland, & Lambert, 1993)	Observational rating scale	Observational rating scale filled out by caregiver in domains of living skills and social behavior
Assessment of Motor and Process Skills (Fisher, 1997)	Objective observation-based	Structured occupation-based tool that evaluates clients during performance of IADL
Canadian Occupational Performance Measure (Law et al., 1998)	Interview	Individualized client-centered interview evaluating self-perception of occupational performance
Functional Independence Measure (*Guide for the Uniform Data Set for Medical Rehabilitation,*1999)	Observation and history taking	Widely used tool that rates level of independence on self-care and social cognition
Functional Performance Record (Mulhall, 1989)	Observation and history taking	Multidisciplinary tool that records observations related to a wide variety of occupational performance areas
Jacobs Pre-Vocational Assessment (Jacobs, 1991)	Structured observation	Instrument that assesses work-related tasks in preparation for employment
Katz Index of ADL; (Katz, Downs, Cash, & Grotz, 1963, 1970)	Observation and interview	Index rating of level of independence in bathing, dressing, toileting, transferring, and eating
Klein–Bell ADL Scale (Klein & Bell, 1982)	Observational rating scale	Comprehensive 170-item scale that rates the level of assistance needed in ADL
Occupational Performance History Interview (Kielhofner et al., 1998)	History taking interview	Instrument that assesses roles, routines, and goals based on the model of human occupation
Oral Function in Feeding (Stratton, 1981)	Structured observation	Instrument that provides a structured format to evaluate oral function during eating
Scales of Independent Behavior–Revised (Bruininks, Woodcock, Weatherman, & Hill, 1996)	Observational rating scale	Scale that provides standardized scores on function and behavior (short-form and long-form versions)
Vineland Adaptive Behavior Scales—Revised (Sparrow, Balla, & Cicchetti, 1984)	Structured interview and rating scale	Interdisciplinary tool that rates clients in ADL, socialization, communication, and motor skills
Vocational Adaptation Rating Scales (Malgady, Davis, Barcher, & Towner, 1982)	Observational rating scale	Scale that emphasizes work-related behaviors in order to assess work readiness

Note. ADL = activities of daily living; IADL = instrumental activities of daily living.

tered during mealtime, and client performance is coded through task analysis in sensory, perceptual, neuromuscular, motor, cognitive, and psychosocial functions. Information from the "Let's Do Lunch" assessment may have implications for occupational performance in other areas of daily living skills.

Client-centered, occupation-based assessments such as the Occupational Performance History Interview (Kielhofner et al., 1998) and the Canadian Occupational Performance Measure (Law et al.,

1998) also are useful in working with clients who have developmental disabilities. Because they yield information about the client's perspective on perceived importance, skill, and function in areas of occupational performance, these tools facilitate client engagement throughout the therapy process. Therapists should consider the client's cognitive ability to engage in this type of assessment and should use information from these tools in conjunction with other assessment methods.

Analyzing the client's environmental context is particularly important in working with adults who have developmental disabilities. Many such clients have limited communication skills and may be difficult to evaluate using formal assessment tools. Traditionally, occupational therapists have examined the client's physical, social, cultural, and temporal contexts. More recently, the *Framework* (AOTA, 2002) has added personal, spiritual, and virtual contexts. Therapists often use ecological environmental assessment tools to identify environmental needs, assess resources, and develop priorities for intervention. Dunn (1998) identified the most important aspects of context-based evaluations as determination of the meaning of occupational performance to the client in a given context, and development of provisions to maximize quality of life within that context. Making an accurate analysis of a client's environmental context requires the therapist to collaborate with the client, the client's family, and the extended care network.

Intervention

The *Framework* defines an *intervention* as "a plan that will guide actions and that is developed in collaboration with the client. It is based on selected theories, frames of reference, and evidence. Outcomes to be targeted are confirmed" (AOTA, 2002, p. 614). Occupational therapists plan the intervention on the basis of the information gained and priorities identified during the evaluation. In carrying out the intervention, the therapist collaborates with the adult client, family, interdisciplinary team, and extended care network to optimize the client's occupational performance and to maximize quality of life. This collaboration may be challenging, particularly when working with people who have severe disabilities. Such clients may have compromised intellect and communication, so alternative strategies may be needed to determine their interests, likes, and dislikes. For example, the therapist may need to rely more on observation and information provided by caregivers.

Renwick (1998) presented the Centre for Health Promotion (CHP) Framework for Quality of Life in providing services to adults with developmental disabilities. The framework proposes three subareas of quality of life: (1) being (physical being, psychological being, and spiritual being), (2) belonging (physical belonging, social belonging, and community belonging), and (3) becoming (practical becoming, leisure becoming, and growth becoming). Renwick's framework may be applied to occupation-based in-

terventions through identification of barriers (areas that detract from quality of life) and development of goals to address such barriers. For example, consider an adult client with severe physical dysfunction who needs 2 hr to dress each morning, which often makes him or her late for work. The client's quality of life could be enhanced through adaptations or physical assistance to help the client dress in less time, leaving more time to enjoy breakfast and get to work. In this example, rather than identifying dressing independently as the end goal of therapy, the intervention focuses on quality of life and occupational balance as priorities. Occupational therapists should consider quality-of-life issues throughout the therapy process.

General Intervention Strategies

Interventions designed for these clients with developmental disabilities (several of which are discussed in other parts of this text) should include the following steps:

1. Determination of barriers to occupational performance
2. Interpretation of evaluation data and application to intervention planning
3. Identification of priorities for intervention
4. Identification of the client's strengths and needs in the targeted areas
5. Development of a plan to address occupational needs
6. Consideration of need for remedial intervention, adaptation, and compensation
7. Development of goals related to health promotion, establishment and restoration of function, maintenance of occupational performance, modification, and prevention (AOTA, 2002)
8. Implementation of learning strategies such as backward and forward chaining; step-by-step directions; use of direct training and practice (if the client has the learning capacity), initially in a familiar environment and gradually in various environments; and use of hand-over-hand techniques, when appropriate
9. Establishment of routines and habits
10. Identification of resource needs, such as assistive technology
11. Implementation of training and education for caregivers and the extended care network.

The following sections provide an overview of basic activities of daily living (BADL), instrumental activities of daily living (IADL), work, education, and play and leisure. Each section identifies general barriers that may be encountered in working with adults who are developmentally disabled and provides examples of strategies that may be used during intervention. The strategies focus not only on the client but also on the training and education that can be provided to caregivers and the extended care network.

Bathing

As a client with a developmental disability advances through the teenage years, he or she may seek greater independence in bathing. If maximizing independence in bathing is determined to be a priority, the occupational therapist should consider the client's current performance, safety issues, and supports needed to achieve the desired outcome.

Remedial Strategies

- If the client can learn and retain information, skill training using videotapes and pictures, discussions, role-plays with clothes or bathing suit on, and direct observation can help ensure that the client fully understands all areas to be washed, how to apply soap, the procedure for shampooing, how to thoroughly rinse the body, and how to get in and out of the bath and shower safely (Box 7.2).
- Underlying postural and balance problems may need to be addressed for the client to bathe in a safe and effective manner.

Adaptive and Compensatory Strategies

- The therapist should consider the level of supervision and assistance needed to ensure safety. For example, the temperature setting at the water heater may need to be set lower to prevent accidental burns.
- Tear-free shampoo may be advisable if the client has difficulty with shampooing hair.
- The environmental assessment should determine whether specialized equipment, such as grab bars, a bath mat, a tub seat, a handheld showerhead, or any other specialized equipment may be needed for positioning.

Dressing

Dressing is a complex activity requiring postural control, motor planning, strength, flexibility, dexterity, cognition, and sensory–perceptual awareness. Value judgments and cultural norms affect clothing style, and climate and activity influence the types of clothing worn. People with develop-

mental disabilities may have difficulties with dressing in any number of areas. People with Fragile X syndrome may have hypotonicity, which causes barriers to dressing and self-caring behavior (Moor, 2000), and people with cerebral palsy often have hypertonicity, which causes different problems. Many people with developmental disabilities become completely independent in dressing; however, people with profound retardation and severe disabilities may remain dependent in this area throughout life.

As the client enters adulthood, size and positioning during dressing must be considered to protect caregivers from injury. If the client can be

---

Box 7.2. Case Example: Michael

Michael, a 34-year-old man with mild mental retardation and depression, was admitted to a group home. Despite daily showers, the group home staff reported that Michael consistently had a strong, offensive body odor. He was referred to the occupational therapist for skill training in grooming and hygiene.

During the evaluation phase of therapy, the therapist asked Michael to demonstrate, with his bathing suit on, his showering procedure. Michael proceeded to stand in the shower, run the water, and turn it off after a couple of minutes. After further exploration, the therapist realized that Michael's concept of a shower was to stand under the water for a few minutes without applying shampoo or soap. Skill and knowledge deficits were determined to be primary barriers to successful occupational performance in this activity.

The therapist chose a combination of behavioral and cognitive–behavioral approaches to take on the role as educator, facilitator, and reinforcer. With Michael wearing his bathing suit, the therapist provided training in how to properly take a shower. After a few sessions, Michael demonstrated the ability to use soap and shampoo independently. Michael also was put on a token program and received weekly points for completion of his grooming and hygiene routines. Michael could redeem his points for items such as magazines, one-to-one time with staff, and food items. Staff members were trained to follow through with Michael's behavior program. After 3 weeks on the program, staff reported a significant decrease in body odor and problems with grooming and hygiene.

trained to help (e.g., by independently moving body parts), the caregiver burden can be eased and the client's dependence on others decreased.

Frequently, another challenge to independent dressing among adults with developmental disabilities stems from sensory-processing difficulties (Baranek et al., 2002; Dunn, Miles, & Orr, 2002). People with sensory-processing difficulties may not want to wear certain types of clothing or may be prone to taking off clothing that feels uncomfortable. Such clients may be helped by using techniques to decrease sensitivities before dressing and by selecting clothes in comfortable fabrics and materials, such as cotton and flannel.

Remedial Strategies

- Provide skill training in clothing selection and dressing techniques using the teaching strategies discussed earlier in this chapter and the text.
- Use hand-over-hand, interactive guiding (the Affolter Approach; Affolter, 1987).
- Address underlying flexibility, strength, dexterity, praxis, sensory, and postural concerns that may pose barriers to dressing.
- Use relaxation, calming, and desensitization techniques before dressing if the client is prone to hypertonicity, sensory defensiveness, or anxiety during dressing.

Adaptive and Compensatory Strategies

- Choose adaptable, loose-fitting, and comfortable clothing. Remember that as young people approach adulthood, clothing style and type may become more important. Some adaptive clothing may be unappealing, and it is important to consider style along with utility.
- Choose attractive, wrinkle-free clothing that is durable, washable, allows ease of movement, and has fasteners that are easy to manipulate.
- Use adaptive dressing aids when appropriate. Clients with cognitive difficulties may have limited capacity to independently use adaptive devices.
- If the client has difficulty with buttons but wants to wear buttoned styles, use hook-and-loop fasteners on the interior of the fabric and attach buttons on the exterior.
- Use tube socks without heels to decrease the likelihood of the heel sliding on the foot and causing discomfort.

Toileting and Bladder and Bowel Management

Several toileting and bladder or bowel concerns may arise in adults with developmental disabilities. Physical problems, dietary concerns, and cognitive problems all interfere with independence in this area. Prescribed medications may cause unwanted side effects, such as constipation, diarrhea, and interference with bladder control. Collaborating with the client's physician and a nutritionist is wise to ensure proper dietary intake and determine whether medical intervention is needed.

Before developing intervention techniques, the occupational therapist must determine whether the client can be trained in toileting and bowel and bladder management. Foxx and Azrin (1973) established a detailed toilet-training procedure for working with people with mental retardation. The authors identified key client requirements for training, which include

- Some level of vision (or visual aids) to navigate to the bathroom;
- The ability to get to the toilet;
- Some level of motor control, including control over hand movements; and
- Some receptive language and ability to understand the training procedures.

The therapist should evaluate client motivation and self-awareness before intervention. People with developmental disabilities may have impaired cognition and self-awareness that significantly delay or even preclude toilet training. To achieve bladder control, clients must have the following abilities (Miller & Bachrach, 1995):

- An awareness that the bladder contracts
- The ability to recognize when the bladder is full
- The ability to inhibit contractions and wait for urination
- An awareness of when the bladder is empty
- The ability to hold urine during stress and overfilling
- The ability to inhibit urination during sleep.

Like bladder control, bowel management requires an internal awareness of the ability to hold and to move the bowels. Intervention techniques that have been identified as key for bowel-management programs include habit training, dietary modifications, biofeedback training, and medical interventions (Mason, Santoro, & Kaull, 1999).

Establishing a toileting routine often helps to maximize independence. Additional adaptive equipment may be needed for toileting in people with physical disabilities or with strength and postural concerns. Intervention plans involving toilet training and bowel and bladder management require collaboration between the client and all caregivers. Consistency is important to maximize the learning process, so caregivers should be trained in specific programs.

Remedial Strategies

- Obtain medical and dietary consultations to address underlying physical and nutritional concerns.
- Begin skill and habit training with daytime hours, and use a routine.
- Use techniques to develop self-awareness of physical sensations related to bowel and bladder control.
- Administer behavioral reinforcement and shaping techniques.
- Implement the use of charts, such as an "accident" chart, to monitor times when incontinence is likely to occur. Such a chart can facilitate development of a plan for intervention in response to the incontinence.
- Use techniques to address underlying postural and strength considerations for toileting.

Adaptive and Compensatory Techniques

- Use disposable training pants and similar products to address bowel and bladder concerns.
- Use easily removable clothing for toileting purposes.
- Use flushable wet wipes or other cleaning pads to assist in the cleaning process.
- Offset physical impairments with adaptive aids, such as raised toilet seats, grab bars, low mirrors to check for hygiene, and accessible, nonslippery surfaces.

Grooming and Hygiene

Cultural norms and personal and familial values influence personal hygiene and grooming. Physical, cognitive, and sensory–perceptual difficulties all may impair a person's ability to successfully participate in grooming activities. Adults with developmental disabilities may need cues and prompts to fully participate in daily grooming procedures. For example, a client with moderate mental retardation may brush the front of her hair daily but forget to brush the back. Less obvious tasks, such as caring for fingernails, may be left undone without cues and assistance. Clients with sen-

sory defensiveness may refuse to brush their teeth, resulting in compromised oral hygiene. Occupational therapists should identify underlying barriers to grooming and hygiene before developing specific intervention strategies.

Remedial Strategies

- Address underlying sensory defensiveness, physical barriers, and knowledge deficits that interfere with grooming.
- Provide skill training through role-plays, videotapes, direct practice, hand-over-hand techniques, and other techniques described in this text.
- Use weighted wrist cuffs and add proprioceptive cues to minimize dyscoordination and enhance motor planning.

Adaptive and Compensatory Strategies

- Textured or electric toothbrushes may be particularly helpful for people with sensory defensiveness.
- Use a toothpaste pump rather than a tube.
- Consider which types of deodorant and personal care items are easiest for the client to handle and use.
- Use liquid soap.
- Guide the caregiver in controlling the amounts used of personal care items like toothpaste and shampoo.
- Use adaptive equipment such as long-handled brushes, suction cups to secure small items like fingernail brushes, and other grooming aids.
- Use checklists, pictures, and cues to prompt completion of the task.

Feeding and Eating

Physical, cognitive, and sensory–perceptual problems may impair a person's ability to feed him- or herself independently and may impair the oral-motor function, causing problems with dysphagia. Food allergies, restrictions, sensitivities, and preferences further confound feeding and eating for people with developmental disabilities. Even before evaluation, occupational therapists may use some indirect strategies with people who have dysphagia. These strategies include

- Using a quiet environment,
- Paying careful attention to positioning,
- Completing oral stimulation before eating,
- Presenting appetizing food in an appealing manner, and

- Using adaptive equipment and feeding utensils as necessary to maximize performance (Avery-Smith, 2001).

Therapists also may apply these techniques during the intervention phase when working with adults who have developmental disabilities. Stratton (1989) stressed the importance of positioning, food presentation, use of adaptive utensils, and careful attention to diet as key areas of concern. Stratton further emphasized that because of difficulty with generalization, skill training of adults with developmental disabilities should occur during mealtimes in the clients' natural context. Additional considerations include the types of foods served and how often they are served. People with oral sensitivities may eat only specific textures of food. Therapists may use oral-motor stimulation programs and gradually introduce foods to enhance dietary variety. For people with attention and task-completion difficulties, sitting at mealtimes may be a challenge. Scheduling shorter but more frequent mealtimes or enhancing small meals with nutritious snacks can alleviate behavior difficulties at mealtimes.

An additional area of difficulty often encountered in clients with developmental disabilities is self-monitoring of intake. Clients may lack the internal controls needed to address the amount of intake. Other clients may lack the cognitive ability to learn about food types and portions. Therapists may therefore find it helpful or necessary to enhance training with external controls on portions and types of foods. A final consideration is training in mealtime manners and common social behaviors that may be required in public settings. Therapists may plan additional interventions to address issues such as maintenance of attention, behavior in public settings, ability to patiently wait for meals in restaurants, and awareness of culturally and contextually specific mealtime manners.

Discussing specific intervention techniques for all of these areas is beyond the scope of this chapter. The following general strategies may be useful in working with adults who have developmental disabilities.

Remedial Strategies

- Address underlying oral-motor or swallowing difficulties and weaknesses through techniques such as vibration, tapping, oral-motor exercises, and stretching (Avery-Smith, 2001).
- Address postural and range-of-motion concerns that inhibit proper feeding and eating.

- Use desensitization, calming, and sensory stimulation techniques to address oral-motor hypo- and hypersensitivities.
- Provide mealtime training regarding proper food portions, social behaviors, and nutrition, possibly using modeling, practice, and role-playing techniques.
- Provide individual and small-group training regarding mealtime manners and public etiquette.

Adaptive and Compensatory Strategies

- Adjust length of mealtimes according to the client's needs. If appropriate, supplement small meals with nutritious snacks.
- Use adaptive equipment, such as built-up and weighted utensils, Dycem plate guards, and adapted cups.
- Select foods by textures and types that meet the client's preferences and needs (e.g., soft foods, liquid-based foods, or food that can be cut into small pieces).
- Schedule visits to public eating places during times when the locations are not busy.
- Provide meaningful activities for the client during waiting periods in public restaurants.

Functional Mobility

As people with developmental disabilities enter adolescence and adulthood, functional mobility extends beyond the home and into the community. An adult with developmental disabilities likely will have established a pattern of mobility throughout childhood and adolescence (see Chapter 6). As the client reaches adulthood, the therapist should reassess his or her occupational needs regarding functional mobility. Expanded occupations and activities outside the place of residence require careful planning to ensure that the necessary supports are available.

The *Framework* (AOTA, 2002) identifies *functional mobility* as relating to mobility of oneself from one position to another, functional ambulation, and transportation of objects. Issues of strength, range of motion, coordination, motor control, and sensory perception may impair the mobility of an adult with developmental disabilities. Additional concerns about cognitive awareness, safety, and judgment may further affect the client's ability to make wise choices about how and where to ambulate. People with epilepsy, for example, will have specific safety concerns in relation to seizures, particularly grand mal seizures, in which clients lose conscious control of motor functions.

Most interventions for adults with developmental disabilities include training for the client, the caregivers, and the extended care network. For example, establishing health maintenance and exercise routines often is crucial to ensure that the client has adequate strength and fitness to manage and maintain functional mobility. Ideally, clients also should be taught proper body mechanics, particularly if muscle imbalances, coordination, and balance issues are matters of concern. Caregivers often need education regarding safe transfers, particularly as an adolescent or young adult client gains height and weight.

Wheelchairs, scooters, walkers, canes, crutches, and other ambulatory devices often are used to enhance functional mobility. Consideration should be given to the environment, equipment demands (i.e., type of wheelchair), occupational needs, and ability of the client to use the equipment or learn the techniques and skills for desired outcomes. If clients expect to increase their independence and motility, a motorized wheelchair may be advantageous, particularly for trips into the community. Bunning, Angelo, and Schmeler (2001) found that use of a motorized wheelchair enhanced occupational performance, adaptability, competence, and self-esteem in a small sample of clients with severe mobility impairments.

Remedial Strategies

- Promote balance, flexibility, and strength training to enhance personal mobility.
- Provide skill training in the use of mobility equipment, the proper way to make transfers, and basic body mechanics.
- Provide skill training using simulated situations, videotapes, pictures, and in vivo training exercises related to safe ambulation in a variety of environments.

Adaptive and Compensatory Strategies

- Use wheelchair bags, walker bags, duffels on wheels, and other provisions for effective and safe carrying of items.
- Provide training for caregivers regarding safety concerns having to do with the client's functional mobility.
- Depending on evaluation findings, recommend ambulatory equipment (if needed) that matches the client's needs and environment.

Sexuality

Occupational therapists should address the topic of sexuality with adolescents and adults who have de-velopmental disabilities. Issues of sexuality include sexual expression, love, and intimacy. Sexual relationships are tied to self-worth, and it is important to educate clients about healthy relationships. Few programs directly address sexuality, however, and teens and young adults may not have adequate knowledge in this area. A Danish survey of people with autistic spectrum disorders revealed increased levels of socially inappropriate expressions of sexuality, social deficits, and deviant sexual behavior (Waltz, 2002). The authors attributed the differences to both unnatural environmental exposure to sexuality (i.e., atypical means of learning about sexuality) and sensory differences. Such deviances may be minimized through carefully planned interventions.

Issues of sexuality in adults with developmental disabilities are complex. For example, people with autism spectrum disorders may be prone to sensory-processing difficulties (Dunn et al., 2002). When such clients exhibit behaviors such as public masturbation, therapists must determine whether the behaviors are due to sexual expression or sensory self-stimulation. Often the question of sexual vulnerability arises, and interdisciplinary teams must work with the client, family, and extended care network to determine means of healthy sexual expression and protect the client from exploitation.

In addition to vulnerabilities and sensory-processing difficulties, people with physical disabilities, such as clients with spina bifida, may experience problems with lubrication or other sexual difficulties (Brei, 1999). Medication side effects may generate additional complications (Waltz, 2002). Along with general education about sexuality and healthy relationships, clients may benefit from education about sexual options for people with disabilities. Chapter 17 provides more information about sexuality and people with developmental disabilities.

Remedial Strategies

- Provide education to the client, caregivers, and extended care network, using techniques such as role-plays, videotapes, group discussions, and contextual training about healthy relationships, sexuality, and boundaries.
- Use health promotion and prevention techniques to educate the client about safe sexual and relationship practices.
- Provide education and intervention specifically related to sexual expression and people with physical disabilities.
- Use intervention strategies to address underlying sensory-processing problems that may

cause inappropriate public sexual stimulation and exposure.

Adaptive and Compensatory Strategies

- Use adaptive sexual aids and techniques (see Chapter 17).
- Provide for an alternative source of stimulation.
- Facilitate environmental accommodations and private spaces for clients with specific sexual needs.
- Implement behavioral plans and vulnerable-adult plans for clients deemed at risk for sexual exploitation.

Sleep and Rest

Client-centered approaches should focus on the client's lifestyle balance and how that is affected by sleep–wake–rest cycles. People with developmental disabilities may have unusual sleeping and waking patterns or may suffer disturbances that affect their daily routines (Waltz, 2002). Sleep difficulties may

affect clients' levels of alertness, productivity, efficiency, and occupational performance. Transitions from an arousing, alerting activity to a restful activity or to bedtime may be difficult, particularly for people who have difficulty regulating their arousal systems. Additional difficulties in sleep–wake–rest cycles, arousal, and energy levels may reflect medications, energy expenditure, stress, and medical conditions. As the occupational therapist considers the client's daily activity profile, problem identification should include any difficulties in sleep or arousal. As problems are reported to the interdisciplinary teams, efforts should be made to determine the underlying cause(s) and develop intervention strategies. In addition to medical interventions, relaxation exercises and calming and alerting techniques may prove helpful, provided they are based on the cognitive level of the client (see Figure 7.1). To promote balanced activities and a healthy transition to bedtime, daily routines, schedules, and transition techniques may help clients with developmental disabilities (Moor, 2000).

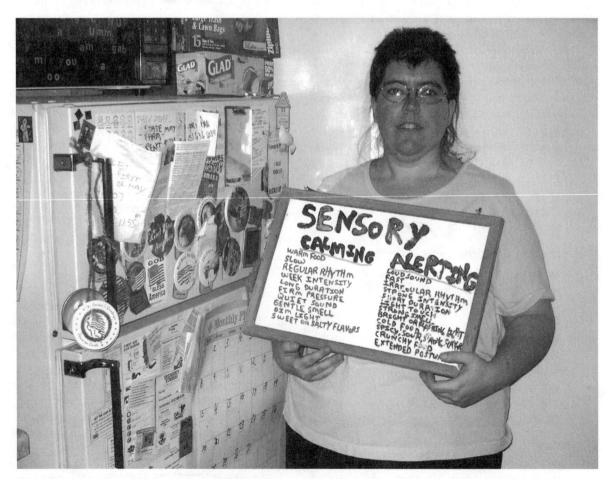

Figure 7.1. Calming and alerting strategies used.

Box 7.3. Case Example: Joy

Joy has developmental disabilities and mental health concerns. Throughout her childhood and adolescence, she received multiple services and lived in structured institutionalized settings. In addition to developmental concerns, barriers to Joy's occupational performance included

- Poor sensory integration, including dyspraxia and sensory defensiveness;
- Cognitive difficulties, such as poor planning, organization, and abstraction; and
- Deficits in living skills and socialization skills.

Joy was totally dependent in all instrumental activities of daily living and required prompts and minimal assistance with basic activities of daily living. Joy had hypo- and hypersensitivity to incoming stimulation and required cues, prompts, and assistance in meeting daily grooming needs. She sought out social relationships, but she frequently was unaware of boundary issues and proper assertiveness. Her difficulties with planning and organization complicated her efforts to meet daily needs, as did her over- and underarousal, which resulted in either hyper- or hypoactivity.

Beginning at 18 years of age, in conjunction with a multidisciplinary approach, Joy received intensive occupational therapy services that included sensory integration therapy, living skills training, social skills training, and modification of her environment. Within a year of intensive intervention, she showed significant gains in occupational performance.

With environmental adaptations and built-in supports, Joy has lived in her own apartment for more than 10 years without rehospitalization. Initially, Joy received fairly intensive case management and therapy services. With a daily routine, development of calming and alerting strategies, and establishment of living and social skills, however, she progressed to the point that she now lives independently without case management assistance. Joy works part-time, maintains active involvement in her church, and engages in socialization through local community events. Examples of the daily adaptations and strategies Joy uses include working part-time on an adapted work schedule; using whiteboards in her apartment to help her stay organized; and scheduling her days to stay busy, manage anxiety, and allow time for relaxation. Joy works part-time during the late morning, her hours of personal peak performance. She uses strategies such as brushing for calming and sour candies for alerting to regulate her arousal state for maximal function (see Figure 7.1). Keeping whiteboards in her apartment helps her maintain a daily routine, schedule her day, and note reminders of important appointments and strategies to meet personal needs (see Figure 7.2). She uses the public transit system, takes weekly trips into the city, and frequently walks to the library and local shopping center. She also manages her routine to allow periods of calming and adjusts her physical environment to help her meet personal goals. For example, Joy enjoys looking out her patio window and will adjust the height of her chair to see over the patio railing (see Figure 7.3).

Remedial Strategies

- Coach the client to use relaxation and calming techniques before bedtime.
- Plan schedules carefully, considering the levels of energy expenditure required by daily activities and adjusting activities to balance out energy expenditures throughout the day (Box 7.3).
- Implement the use of stress-reducing and self-awareness techniques to address underlying stress and anxiety.
- Plan interventions using a holistic approach that includes health promotion, good nutrition, and exercise.

Adaptive and Compensatory Strategies

- Establish a routine for the client that includes careful transition plans before bedtime.

- Adjust the client's schedule and daily activity requirements on the basis of his or her natural sleep–wake–rest cycles. For example, if the client naturally goes to bed late and gets up late in the morning, then do not schedule appointments in early morning (Figure 7.2).
- Adapt the environment to promote rest and sleep (e.g., encourage a restful, rather than overstimulating, design for the client's bedroom).

Assistive Technology and Use of Personal Devices

Assistive technology often facilitates occupational performance and increases the level of independence in clients with developmental disabilities. Cook and Hussey (2002) defined *assistive technology* as "a broad range of devices, services, strategies, and practices

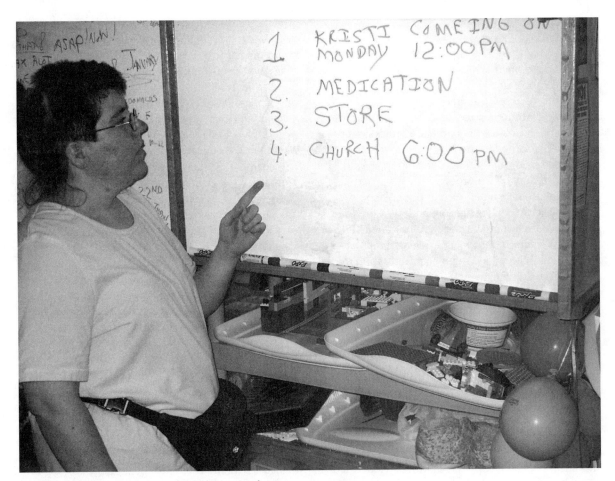

Figure 7.2. Daily schedule and routine organizer.

that are conceived and applied to ameliorate the problems faced by individuals who have disabilities" (p. 5). This definition broadens the scope of assistive technology to include not only physical devices but also the application of knowledge and the development of strategies to enhance client function. A comprehensive discussion of this topic is beyond the scope of this chapter, but some basic considerations in using assistive technology with clients who have developmental disabilities are presented below.

Two notable models have been proposed to guide evaluation and intervention using assistive technology: Mann and Beaver's (1995) identification of areas for assessment in assistive technology, which emphasizes the interaction between the person, environment, tasks, and devices, and Cook and Hussey's (2002) Human Activity Assistive Technology (HAAT) model.

Within Mann and Beaver's assessment approach, the interactions are considered simultaneously to provide a comprehensive analysis of the needs of the client. In using this approach with

adults who have developmental disabilities, occupational therapists need to consider the client's current function, desired outcome, requirements of the task, environmental context, and a selection of technology appropriate to the client. An important technology consideration is whether the client can learn to use the device. Additional selection criteria identified by Mann and Beaver include

- The appearance of the device,
- The cost–benefit ratio of the device,
- The ability of the device to complete the desired task, and
- The availability of a selection of custom-made versus off-the-shelf items (Mann & Beaver, 1995).

Cook and Hussey's (2002) HAAT model emphasizes the interaction between human being, activity, and technology within the client's environmental, social, cultural, and physical contexts. In the HAAT model, the client's skills and abilities are identified as intrinsic enablers that allow the client to complete the task. Assistive technologies, by contrast, are identified as extrinsic enablers. The client and the technology interface within the given contexts, which is key to implementing assistive technology for successful outcomes.

Types of assistive technology range from low-technology items, such as basic assistive devices without major electronic components, to high-technology devices that may include sophisticated computer and electronic applications. Assistive technologies often used with adults who have developmental disabilities include keyboard and computer technologies, communication systems, devices for functional and transportation mobility, robotic aids, and sensory aids.

Trefler and Hobson (1997) discussed the Symm and Ross hierarchy of assistive technology. According to Symm and Ross, therapists considering assistive technology should follow the following hierarchy:

1. Modification or revision of the job or task
2. Use of commercially available products by people with no disabilities
3. Use of commercially available rehabilitation products
4. Combinations of existing technologies not typically used together
5. Modifications of existing commercial devices and (if no other option is feasible) fabrication of new devices.

The therapist must consider the nature and purpose of each device being considered and how well it fits in the client context. Trefler and Hobson (1997) recommended that clients with developmental disabilities be given a chance to try a particular technology to assess whether it is an appropriate fit for them. Some clients may be resistant to using specific types of technology, so before recommending an expensive item, the occupational therapist should assess client motivation and ability to use the technology. The client's training needs also must be determined. Trefler and Hobson recommended that this training occur in the context in which the client will use the technology. Providing training in the proper context is especially important for adult clients with developmental disabilities, given potential concerns about such clients' ability to transfer learning from one environment to another. In addition, training of the client's family, caregivers, and extended care network often is necessary to ensure consistency of skill training and reinforcement among the people who interact with the client.

Home Management, Self-Care, and Care of Others and Pets

Many adults with developmental disabilities lead healthy, satisfying lives and have nurturing relationships. Some clients, however, encounter barriers to maintaining their household responsibilities and developing strategies to take care of themselves and others. For example, relatively subtle disabilities like Fetal Alcohol Effects (FAE), borderline retardation, or learning disabilities initially may go unrecognized by people outside the client's family and circles of close associates. People with less obvious disabilities may perform fairly independently on BADL but struggle to execute other tasks, such as writing a paper, managing a checkbook, or filling out a job application. They also may struggle to meet the level of expectations placed on them at school, at work, or in other external settings. A holistic approach to intervention considers the client's interactions with other people, including the client's ability to maintain a household.

According to Mulcahey (1999), a healthy, well-adjusted adult has the ability to interact comfortably with others, respect authority, respect him- or herself, solve problems with confidence, and ask for help when it is needed. Strategies to maintain daily chores and responsibilities involve using skill training, adaptive equipment, and development of daily routines. Some clients hire personal care attendants or other helpers to assist with daily chores, cleaning, and cooking responsibilities. One area of concern, particularly with cognitively impaired clients, is the client's ability to use good judgment and adhere to safety procedures when completing daily routines. Using both formal and informal evaluations of living skills in the client's place of residence often helps the occupational therapist evaluate client needs and develop intervention strategies.

Parenting may be one of the most underused areas of skill training in occupational therapy. A review of the literature (Cohn, 2001; Cohn, Miller, & Tickle-Degnen, 2000; Humphry & Thigpen-Beck, 1998) reveals that therapists readily focus on parenting from the perspective of a parent whose child has disabilities, but little on the challenges of being a parent who has disabilities. Parents with physical disabilities may require compensatory techniques and household adaptations, and parents with cognitive deficits often require basic training in child development and parenting skills. In cases of more severe developmental disabilities, issues of competence and safety may be of concern, in which case care must be taken to involve the family and extended care network in determining supports needed to ensure the well-being of the client, the spouse (if the client is married), and children.

Remedial Strategies

- Provide skills training in household maintenance and caring for the self, for others, and for pets.
- Provide education for the entire family on safety, adaptation, and home management techniques.
- Pursue remediation of underlying strength, endurance, and range-of-motion difficulties to ease the client's physical burden.
- Conduct interactive parenting sessions and training in child development and parenting skills.

Adaptive and Compensatory Strategies

- Use adaptive equipment, such as long-handled brooms, reachers, and mops (Figure 7.3).
- Use a selection of small, lightweight appliances.
- Use daily reminders, schedules, and whiteboards for self-organization.
- Add necessary support systems, such as a nanny or housekeeper.
- Use sensory aids, such as talking clocks, visual aids, and teletype systems.
- Provide training in energy conservation and efficiency techniques (i.e., use of schedules, ergonomics, establishment of routines, and so forth).

Shopping, Meal Preparation, Safety, and Emergency Management

Shopping and meal preparation require a high level of cognitive ability. These activities involve community mobility, budgeting, planning, organization, and adherence to safety procedures. Accurate evaluation of the client's safety and judgment are important to ensure that the client understands the proper and safe use of appliances and to identify the supports needed to minimize risks. Clients with physical and sensory impairments may benefit from using adapted appliances and utensils, such as enlarged stove knobs, high-contrast items (for people with low vision), and ergonomic aids. Clients with subtle cognitive disabilities and safety concerns may learn to prepare meals primarily in a microwave to lessen the risk of fire and other safety hazards. Emergency response and crisis management preparations should include clear displays of

emergency telephone numbers and training in a few important first-aid and safety principles. Some adult clients with developmental disabilities may have limited ability to generalize emergency procedures to other environments, so occupational therapists should evaluate needed supports and experiential training using role-plays and scenario simulations.

Remedial Strategies

- Use skill training in shopping and meal preparation in the client's community and place of residence.
- Use skill training, including role-plays, videotapes, training aids, and simulated situations, to educate the client in emergency response practices in the client's community and place of residence.
- Provide repeated practice in preparation of a few nutritious meals.

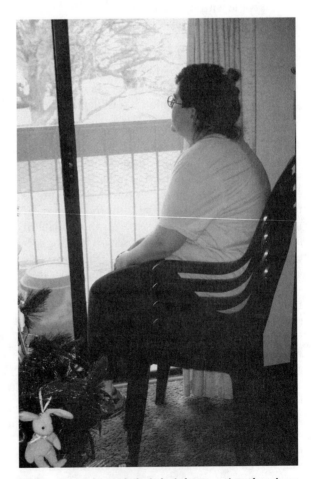

Figure 7.3. Adapted chair height to enjoy the view during a calming period.

- Pursue therapeutic interventions to remediate underlying physical and sensory deficits that impair client occupational performance in this area.

Adaptive and Compensatory Strategies

- Use adapted appliances and ergonomic aids.
- Use safer cooking methods, such as microwave cooking, if safety is a concern.
- Recommend shopping at smaller stores and accessible stores in close proximity to the client's place of residence.
- Provide for external supports, such as a housekeeper or aide, to prepare meals.
- Use charts and visible aids to cue the client regarding safety and emergency procedures and important emergency telephone numbers.

Financial Management

Decisions regarding finances should involve the client to the extent possible given the client's cognitive ability. Various levels of independence are possible in financial management. As an adolescent with developmental disabilities enters adulthood, the client and the client's family must make decisions about his or her level of competence and financial management ability. Parents may continue to manage the client's finances, a conservator may be appointed, the client may obtain assistance through external supports, or the client may manage his or her finances independently.

Basic money management skills include counting change, making change from a transaction, budgeting, and banking. People with developmental disabilities are at risk for financial exploitation and must have protection from exploitation as prescribed by "vulnerable adult" laws. People with cognitive and attention disorders also may be prone to impulse-control issues that may affect spending habits. In people with attention deficit disorders, impulsivity and inattention may impair occupational functioning (Weiss, 1997), which in turn affects advanced living skills such as money management. Other developmental disabilities, such as autism spectrum disorders, affect executive functions and can result in problems with organization, inability to think flexibly, issues with impulse control, and inefficient memory (Bolick, 2001). All of these symptoms affect a person's ability to effectively manage finances and make responsible spending decisions. In addition to external assistance, the following strategies may prove effective in promoting money management skills and financial responsibility in clients with developmental disabilities.

Remedial Strategies

- Allow for mastery of money management skills on a developmental level, starting with basic tasks, such as counting change and making change before working toward more complex banking skills.
- Use role-plays and experiential sessions to practice assertive behaviors and social responsibility to prevent financial exploitation.
- When possible, work with parents of adolescents who have developmental disabilities regarding estate and financial planning before the client reaches adulthood.
- Provide opportunities for the client to practice basic money management skills through use of vocational programs and at the hospital, clinic, day treatment, and program-based stores, and through trips into the community.
- Teach the client the value of items to promote wise decision making regarding spending.

Adaptive and Compensatory Strategies

- Provide for a financial conservator and external supports as needed.
- Use simplified weekly budgets (e.g., the client may have a conservator but is given responsibility to budget for a nominal amount on a daily or weekly basis).
- Have the client manage only one account (e.g., a savings account) and another individual manage the checking account.
- Use accounts that require cosignatures.
- Arrange with the client's employer to pay the client on a weekly basis, if possible, or develop external supports so that the client receives a weekly check as opposed to a biweekly or monthly check. Weekly payment schedules often are easier to manage.

Health Management and Maintenance

Health management and maintenance involve health promotion, health-enhancing behaviors, and prevention of illnesses and injuries. Problems occur when clients do not follow through with health maintenance and management or engage in health-compromising behaviors such as smoking, drug use, or other negative behaviors (Taylor, 1999). Further difficulties can result when clients have additional concerns related to disabilities, such as special nutritional requirements, daily medications, and exercise regimens designed to preserve and enhance physical and emotional functioning. For therapeutic interventions to be of benefit, the client must be willing and motivated to adhere to the therapy program and recommendations. The therapy must fit the needs of the client. It also must be presented at a level the client can fully understand in order to follow through with the recommendations. Key need areas in developmental disabilities include proper use of assistive technology, maintenance of exercise programs, adherence to nutritional recommendations, and medication compliance.

Many adult clients with developmental disabilities receive multiple medications. Haynes, McKibbon, and Kanani (1996) found that in the general population, follow-through with prescriptions and health advice was about 50%. Clients with compromised cognition often struggle with compliance, not only because of motivational issues but also because of a lack of understanding and ability to follow the medication regimen. More complex treatments have been found to lower compliance rates (Brannon & Feist, 2000). The use of external supports and assistance in conjunction with pill boxes and other aids can help ease the burden of medication compliance. Additional strategies to encourage health-promoting behaviors include establishing norms within group facilities (i.e., group exercises), developing routines and habits, and using positive educational and behavioral strategies.

Remedial Strategies

- Educate the client, family, and extended care network regarding medication management, nutritional requirements, and therapy regimens.
- Provide group and individual therapy sessions to create opportunities for the client to practice health-promoting skills and develop healthy habits and routines (e.g., cooking nutritious meals within specialized or diabetic diets).
- Use behavioral techniques and reinforcement to establish healthy behaviors.
- Use peer support to promote healthy behaviors.

Adaptive and Compensatory Strategies

- Use external supports, such as a visiting nurse or attendant to assist with follow-through.
- Use adaptive strategies and equipment (e.g., pill boxes, premeasured food, or talking clocks).
- Post reminders regarding daily health routines on a bulletin board or white board.

- Adjust schedules to provide the client cues (e.g., taking medications before each meal, receiving a phone call to remind the client about an appointment).

Community Mobility

As an adolescent with developmental disabilities enters adulthood, community mobility becomes increasingly important for educational, vocational, and social reasons. In addition to mobility provided from wheelchairs and ambulatory equipment, issues of transportation, driving, and travel aids should be addressed with the client. Depending on state requirements, driving evaluations may be recommended to ensure that the client can drive safely. Occupational therapists may evaluate clients' abilities in the clinic before formal evaluation by the state. Cook and Hussey (2002) identified a set of predriving evaluation items that included visual and perceptual skills, hearing, reaction time, cognitive skills, and physical skills. The predriving evaluation should determine needs related to competence, special vehicle modifications, vehicle selection, and vehicle access. For clients who are unable to drive, medical transportation systems and training in using public transit systems may be useful.

Remedial Strategies

- Reassess and prescribe any changes in ambulatory aids. Some clients may need electric wheelchairs or scooters to enhance community mobility; others may require a lighter, more easily propelled wheelchair.
- Use driver simulation training before the actual state driving test.
- Implement bus training, including how to use public transit systems and medical transportation systems. For clients with cognitive issues, training should begin with only one route and involve repeated practice under therapist supervision before generalizing to other routes.

Adaptive and Compensatory Strategies

- Use adaptive aids such as secondary vehicle controls, lifts, wheelchair restraint systems, and adapted driving controls (adapted handles, blinkers, and brakes).
- Use restricted licenses as available in some states (e.g., the client can drive only during daytime hours or within a certain distance from home).
- Use volunteer drivers and other assistive transportation systems.

Communication

Clients with cognitive impairments or autism spectrum disorders often have compromised language capabilities. Other people with central nervous system involvement of the speech centers, such as clients with cerebral palsy, may have disjointed or difficult-to-understand speech. As these clients age, traditional low-technology communication aids may no longer suit their needs, at which point the team must determine the best communication system to maximize performance. The first decision in this regard should be to determine the client's primary mode of communication (Harden, 2001) so that the team, family, and extended care network can work consistently with the communication program. Additional decisions include where communication needs to occur, how effective the technology will be within the environment, the client's ability and motivation to use the system, and the ability for other people to use the communication system with the clients.

Clients with developmental disabilities often need to learn communication skills related to social interaction, assertiveness training, and the differences between private and public conversations. Because of difficulties with generalization, a client may need repeated practice, both at home and in the community, to master communication and social skills. Additional strategies that may help include using role-plays, videotapes, and feedback following social interaction.

Remedial Strategies

- Use social skills training groups and therapy techniques to enhance the client's ability to communicate in a variety of public situations.
- Use role-plays, modeling, practice, and feedback to enhance verbal and written communication skills.
- Provide skill training to the client, family, and extended care network in the use of communication devices in multiple contexts.

Adaptive and Compensatory Strategies

- Use communication devices, picture boards, and sign language.
- Use simplified language, yes or no questions, and brief sentences.
- Use adapted household equipment, such as teletype systems, telephones with enhanced volume, hearing aids, and voice recognition software.

Play, Leisure, and Social Participation

Development of social skills affects every area of a person's life, including the ability to secure employment, participate in community events, and engage in play and leisure activities with others. Several developmental disorders have accompanying symptoms that can interfere with social interactions and participation. The *Diagnostic and Statistical Manual of Mental Disorders* (American Psychiatric Association [APA], 2000) includes the following diagnostic criteria for autistic and Asperger's disorders:

- Marked impairment in the use of nonverbal behaviors, such as eye-to-eye gaze, facial expression, body postures, and gestures to regulate social interaction
- Failure to develop peer relationships appropriate to developmental level
- Lack of spontaneous seeking to share enjoyment, interests, or achievements with other people
- A lack of social or emotional reciprocity.

Other disorders, such as childhood disintegrative disorder, Rett's disorder, and attentional disorders all have criteria that indicate potential difficulties in social interactions or difficulty with engagement in leisure and social activities. Clients with cognitive deficits may encounter even more occupational barriers because their ability to explore and identify meaningful activities may be impaired.

Intervention techniques designed to enhance social skills and social participation may include the use of social skills curricula, social stories, and activity groups. Greene (2001) presented social modeling as an effective tool in teaching social skills. The author identified modeling as a cognitive–behavioral approach that includes verbal modeling, skill performance, practice, and feedback. Programs that incorporate social modeling often include the use of role-plays, stories, and discussions. Social skills also can be practiced during activities and goals related to play and leisure. Games, community outings, and exploration of interests are suitable activities for intervention and serve a dual purpose, as they provide the client opportunities to work on social skills. Clients may need cues and reminders regarding social behaviors in a variety of situations, such as personal versus public social interaction, maintenance of boundaries, and use of personal space. Occupational therapists should emphasize developing leisure interests that are appropriate to the client's skill level, interests, and context.

Remedial Strategies

- Provide social skills training using psychoeducation, behavioral modification, and cognitive–behavioral programs.
- Use interest checklists and opportunities to explore and develop play and leisure interests.
- Use activity groups, task groups, community outings, and structured play opportunities.

Adaptive and Compensatory Strategies

- Provide education to caregivers and the client's extended care network regarding modification of communication and social interaction to facilitate social exchange.
- Focus on mastery of one or two social skills at a time.
- Use adapted play and leisure equipment (e.g., adapted sports equipment, bicycles, and games).
- Modify rules to match the cognitive level of the client.
- Use schedules to promote daily leisure time.

Education and Work

Young adults with developmental disabilities who are involved in meaningful activities, such as work or volunteer opportunities, report a higher level of life satisfaction (Salkever, 2000). Transition planning for the client with developmental disabilities occurs as the adolescent enters adulthood, and decisions must be made regarding whether the client will pursue vocational training, education toward a degree, or employment directly following high school. Many students with developmental disabilities do well in vocational training programs, and these programs often result in increased attendance, provide practical experience toward a vocation, and facilitate exploration of a particular type of career or job (American Academy of Pediatrics, 2000). Other people, especially those with milder forms of disabilities and higher cognitive abilities, choose college. For clients who are unlikely to pursue education beyond high school, the client and team must work together in determining a plan to pursue vocational goals.

Therapists selecting the appropriate work and educational environment for a client with developmental disabilities should consider the client's interests, skills, performance level, and occupational needs. The American Academy of Pediatrics (2000) recommended that occupational therapy for adolescents and young adults with developmental disabilities emphasize the following:

- Education regarding public laws (i.e., Americans With Disabilities Act [ADA] and Individuals With Disabilities Education Act [IDEA]) and their implications for education and career opportunities
- Opportunities for volunteer work and internships
- Opportunities for career exploration
- Emphasis on independence at place of residence
- Opportunities for meaningful employment.

Intervention for work and educational goals should focus not only on vocational skill training but also on the ability to search and apply for employment, engage in the interview process, and determine applicability to the client's skills and interests. Dolyniuk et al. (2002) suggested the importance of training the individual in social skills along with vocational and educational skills to promote self-efficacy and increased awareness of social context in vocational and educational settings. The authors stressed the value of role-playing, perspective taking, and direct experience in social settings in order to develop skills necessary for successful experience in vocational settings.

Remedial Strategies

- Direct training in educational and vocational skill areas, including getting to and from school or work, social behaviors, study and work habits, work routines, understanding rules and regulations, ability to take feedback and make changes as necessary, follow-through with safety procedures, and ability to obtain necessary resources and external supports for success in the work and school environments.
- Use social stories, role-plays, videotapes, and direct practice to teach problem solving and adaptive behaviors in the work and school settings.
- Use internships and volunteer experiences to develop work skills.

Adaptive and Compensatory Strategies

- Match the work or education setting to the client's skills (ranging, e.g., from sheltered workshops to enclaves, to supported employment, to transitional employment, and to competitive employment)
- Educate the academic and vocational staff working with the client (in conformity with the ADA, IDEA, and other regulatory practices).
- Develop prevocational skills.

- Use adaptive equipment as needed (e.g., adaptive keyboards, voice recognition software, or ergonomic aids).
- Adapt the client's daily routine to accommodate the disability by incorporating extended or more frequent breaks, extended test-taking time, extended deadlines, or a shorter work day.
- Adapt the work environment and job tasks to the skills and needs of the client.

Summary

Occupational therapists apply diverse approaches to evaluation and intervention for adults with developmental disabilities. The selection of an approach requires clinical reasoning that is based on the needs and therapeutic goals of the client. Therapists should use client-centered, holistic practices to focus on quality of life in working to maximize occupational performance for the client. This chapter presented a framework for approaching clients with developmental disabilities along with strategies for evaluation and intervention. Additional resources regarding specific disorders are provided in the appendixes.

Study Questions

1. What are some of the categories of developmental disabilities?
2. What is a client-centered occupation-based approach? How is it used with people with developmental disabilities?
3. What are some common reasons for evaluation in developmentally disabled populations?
4. What measurement tools are available for assessing ADL skills in adults with developmental disabilities?
5. What is the difference between remedial and adaptive approaches? When would you use these approaches in treating a client with developmental disabilities?
6. List examples of intervention techniques using remedial and adaptive strategies for adults with developmental disabilities.
7. How would you involve the family and extended care network in caring for a person with developmental disabilities?

References

Abreu, B. C. (1992). The quadraphonic approach: Management of cognitive-perceptual and postural control dysfunction. *Occupational Therapy Practice, 3,* 12–29.

Abreu, B. C. (1998). The quadraphonic approach: Holistic rehabilitation for brain injury. In N. Katz (Ed.), *Cognition and occupation in rehabilitation: Cognitive models for intervention in occupational therapy* (pp. 51–123).

Bethesda, MD: American Occupational Therapy Association.

Affolter, F. D. (1987). *Perception, interaction and language; Interaction of daily living: The root of development.* Berlin: Springer-Verlag.

Allen, C. D., & Blue, T. (1998). Cognitive disabilities model: How to make clinical judgments. In N. Katz (Ed.), *Cognition and occupation in rehabilitation: Cognitive models for intervention in occupational therapy* (pp. 225–279). Bethesda, MD: American Occupational Therapy Association.

Allen, C. K. (1985). *Occupational therapy for psychiatric diseases: Measurement and management of cognitive disabilities.* Boston: Little, Brown.

American Academy of Pediatrics. (2000). The role of the pediatrician in transitioning children and adolescents with developmental disabilities and chronic illnesses from school to work or college. *Pediatrics, 106,* 854–856.

American Occupational Therapy Association. (2002). Occupational therapy practice framework: Domain and process. *American Journal of Occupational Therapy, 56,* 609–639.

American Psychiatric Association. (2000). *Desk reference to the diagnostic criteria from DSM–IV–TR.* Washington, DC: Author.

Avery-Smith, W. (2001). Dysphagia. In C. A. Trombly & M. V. Radomski (Eds.), *Occupational therapy for physical dysfunction* (5th ed., pp. 1091–1109). Philadelphia: Lippincott Williams & Wilkins.

Ayres, A. J. (1972). *Sensory integration and learning disorders.* Los Angeles: Western Psychological Services.

Ayres, A. J. (1979). *Sensory integration and the child.* Los Angeles: Western Psychological Services.

Babola, K. T. (2000). Independent living strategies for adults with developmental disabilities. In C. Christiansen (Ed.), *Ways of living* (2nd ed., pp. 123–140). Bethesda, MD: American Occupational Therapy Association.

Bachner, S. (1998). Let's Do Lunch: A comprehensive nonstandardized assessment tool. In M. Ross & S. Bachner (Eds.), *Adults with developmental disabilities: Current approaches in occupational therapy* (pp. 263–306). Bethesda, MD: American Occupational Therapy Association.

Baranek, G. T., Chin, Y. H., Hess, L. M., Yankee, J. G., Hatton, D. D., & Hooper, S. R. (2002). Sensory processing correlates of occupational performance in children with fragile X syndrome: Preliminary findings. *American Journal of Occupational Therapy, 56,* 538–546.

Bass Haugen, J. B., & Mathiowetz, V. (1995). Contemporary task oriented approach. In C. A. Trombly (Ed.), *Occupational therapy for physical dysfunction* (4th ed., pp. 510–527). Baltimore: Williams & Wilkins.

Berger, K. (2001). *The developing person through the life span* (5th ed.). New York: Worth.

Bolick, T. (2001). *Asperger syndrome and adolescence: Helping preteens and teens get ready for the real world.* Gloucester, MA: Fair Winds Press.

Brannon, L., & Feist, J. (2000). *Health psychology: An introduction to behavior and health.* Stamford, CT: Wadsworth.

Brei, T. (1999). The adult with spina bifida. In M. Lutkenhoff (Ed.), *Children with spina bifida: A parent's guide* (pp. 313–328). Bethesda, MD: Woodbine House.

Bruce, M. A., & Borg, B. (2002). *Psychosocial frames of reference: Core for occupation-based practice.* Thorofare, NJ: Slack.

Bruininks, R. H., Woodcock, R. W., Weatherman, R. F., & Hill, B. K. (1996). *SIB-R: Scales of Independent Behavior—Revised.* Itasca, IL: Riverside.

Bundy, A. C., Lane, S. J., & Murray, E. A. (2002). *Sensory integration: Theory and practice.* Philadelphia: F. A. Davis.

Bunning, M. E., Angelo, J. A., & Schmeler, M. R. (2001). Occupational performance and the transition to powered mobility: A pilot study. *American Journal of Occupational Therapy, 55,* 339–344.

Burns, T. (1992). Cognitive performance test. In C. K. Allen, C. A. Earhart, & T. Blue (Eds.), *Occupational therapy treatment goals for the physically and cognitively disabled* (pp. 46–50). Bethesda, MD: American Occupational Therapy Association.

Christiansen, C., & Baum, C. (1997). Person-environment occupational performance: A conceptual model for practice. In C. Christiansen & C. Baum (Eds.), *Occupational therapy: Enabling function and well being* (2nd ed., pp. 47–70). Thorofare, NJ: Slack.

Cohn, E. S. (2001). From waiting to relating: Parents' experiences in the waiting room of an occupational therapy clinic. *American Journal of Occupational Therapy, 55,* 167–174.

Cohn, E. S., Miller, L. J., & Tickle-Degnen, L. (2000). Parental hopes for therapy outcomes: Children with sensory modulation disorders. *American Journal of Occupational Therapy, 54,* 36–43.

Cook, A. M., & Hussey, S. M. (2002). *Assistive technologies: Principles and practice* (2nd ed.). St. Louis, MO: Mosby.

Developmental Disabilities Assistance and Bill of Rights Act of 2000, Pub. L. No. 106–402, 114 Stat. 1677 (2000).

Dolyniuk, A., Kamens, M. W., Corman, H., Dinardo, P. O., Totaro, R. M., & Rockoff, J. C. (2002). Students with developmental disabilities go to college: Description of a collaborative transition project on a regular college campus. *Focus on Autism and Other Developmental Disabilities, 17*(4), 236–239.

Dunn, W. (1998). Person centered and contextually relevant evaluation. In J. Hinojosa & P. Kramer (Eds.), *Evaluation: Obtaining and interpreting data* (pp. 47–76). Bethesda, MD: American Occupational Therapy Association.

Dunn, W., Brown, C., & McGuigan, A. (1994). The ecology of human performance: A framework for considering the effect of context. *American Journal of Occupational Therapy, 48,* 595–607.

Dunn, W., Miles, S. M., & Orr, S. (2002). Sensory processing issues associated with Asperger's syndrome: A preliminary investigation. *American Journal of Occupational Therapy, 56,* 97–102.

Earhart, C. A. (1992). Analysis of activities. In C. K. Allen, C. A. Earhart, & T. Blue (Eds.), *Occupational therapy treatment goals for the physically and cognitively disabled* (pp. 125–305). Bethesda, MD: American Occupational Therapy Association.

Fanchiang, S. C. (1996). The other side of the coin: Growing up with a learning disability. *American Journal of Occupational Therapy, 50,* 277–285.

Fearing, V. G., Law, M., & Clark, J. (1997). An occupational performance process model: Fostering client and therapist alliances. *Canadian Journal of Occupational Therapy, 64*(1), 7–15.

Fertel-Daly, D., Bedell, G., & Hinojosa, J. (2001). Effects of a weighted vest on attention to task and self-stimulatory behaviors in preschoolers with pervasive developmental disorders. *American Journal of Occupational Therapy, 55,* 629–640.

Fisher, A. G. (1997). *Assessment of motor and process skills* (2nd ed.). Ft. Collins, CO: Three Star Press.

Foxx, R. M., & Azrin, N. H. (1973). *Toilet training the retarded: A rapid program for day and nighttime independent toileting.* Champaign, IL: Research Press.

Greene, S. (2001). Social skills intervention for children with autism and Asperger's disorder. In H. Miller-Kuhaneck (Ed.), *Autism: A comprehensive occupational therapy approach* (pp. 153–171). Bethesda, MD: American Occupational Therapy Association.

Guide for the Uniform Data Set for Medical Rehabilitation (FIM™ Instrument), Version 5: Australia. (1999). Buffalo, NY: University at Buffalo.

Hale, S. (2000). Naming strengths and resources of the client and therapist. In V. G. Fearing & J. Clark (Eds.), *Individuals in context: A practical guide to client-centered practice* (pp. 69–78). Thorofare, NJ: Slack.

Hanschu, B. (1998). Using a sensory approach to serve adults who have developmental disabilities. In M. Ross & S. Bachner (Eds.), *Adults with developmental disabilities: Current approaches in occupational therapy* (pp. 165–211). Bethesda, MD: American Occupational Therapy Association.

Harden, B. (2001). Assistive technology for students with autism. In H. Miller-Kuhaneck (Ed.), *Autism: A comprehensive occupational therapy approach* (pp. 201–223). Bethesda, MD: American Occupational Therapy Association.

Harjamaki, K. (2000). *Assessing cognitive abilities of adults with developmental disabilities: A survey of current practice.* Unpublished master's thesis, College of St. Catherine, St. Paul, MN.

Haynes, R. B., McKibbon, K. A., & Kanani, R. (1996). Systematic review of randomized trials of interventions to assist patients to follow prescriptions for medications. *Lancet, 348,* 383–386.

Hirama, H. (1989). *Self-injurious behavior: A somatosensory treatment approach.* Baltimore: Chess Publications.

Humphry, R., & Thigpen-Beck. (1998). Parenting values and attitudes: View of therapists and parents. *American Journal of Occupational Therapy, 52,* 835–842.

Jackson, J., Gray, J. M., & Zemke, R. (2001). Optimizing abilities and capacities: Range of motion, strength, and endurance. In C. A. Trombly & M. V. Radomski (Eds.), *Occupational therapy for physical dysfunction* (5th ed., pp. 463–480). Philadelphia: Lippincott Williams & Wilkins.

Jackson, J. P., & Schkade, J. K. (2001). Occupational adaptation model versus biomechanical-rehabilitation model in the treatment of patients with hip fracture. *American Journal of Occupational Therapy, 55,* 531–537.

Jacobs, K. (1991). *Occupational therapy: Work-related programs and assessment* (2nd ed.). Boston: Little, Brown.

Katz, S., Downs, T. D., Cash, H. R., & Grotz, R. C. (1970). Progress in development of index of ADL. *Gerontologist, 10,* 20–30.

Kellogg, H. A. (1998). An OTR's description of the legacy, current environment, and clinical issues characterizing adults with profound disabilities. In M. Ross & S. Bachner (Eds.), *Adults with developmental disabilities: Current approaches in occupational therapy* (pp. 90–122). Bethesda, MD: American Occupational Therapy Association.

Kielhofner, G. (1995). *A model of human occupation: Theory and application* (2nd ed.). Baltimore: Williams & Wilkins.

Kielhofner, G., Mallinson, T., Crawford, C., Nowak, M., Rigby, M., Henry, A., et al. (1998). *A user's manual for the Occupational Performance History Interview* (Version 2.0). Chicago: University of Illinois, Model of Human Occupation Clearinghouse.

Kinnealey, M., Oliver, B., & Willbarger, P. (1995). A phenomenological study of sensory defensiveness in adults. *American Journal of Occupational Therapy, 49,* 444–451.

Klein, R. M., & Bell, B. (1982). Self care skills: Behavioral measurement with Klein-Bell ADL Scale. *Archives of Physical Medicine and Rehabilitation, 63,* 335–338.

Law, M., Baptiste, S., Carswell, A., McColl, M., Polatajko, H., & Pollock, N. (1998). *Canadian Occupational Performance Measure* (3rd ed.). Ottawa, Ontario: Canadian Association of Occupational Therapy.

Malgady, R. G., Barcher, P. R., Davis, J. D., & Towner, G. *Vocational Adaptation Rating Scales.* Los Angeles: Western Psychological Services.

Malone, D. M., McKinsey, P. D., Thyer, B. A., & Straka, E. (2000). Social work early intervention for young children with developmental disabilities. *Health and Social Work, 25,* 169–180.

Mann, W. C., & Beaver, K. A. (1995). Assessment services: Person, device, family, and environment. In W. C. Mann & J. P. Lane (Eds.), *Assistive technology for persons with disabilities* (2nd ed., pp. 219–317). Bethesda, MD: American Occupational Therapy Association.

Mason, D. B., Santoro, K., & Kaull, A. (1999). Bowel management. In M. Lutkenhoff (Ed.), *Children with spina bifida: A parent's guide* (pp. 87–105). Bethesda, MD: Woodbine House.

Mathiowetz, V., & Bass Haugen, J. (1994). Motor behavior research: Implications for therapeutic approaches to central nervous system dysfunction. *American Journal of Occupational Therapy, 48,* 733–745.

Miller, F., & Bachrach, S. J. (1995). *Cerebral palsy: A complete guide for caregiving.* Baltimore: Johns Hopkins University Press.

Moor, D. Y. (2000). Daily care. In J. D. Weber (Ed.), *Children with fragile X syndrome: A parent's guide* (pp. 121–154). Bethesda, MD: Woodbine House.

Mulcahey, M. A. (1999). Nurturing an emotionally healthy child. In M. Lutkenhoff (Ed.), *Children with spina bifida: A parent's guide* (pp. 257–271). Bethesda, MD: Woodbine House.

Mulhall, D. (1989). *Functional performance record.* Windsor, England: Darville House.

Neistadt, M. E. (1990). A critical analysis of occupational therapy approaches for perceptual deficits for adults with brain injury. *American Journal of Occupational Therapy, 44,* 299–304.

Nihira, K., Leland, H., & Lambert, N. (1993). *AAMR Adaptive Behavior Scale—Residential and Community* (2nd ed.). Austin, TX: PRO-ED.

Oetter, P., Laurel, M., & Cool, S. (1991). Sensory motor foundations of communication. In C. B. Royeen (Ed.), *Neuroscience foundations of human performance* Rockville, MD: American Occupational Therapy Association.

Oetter, P., Richter, E., & Frick, S. (1993). *M.O.R.E.: Integrating the mouth with sensory and postural functions* (2nd ed.). Hugo, MN: PDP Publications.

Pierce, D. E. (2003). *Occupation by design: Building therapeutic power.* Philadelphia: F. A. Davis.

Portwood, M. (1996). *Developmental dyspraxia: A practice manual for parents and professionals* (2nd ed.). Durham, England: Educational Psychology Service.

Reisman, J. E., & Hanschu, B. (1992). *Sensory Integration Inventory—Revised for Individuals With Developmental Disabilities.* Hugo, MN: PDP Press.

Renwick, R. (1998). Quality of life: A guiding framework for practice with adults who have developmental disabilities. In M. Ross & S. Bachner (Eds.), *Adults with developmental disabilities: Current approaches in occupational therapy* (pp. 23–41). Bethesda, MD: American Occupational Therapy Association.

Rogers, J. C., & Holm, M. B. (1989). The therapist's thinking behind functional assessment I. In C. Royeen (Ed.), *AOTA self study series: Assessing function.* Rockville, MD: American Occupational Therapy Association.

Salkever, D. S. (2000). Activity status, life satisfaction, and perceived productivity for young adults with developmental disabilities. *Journal of Rehabilitation, 66,* 4+. Retrieved September 9, 2003, from InfoTrac database.

Sonander, K. (2000). Early identification of children with developmental disabilities. *Acta Paediatrica, 89,* 17–23.

Sparrow, S. S., Balla, D., & Cicchetti, D. V. (1984). *Vineland Adaptive Behavior Scales.* Circle Pines, MN: American Guidance Service.

Spencer, K. C., & Sample, P. L. (1993). Transition planning services. In C. B. Royeen (Ed.), *AOTA self study series: Classroom applications for school based practice* (Lesson 10). Rockville, MD: American Occupational Therapy Association.

Spitzer, S., & Roley, S. S. (2001). Sensory integration revisited: A philosophy of practice. In S. S. Roley, E. I. Blanche, & R. C. Schaaf (Eds.), *Understanding the nature of sensory integration with diverse populations* (pp. 3–27). San Antonio, TX: Therapy Skill Builders.

Stancliff, B. L. (1998, October.). Play with a purpose: Sensory integration treatment and developmental disabilities. *OT Practice, 3*(9), 34–40.

Stratton, M. (1981). Reliability of the behavioral assessment scale of oral functions in feeding. *American Journal of Occupational Therapy, 39,* 436–440.

Stratton, M. (1989). Clinical management of dysphagia in the developmentally disabled adult. In J. A. Johnson & D. A. Ethridge (Eds.), *Developmental disabilities: A handbook for occupational therapists.* New York: Haworth.

Taylor, S. (1999). *Health psychology* (4th ed.). Boston: McGraw-Hill.

Toglia, J. P. (1991). Generalization of treatment: A multi-context approach to cognitive perceptual impairment in adults with brain injury. *American Journal of Occupational Therapy, 45,* 505–516.

Toglia, J. P. (1998). A dynamic interactional model to cognitive rehabilitation. In N. Katz (Ed.), *Cognition and occupation in rehabilitation: Cognitive models for intervention in occupational therapy* (pp. 5–50). Bethesda, MD: American Occupational Therapy Association.

Trefler, E., & Hobson, D. (1997). Assistive technology. In C. Christiansen & C. Baum (Eds.), *Occupational therapy: Enabling function and well being* (2nd ed., pp. 483–506). Thorofare, NJ: Slack.

Waltz, M. (2002). *Autistic spectrum disorders: Understanding the diagnosis and getting help* (2nd ed.). Sebastopol, CA: O'Reilly.

Weiss, L. (1997). *Attention deficit disorder in adults: Practical help and understanding.* Dallas, TX: Taylor.

Willbarger, P. (1995, June). The sensory diet: Activity programs based on sensory processing theory. *Sensory Integration Special Interest Section Newsletter, 18*(2), 1–4.

Willbarger, P. & Willbarger, J. (1991). *Sensory defensiveness in children aged 2–12.* Santa Barbara, CA: Avanti Educational Publications.

Williams, M. S., & Shellenberger, S. (1994). *How does your engine run? A leader's guide to the Alert Program for self-regulation.* Albuquerque, NM: Therapy Works.

Appendix 7.A.

Performance Inventory
Performance Domain: *Domestic/Home*

School: _____   Student: _____

Age: _____ Date: _____

Directions: Address the following areas through interviews with the student, family members, or others as appropriate, or through student observation.

Goal Area	Activity	Current Level of Functioning
Eating and food preparation	1. Meal planning	
Interview with parents and school cafeteria staff	2. Preparing meals and snacks • gathers ingredients and equipment • opens containers (i.e., soda cans, milk cartons, cereal box) • follows recipes • uses microwave • uses stove top • uses oven • users other appliances	
Observation of student's home kitchen layout	3. Eating a meal/snack • oral motor skills (i.e., swallowing, chewing) • uses utensils • uses manners	
	4. Preparing eating area • sets table • gets condiments	

	5. Cleaning up after meal
	• puts away leftovers
	• wipes off work surface
	• washes dishes
	  – handwashing
	  – using dishwasher	

	6. Accessibility to kitchen • uses adaptive equipment	
Grooming and dressing	1. Grooming • brushes teeth • uses mouthwash • brushes/combs hair • styles hair • skin care • maintains appearance	
Interview with parents/ caregivers and student	2. Dressing/undressing • undresses self • chooses appropriate clothes • dresses self • dresses appropriate for season/weather conditions	
Priorities:		
Hygiene and toileting Interview with parents/ caregivers and student	1. Uses private and public toilets • wipes self • flushes toilet • washes hands 2. Washing hands and face 3. Bathing/showering 4. Shampooing/rinsing hair 5. Shaving • men 6. Using deodorant	
Priorities:		

Domestic/Home Domain (continued)

Goal Area	Activity	Current Level of Functioning
Houshold maintenance	1. Keeping room neat • makes bed • changes bed linens • straightens room	
Interview with parents/ caregivers	2. Handling household chores • does laundry • vacuums/dusts • cleans bathroom • sweeps	
	3. Maintaining outdoors • rakes leaves • mows lawn • weeds • waters lawn • cleans up after animals	
Priorities:		
Social skills	1. Telephone use • telephone etiquette • takes message • dials telephone • can use telephone for emergency • can use assistive devices if necessary • can use telephone directory	
Interview with parents/ caregivers	2. Caring for others • pet care • sibling care • babysitting • care of elderly	
	3. Reciprocal relationships • gift giving • remembers birthdays • sends thank you cards	
Priorities:		
Sexuality/health/safety Hygiene and toileting	1. Awareness of public versus private sexual activities • closes door for bathing, toileting, dressing, etc. • chooses appropriate place to masturbate	
Interview with parents/ caregivers	2. Appropriate show of affection	
	3. Awareness of bodily and sexual functions	
	4. Knowledge and use of birth control methods	
	5. Knowledge of sexually transmitted diseases	
	6. Knowledge of general health concerns • disease transmission (i.e., covers mouth when sneezing, coughing, controls drooling, blows nose, etc.) • health concerns specific to disability (i.e., skin care, range of motion, positioning of weight) • takes medication (i.e., knows medication schedule, ability to swallow, related behavioral concerns) • cares for minor injury	
	7. Awareness of home hazards and emergency procedures • poisons • fire • accidents	
Priorities:		

Performance Inventory
*Performance Domain: **General Community***

School: _____   Student: _____
                                                                            Age: _____ Date: _____

Directions: Address the following areas through interviews with the student, family members, or others as appropriate, or through student observation.

Goal Area	Activity	Current Level of Functioning
Travel	1. "Walking" (wheeling) to and from destination • safety when crossing streets • arrives at destination	
	2. Riding bicycle • knows safety rules • able to find way • locks bicycle	
	3. Riding school bus/city bus • demonstrates appropriate behavior when on bus • communicates with bus driver • can find appropriate bus • can read bus map • can make a transfer • knows how to pay an appropriate amount • shows bus pass	
	4. Driving own vehicle • knows laws • demonstrates safe and defensive technique • can physically handle task • uses appropriate adaptive equipment • uses seat belts	
	5. Orienting skills • identifies signs • carries identification • asks for help • responsible for possessions • uses caution with strangers • reads maps	
Priorities:		
General shopping	1. Handling money/budgeting • makes shopping lists • recognizes budget constraints • handles money exchanges	
	2. Locating/getting items • pushes cart • uses store directory • asks for help • follows list • makes choices • does cost comparisons	
	3. Clothes/personal items • plans for trip • selects appropriate store • selects items within budget • makes wise choices • handles money exchanges	
Priorities:		
Restaurant	1. "Reads" menu (or alternative) 2. Communicates to wait person 3. Uses manners 4. Locates restrooms 5. Tallies bill (including tip) 6. Handles money exchanges	
Priorities:		

General Community Domain (continued)

Goal Area	Activity	Current Level of Functioning
Using services	1. Uses pay telephone 2. Uses relay system (if hearing impaired) 3. Uses beauty parlor 4. Makes appointments 5. Uses banking services 6. Uses/communicates with dentist, doctor, etc. 7. Uses laundromat/drycleaner	
Priorities:		

Note. From "Transition Planning Services", by K. C. Spencer and P. L. Sample, 1993, in C. B. Royeen (Ed.), *AOTA Self Study Series: Classroom Applications for School-Based Practice* (Lesson 10), Rockville, MD: American Occupational Therapy Association. Copyright 1993 by the American Occupational Therapy Association. Reprinted with permission.

Appendix 7.B.

Resident: _____*Helen*_____   Therapist: ___*S. Bachner, OTR/L*___   Date: _____*11/13/96*_____

"Let's Do Lunch" Assessment Tool
Task Analysis: Eating in the Lodge

Scoring Codes:
S = Sensory = tactile, proprioceptive, vestibular, visual, auditory, gustatory, olfactory
P = Perceptual = stereognosis, pain response, body scheme, visual perceptual, visual acuity
N = Neuromuscular = reflex, ROM, muscle tone, endurance, postural control
M = Motor = gross coordination, crosses midline, laterality, praxis, oral motor control
C = Cognitive Integration = level of arousal, attention span, initiation, problem solving
p = Psychosocial = social conduct, self-expression, self-management

TASK 0 = independent, 1 = verbal cue, 2 = physical assist, 3 = total assist	S	P	N	M	C	p
1. Enters Dining Room · 0 1 ②3	✔	✔				
2. Locates End of Line · 0 1 2 ③	✔	✔				
3. Stands on Line · ⓪1 2 3						
4. Collects a Tray · 0 1 2 ③		✔			✔	
5. Puts Tray on Counter · 0 1 2 ③		✔			✔	
6. Faces Correct Direction · 0 1 2 ③						
7. Moves "Forward" · 0 ① 2 3						
8. Balances on Two Feet · ⓪1 2 3						
9. Sees Food Items · 0 1 2 ③		✔				
10. Reaches for Food Items · 0 1 2 ③		✔			✔	
11. Inhibits Impulse to Take All Food · ⓪1 2 3						
12. Makes Food Choice Decisions *N.A.* · 0 1 2 ③					✔	
13. Holds Loaded Tray With Two Hands · 0 1 2 ③					✔	
14. Navigates Turn Off of Line to Seating Area · 0 1 2 ③		✔			✔	
15. Ambulates Efficiently With Tray and Contents · 0 1 2 ③	✔	✔				
16. Visually Scans Room *Only responds to stimuli in central visual field* · 0 1 2 ③		✔				
17. Visually Targets an Available seat *Guided to table c̄ available seat* · 0 1 ② 3						
18. Visually Targets an Available Seat With Friends *Stands beside chair per escort #17* · 0 1 ② 3						
19. Gets to a Targeted Seat · 0 1 ② 3						
20. Puts Tray on Table · 0 1 2 ③						
21. Pulls Chair Out *Refuses* · 0 1 2 3						
22. Sits Down and Positions Legs Under the Table *Refuses to sit* · 0 1 2 3						
23. Achieves Good Upper Body Posture in Seat *N.A.* · 0 1 2 3						
24. Achieves Good Lower Body Posture in Seat *Wants to eat while standing* · 0 1 2 3						
25. Aligns Self With Tray at Midline *Continues to resist sitting in chair* · 0 1 2 3						
26. Acknowledges Peers at Table (or nearby) *Smiles at peers if in her central vision (20"–30" central)* · 0 1 2 3		✔				

Appendix 7.B *(continued)*

		S	P	N	M	C	p
27. Visually Attends to Tray/Contents *Moves visual target to 4" from eyes*	0 1 2 ③						
28. Reaches for Utensils (Wrapped in napkin)	0 1 2 ③						
29. Uses Two Hands to Unwrap Utensils *If given to her*	⓪ 1 2 3						
30. Places Napkins in Lap *Still standing—N.A.*	0 1 2 3						
31. Uses Bilateral Hand Movements to Open Packets *Fine-motor O.K.—Doesn't coordinate c̄ eyes*	0 1 ② 3						
32. Seasons Food With Salt and Pepper *N.A.*	0 1 2 3						
33. Holds Knife by the Handle *Only uses spoon*	⓪ 1 2 3						
34. Spreads Butter With Knife *N.A.*	0 1 2 3						
35. Cuts Food With Knife *N.A.*	0 1 2 3						
36. Grasps Eating Utensils With Functional Grip (Ⓡor L) *Only briefly—prefers to use fingers*	⓪ 1 2 3						
37. Visually Targets Desired Food Items *Seems to need high contrast, central 20"–30", 4" from eyes*	0 1 2 3						
38. Initiates Movement of Utensils Toward Food Item *Prefers fingers for food exploration*	⓪ 1 2 3						
39. Loads Spoon/Pieces With Fork *Can use spoon but likes fingers*	⓪ 1 2 3						
40. Contains Food Items on Plate/Bowl *Given hi-sided plate to assist c̄ containment— did better*	0 1 ② 3		✔				
41. Brings Food to Mouth With Utensil *Holds bowl at 4" from face c̄ Ⓛ hand*	⓪ 1 2 3		✔				
42. Closes Lips to Contain Food in Mouth	⓪ 1 2 3						
43. Chews Bolus With Teeth *Needs mechanical-soft/ground meat for safety*	0 1 2 3						
44. Swallows Bolus	⓪ 1 2 3						
45. Safe Chewing and Swallowing—*Not when eating regular diet (consistency)*	0 1 2 3						
46. Wipes Mouth as Needed	⓪ 1 2 3					✔	
47. Targets Drinking Glass *Having Trouble Locating it*	0 1 2 ③		✔				
48. Crosses Midline (R/L) With Hands as Needed	⓪ 1 2 3						
49. Reaches/Grasps/Lifts Glass to Mouth *Needs to be placed in her hand*	0 1 2 ③		✔				
50. Drinks Liquid With a Safe Pace and Adequate Swallow *Doesn't tip head back. Why?*	⓪ 1 2 3						
51. Finishes All Food Items on Plate *Required verbal and physical prompts to locate food*	0 1 2 ③		✔				
52. Pushes Chair Back *N.A.*	0 1 2 3						
53. Sitting to Standing With Adequate Balance	⓪ 1 2 3						
54. Reaches To Table and Picks Up Tray	0 1 2 ③						

Appendix 7.B *(continued)*

		S	P	N	M	C	p
55. Re-Aligns Body for Ambulation	⓪ 1 2 3						
56. Carries Tray Without Spilling	0 1 2 ③						
57. Determines Where to Return Tray	0 1 2 ③		✔			✔	
58. Reaches Location for Tray Deposit	0 1 2 ③						
59. Deposits Tray in Return Window	0 1 2 ③						
60. Locates Exit Door From Dining Room	0 1 2 ③						

Summary of Components:		S	P	N	M	C	p
	Lack of Familiarity		✔				
	Needs (Least Functional)					✔	
	Strengths (Most Functional)	✔		✔	✔		✔

Item Numbers Identified for TX: _____

COMMENTS: *If bowl remains on tray, client stretches head forward—obvious muscle strain, tension. Tension disappeared when bowl lifted 4" from eyes/mouth. Needs eye exam. ••previous socialization to people ••*

Chapter 8

Adaptive Strategies for Rheumatic Diseases

CATHERINE L. BACKMAN, PHD, OT(C)

KEY TERMS

ankylosing spondylitis

fibromyalgia

hand function

joint-protection and energy-
conservation principles

juvenile rheumatoid arthritis

osteoarthritis

osteoporosis

rheumatoid arthritis

scleroderma

self-management principles

systemic lupus erythematosus

systemic sclerosis

OBJECTIVES

Upon completion of this chapter, the reader will be able to

• Describe the impact of several different rheumatic diseases on occupational performance;

• Explain the factors to consider when recommending adaptive techniques, equipment, and environmental modifications for clients with rheumatic diseases;

• Describe adaptive strategies, equipment, and environmental modifications for maintaining, restoring, or improving performance in ADL, IADL, work, play, leisure, and social participation;

• Given a case example, apply joint-protection and energy-conservation principles to specific adaptive strategies to enhance the client's occupational performance; and

• Summarize principles incorporated into arthritis self-management programs.

The term *rheumatic diseases* refers to more than 100 different acute and chronic illnesses affecting the musculoskeletal system of bones, joints, muscles, tendons, and ligaments. Similarly, *arthritis* is a general term referring to the predominant characteristic in many rheumatic diseases: joint inflammation (arthro = joint, itis = inflammation). Rheumatic diseases affect people of all ages, from infancy to old age. Although some rheumatic conditions are self-limiting and result in short-term, isolated problems, many are chronic, systemic illnesses resulting in lifelong functional limitations to various degrees. Arthritis disability reduces participation in employment, leisure, and social activities (Badley & DesMeules, 2003). Because arthritis is common, even practitioners who do not work in programs "specializing" in rheumatic diseases will encounter clients with these conditions. Occupational therapy is appropriate at any stage of disease activity, whenever clients experience difficulties in occupational performance.

Epidemiology

Rheumatic and musculoskeletal conditions are among the most prevalent chronic conditions and a leading cause of disability in both the United States (Hannan, 2001) and Canada (Badley & DesMeules, 2003). The prevalence is approximately 15% to 16% (Hannan, 2001; Lagace, Perruccio, DesMeules, & Badley, 2003). About two-thirds of those affected by rheumatic diseases are girls and women. At approximately 19%, the prevalence is higher in Aboriginal peoples; prevalence increases to 27% when age standardized (Lagace et al., 2003). Because many rheumatic diseases are chronic, prevalence increases with age, and arthritis is the most common reason men and women age 65 and older visit a physician (Hannan, 2001). Put another way, more than 37 million Americans and more than 4 million Canadians have rheumatic disorders, and those numbers are expected to increase to close to 60 million and 6 million, respectively, by 2020. Moreover, if arthritis were eradicated, the average life expectancy of the population would increase by almost 1 full year (Manuel, Lagace, DesMeules, Cho, & Power, 2003).

Rheumatic diseases create a large economic burden on individuals and society. In 1995 dollars, the cost of rheumatic diseases in the United States was estimated at $82.5 billion (Callahan, 2001); the majority of costs are indirect (predominantly lost employment income), and slightly less than half the costs are attributed to the direct costs of managing the illness (e.g., hospitalizations, medications,

equipment and assistive devices). In 1998, the economic burden of arthritis in Canada was estimated at CAD$4.4 billion (Stokes, Desjardins, & Perruccio, 2003). The costs are substantial for individuals, families, insurers, and society. Given that more than half the costs are attributed to lost income, interventions that enable people with rheumatic diseases to maintain, improve, or restore their ability to participate in productive activities will decrease the economic burden.

Types of Rheumatic Conditions

The following sections summarize pertinent features for a handful of major types of rheumatic conditions and provide examples of issues that occupational therapists may address.

Osteoarthritis

Osteoarthritis (OA) is the most common of the rheumatic conditions. It affects about 10% of the adult population (Badley & DesMeules, 2003) and has a typical onset after age 45. Prevalence increases with age (Hannan, 2001). OA is characterized by joint pain, aching, stiffness, and decreased range of motion. It is mainly a disease of the cartilage, although the precise mechanism is not known, and there is currently no cure. The most commonly affected joints are those that bear weight (hips, knees, feet, and spine) and the small joints of the hand (i.e., the carpometacarpal joint of the thumb and the proximal interphalangeal and distal interphalangeal joints of all fingers). Risk factors include being female, older age, history of joint trauma (from injury, sports, or occupations with repetitive or heavy joint stress), and obesity. For unknown reasons, African-Americans have a greater incidence of knee OA than Caucasians (Hannan, 2001). Occupational therapists may play a preventative role in the development of OA when they help clients minimize repetitive stress to joints at work or in sports, play, and recreational activities.

Severe joint damage may be treated with reconstructive surgery. For example, hip and knee joint arthroplasties (total joint replacements) are a common and successful intervention to alleviate pain and restore function. Other surgical procedures include joint resurfacing, osteotomies, and joint fusions. Occupational therapy is indicated in both conservative and postoperative management of OA when joint pain and limited mobility hamper activities of daily living (ADL) or threaten participation in instrumental activities of daily living (IADL), work, and leisure.

Rheumatoid Arthritis

Rheumatoid arthritis (RA) is a chronic, systemic, inflammatory disease of unknown cause that is characterized by exacerbations and remissions. It is less common than OA (affecting just under 1% of the population; Badley & DesMeules, 2003; Hannan, 2001), although it can be much more disabling. The peak age of onset is in the 30s and 40s, although it may occur at any time from the late teens onward. RA is a disorder of the immune system that has no known cure. It features symmetrical involvement of the synovial joints, especially metacarpophalangeal joints, wrists, elbows, knees, and feet, although any synovial joint may be affected. During exacerbations, joints are swollen and painful due to inflammation of the synovial lining of the joint capsule. Prolonged periods of inflammation lead to thickening of the synovial cells (pannus formation), thinning cartilage, lax ligaments and capsule, muscle weakness, and instability of the joint. The systemic nature of RA means that other organs, such as the heart, eyes, and lungs, may be involved. People with RA feel a general malaise during exacerbations and may have a fever, fatigue, and long periods of morning stiffness. When the disease is well-controlled with medications or during remissions, however, people may resume many of the activities they ceased during an exacerbation. These "ups and downs" in ability to perform daily activities can be frustrating and may influence mood and well-being.

Hormonal factors are suspected to play a role in RA because the disease is more common in women and tends to remit during pregnancy and flare after delivery. Men with RA tend to have low levels of circulating testosterone (Hannan, 2001). A genetic predisposition exists; risk is 3 to 4 times greater in people with a first-degree relative with the disease, and a genetic marker may be predictive of disease severity (Khani-Hanjani et al., 2000). RA may run a mild course that is easily controlled, or it may be severe and result in progressive joint destruction and disability.

A range of medications is available for RA, including nonsteroidal anti-inflammatory drugs, corticosteroids, disease-modifying antirheumatic drugs, and biologic response modifiers. Some medications are taken orally; others are administered by injection. Managing medications, staying informed, and being alert to potentially harmful side effects is part of the lifelong self-management of this illness.

RA may restrict people's ability to participate in both paid and unpaid work. Recent estimates of work disability (i.e., cessation of paid employment) due to RA range from 22% to 38% (Allaire, Anderson, & Meenan, 1996; Lacaille, Sheps, Spinelli, & Esdaile, 1999; Wolfe & Hawley, 1998), and RA also limits performance of household work, home maintenance, caregiving, volunteer work (Backman, Kennedy, Chalmers, & Singer, 2004), and leisure and social activities (Katz & Yelin, 1994).

Most people with RA will experience reduced strength and dexterity in the hands and wrists. This weakness may be the cause of their difficulties with occupational performance, so occupational therapists give particular attention to assessment and treatment of hand function. Occupational therapy interventions have the potential to minimize the pain and inflammation that restrict participation and enhance function in all aspects of daily living.

Fibromyalgia

Fibromyalgia (FM) is a syndrome of widespread, chronic pain. The diagnostic criteria established by the American College of Rheumatology (ACR) include a history of widespread pain for more than 3 months duration and presence of pain when direct pressure is applied to at least 11 of 18 specific tender points in the body (Wolfe et al., 1990). No laboratory tests currently contribute to the diagnosis. About 3% to 5% of women and 0.5% of men in the United States have FM; although the typical person with FM is a middle-aged woman, the syndrome also affects children (Burckhardt, 2001). A number of theories exist regarding the cause of FM, and it is likely a complex phenomenon. In general, it is understood to be a hypersensitivity to pain or lowering of the pain threshold. Possible biological explanations include disordered central processing of pain stimuli; changes in the neurotransmitter systems of substance P and serotonin; low levels of growth hormone; and decreased blood flow in the thalamus and caudate nuclei, which are involved in processing pain stimuli (Burckhardt, 2001).

Characteristic features of FM include complaints of aches, pain, and tenderness throughout the body, near but not in the joints. Pain is usually worse in the neck and shoulders. Clients report sleep disturbances and persistent fatigue. Headaches, parethesias, and irritable bowel and bladder frequently are reported. Because of the difficulty diagnosing FM, many people spend considerable time and frustration trying to identify the source of their pain. The diagnosis may come as a relief, particularly for clients who have been told they had any number of other diagnoses or, worse, that it was "all in their heads." Once diagnosed, some clients may be anxious about how to manage their illness.

Pain and fatigue may limit physical activity, leading to decreased muscle strength and endurance. Clients with FM who are referred for rehabilitation interventions often are deconditioned and may be reluctant to engage in even modest amounts of physical activity. One of the cornerstones of managing fibromyalgia is exercise or physical activity, however, which should be carefully graded to match the interests and physical capacity or fitness of the client. It generally is best to begin at a level below that which the client feels is achievable and build on success. This concept of the "just right challenge" is common in grading activities in occupational therapy and contributes to maintaining motivation and developing new habits. FM does not appear to progress over time, so management strategies learned early in the course of the illness will enable clients to effectively manage their symptoms and participate in life. Unlike most other rheumatic conditions, no joint or tissue damage results from FM.

Juvenile Rheumatoid Arthritis

Juvenile rheumatoid arthritis (JRA) is one classification of several rheumatic diseases arising in childhood. Other such diseases include connective tissue disorders such as juvenile polymyositis; overuse syndromes like chondromalacia patellae; and systemic illnesses with musculoskeletal manifestations, such as hemophilia (Cassidy & Petty, 2001). It is beyond the scope of this chapter to address so many conditions; however, many of the principles that apply to JRA may be applied to or adapted for children with related arthropathies. Like RA, JRA is characterized by exacerbations and remissions of joint pain and inflammation. To be classified as a juvenile disease, the onset must occur by age 16.

JRA takes three forms (Cassidy & Petty, 2001; Taylor & Erlandson, 2001):

1. At onset, *polyarticular* JRA involves five or more joints, usually in a symmetrical pattern, similar to adult RA. Systemic features such as fever and anemia may occur. Prevalence is greater among girls than among boys. The course of the disease may be severe, resulting in joint damage requiring reconstructive surgery in young adulthood. About 30% of children with JRA have polyarticular disease.
2. *Pauciarticular* JRA presents as arthritis in one to four joints. It is usually asymmetrical and without systemic features. The knee, ankle, and elbow commonly are affected. There are subtypes, including early onset pauciarticular JRA, which occurs before 5 years of age and is more common among girls, and later onset pauciarticular JRA, which is more common among boys ages 10–12 and affects weight-bearing joints (Taylor & Erlandson, 2001). Pauciarticular JRA is associated with a risk of uveitis (inflammation of the vascular area of the eye) and iritis (inflammation of the iris), so regular ophthalmology examinations are important. About 50% of children with JRA present with pauciarticular disease.
3. *Systemic onset* JRA is characterized by daily or twice-daily fever spikes, a classic pink rash, and inflammation in one or more joints. The fever and fatigue associated with systemic onset JRA may prevent children from feeling well enough to participate in school and play. Other organ systems may be involved, including the liver, spleen, heart, and lungs. Approximately 20% of children with JRA present with systemic JRA.

All forms of JRA affect normal growth and development. The inflammation of joints and tendons may affect bone growth; pain, stiffness, decreased mobility, and fatigue limit participation in some age-appropriate activities. Joint contractures or subluxation are not uncommon and may require splinting, a visible sign of illness. Hospitalizations, outpatient treatments, and medications all affect children's schedules. When possible, therapy should be playful and integrated into the child's routine with the help of parents and other family members. At school, the occupational therapist may consult with teachers regarding ways to facilitate the child's participation in classroom and extracurricular activities.

Ankylosing Spondylitis

Ankylosing spondylitis (AS) affects children and adults. About 5% of cases begin in adolescence (Hannan, 2001). AS is the primary disorder of the group of rheumatic conditions classified as *spondyloarthropathies* (Helewa & Stokes, 2001); this group includes psoriatic arthritis and Reiter's syndrome. All the disorders in this group tend to run in families, and the histocompatibility antigen HLA-B27 is positive for most people with spondyloarthropathies (Helewa & Stokes, 2001). The prevalence of AS is about 1%, and men are affected 3 times more often than women (Badley & DesMeules, 2003; Helewa & Stokes, 2001). The prevalence is higher among North American Aboriginal peoples, especially among Haida and Pima First Nations (Hannan, 2001). The onset is insidious and typically begins as hip pain (from inflammation of the sacroiliac joint) between ages 16 and 35. AS affects the sacroiliac joint and spine. The primary site of inflammation is at the insertion of ligaments to bones. Like other inflammatory rheumatic conditions, AS is characterized by exacerbations and remissions, and the severity of the disease varies widely (Badley & DesMeules, 2003). The pain and stiffness associated with AS is worse after a period of rest and improves after exercise or a hot bath (Helewa & Stokes, 2001). Bony ankylosis, which severely limits flexion and extension of the spine, may occur in later disease. Peripheral joints, such as the ankle or wrist, are sometimes inflamed, and heel spurs are not uncommon.

The disabilities associated with AS include difficulty reaching the feet or floor; maintaining an effective posture at work and rest; and doing physically demanding activities at work, home, or recreation. Occupational therapy therefore includes the provision of long-handled assistive devices, advice on positioning devices such as chairs and pillows, and problem-solving strategies specific to the client's daily occupations. Therapeutic exercise to maintain strength and mobility and an erect posture if ankylosis occurs are mainstays of treatment.

Systemic Lupus Erythematosus and Systemic Sclerosis

Two of the main connective tissue diseases that occupational therapists may see are systemic lupus erythematosus (SLE) and systemic sclerosis (SSc; commonly called *scleroderma*). SLE is a chronic autoimmune disease that occurs primarily in women during their childbearing years (Ramsey-Goldman, 2001). It ranges from a fairly mild disease characterized by a rash, arthritis, and fatigue to a severe, life-threatening illness involving the kidneys, lungs, heart, and central nervous system. The prevalence of SLE is about 0.05% in North America, and the disease affects women 10 times more frequently than it does men (Badley & DesMeules, 2003; Ramsey-Goldman, 2001). Children also may have SLE. The course of SLE is marked by exacerbations and remissions of skin rashes, joint and muscle swelling, and pain. Joint involvement is symmetrical and similar in distribution to RA, but rarely do people with SLE develop severe arthritis limitations (Nalebuff & Melvin, 2000). They may demonstrate some instability at the joints, but they tend not to develop contractures or fixed deformities. Medical management can be quite complex, and it is essential that patients be regularly followed by a rheumatologist. Clients may have to cope with multiple medical challenges, such as kidney disease, along with

rashes and joint pain. People with SLE are photosensitive and require sunblock to prevent sunburn and exacerbation of skin rashes, even when the sun does not appear to be intense. Occupational therapy addresses individual occupational performance problems within the context of managing a chronic illness; it also focuses on maintaining joint mobility and alignment.

SSc is characterized by inflammatory, fibrotic, and degenerative changes of the skin, blood vessels, tendons, skeletal muscle, gastrointestinal tract, heart, lungs, and kidneys (Ramsey-Goldman, 2001). Colloquially, it is referred to as "hardening of the skin," because that is the disease's most apparent feature. The skin appears edematous and shiny, and it feels rigid (i.e., it is hard to pinch the skin and subcutaneous tissue). Approximately 0.02% of the population is affected with scleroderma, women at a rate about 5 times more frequently than men. Two subtypes exist: *Diffuse cutaneous* SSc has a higher likelihood of pulmonary fibrosis, myopathy, tendon friction rubs, and renal crises and lower survival rates than limited *cutaneous* SSc. Both types present with Raynaud's phenomenon, joint contractures, and gastrointestinal problems. Particular occupational performance issues arising as a result of SSc include difficulty eating and managing oral care (which is secondary to decreased ability to swallow and to fully open the mouth) and decreased ability to grasp and manipulate objects required in everyday activities (which is secondary to joint contractures, hardening of the skin in the hands, and Raynaud's symptoms). Warmth, including use of thermal gloves, socks, and small heat packs or pocket warmers found among hiking and skiing equipment in stores, relieves the discomfort associated with mild Raynaud's symptoms.

Osteoporosis

Osteoporosis (OP) is characterized by low bone-mineral density and increased bone fragility; those conditions, in turn, lead to an increased risk of fractures (Maricic, 2001). OP affects more women than men and has higher prevalence among Caucasian and Asian women than among other ethnic groups. Peak bone mass is attained in the third decade of life and is typically higher in men than women. It slowly declines with age in both sexes, but a rapid decline occurs in women during the first few years after menopause (Maricic, 2001). A genetic predisposition exists for low bone mass, but other risk factors are potentially modifiable, including a dietary intake low in calcium, chronic alcohol and nicotine use, immobilization, and long-term corticosteroid use. Because corticosteroids are used to treat other rheumatic conditions (at higher doses in the past than are used today), OP may be secondary to a primary rheumatic disease diagnosis that initiated the referral to occupational therapy.

The risk of osteoporotic fractures is high. Caucasian women age 45 and older have about a 40% to 50% chance of sustaining an osteoporotic fracture during their lifetime, and the risk of hip fracture doubles every 5 years after age 45 (Maricic, 2001). OP is treated with medications aimed at decreasing the rate of bone resorption. Estrogen replacement therapy may be considered for some postmenopausal women, depending on their risk factors for other conditions associated with estrogen, such as breast cancer and heart disease. Calcium and vitamin D supplements and dietary advice also are recommended. Occupational therapy for people with OP addresses fall prevention, increased physical activity (especially weight-bearing activities), and reinforcement of nutritional guidelines (e.g., when assessing and intervening with meal preparation or kitchen safety).

Occupational therapy clients also present with *periarticular rheumatic conditions,* including Dupuytren's contracture (which typically presents as flexion contractures of the fourth and fifth digits), tendinitis or tenosynovitis (i.e., tennis elbow, golfer's elbow, or local inflammation of the tendon sheaths surrounding the tendons to the fingers and thumbs), carpal tunnel syndrome (i.e., impingement of the median nerve affecting sensation in the hand and strength of the thenar muscles), and bursitis (i.e., inflammation of the bursa in joints such as the shoulder and knee). Any of those conditions may result in pain and motor impairment and, thus, difficulty managing everyday activities.

Role of Occupational Therapy in Rheumatic Diseases

As in many areas of practice, the role of the occupational therapist is to maintain, restore, and improve clients' abilities to manage their daily activities and enable full participation in life. In rheumatology, some occupational therapy interventions address the underlying pathology of the condition (e.g., resting splints to decrease joint pain and inflammation) or improve the biomechanics of a specific motion (e.g., carpometacarpal [CMC] splint to stabilize a thumb and improve grasp). Some interventions target tasks that are necessary to effective occupational performance (e.g., strategies to enable note taking at school). Adaptive strategies, equipment,

and environmental modifications incorporate joint-protection and energy-conservation principles to help clients manage the main symptoms of most rheumatic diseases: pain and fatigue. It is essential that principles be illustrated with practical examples that directly apply to the client's roles and occupations; otherwise, routines and behaviors are unlikely to change.

Growing evidence supports the effectiveness of occupational therapy in the management of rheumatic diseases. In a systematic review of occupational therapy interventions in managing RA, Steultjens and colleagues (2002) reported on one high-quality randomized controlled trial (Helewa et al., 1991) and three additional trials and found that comprehensive occupational therapy services improve functional abilities. They also noted that joint-protection and energy-conservation strategies improve functional ability, that wrist splints decrease pain and improve grip strength, and that insufficient data were available to evaluate the effects of assistive devices. This rigorous review was based on a quantitative research paradigm, which requires quantitative data collection under controlled circumstances. Qualitative reports—evidence that is not readily captured in controlled trials—also provide compelling support for the positive effects of occupational therapy on participation in valued activities. One such example is Moss's (1997) description and interpretation of how older women with arthritis manage their home environments. Her study illustrated the role of assistive devices (e.g., enlarged key grips and long-handled reachers) and environmental modifications (e.g., an electric stair glider) in maintaining participation in household activities and social networks.

Occupational therapy is part of an interdisciplinary team approach to managing rheumatic diseases (ACR Subcommittee on Rheumatoid Arthritis Guidelines, 2002). All team members contribute to client education and self-management in addition to discipline-specific interventions; all efforts are aimed at helping clients manage their illness and minimize its impact on participation in life activities. Consumer education programs improve functional status, at least in the short term (Riemsma, Kirwan, Taal, & Rasker, 2002). The Arthritis Self-Management Program, a series of educational sessions offered in small groups by trained lay leaders, enhances self-efficacy, reduces pain, and decreases the number of physician visits (Superio-Cabuslay, Ward, & Lorig, 1996). The comprehensive education programs in these sessions include content typically provided in occupational therapy, such as application of joint-protection and energy-conservation principles, use of assistive devices, and modification of tasks.

Performance Component Impairments Associated With Rheumatic Diseases

Rheumatic diseases may affect all performance components, but the *sensorimotor component* typically is most limited. Depending on the natural course of the disease and how well it is managed by medications, damage to joint surfaces, cartilage, bone, and the soft tissue surrounding the joint may result. These changes lead to decreased range of motion, joint instability when ligaments are stretched, or joint stiffness when swelling is profuse or soft tissues contract. Joint biomechanics are compromised, and joint deformities or malalignment may occur. Strength, endurance, and hand function may be impaired. Subsequent to pain and periods of inactivity, many people with rheumatic diseases are deconditioned. Clients may report difficulty with standing, walking, transferring, bending, rising, reaching, grasping, holding, and carrying. Even resting and sleeping become problematic in the presence of pain and difficulty positioning joints and moving in bed.

Surgical procedures, after a period of healing and rehabilitation, reduce pain and restore joint function, but during the postoperative phase, patients need occupational therapy to address occupational performance difficulties arising from pain and limitations in range of motion and strength. Occupational therapists also assist patients with adherence to postoperative precautions.

The central nervous system usually is not involved in most rheumatic diseases, but systemic conditions, especially the connective tissue diseases, may affect central nervous system processing and manifest in sensory or cognitive problems. Peripheral nerves are involved when inflammation compresses nerves passing through soft-tissue compartments, as happens with the median nerve in carpal tunnel syndrome. Paresthesias and decreased sensation may result.

Rheumatic diseases affect psychosocial components including the client's coping skills: that is, his or her response to pain and ability to manage the sequelae of pain, fatigue, and motor impairment. It is not unusual to experience changes in mood as a result of rheumatic diseases, and depression and anxiety are frequently associated with the loss of valued activities (Katz & Yelin, 1993, 1994). Dealing with chronic pain and changes in mood may affect concentration and memory. Social support appears to mediate the effects of rheumatic diseases in fulfilling roles such as parent (Backman & Mitchell, 2003) and employee (Allaire et al., 1996). Self-efficacy also appears to be related to effective management of chronic illness (Boutaugh & Brady, 1998).

The performance limitations associated with rheumatic diseases may be short-term, in the case of localized inflammatory conditions, an exacerbation of symptoms, or postoperative recovery. In chronic diseases, limitations may progress over time and lead to increasing levels of disability. Yet, many people with apparently severe physical impairments are able to effectively manage their daily activities, whereas others who have relatively mild impairments have great difficulty performing the tasks necessary to their life roles and expectations. It is therefore necessary to continually evaluate the interaction of performance components with the demands of the client's occupations and the context in which the client performs each occupation.

Common Occupational Performance Challenges Associated With Rheumatic Diseases

Collectively, rheumatic diseases affect all areas of occupational performance and participation in life. Precise effects vary across and within rheumatic diseases as well as across clients. Exacerbations and remissions in RA and JRA, for example, mean that clients are able to manage ADL, IADL, work, and school activities on some days, but not on others. Systemic effects associated with exacerbations include feelings of general malaise that contribute to fatigue and lack of endurance. This pattern affects interpersonal relationships because the course of the illness is unpredictable.

Limitations in hand strength and dexterity result in problems across the spectrum of ADL, IADL, school or employment, and leisure, because almost every activity requires that objects be grasped, manipulated, moved, smoothed, or pressed. Consider a typical parent's day and the possible difficulties encountered if arthritis limits her hand strength and dexterity: Holding a toothbrush, opening a box of cereal, buttoning clothes, picking up a child, opening doors, reaching for groceries, opening a jar of peanut butter, and doing laundry all may present difficulties that need to be addressed in occupational therapy.

When OA, RA, or JRA affects the hips or knees, mobility is impaired. Common ADL challenges include standing, walking, managing stairs, rising from a chair, putting on shoes and socks, and getting on and off the toilet and in and out of the bathtub. It can be difficult, if not impossible, to get down to the floor to play with children or pick up items; a young child with JRA may not be able to sit on the floor at school for reading circles or other classroom activities. Similar difficulties may be present when AS limits movement in the spine and hips. Depending on workplace demands, employment may be adversely affected by limitations in mobility.

Reconstructive surgery presents a need for preparation as well as a need to follow precautions to promote healing; those needs affect all occupational performance areas. For example, metacarpal-phalangeal joint replacement surgery requires use of a splint to maintain the alignment of the fingers, so one-handed techniques are used for basic ADL for a short time during the postoperative period. Total hip arthroplasty requires avoidance of excessive hip flexion and adduction (and, perhaps, other motions, depending on the surgeon's approach); thus, a raised toilet seat, bath bench, and cushion to raise the height of car seats or chairs typically are used for a postoperative period of up to 3 months. A long-handled reacher, dressing stick, and sock aid also may enable ADL while hip flexion is restricted, whether due to surgery or the effects of the disease.

Focus of Occupational Therapy Evaluation

The purpose of the occupational therapy evaluation is to understand the impact of rheumatic disease on everyday living in order to help clients use strategies to maintain participation in their chosen activities while managing their condition and health. In today's health care context, it is difficult to find time for comprehensive evaluation of clients with complex conditions. Therefore, the initial interview in occupational therapy seeks to identify the most pressing occupational performance issues or problems for the client. Additional assessment tools may then be selected, depending on the nature of the priority problems (Backman, 1998; Backman, Fairleigh, & Kuchta, 2004). For example, the Canadian Occupational Performance Measure (Law, Baptiste, Carswell, Polatajko, & Pollack, 1998) is a semistructured interview that addresses all areas of occupational performance. It has the additional advantage of a scoring system that will measure the outcome of occupational therapy interventions when readministered at a later date. Regardless of the interview format used, it should identify which occupations, tasks, or activities are problems that require attention.

Once priority occupational performance issues are identified, a variety of cues will guide the choice of additional evaluation methods to determine the underlying performance components or environmental conditions that contribute to the problem (Backman & Medcalf, 2000). Evaluation procedures may include the following elements:

- Goniometry to measure joint range of motion (ROM)
- Manual muscle testing and dynamometry (e.g., grip strength)
- Hands-on evaluation of soft-tissue integrity
- Measurement of hand dexterity (e.g., pegboard tests)
- Measurement of hand function (see Table 8.1)
- Measurement of symptoms affecting occupational performance, such as pain and fatigue using the National Institutes of Health Activity Record (Gerber & Furst, 1992)
- Specific ADL, IADL, work, or leisure assessments, as indicated by the client's occupational performance issues and priorities.

Two promising tools specific to the effects of arthritis on work participation are the Work Limitations Questionnaire (Lerner et al., 2001) and the Work Instability Scale (Gilworth et al., 2003).

As part of the interdisciplinary team, the occupational therapist may administer or have access to the results of outcome measures that are used to track clients' progress and program effectiveness. Examples of commonly used tools are listed in Table 8.2. An excellent review of a comprehensive range of rheumatology patient outcome measures is available in an October 2003 special supplement to the journal *Arthritis and Rheumatism (Arthritis Care and Research)* (Katz, 2003). The supplement summarizes pediatric and adult measures in the areas of function, pain, quality of life, psychological status and well-being, fatigue and sleep, and specific diseases.

The initial administration of outcome measures is a useful screening process for referral to appropriate health professionals. For example, a referral to occupational therapy may be initiated by another health professional on the basis of scores from the Health Assessment Questionnaire Disability Index (Fries, Spitz, Kraines, & Holman, 1980) or Western Ontario and McMaster Universities Osteoarthritis Index (Bellamy, Buchanan, Goldsmith, Campbell, & Stitt, 1988). Although many outcome measures provide content pertinent to occupational therapy, many do not have enough information to help therapists identify precise occupational performance issues and set goals. A combination of interview, standardized measures, and observation usually is required for a comprehensive evaluation.

Table 8.1. Selected Tests of Hand and Upper Limb Function for Clients With Rheumatic Diseases

Test	Description	Reference(s)
Arthritis Hand Function Test (AHFT)	Performance-based test of hand strength, dexterity, and functional tasks for adults with rheumatoid arthritis, osteoarthritis, and scleroderma	Backman, Mackie, & Harris, 1991; Poole, Gallegos, & O'Linc, 2000
Cochin Rheumatoid Hand Disability Scale	Self-report questionnaire evaluating level of difficulty performing 18 functional tasks	Duruoz et al., 1996
Disabilities of the Arm, Shoulder, and Hand (DASH) Questionnaire	Self-report questionnaire (30 items) evaluating level of pain and difficulty with functional tasks, with optional modules for sports, work, and musicians; for any diagnosis	Beaton et al., 2001 (includes entire questionnaire)
Hand Mobility in Scleroderma (HAMIS) Test	Observational test of functional hand range of motion specific to scleroderma	Sandqvist & Eklund, 2000
Michigan Hand Outcomes Questionnaire (MHQ)	Self-report questionnaire evaluating symptoms, function, and aesthetics for pre- and postoperative evaluations	Chung, Pillsbury, Walters, & Hayward 1998 (includes entire questionnaire)
Sequential Occupational Dexterity Assessment (SODA)	Performance-based assessment of ability to do 12 functional tasks, with difficulty scored by both occupational therapist and client	van Lankveld et al., 1996

Note. All tests listed in this table have satisfactory psychometric properties.

Table 8.2. Selected Rheumatology Outcome Measures

Test	Description	Reference
Arthritis Impact Measurement Scales 2 (AIMS–2)	Self-report of mobility, physical, household and social activities, ADL, pain, depression, and anxiety	Meenan, Mason, Anderson, Guccione, & Kazis, 1992
Bath Ankylosing Spondylitis Functional Index (BASFI)	Self-report of ability to perform 10 functional activities frequently limited in ankylosing spondylitis	Garrett, Jenkinson, Kennedy, Whitelock, Gaisford, & Calin, 1994
Child Health Assessment Questionnaire (CHAQ)	Interview or self-report for children age 8 and older; includes eight ADL subscales	Singh, Athreya, Fries, & Goldsmith, 1994
Fibromyalgia Impact Questionnaire	Self-report of physical function, symptoms, and well-being	Burckhardt, Clark, & Bennett, 1991
Juvenile Arthritis Functional Status Index (JASI)	Self-report of functional activities for children ages 8 to 17; computer and interview; ranks five priority activities	Wright, Law, Crombie, Goldsmith, & Dent, 1994
Health Assessment Questionnaire (HAQ) Disability Index	Self-report of difficulties performing in eight categories of ADL	Fries, Spitz, Kraines, & Holman, 1980
Western Ontario and McMaster Universities Osteoarthritis Index (WOMAC)	Self-report of pain, stiffness, and function for adults with osteoarthritis affecting hips or knees	WOMAC User Guide, www.womac.org

Note. ADL = activities of daily living.

Factors to Consider When Recommending Adaptive Strategies, Equipment, or Environmental Modifications

The primary factor to consider when making recommendations is the client: Not all strategies, equipment, and modifications work for all people, even when they have similar joint involvement and similar problems. Collaborative problem solving between the occupational therapist and client leads to recommendations that best fit the client's priorities, contextual limitations, and opportunities (Law, 1998). Finding the most appropriate solution to an occupational performance problem often involves trial and error; encouragement and perseverance are necessary. Feasibility of recommendations will vary according to the context and the anticipated duration of the limitation. For example, someone who is renting an apartment is less likely than a home owner to be able to make structural changes to a kitchen or bathroom. The cost of a recommendation is a consideration for most people, and even when insurance is expected to cover the costs, the client may face restrictions regarding the circumstances under which devices or modifications are reimbursable or a "lifetime limit" on total rehabilitation expenditures. Large corporations may have more resources available than small businesses do to facilitate adjustment at work. Some clients will choose to disclose their arthritis to supervisors and coworkers, and others will not. These contextual factors dictate careful planning.

Group support influences the acceptability of many recommendations. Consider this example:

> In a group session on joint-protection and energy-conservation principles for people with RA, Cathy, the occupational therapist, responds to a comment from Alisha about the difficulty in delegating work to others to accommodate fatigue or mobility limitations by saying, "You can ask your children to pick up after themselves."
>
> "I don't want my RA to ruin my kids' childhoods," says Alisha, who has two young children. "It's not fair that they should have to clean up after themselves just because it's hard for me to do it."
>
> "There's nothing unfair about it," interjects Leona, another client in the group. "It's got nothing to do with your arthritis; part of your role as a parent is to teach your kids to be responsible and pick up after themselves."
>
> Alisha asks Leona several more questions and is pleased to hear Leona say that RA did

not have a "detrimental" effect on raising her children.

In the preceding example, Leona has more credibility than the occupational therapist because she has both RA and children, and the occupational therapist has neither. The sharing of experiences and strategies among people who have similar issues is an important part of planning effective interventions.

Consider involving family members, as appropriate, when negotiating recommendations. Home modifications, such as adding handrails to staircases or hallways, changing furnishings, installing lever handles on faucets, or a raised toilet seat, affect the entire family. Some clients may be reluctant to adopt such modifications. An open discussion of options with the client's spouse, parents, or children, facilitated by the occupational therapist, may be useful.

The appearance of assistive devices and modifications is important to some people. Fortunately, many devices are now less visible, because they are readily available in the general marketplace rather than medical supply stores alone. Cooking utensils sold in gourmet cooking stores may have large handles that are easy to grasp, yet stylish; casual clothing often has features such as rings or pull tabs on zippers. Some children find neon-colored spiral elastic shoelaces to be a "cool" accessory—the fact that they eliminate the need to tie laces is secondary.

Adaptive Strategies, Equipment, and Environmental Modifications

Joint-protection and energy-conservation principles guide the recommendation of adaptive strategies and equipment for all occupational performance areas. Clients are more likely to incorporate joint protection and energy conservation principles if the occupational therapist provides clear and relevant examples of how to apply the principles to the client's daily routines. Some examples are presented in Table 8.3. Recent studies suggest that practice with applying joint-protection principles improves functional ability (Hammond & Freeman, 2001; Steultjens et al., 2002). Splints help stabilize joints, address underlying biomechanics of motion, reduce pain during activity, and improve hand strength and function (Harrell, 2001; Haskett, Backman, Porter, Goyert, & Palejko, in press). Energy-conservation principles involve prioritizing activities; planning and pacing activities over the day, week, or month; and regular physical activity as a mainstay for sustaining endurance for daily activities (Cordery & Rocchi, 1998). Regular physical activity

Table 8.3. Joint-Protection and Energy-Conservation Principles and Sample Techniques

Principle	Sample Techniques or Application
Respect your pain.	Reduce time and/or effort spent on an activity if pain occurs and lasts for more than 2 hours after the activity has been discontinued. Avoid nonessential activities that aggravate your pain.
Balance rest and work.	Take short breaks during your work. For example, take a 5-minute rest at the end of an hour of work. Intersperse more active tasks with more passive or quiet work.
Reduce the amount of effort needed to do the job.	Use assistive devices such as a jar opener or lever taps. Slide pots across the counter instead of lifting. Use a trolley to transport heavy items. Use a raised toilet seat and seat cushion to reduce stress on hips, knees, and hands. Use frozen vegetables to minimize peeling and chopping.
Avoid staying in one position for prolonged periods of time.	Change position frequently to avoid joint stiffness and muscle fatigue. For example, take a 30-second range of motion break after 10–20 minutes of typing or holding a tool; after standing for 20 minutes perch on a stool for the next 20 minutes; walk to the mailroom after 20–30 minutes sitting at your desk.
Avoid activities that cannot be stopped immediately if you experience pain or discomfort.	Plan ahead. Be realistic about your abilities so you don't walk or drive too far, or leave all your shopping and errands to a single trip.
Reduce unnecessary stress on your joints while sleeping.	Use a firm mattress for support. Sleep on your back with a pillow to support the curve in your neck. If you prefer to lay on your side, place a pillow between your knees and lay on the least painful side.
Maintain muscle strength and joint range of motion.	Do your prescribed exercises regularly. Strong muscles will help support your joints. Regular exercise will reduce fatigue.
Use a well-planned work space.	Organize your work space so that work surfaces and materials are at a convenient height for you, to ensure good posture. Place frequently used items within close reach. Reduce clutter by getting rid of unnecessary items, or storing less frequently used items away from the immediate work space.

Note. From "Occupational Therapy," by C. L. Backman, A. Fairleigh, & G. Kuchta, 2004. In *RA: Rheumatoid Arthritis,* by B. Hayes, D. S. Pisetsky, & B. St. Clair (Eds.), Philadelphia: Lippincott Williams & Wilkins. Reprinted with permission from Lippincott Williams & Wilkins.

reduces pain and fatigue regardless of the type of rheumatic disease. Occupational therapists must find physical activities that the client will enjoy and maintain.

Self-management strategies also contribute to improved occupational performance. Self-management has been defined as "learning and practicing the skills necessary to carry on an active and emotionally satisfying life in the face of chronic illness" (Lorig, 1993, p. 11). Helping clients acquire self-management skills requires an interactive approach that focuses on skill development, thereby increasing clients' confidence and their ability to cope with their arthritis (Boutaugh & Brady, 1998). Approaches that are based on cognitive–behavioral principles, self-efficacy theory, and other learning theories include strategies such as setting goals and making contracts, problem-solving discussions,

role-modeling (i.e., learning from others in similar circumstances), and experiential learning (i.e., practicing techniques). These strategies, which are offered in a range of consumer education packages including the Arthritis Self-Management Program, Fibromyalgia Self-Help Course, and Bone-up on Arthritis Course (available through local chapters of the Arthritis Foundation) have been shown to increase knowledge, self-efficacy, self-care behaviors, functional status, and quality of life; they also decrease perceived pain, depression, helplessness, and health care utilization (i.e., visits to physicians and specialists; Boutaugh & Brady, 1998).

ADL

Morning stiffness may limit a client's ability to manage morning ADL. Laying out clothes the night before, setting timers on appliances like the coffee maker at bedtime, and doing gentle ROM exercises in bed before rising minimize the effect of morning stiffness on task performance. Assistive devices facilitate many personal care activities related to dressing, bathing, grooming, and eating (Mann, 1998; Mann, Tomita, Hurren, & Charvat, 1999). Common examples are illustrated in Figure 8.1. With increasing interest in universal accessibility, useful equipment is readily available in housewares and hardware stores. Many devices are attractive as well as functional, but no one device suits all people. Enlarged or curved handles on eating and cooking utensils accommodate limited ROM and facilitate alternative grasping patterns (Luck, 2001). Some clients, however, will manage better with a smooth, flat utensil that fits more easily into the webbed space between thumb and forefinger or several fingers. The effect of devices on joint biomechanics requires careful attention: In some cases, devices will increase joint stress, require more strength, or make tasks more difficult to perform.

Purchasing two long-handled sponges facilitates bathing; one sponge is reserved for hard-to-reach body parts, and the second is used for cleaning the tub. Extended handles on combs and styling aids are useful for hair care when shoulder motion is restricted. Sitting in the bathroom and resting the elbow on the vanity can accommodate reduced strength and endurance. Mounting the blow-dryer on a wall bracket eliminates the need for holding the dryer overhead.

Mobility may be facilitated with the use of a cane or walking stick when hips, knees, and feet are painful or weak. It is important to consider all the joints when recommending a cane: If hands and wrists are involved, a modified or custom-molded grip on the cane or walking stick may be required. A wheeled walker with a basket for holding parcels and a fold-down seat for waiting in line or taking brief rests may enable people who are otherwise limited to walking very short distances to manage errands.

Environmental modifications such as installing a walk-in shower and lever taps may be expensive, but some people will incorporate such changes into home renovations over the years. Grab bars to facilitate tub and toilet transfers should be installed by a qualified tradesperson to ensure that they are adequately anchored to wall studs and sustain body weight. Towel racks were designed to hold towels, not people, and are not a safe alternative. Limitations in upper limb ROM and strength may prevent adequate perineal care and toilet hygiene. A curved toilet tissue holder is a portable and simple aid; an attachable bidet-style toilet seat that washes and dries the perineal area is a more expensive, home-based option. Additional suggestions are presented in Table 8.4.

IADL

Shopping can be tiring. One option is to delegate shopping to family members or friends in exchange for doing other tasks that can be more easily paced. Shopping by phone or Internet is relatively stress-free; even groceries can be ordered over the Internet in many cities. If clients prefer to choose their own products, shopping in person but requesting delivery eliminates the need to carry parcels. Some stores provide delivery services for a reduced fee on specific days of the week. These options may be more readily available in urban areas than in rural areas. Exchanging services with friends and family members may be an option in some communities.

The huge volume of cookbooks and magazines on the market are full of suggestions for making meal preparation quick and easy. One-pot meals, slow-cookers, or bamboo steamers cook the entire meal in one pot, reducing the cleanup afterwards. Partially prepared ingredients save time and energy or compensate for weak or painful hand joints; they include cleaned and chopped salads in a bag, deli-prepared meats, and frozen vegetables and main dishes. Although sometimes more expensive, prepared foods nevertheless may be an option suitable for some clients or may serve as a backup on a "bad day." Clients can also strive to "cook once, eat twice": Large casseroles, soups or stews, and leftovers can be frozen for later use (in individual containers for school or work lunches). Opening packages and containers can be difficult for people with arthritis that affects the hands. Box openers, jar openers, a sharp knife, nonskid mats, and electric scissors are examples of helpful kitchen equipment. Lightweight pots, sliding pots along counters, or cooking food inside a steamer basket to avoid the need to lift and drain a heavy pot are additional suggestions. A pull-out breadboard—or having two pull-out boards at different work heights—provides multiple height work surfaces in one kitchen to facilitate effective work postures, whether sitting or standing (Figure 8.2). A trolley is useful for transporting items when unpacking groceries or setting and clearing the table. For clients who attribute strong meaning to cooking or value it as a leisure activity, some suggestions may be unacceptable, even if they "make sense." It is a matter of setting priorities and making choices within the client's entire routine and roles. Often just presenting a few exam-

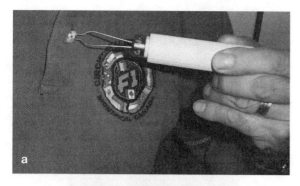

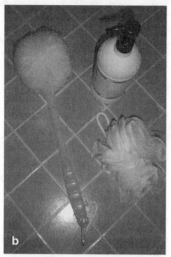

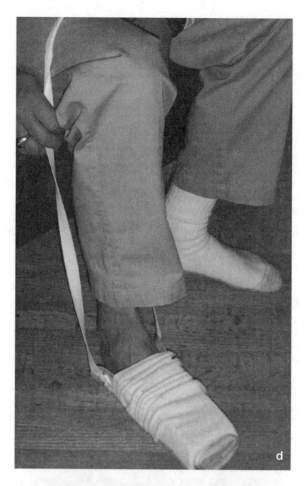

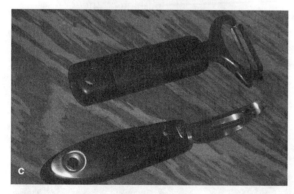

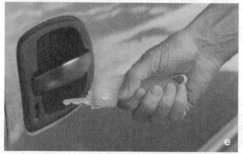

Figure 8.1. Aids to daily living: (a) button hook to compensate for inability to pinch or manipulate small objects; (b) bathing aids to compensate for limited grasp or reach; (c) two examples of vegetable peelers, each promoting different grasp patterns; (d) sock aid in use, to compensate for inability to reach feet; (e) key extension to improve leverage and compensate for limited strength, limited pronation, or supination.

ples facilitates the problem-solving process, and the client then can generate additional ideas for managing his or her most important tasks. Other suggestions are listed in Table 8.5.

Work

Many people with rheumatic disease will already have an established career or job at the time they are diagnosed. Depending on the task demands of work and their disease status, they may be able to continue working at the same job with minor modifications and equipment. Sometimes, however, it is necessary to consider changes in employment. One frustration for some workers is the assumption that they need a sedentary job; however, many sedentary jobs require static postures or repetitive mo-

Table 8.4. Sample Difficulties Performing Activities of Daily Living and Potential Solutions

Task	Underlying Performance Components	Potential Solutions
Difficulty holding toothbrush	Pain in thumb and finger joints Stiffness and decreased ROM in hand joints	Enlarged handle on standard toothbrush Electric toothbrush with easy-to-manage switch (handle is larger, powered brush does all the work)
Difficulty pinching and managing small objects (e.g., buttons and zippers, foil lids on yogurt and similar containers)	Pain in CMC joint of thumb, together with decreased joint stability and strength	CMC splint or orthosis to stabilize thumb Assistive devices specific to task (e.g., button hook, zipper pull) Alternative strategies specific to task (e.g., stab center of foil lid with knife and peel back from center)
Difficulty bathing: transferring to and from tub	Pain and decreased range of motion in hips and knees Fear of falling	Bath bench or bath stool and handheld shower attachment Water-powered bath seat that lowers into tub Walk-in shower and bath seat Bath safety rails or bars Nonskid mat
Difficulty bathing: holding soap and reaching body parts	Limited ROM in multiple joints Decreased grasp	Long-handled sponge or loofah Soap-on-a-rope Nylon "poofy" sponge with wrist strap and bath gel in pump dispenser
Difficulty putting on and removing socks and shoes	Limited ROM in hips and knees	Sock or stocking aid Long-handled shoehorn and elastic laces in shoes Dressing stick for pushing off shoes and socks Bootjack for pushing off shoes

Note. CMC = carpometacarpal; ROM = range of motion.

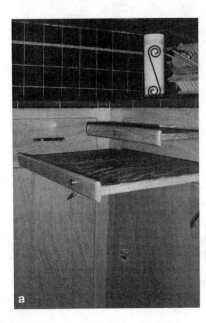
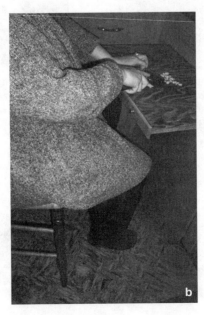
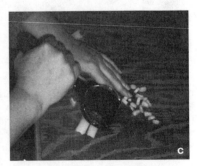

Figure 8.2. (a) Pull-out breadboards offer "adjustable" work heights. (b) Sitting to work in the kitchen takes stress off knees. (c) Close-up view of alternate grasp using large-handled rolling cutter for vegetables and herbs.

Table 8.5. Sample Difficulties With Performing Instrumental Activities of Daily Living and Potential Solutions

Task	Underlying Performance Components	Potential Solutions
Difficulty preparing meals: chopping vegetables, lifting pots	Pain or decreased grasp Decreased upper limb strength Fatigue	Purchase prewashed and chopped vegetables. Use lightweight, large-handled utensils. Use cutting boards with food spikes to stabilize vegetables. Use food processor and lightweight pots. Slide pots on counters. Use spray hose from sink to fill pots without lifting.
Difficulty turning taps on and off or turning doorknobs	Decreased hand strength	Replace taps and doorknobs with lever fixtures. Carry removable tap turner when visiting or traveling. Use rubber disk jar opener to improve friction when grasping door knobs or taps.
Carrying books, bags, parcels when shopping, going to or from work or school	Pain in hands and/or wrists Decreased hand and wrist strength Desire to protect small joints from strong forces	Use backpack, if shoulder range of motion permits, with padded shoulder straps. Carry lightweight nylon briefcase with shoulder strap diagonally across trunk. Use wheeled briefcase or luggage.
Difficulty turning keys (car door, ignition, house door)	Decreased pronation and supination Limited hand strength	Use key extension, commercial or custom-made. Where feasible, change locks to key cards or push-button codes (use eraser end of pencil or dowel rod to push buttons).
Difficulty vacuuming and other heavy housecleaning	Decreased strength Limited reach Fatigue	Delegate some tasks to others in household. Use lightweight stick vacuum or carpet sweeper in-between heavy cleanings. When feasible, choose hard surface floors and lightweight dust mops. Purchase selected services.

tions that are just as difficult to manage as physically demanding jobs. Vocational rehabilitation services may assist with job retraining or re-entry. Self-employment is an attractive option for those who have a well-defined skill set and the desire for autonomy.

For children who have rheumatic diseases, the transition to adulthood and employment presents different issues. Identifying career options, attaining skills through postsecondary education, and seeking and securing employment are concerns to be addressed with young adults. By young adulthood, some people no longer will have active arthritis, some will have residual physical impairments, and some will continue to manage the active disease. People may need occupational therapy to enable task performance that is specific to their training and employment goals.

Computer workstations are part of many work environments. They should be adjustable to the needs of the client. The occupational therapist may suggest modifications to the typical baseline ergonomic recommendations (which are designed with population health needs in mind) to accommodate restricted reach, a painful hip or knee, or a stiff neck. For example, if the feet dangle when the office chair is adjusted to optimal height, a footstool is recommended. Although a tilted footstool may provide adequate support for some people, a flat footstool is appropriate if the client has inflammation or limited ankle dorsiflexion. A document holder set at eye level can accommodate a stiff or painful neck. An angled drafting table may be a better desk choice for those who read and write rather than use the computer. Other work modifications are listed in Table 8.6.

Table 8.6. Sample Occupational Performance Problems at Work and Potential Solutions

Task	Underlying Performance Components	Potential Solutions
Computer mouse and keyboard at work exacerbate wrist symptoms.	Wrist pain and swelling Limited strength and endurance	Use resting splints at night and/or rest periods. Do an ergonomic evaluation and make adjustments to workstation to maintain optimal posture and arm position. Take frequent brief pauses to move limbs through full range of motion. Consider feasibility of arm rests or wrist splints.
Talking on phone and taking notes exacerbate neck and back pain.	Painful cervical spine and shoulders	Use lightweight telephone headset (maintains privacy) or speakerphone (less private). Explore options available from telephone company.
Writing on blackboard, whiteboard, or flipcharts (teachers, facilitators, consultants) is difficult.	Decreased grasp Limited hand strength and dexterity Limited shoulder or elbow range of motion and strength	Invite students or participants to record information. Anticipate key points and prepare overheads or charts in advance. Use adapted chalk holder or marker.
Standing for long periods at work is difficult.	Decreased endurance Foot and ankle pain	Wear supportive shoes and foot orthoses. Use anti-fatigue mats (if standing in a single workstation). Have a high stool to perch on periodically. Have a footstool or ledge to support one foot for short periods in alternate posture. Lie, sit, and stretch during breaks.
Reading for sustained periods at work or school is difficult.	Difficulty grasping book Neck pain and upper-limb pain and weakness	Try various bookstands: wire book holder on stack of books to hold book at eye level, cookbook stand on desk, drafting table in place of desk, lap desk to support book while seated in easy chair, adjustable music stand in office or study area.

One of the predictors of retaining employment among people with RA or AS is autonomy over pace of work (Allaire et al., 1996; Chorus, Boonen, Miedema, & van der Linden, 2002). Occupational therapists may review work duties and advise clients on pacing or rotating activities to accommodate arthritis limitations or symptoms. Simple strategies integrated into work habits, such as standing up to answer the phone, reduce static postures that lead to discomfort. Clients may be reluctant to incorporate suggestions in the workplace, especially if they have not disclosed their arthritis. Many ergonomic suggestions, however, improve productivity and reduce complaints and absenteeism for all workers. Clients should be encouraged to share ideas with coworkers and take advantage of occupational health nurses or ergonomists when available, as is the case with some large corporate employers. With the client's consent, the occupational therapist may find an on-site visit the most efficient way to evaluate work du-ties and make feasible suggestions. Consulting with employers also may facilitate the acquisition of appropriate equipment or modifications.

Up to one-third of people with RA will stop work prematurely, before retirement age. Exploring alternative activities, such as volunteer work or leisure activities, to facilitate the transition to retirement may be appropriate. After many years of managing arthritis, sharing their knowledge as a volunteer lay leader for an arthritis education course or as a telephone service volunteer may appeal to some clients. People who have done so appear to have better health outcomes (Hainsworth & Barlow, 2001). Others may serve as Patient Partners (a program sponsored by the pharmaceutical company Searle) to educate health professional students or as volunteer consumer advisors to research projects. The Arthritis Foundation (USA) and The Arthritis Society (Canada) are key resources for such volunteer opportunities.

For other clients, the transition to retirement may present the opportunity for a greater focus on leisure activities. Exploring interests and suggesting community resources encourage people to maintain a physically active lifestyle: Gardening, swimming, Tai Chi, and dancing are just a few examples.

School and Play

When children are feeling good, they will participate in the play activities that interest them (Taylor & Erlandson, 2001). When their arthritis is holding them back, they may benefit from specific suggestions to encourage active and quiet play activities at home and school. To protect vulnerable joints, low-impact sports (e.g., swimming and bicycle riding) are generally favored over high-impact sports (e.g., running) and body contact sports (e.g., hockey and football). Summer camps for children with JRA present opportunities to explore interests and try out new play activities in a supported environment.

Although it may be possible to modify games and school activities to enable children to participate, they may not wish to stand out among their peers as being different. It is therefore important to involve even the youngest child in problem solving to find out what is acceptable or "cool" in his or her eyes, and plan accordingly. Many "fat" pens are on the market; encouraging a child to try a variety of styles and colors to determine the easiest pens to write with and select his or her favorite is likely to be more successful than prescribing a writing aid to accommodate poor grip. Inviting children to choose their favorite color of splint material for orthoses, supportive running shoes, or assistive devices involves them in the process. Obtaining two sets of textbooks—one for home and one for school—minimizes carrying heavy loads and accommodates both fatigue and painful joints. Consultation with teachers is also useful to help integrate joint-protection principles in the classroom. For example, once the child has established a skill, such as handwriting or solving arithmetic problems, then repetitive pencil-and-paper exercises are not necessary. Instead, the child can take a brief period to rest her hand joints while classmates continue with repetitive practice. Coping with pain affects concentration and mood and, therefore, the child's interaction with peers. Finding ways to incorporate short rest periods or minimize activities that exacerbate pain will facilitate function.

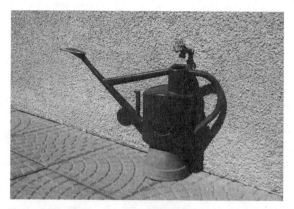

Figure 8.3. Items readily available can become assistive devices. This inverted flowerpot positions the watering can close to the faucet and supports the weight while it is filled with water. It can then be carried with two hands to plants.

Leisure

Gardening is a popular leisure activity for which a wide range of tools and methods can accommodate limitations secondary to arthritis. Lightweight, flexible hoses with easy-to-manage trigger nozzles decrease the strain of watering gardens. Lightweight, long-handled, and wide-handled rakes, trowels, hoes, and shears provide the "right tool for the job" so that gardening maintenance is both achievable and enjoyable. Other gardeners, who may be found through garden shops, clubs, or botanical display gardens, are a source of wise advice on tools, garden designs, and plant selection for easy care as well as tips on how readily available objects can serve as assistive devices; see Figure 8.3. Sailing, golfing, dancing, crafts, woodworking, and reading for pleasure all can be enjoyed when the "tools of the trade" are adapted to accommodate physical limitations.

It is important to stay involved and connected with family, friends, and community activities. The "inability to perform integrated life activities, such as housework, leisure and recreational activities, or social activities, appears to be more closely linked to poor psychological outcomes than does difficulty with performing basic ADLs" (Katz & Alfieri, 1997, p. 90). Therefore, to have the greatest impact on health and well-being, it is highly recommended that occupational therapy practitioners take time to evaluate the occupations of greatest value to the client and focus on improving participation in those occupations. Suggestions for modifications to some leisure activities are listed in Table 8.7.

Table 8.7. Sample Difficulties Performing Leisure Occupations and Potential Solutions

Task	Underlying Performance Components	Potential Solutions
Inability to maintain garden	Limited range of motion prevents reaching to ground Unable to grasp some tools Painful knees Fatigue	Explore garden designs such as raised beds and terraced gardens and containers set at accessible heights. Select low-maintenance plants. Use long-handled tools (for leverage), lightweight tools, enlarged handles. Use knee pads or kneeling bench with handles. Pace tasks.
Difficulty walking for pleasure	Hip and knee pain and weakness Foot pain	Wear supportive shoes and orthoses, or shock-absorbing insoles. Develop graded exercise program to build up endurance. Use cane or walking stick to minimize load on hip and knee. Wear knee support or orthosis.
Difficulty playing musical instrument	Joint pain and instability Muscle weakness, decreased hand dexterity	Wear custom-designed orthoses. Adapt instruments to compensate for limited movement. Pace activities. Select music to match abilities. Create nontraditional fingering pattern.

Summary

More than 100 rheumatic diseases have been identified, and many of them have progressive symptoms that lead to impairment of joint motion, muscle strength, endurance, and subsequent disability. Occupational therapy offers a range of strategies, orthoses, assistive devices, and environmental modifications to enhance clients' occupational performance and help them overcome many of the limitations caused by arthritis. The increasing prevalence of arthritis, and the fact it is one of the leading causes of long-term pain and disability, led to the current decade (2000–2010) being named the Bone and Joint Decade by the United Nations with the support of dozens of organizations worldwide. The goal is to improve the health-related quality of life for people with musculoskeletal disorders throughout the world. Occupational therapy practitioners actively contribute to achieving this goal every time they work to improve the occupational performance of people living with arthritis.

Acknowledgments

The author acknowledges the occupational therapists at the Mary Pack Arthritis Program, Vancouver Hospital and Health Sciences Centre, for inspiring and contributing many of the ideas presented in this chapter. The contributions of Jeanne Melvin, who authored this chapter for earlier editions of this book, are also kindly acknowledged.

Study Questions

1. Compare and contrast the effects of OA and RA on occupational performance and performance components.
2. Gary is a 65-year-old man with OA in his right knee, secondary to injuries sustained during his college football years. Jenny is a 67-year-old woman who has had RA for 23 years, affecting her wrists, hands, knees, and feet. Both Gary and Jenny are having knee replacement surgery. Anticipate the occupational performance problems for both Gary and Jenny in the 3 months following surgery, and propose strategies and equipment for resolving those problems.
3. List five principles of joint protection. Give an example of how each one can be applied to a specific limitation in occupational performance.
4. Write down three of the most important tasks you must complete this week. If your metacarpal-phalangeal (knuckles) and wrist joints were painful, your grip strength were reduced, and feelings of fatigue made you want to rest just 5 hours after you got out of bed, what impact would that have on your ability to complete those tasks?

Box 8.1. Sources for Assistive Devices

Photographs of the assistive devices commonly used by people with rheumatic diseases can be found at the Arthritis Storefront, on the Canadian Arthritis Society's Web site at www.arthritis.ca. Equipment may be ordered worldwide, with payment in Canadian or American dollars, through a direct consumer link to Sammons Preston. The Wright Stuff Arthritis Supplies is a similar site at www.arthritissupplies.com. Hundreds of assistive devices and technologies are described at www.abledata.com. Consumer magazines like *Arthritis Today* (available through the Arthritis Foundation [AF]) or *Arthritis News* (available through The Arthritis Society [TAS]) also provide ongoing information about useful devices, strategies, and ways to promote health and well-being. The AF and TAS also provide information about community-based self-management and exercise programs.

5. Propose alternative strategies, assistive devices, or environmental modifications that might help you do the tasks you listed in response to Question 4. Critically evaluate each one, and state whether you would accept those suggestions. Why or why not?

References

Allaire, S. H., Anderson, J. J., & Meenan, R. F. (1996). Reducing work disability associated with rheumatoid arthritis: Identification of additional risk factors and persons likely to benefit from intervention. *Arthritis Care and Research, 9,* 349–357.

American College of Rheumatology Subcommittee on Rheumatoid Arthritis Guidelines. (2002). Guidelines for the management of rheumatoid arthritis: 2002 update. *Arthritis and Rheumatism, 46,* 328–346.

Backman, C. (1998). Functional assessment. In J. Melvin and G. Jensen (Eds.), *Rheumatologic rehabilitation series: Vol. 1. Assessment and management* (pp. 157–178). Bethesda, MD: American Occupational Therapy Association.

Backman, C. L., Fairleigh, A., & Kuchta, G. (2004). Occupational therapy. In B. Hayes, D. S. Pisetsky, & B. St. Clair (Eds.), *RA: Rheumatoid arthritis* (pp. 431–439). Philadelphia: Lippincott Williams & Wilkins.

Backman, C. L., Kennedy, S. M., Chalmers, A., & Singer, J. (2004). Participation in paid and unpaid work by adults with rheumatoid arthritis. *Journal of Rheumatology, 31*(1), 47–56.

Backman, C., Mackie, H., & Harris, J. (1991). Arthritis Hand Function Test: Development of a standardized assessment tool. *Occupational Therapy Journal of Research, 11,* 245–256.

Backman, C., & Medcalf, N. (2000). Identifying components and environmental conditions contributing to occupational performance issues. In V. G. Fearing & J. Clark (Eds.), *Individuals in context: A practical guide to client-centered practice* (pp. 55–67). Thorofare, NJ: Slack.

Backman, C., & Mitchell, A. (2003, May 30). *A day in the life of mothers with rheumatoid arthritis.* Paper presented at the Annual Meeting of the Canadian Association of Occupational Therapists, Winnipeg, Manitoba.

Badley, E., & DesMeules, M. (2003). Introduction. In Health Canada, *Arthritis in Canada: An ongoing challenge* (Cat. No. H39-4/14-2003E, pp. 1–6). Ottawa, Ontario: Health Canada.

Beaton, D. E., Katz, J. N., Fossel, A. H., Wright, J. G., Tarasuk, V., & Bombardier, C. (2001). Measuring the whole or the parts? Validity, reliability, and responsiveness of the disabilities of the arm, shoulder, and hand outcome measure in different regions of the upper extremity. *Journal of Hand Therapy, 14,* 128–146.

Bellamy, N., Buchanan, W. W., Goldsmith, C. H., Campbell, J., & Stitt, L. W. (1988). Validation study of WOMAC: A health status instrument for measuring clinically important patient relevant outcomes to antirheumatic drug therapy in patients with osteoarthritis of the hip or knee. *Journal of Rheumatology, 15,* 1833–1840.

Boutaugh, M. L., & Brady, T. J. (1998). Patient education for self-management. In J. Melvin & G. Jensen (Eds.), *Rheumatologic rehabilitation series: Vol. 1. Assessment and management* (pp. 219–258). Bethesda, MD: American Occupational Therapy Association.

Burckhardt, C. S. (2001). Fibromyalgia. In L. Robbins, C. S. Burckhardt, M. T. Hannan, & R. J. DeHoratius (Eds.), *Clinical care in the rheumatic diseases* (2nd ed., pp. 135–139). Atlanta, GA: Association of Rheumatology Health Professionals.

Burckhardt, C. S., Clark, S. R., & Bennett, R. M. (1991). The Fibromyalgia Impact Questionnaire: Development and validation. *Journal of Rheumatology, 18,* 728–733.

Callahan, L. F. (2001). Impact and economic burden on society. In L. Robbins, C. S. Burckhardt, M. T. Hannan, & R. J. DeHoratius (Eds.), *Clinical care in the rheumatic diseases* (2nd ed., pp. 21–23). Atlanta, GA: Association of Rheumatology Health Professionals.

Cassidy J. T., & Petty, R. E. (2001). *Textbook of pediatric rheumatology* (4th ed.). Philadelphia: Saunders.

Chorus, A. M. J., Boonen, A., Miedema, H. S., & van der Linden, S. (2002). Employment perspectives of patients with ankylosing spondylitis. *Annals of Rheumatic Diseases, 61,* 693–699.

Chung, K. C., Pillsbury, M. S., Walters, M. R., & Hayward, R. A. (1998). Reliability and validity testing of the Michigan Hand Outcomes Questionnaire. *Journal of Hand Surgery* [Am], *23,* 575–587.

Cordery, J., & Rocchi, M. (1998). Joint protection and fatigue management. In J. Melvin & G. Jensen (Eds.), *Rheumatologic rehabilitation series: Vol. 1: Assessment and management* (pp. 279–322). Bethesda, MD: American Occupational Therapy Association.

Duruoz, M. T., Poiraudeau, S., Fermanian, J., Menkes, C., Amor, B., & Dougados, M. (1996). Development and validation of a rheumatoid hand functional disability scale that assesses functional handicap. *Journal of Rheumatology, 23,* 1167–1172.

Fries, J. F., Spitz, P., Kraines, R. G., & Holman, H. R. (1980). Measurement of patient outcome in arthritis. *Arthritis & Rheumatism, 23*, 137–145.

Garrett, S., Jenkinson, T., Kennedy, L. G., Whitelock, H., Gaisford, P., & Calin, A. (1994). A new approach to defining disease status in ankylosing spondylitis: The Bath Ankylosing Spondylitis Disease Activity Index. *Journal of Rheumatology, 21*, 2286–2291.

Gilworth, G., Chamberlain, M. A., Harvey, A., Woodhouse, A., Smith, J., Smyth, M. G., et al. (2003). Development of a work instability scale for rheumatoid arthritis. *Arthritis and Rheumatism, 49*, 349–354.

Hainsworth, J., & Barlow, J. (2001). Volunteers' experiences of becoming arthritis self-management lay leaders: "It's almost as if I've stopped aging and started to get younger!" *Arthritis & Rheumatism, 45*, 378–383.

Hammond, A., & Freeman, K. (2001). One-year outcomes of a randomized controlled trial of an educational-behavioural joint protection programme for people with rheumatoid arthritis. *Rheumatology, 40*, 1044–1051.

Hannan, M. T. (2001). Epidemiology of rheumatic diseases. In L. Robbins, C. S. Burckhardt, M. T. Hannan, & R. J. DeHoratius (Eds.), *Clinical care in the rheumatic diseases* (2nd ed., pp. 9–14). Atlanta, GA: Association of Rheumatology Health Professionals.

Harrell, P. B. (2001). Splinting of the hand. In L. Robbins, C. S. Burckhardt, M. T. Hannan, & R. J. DeHoratius (Eds.), *Clinical care in the rheumatic diseases* (2nd ed., pp. 191–196). Atlanta, GA: Association of Rheumatology Health Professionals.

Haskett, S., Backman, C., Porter, B., Goyert, J., & Palejko, G. (in press). A crossover trial of commercial versus custom-made wrist splints in the management of inflammatory polyarthritis. *Arthritis and Rheumatism.*

Helewa, A., Goldsmith, C. H., Lee, P., Bombardier, C., Hanes, B., Smythe, H. A., et al. (1991). Effects of occupational therapy home service on patients with rheumatoid arthritis. *Lancet, 337*, 1453–1456.

Helewa, A., & Stokes, B. (2001). Spondyloarthropathies. In L. Robbins, C. S. Burckhardt, M. T. Hannan, & R. J. DeHoratius (Eds.), *Clinical care in the rheumatic diseases* (2nd ed., pp. 105–112). Atlanta, GA: Association of Rheumatology Health Professionals.

Katz, P. P. (Ed.). (2003). Patient outcomes in rheumatology: A review of measures. *Arthritis and Rheumatism, 49*(5) (supplement).

Katz, P. P., & Alfieri, W. S. (1997). Satisfaction with abilities and well-being: Development and validation of a questionnaire for use among persons with rheumatoid arthritis. *Arthritis Care and Research, 10*, 89–98.

Katz, P. P., & Yelin, E. H. (1993). Prevalence and correlates of depressive symptoms among persons with rheumatoid arthritis. *Journal of Rheumatology, 20*, 790–796.

Katz, P. P., & Yelin, E. H. (1994). Life activities of persons with rheumatoid arthritis with and without depressive symptoms. *Arthritis Care and Research, 7*, 69–77.

Khani-Hanjani, A., Lacaille, D., Hoar, D., Chalmers, A., Horsman, D., Anderson M., et al. (2000). Association between dinucleotide repeat in non-coding region of interferon-gamma gene and susceptibility to, and severity of, rheumatoid arthritis. *Lancet, 356*, 820–825.

Lacaille, D., Sheps, S., Spinelli, J., & Esdaile, J. M. (1999). Work-related factors that determine risk of work disability (WD) in rheumatoid arthritis (RA) [Abstract]. *Arthritis and Rheumatism, 42*(Suppl.), S238.

Lagace, C., Perruccio, A., DesMeules, M., & Badley, E. (2003). The impact of arthritis on Canadians. In Health Canada, *Arthritis in Canada: An ongoing challenge* (Cat. No. H39-4/14-2003E, pp. 7–34). Ottawa, Ontario: Health Canada.

Law, M. (1998). Does client-centered practice make a difference? In M. Law (Ed.), *Client-centered occupational therapy* (pp. 19–27). Thorofare, NJ: Slack.

Law, M., Baptiste, S., Carswell, A., Polatajko, H., & Pollack, N. (1998). *Canadian Occupational Performance Measure* (3rd ed.). Ottawa, Canada: Canadian Association of Occupational Therapists.

Lerner, D., Amick, B. C., Rogers, W. H., Malspeis, S., Bungay, K., & Cynn, D. (2001). The Work Limitations Questionnaire. *Medical Care, 39*, 72–85.

Lorig, K. (1993). Self-management of chronic illness: A model for the future. *Generations, 17*(3), 11–14.

Luck, J. N. (2001). Enhancing functional ability. In L. Robbins, C. S. Burckhardt, M. T. Hannan, & R. J. DeHoratius (Eds.), *Clinical care in the rheumatic diseases* (2nd ed., pp. 196–202). Atlanta, GA: Association of Rheumatology Health Professionals.

Mann, W. (1998). Assistive technology for persons with arthritis. In J. Melvin & G. Jensen (Eds.), *Rheumatologic rehabilitation series: Vol. 1. Assessment and management* (pp. 369–392). Bethesda MD: American Occupational Therapy Association.

Mann, W. C., Tomita, M., Hurren, D., & Charvat, B. (1999). Changes in health, functional and psychosocial status and coping strategies of home-based older persons with arthritis over three years. *Occupational Therapy Journal of Research, 19*, 126–146.

Manuel, D., Lagace, D., DesMeules, M., Cho, R., & Power, J. D. (2003). Life expectancy and health-adjusted life expectancy (HALE). In Health Canada, *Arthritis in Canada: An ongoing challenge* (Cat. No. H39-4/14-2003E, pp. 40–41). Ottawa, Ontario: Health Canada.

Maricic, M. J. (2001). Osteoporosis. In L. Robbins, C. S. Burckhardt, M. T. Hannan, & R. J. DeHoratius (Eds.), *Clinical care in the rheumatic diseases* (2nd ed., pp. 121–126). Atlanta, GA: Association of Rheumatology Health Professionals.

Meenan, R. F., Mason, J. H., Anderson, J. J., Guccione, A. A., & Kazis, L. E. (1992). AIMS2: The content and properties of a revised and expanded Arthritis Impact Measurement Scales health status questionnaire. *Arthritis and Rheumatism, 35*, 1–10.

Moss, P. (1997). Negotiating spaces in home environments: Older women living with arthritis. *Social Sciences and Medicine, 45*, 23–33.

Nalebuff, E. A., & Melvin, J. L. (2000). Orthotic treatment for arthritis of the hand. In J. L. Melvin & E. A. Melvin (Eds.), *Rheumatologic rehabilitation series: Vol. 4. The hand: Evaluation, therapy and surgery.* Bethesda, MD: American Occupational Therapy Association.

Poole, J. L., Gallegos, M., & O'Linc, S. (2000). Reliability and validity of the Arthritis Hand Function Test in adults with systemic sclerosis (scleroderma). *Arthritis Care and Research, 13*, 69–73.

Ramsey-Goldman, R. (2001). Connective tissue diseases. In L. Robbins, C. S. Burckhardt, M. T. Hannan, & R. J. DeHoratius (Eds.), *Clinical care in the rheumatic diseases* (2nd ed., pp. 97–103). Atlanta, GA: Association of Rheumatology Health Professionals.

Riemsma, R. P., Kirwan, J. R., Taal, E., & Rasker, J. J. (2002). Patient education for adults with rheumatoid arthritis (Cochrane Review). *Cochrane Library*, Issue 2.

Sandqvist, G., & Eklund, M. (2000). Hand Mobility in Scleroderma (HAMIS) test: The reliability of a novel hand function test. *Arthritis Care and Research, 13*, 369–374.

Singh, G., Athreya, B. H., Fries, J. F., & Goldsmith, D. P. (1994). Measurement of health status in children with juvenile rheumatoid arthritis. *Arthritis and Rheumatism, 37*, 1761–1769.

Steultjens, E. M. J., Dekker, J., Bouter, L. M., van Schaardenburg, D., van Kuyk, M. A., & van den Ende, C. H. (2002). Occupational therapy for rheumatoid arthritis: A systematic review. *Arthritis and Rheumatism, 47*, 672–685.

Stokes, J., Desjardins, S., & Perruccio, A. (2003). Economic burden. In Health Canada, *Arthritis in Canada: An ongoing challenge* (Cat. No. H39-4/14-2003E, pp. 42–46). Ottawa, Ontario: Health Canada.

Superio-Cabuslay, E., Ward, M. M., & Lorig, K. R. (1996). Patient education interventions in osteoarthritis and rheumatoid arthritis: A meta-analytic comparison with non-steroidal anti-inflammatory drug treatment. *Arthritis Care and Research, 9*, 292–301.

Taylor, J., & Erlandson, D. M. (2001). Pediatric rheumatic diseases. In L. Robbins, C. S. Burckhardt, M. T. Hannan, & R. J. DeHoratius (Eds.), *Clinical care in the rheumatic diseases* (2nd ed., pp. 81–88). Atlanta, GA: Association of Rheumatology Health Professionals.

van Lankveld, W., van't Pad Bosch, P., Bakker, J., Terwindt, S., Franssen, M., & van Riel, P. (1996). Sequential Occupational Dexterity Assessment (SODA): A new test to measure hand disability. *Journal of Hand Therapy, 9*, 27–32

Wolfe, F., & Hawley, D. J. (1998). The longterm outcomes of rheumatoid arthritis: Work disability: A prospective 18 year study of 823 patients. *Journal of Rheumatology, 25*, 2108–2117.

Wolfe, F., Smythe, H. A., Yunus, M. B., Bennett, R. M., Bombardier, C., Goldenberg, D. L., et al. (1990). The American College of Rheumatology 1990 criteria for the classification of fibromyalgia: A report of the Multicenter Criteria Committee. *Arthritis and Rheumatism, 33*, 160–172.

Wright, F. V., Law, M., Crombie, V., Goldsmith, C. H., & Dent, P. (1994). Development of a self-report functional status index for juvenile rheumatoid arthritis. *Journal of Rheumatology, 21*, 536–544.

Chapter 9

Adaptive Strategies Following Spinal Cord Injury

SUSAN L. GARBER, MA, OTR, FAOTA, FACRM

THERESA L. GREGORIO-TORRES, MA, OTR

KEY TERMS

ASIA impairment scale

autonomic dysreflexia

intermittent catheterization

paraplegia

pressure ulcer

tenodesis grasp

tetraplegia

OBJECTIVES

Upon completion of this chapter, the reader will be able to

- Distinguish between paraplegia and tetraplegia;
- Discuss the prevalence of spinal cord injury (SCI), the potential secondary health complications, and innovative treatment strategies;
- Understand how SCI affects every aspect of a person's daily life;
- Describe the performance limitations experienced by people with various levels of SCI; and
- Describe adaptive strategies, equipment, or environmental modifications for activities of daily living (ADL), instrumental activities of daily living (IADL), work, play, and leisure for people with SCI.

The term *spinal cord injury* (SCI) refers to a disruption of the spinal cord secondary to trauma that results in the loss of sensory and motor function below the level of the injury. SCI is a life-altering event that can interfere with every aspect of occupational performance and quality of life. Unlike injuries to the extremities, SCI is complex and often results in an overwhelming loss of function, thereby presenting enormous, often insoluble, problems and challenges for patients and therapists alike.

Prevalence of SCI

Not until the 1940s, following World War II, were rehabilitation programs developed for people with SCI. These programs created a new philosophy of care for people with SCI (Clifton, Donovan, & Frankowski, 1985). Today, more than 200,000 people in the United States live with SCI, and approximately 11,000 new cases are reported every year (National Spinal Cord Injury Statistical Center, 2002). The veteran population makes up 22% of people with SCI (Lasfargues et al., 1995).

The most frequent causes of SCI are motor vehicle crashes (44.5%), falls (18%), acts of violence (17%), and recreational sporting activities (13%). SCI occurs most frequently in males (80%) between 16 and 30 years of age (55%). Today, the average age at injury is 35.3 years (James & Cardenas, 2003). Among patients injured since 1990, 59% are Caucasian, 28% are Black, 8% are Hispanic, and 3% belong to other ethnicities. Almost half of people with SCI had completed high school as of the time of injury, more than half were unmarried, and—although most were employed at the time of their injury—more than 14% were unemployed (Go, DeVivo, & Richards, 1995).

Pulmonary complications are the most common cause of death following SCI and may occur during both the acute and chronic phases (Ragnarsson, Hall, Wilmot, & Carter, 1995). Other complications that may arise soon after injury and that can become lifelong problems are fractures, heterotopic ossification, osteoporosis, pressure ulcers, and urinary tract infections.

Autonomic dysreflexia (also called *autonomic hyperreflexia*) is a sudden and severe rise in blood pressure. It is a potentially life-threatening condition that affects people with SCI above T-6. Caused by various noxious stimuli that trigger sympathetic hyperactivity, autonomic dysreflexia can result from bladder or bowel distension, suppository insertion, skin irritation, clothing or legbag straps that are too tight, or pressure ulcers. It can lead to a cerebrovascular accident or death if not relieved (Linsenmeyer et al., 1997). People with SCI must be familiar with how to manage autonomic dysreflexia and be able to instruct others, such as their caregivers, in what to do should this condition occur.

Role of Occupational Therapy

The role of occupational therapy in the evaluation and treatment of people with SCI has evolved into a complex array of intervention categories. Therapists assume responsibility for evaluation and training in all aspects of occupational performance, including

- Activities of daily living (ADL);
- Designing and fabricating assistive devices that maximize independence;
- Strengthening innervated musculature, particularly in the upper extremities;
- Exploring avocational and vocational interests and skills; and
- Applying the latest approaches and technology that promote maximum independence (Garber, 1985).

Therapies primarily focus on applying adaptive strategies, including equipment and environmental modifications, to ADL, instrumental activities of daily living (IADL), work, education, play, leisure, and social participation.

Rehabilitation of persons with spinal cord injury depends on these traditions and identifies innovative evaluation and treatment methods in such areas as environmental control, pressure ulcer prevention, mobility, assistive technology, adaptive skills training, and sexuality (Garber, 1985). New challenges include the reduced length of hospital stay and community-based programs for people with severe disabilities in concert with new developments in vocational rehabilitation and independent living (Tate et al, 1998).

Objective documentation of occupational performance following SCI and of progress throughout the intervention are accomplished most often using the Functional Independence Measure (FIM™), supplemented by other objective scales that provide necessary sensitivity and detail (Watson, Kanny, White, & Anson, 1995).

This chapter describes the occupational performance challenges faced by people with SCI in the context of the major categories of injury level:

- High-level tetraplegia (C-1–C-4);
- Tetraplegia (C-5–C-6, C-7–C-8);
- Paraplegia (T-1–T-6); and
- Paraplegia (T-7–S-5).

The neurological levels of the spinal cord form the basis of this chapter. The cervical spinal cord and its associated muscles and functional levels are described in Table 9.1. In addition to describing the neurological levels of the spinal cord, therapists determine the neurological completeness of an injury as well. The American Spinal Injury Association (ASIA; 2000) recommends that therapists use the International Standards for Neurological and Functional Classification of Spinal Cord Injury as the standard measure of impairment among people with SCI (Cohen, Sheehan, & Herbison, 1996). ASIA has adopted the ASIA Motor and Sensory Scale (modified and updated from the Frankel grading system), which defines the level of injury as the last caudal segment with intact motor and sensory innervations (Table 9.2; ASIA, 2000). Examination components (i.e., motor and sensory testing) are reliable, but confident and competent interpretation of the results requires thorough training and experience.

Among people with SCI, injuries to the cervical spine often result in greater loss of occupational performance. Table 9.3 provides an overview of the expected performance outcomes in ADL for different levels of injury. Not all lesions are complete, however, so the actual abilities and levels of independence achieved by clients with injuries at different levels will vary. The client's age, motivation, preinjury lifestyle and circumstances, and the presence of other injuries all influence rehabilitation outcomes and occupational therapy efforts.

Traumatic SCI not only causes sensorimotor impairment but also affects all body systems. Members of the rehabilitation team (physicians, therapists, nurses) assess the client's neurological status in conjunction with comprehensive and systematic assessments of the musculoskeletal, pulmonary, cardiovascular, gastrointestinal, genitourinary, and integumentary systems (James & Cardenas, 2003). Spasticity, bowel and bladder dysfunction, and respiratory and circulatory complications can significantly interfere with rehabilitation, participation in occupational therapy, and quality of life. Because people with SCI are living longer than even a decade ago, they are at risk to develop some of the medical conditions that affect the general population such as diabetes, heart disease, arthritis, and cancer.

Therapists should not overlook cognitive and psychosocial problems associated with SCI. Although cognition usually remains intact unless concomitant brain injury occurred, standardized assessment tools should be used to determine cognitive status. Depression, adaptation to disability, family dynamics and support, sexuality, and the risk of secondary complications all must be evaluated.

High-Level Tetraplegia: Levels C-1–C-4

High-level tetraplegia is paralysis resulting from an injury to the spinal cord at any segmental level between the C1 and C4 vertebrae. For the purpose of this chapter, this term describes any of the following conditions:

- A neurological level of C-4 or above (complete motor and sensory deficits bilaterally)
- Total or partial dependence on breathing aids
- Long-term medical and personal care needs
- Limited expected functional recovery (Garber, Lathem, & Gregorio, 1988).

Although people with high-level SCI usually are dependent on others for self-care, they learn to verbally instruct others in their care, thereby attaining some control in their life. The three major objectives in the rehabilitation of clients with C-1 through C-4 tetraplegia are

- Education regarding their care,
- Exposure to occupational performance activities, and
- Adaptation through the use of assistive technology.

Clients with SCI at the C-1 and C-2 level are ventilator dependent. The primary innervated muscle is the sternocleidomastoid, which controls neck flexion and head rotation. At the C-4 level, the significant innervated muscles are the diaphragm and the upper trapezius. A client with SCI at this level may need a ventilator at first, but he or she usually can be weaned from the ventilator over time. Active movement includes full neck rotation, neck extension and flexion, and some scapular elevation. Little or no scapular depression exists (Trombly, 1995b).

Clients with SCI at the C-1–C-4 level need stable head support for safety and comfort when washing or shaving the face, combing hair, and applying makeup. A caretaker must perform those tasks along with those related to feminine hygiene and bowel and bladder care. Clients with tetraplegia naturally will have preferences regarding how those tasks should be performed. They must be able to give accurate directions to caregivers to ensure that the tasks are completed in the preferred manner.

Dental Care

To brush and floss their teeth, rinse their mouths, use mouthwash, or clean dentures, clients with C-

Table 9.1. Functional Levels of the Cervical Spinal Cord

Roots	Muscles	Function
C-2, C-3	Sternocleidomastoid	Neck flexion and head rotation
C-3, C-4	Trapezius	
	Superior	Neck extension and scapular elevation
	Middle	Scapular adduction
	Inferior	Scapular adduction and depression
C-3, C-4, C-5	Diaphragm	Respiration
C-4, C-5	Rhomboids	Scapular medial adduction, retraction, and elevation
C-5, C-6	Deltoid	
	Anterior	Shoulder flexion to 90°
	Middle	Shoulder abduction to 90°
	Posterior	Shoulder extension and horizontal abduction
	Supraspinatus	Shoulder abduction
	Infraspinatus	Shoulder lateral rotation
	Teres minor	
	Subscapularis	Shoulder medial rotation
	Teres major	
	Biceps brachii	Elbow flexion and forearm supination
	Brachialis	Elbow flexion
	Brachioradialis	
	Extensor carpi radialis longus	Wrist flexion and abduction
C-5, C-6, C-7	Serratus anterior	Shoulder forward thrust; scapular rotation for shoulder abduction
C-5, T-1	Pectoralis major	Shoulder adduction, flexion, and medial rotation
	Pectoralis minor	Shoulder forward and downward
C-6, C-7	Supinator	Forearm supination
	Pronator teres	Forearm pronation
C-6, C-7, C-8	Latissimus dorsi	Shoulder medial rotation
	Triceps brachii	Elbow extension
	Extensor digiti communis	MCP extension
	Extensor digiti minimus	Little finger extension
C-7, C-8	Extensor indicis proprius	Index finger MCP extension
	Extensor carpi ulnaris	Wrist extension
	Extensor pollicis longus	Thumb IP extension
	Extensor pollicis brevis	Thumb MCP extension
	Abductor pollicis longus	Thumb abduction
C-7, C-8, T-1	Flexor digitorum superficialis	IP flexion
	Flexor digitorum profundus	DIP flexion
C-8, T-1	Flexor carpi ulnaris	Wrist flexion and adduction
	Interossei	MCP flexion
	Dorsales	Finger abduction
	Palmares	Finger adduction
	Flexor pollicis longus	Thumb IP flexion
	Flexor pollicis brevis	Thumb MCP flexion
	Abductor pollicis	Thumb abduction
	Adductor pollicis brevis	Thumb adduction
	Opponens pollicis	Thumb opposition
	Lumbricales	MCP flexion

Note. DIP = distal interphalangeal; IP = interphalangeal; MCP = metacarpophalangeal. From *Specialized Occupational Therapy for Persons With High Level Quadriplegia* by S. L. Garber, P. Lathem, and T. L. Gregorio, 1988, Houston: TIRR. Copyright © 1988 by TIRR. Reprinted by permission. There may be some variation among references regarding actual nerve roots and innervated muscles (Burke & Murray, 1975; Chusid, 1985; *Dorland's Medical Dictionary,* 1962; Hoppenfeld, 1977; Sharrard, 1964).

Table 9.2. International Standards for Neurological Classification of Spinal Cord Injury (ASIA Impairment Scale)

A = *Complete:* No motor or sensory function is preserved in the sacral segments S4–S5.

B = *Incomplete:* Sensory but not motor function is preserved below the neurological level and includes the sacral segments S4–S5.

C = *Incomplete:* Motor function is preserved below the neurological level, and more than half of key muscles below the neurological level have a muscle grade less than 3.

D = *Incomplete:* Motor function is preserved below the neurological level, and at least half of key muscles below the neurological level have a muscle grade of 3 or more.

E = *Normal:* Motor and sensory function are normal.

1–C-4 tetraplegia must rely on a caretaker. Because people with this level of injury may use a mouth stick to perform certain tasks, dental hygiene is extremely important. The structure and health of teeth and gums can affect their ability and ease in using a mouth stick (Figure 9.1). Clients should be encouraged to obtain dental evaluations at least annually to ensure healthy oral hygiene.

Bathing

Although people with C-1–C-4 tetraplegia are totally dependent in bathing, options are available to allow caregivers to accomplish this activity efficiently and effectively. Bathing often takes place in bed because the bathroom is inaccessible or appropriate equipment is not available. Some type of plastic covering can be used under the client to protect the bedding from getting wet, or a commercially available inflatable bathtub can be used on top of the bed to hold water. The inflatable bathtub is portable, which enables bathing while traveling. A basin of water and all necessary items (e.g., soap, washcloth and towels, shampoo, and a razor) should be brought to the bedside before the bath begins to reduce the time the client is exposed to the water and the possibly cool room air. An inflatable shampoo basin also can be used for washing hair while the client is in bed.

If the bathroom is accessible, a tall-back shower lift sling with head and neck support may be used to support the client while he or she sits in a padded, tilted, or reclined shower/commode chair. The sling helps ensure safe transfer and body support under wet conditions (Whiteneck et al., 1999). A client who uses a ventilator also must be protected from the possibility of water entering the trachea and coming in contact with the ventilator.

Bowel and Bladder Care

Clients with C-1–C-4 tetraplegia require assistance in all bowel and bladder management and feminine hygiene tasks except for emptying legbags. Legbags can be emptied using a special electric device powered by the electric wheelchair battery. The emptying device is connected to the clamp that surrounds the legbag tubing. The client uses a breath control or lever switch mounted in an accessible place to activate the device. When not activated, the tube is held closed by pressure and does not allow urine to pass. When the electric switch is activated, the pressure is released from the tube, allowing the urine to leave the legbag. This device limits a person to emptying the legbag into a floor drain, basin, or outdoors. Nonetheless, particularly for clients who are active in the community, the device can be liberating because it frees them from having to ask others to perform this personal task for them. Urine also can be collected by mounting a sealed container onto the wheelchair. The legbag tubing reaches around the wheelchair and into the container, which must be emptied daily by a caregiver or other person. The container also must be cleaned regularly to avoid odor.

Maintaining a sitting position can assist clients in bowel evacuation. A commode chair with a high back and head positioner is needed to give proper body support during this daily activity.

Ovulation and fertility usually are not altered in women with SCI once spinal shock resolves. Women with C-1–C-4 tetraplegia depend on caregivers to manage menstrual needs and birth control. Therapists and caregivers should respect clients' choices in these intimate, personal matters.

Eating

Head position and sitting angle may affect a client's ability to chew and swallow food or medications, especially if the SCI includes any involvement of the brain stem. For both safety and enjoyment, clients must be able to independently direct another person in proper positioning when eating.

Table 9.3. Expected Performance Outcomes for Individuals With Complete Spinal Cord Injury

Location of Injury	Mobility	Orthotic Devices	Community Transport	Communication	Feeding	Grooming	Bathing	Dressing	Toilet Needs
C-3–C-4	Can use pneumatic or chin-control power wheelchair with power recliner	U/E externally powered orthosis, dorsal cock-up splint, BFOs	Needs assistance of others in accessible van with lift, cannot drive	Can use phone and typewriter with adapted equipment	Usually needs feeding assistance; may use BFOs with universal cuff and adapted utensils; drinks with long straw after set-up	Must rely on personal care assistance	Must rely on personal care assistance	Must rely on personal care assistance	Must rely on personal care assistance
C-5	Can use powered W/C indoors and outdoors; can travel short distances in manual W/C with adapted hand rims indoors	U/E externally powered orthosis, dorsal cock-up splint, BFOs	Can drive with specially adapted van	Can use phone and typewriter with adapted equipment	Can self-feed with specially adapted equipment for feeding after set-up	Can be independent with adapted equipment	Must rely on personal care assistance	Requires assistance with U/E dressing; dependent for L/E dressing	Needs assistance from others and by equipment
C-6	Can travel short distances with manual W/C with adaptations; assistance needed outdoors; independent in hand-driven W/C	Wrist-driven orthosis, universal cuff, writing devices, built-up handles	Independent driving in specially adapted van	Can use phone, can also type and write with adapted equipment; can turn pages without assistance	Can be independent with adapted equipment; can drink from glass	Can be independent with adapted equipment	Independent in U/E and L/E bathing with adapted equipment	Independent with U/E dressing; assistance needed for L/E dressing	Independent for bowel routine; needs assistance with bladder routine
C-7	Can use manual W/C indoors and outdoors, except stairs	None	Independent driving in car with hand controls or specially adapted van; can independently place W/C in car	Independent with adapted equipment for phone, typing and writing; independent in turning pages	Independent	Independent	Independent with equipment	Independent	Independent
C-8–T-1	Can use manual W/C indoors with curbs, escalators	None	As above	Independent	Independent	Independent	Independent	Independent	Independent
T-2–T-10	Independent	KAFO with forearm crutches or walker	As above	Independent	Independent	Independent	Independent	Independent	Independent
T-11–L-2	Independent	KAFO or AFO with forearm crutches	As above	Independent	Independent	Independent	Independent	Independent	Independent
L-3–S-3	Independent	KAFO or AFO with forearm crutches or canes	As above	Independent	Independent	Independent	Independent	Independent	Independent

Note. AFO = ankle-foot orthosis; BFO = ballbearing forearm orthosis; KAFO = knee-ankle-foot orthosis; L/E = lower extremity; U/E = upper extremity; W/C = wheelchair.

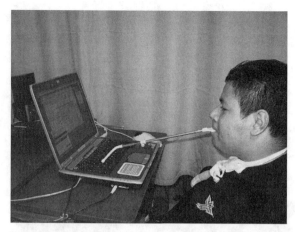

Figure 9.1. Person with high-level tetraplegia using a mouth stick.

Meal Preparation

People with C-1–C-4 tetraplegia use verbal instructions to fulfill family life roles, such as instructing a child to prepare a simple meal or use household appliances. During rehabilitation, a goal of occupational therapy for a client with C-1–C-4 tetraplegia is for the person to learn to effectively direct someone to prepare a simple food item, such as a sandwich, and to use the microwave. The therapist's responsibility is to give the client direct feedback regarding the effectiveness of the instructions. Because difficulties with voice volume and word choice can decrease others' willingness to listen to and assist the client, these aspects of verbal direction are considered as important as accuracy.

Medication

All people with SCI should be knowledgeable about the prescribed dosage and frequency of all their medications. Clients with C-1–C-4 tetraplegia should be able to identify their medications visually and know the dosage, purpose, and side effects of each medication so that, in an emergency, they can let others know their medication history. Therapists can provide clients, their families, and caretakers with notebooks that are organized according to the client's current medications. Clients and caregivers not only must keep track of this information but also must commit it to memory; occupational therapists should test them on the accuracy of the details.

Dressing and Undressing

Clients with C-1–C-4 tetraplegia will depend on others for dressing and undressing, but they can retain control over this task by making daily clothing se-

lections. Consideration should be given to purchasing clothing designs that reduce the effort needed to dress and undress. Some suggestions are loose-fitting clothing, stretchable fabrics, touch-fastener closures, slip-on shoes, minimal zippers and buttons, and elastic sleeves and waistbands (Farmer, 1986).

Because clients with SCI at C-1–C-4 have impaired sensation, fabrics should be selected that do not irritate the skin. Breathable materials, such as cotton, are best for air exchange between the atmosphere and the skin. Pants with double-welted seams and studs or rivets should be avoided because they can cause excessive pressure. Removing the rear pockets of pants reduces the risk of pressure from seams. Jewelry should be carefully selected for size because tight bracelets, necklaces, watchbands, and rings can restrict circulation. If swelling occurs, it might be necessary to cut off the jewelry.

The caregiver performs upper-body dressing using one of three methods: overhead, side-to-side, or around-the-back. People with C-1–C-2 injury will need assistance to extend the neck; people with C-3–C-4 injury can assist by flexing the neck forward. Nonrestrictive front access means that bras with front-touch fasteners or hooks will be easier to put on using the around-the-back method. Bras with back closures can be fastened first and then slipped over the head, much as one would put on a T-shirt. Clip-on ties or ties knotted partway are the easiest for a caregiver to put on someone with a C-1–C-4 injury.

To undress the person's upper body, the caregiver performs the same techniques in reverse. If the client is sitting in a wheelchair, he or she must be well supported during dressing and undressing to maximize trunk balance.

Lower-body dressing presents additional concerns. For example, the thick border seams at the leg openings of brief-style underpants sometimes cause pressure-induced skin breakdown over the ischial tuberosities. The seams of boxer shorts do not fall directly over these sensitive areas, so they may be a safer underwear choice. Excess cloth should be smoothed against the buttocks and upper legs, however, so that the underwear does not become wadded and cause undue pressure. Dressing technique also makes a difference: If the client is rolled side-to-side so that garments can be pulled up over the hips, shearing and friction can occur and damage the skin. A safer technique is to place one leg in both the underwear and pants leg openings simultaneously and pull the garment to knee level. Next, the other leg's underwear and pants leg openings are put on and pulled up to knee level. Then the client is rolled to one side and the underwear and pants leg on that side are pulled up into place. Finally, the client is rolled to the opposite side and the underwear and pants leg on that side are pulled into place. This method minimizes excessive rolling, decreasing the likelihood of skin shearing and friction to the buttocks.

Loose-fitting socks are much easier to pull over the foot than are tight, elasticized socks. Slip-on shoes or shoes with self-fastening closures also are recommended.

Dressing and undressing tasks provide caregivers with convenient opportunities to thoroughly inspect the client's skin. Pressure ulcers or other lesions should be noted carefully and treated promptly.

Functional Mobility

Transfers with clients with C-1–C-4 tetraplegia can be accomplished in any of the following ways: a mechanical or electric lift transfer, a three-person lift, or a dependent sliding-board transfer. Therapists should take into account the client's size and the caregiver's strength in determining the safest and most effective transferring method. Also, the client must be prepared to verbally direct each step of the transfer using complete and accurate instructions.

Most people with C-1–C-4 tetraplegia use a motorized (power) wheelchair for independent mobility. Appropriate driving mechanisms depend on the exact level of injury and may include sip-and-puff control, chin control, fiber-optic head array, or remote proportional joystick or head control. A manual wheelchair is recommended as a backup to the power wheelchair. The frame style of the manual wheelchair may be upright, tilted, or reclining, depending on the client's needs. A pressure-reducing seat cushion is required to distribute weight across the buttocks and provide pelvic stability while sitting (Garber, Biddle, et al., 2000).

To activate the sip-and-puff control switch, the operator seals his or her lips around a strawlike tube and either softly or forcefully blows or sucks air into the tube to trigger the motors in the chosen direction. The chin control is operated by moving the jaw to direct a small, remote, proportional-drive joystick positioned on a midline mount under the person's chin. A fiber-optic head array or a remote proportional joystick mounted behind the person's head are additional options. Optimal positioning of the head array or remote proportional joystick is crucial for safe and reliable head placement and control. It is imperative that an emergency kill switch be mounted in a reliable and accessible location. The kill switch will allow the wheelchair to be

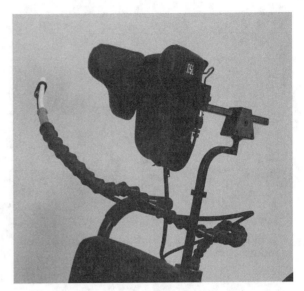

Figure 9.2. Powered mobility options for people with high-level tetraplegia: Sip-and-puff switch.

stopped should the drive switch that normally is used become dislodged or out of the reach of the person in the chair (Figure 9.2 and Figure 9.3).

A power-tilt or reclining system on a power wheelchair will allow the client to perform independent weight shifting to reduce the risk of pressure ulcers. A power-reclining system offers the most effective weight shifting because more body weight is distributed over a larger body surface during the maneuver. For people who experience postural problems from spasticity, changing the hip angle can cause them to sit out of alignment after a weight shift is performed. If spasticity is a significant problem, a power-tilt system would allow for shift-

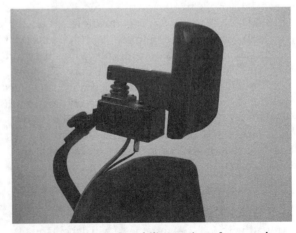

Figure 9.3. Powered mobility options for people with high-level tetraplegia: Remote proportional head control.

ing weight 45 degrees to 60 degrees, depending on the manufacturer of the system (Goossens et al., 1997; Lathem, Gregorio, & Garber, 1985). A power-tilt system preserves the hip-to-back angle at a constant position during a weight shift, thus maintaining pelvic positioning (Garber, Biddle, Click, Cowell, Gregorio-Torres, Hansen, 2000).

Community Mobility

The client with C-1–C-4 tetraplegia will require assistance with all community mobility. The therapist must discuss information about adapted vans with wheelchair lifts and tie-down systems with the client and caregivers. The wheelchair must have adequate positioning devices to support the client's body and to maintain stability while the van is in motion. These devices may include head supports, chest straps, seatbelts, and lateral supports.

Clearance through the van door is important, because wheelchair backs with head supports tend to be higher than a conventional van doorway opening. The safest position for securing the wheelchair to the floor is facing forward. Visual restriction from the van's headliner sometimes is a problem. This may be resolved by raising the van's roof or dropping its floor.

Clients who are unable to afford a modified van for personal transportation need education about how to use public transportation systems. Supervised outings provide the best preparation for clients who are learning how to access public transportation.

Communication

People with C-1–C-2 tetraplegia have limited head and neck control, so using electronic equipment helps them be more successful at completing tasks such as turning pages, typing, and activating a tape recorder or telephone. People with C-3–C-4 tetraplegia may use electronic devices or a mouth stick to achieve such tasks (Figure 9.4). People with SCI at this level often use mouth sticks to participate in leisure and avocational activities, such as board games or games activated by remote control. Other frequently used communication-enhancing equipment includes

- Bookholders
- Computers with modified input devices
- Electric page turners
- Elevating tables
- Electronic aids to daily living (EADL)
- Keyboard keyguards
- Modified work stations
- Mouth stick holders

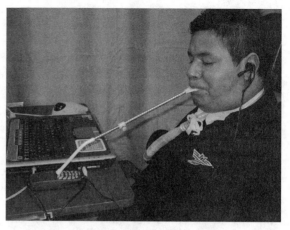

Figure 9.4. Person with high-level tetraplegia using cellular phone with earpiece.

- Phone enhancements, like gooseneck supports, cellular phones, phone flippers, and speaker phones (Figure 9.5).

Electronic aids to daily living and computer input devices now operate reliably with voice commands. Access to phone systems may require a combination of mouth stick skills, voice activation, and setup by another person.

Tetraplegia: Levels C-5–C-6

People with C-5 tetraplegia have functional biceps. They can feed themselves and perform simple grooming tasks using adapted equipment. At level C–6, wrist extension is preserved, enabling the person to require only minimal to moderate assistance in grooming, bathing, and meal preparation (Stover & Fine, 1986). People with C-5–C-6 tetraplegia sometimes undergo tendon transfer surgery to improve hand and arm performance. Upper-extremity tendon transfer surgery can improve clients' quality

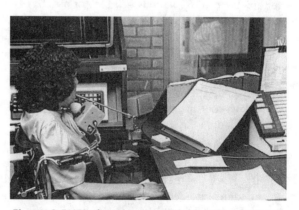

Figure 9.5. Workstation modified for the person with high-level tetraplegia.

of life by increasing their independence in performing ADL (Wuolle et al., 2003).

In tendon transfer surgery, an innervated but nonessential muscle is used to replace a muscle that has lost its function. This type of surgery has been perfected more for the upper extremities than the lower extremities. Typically, it is not considered until a year following the SCI to allow time for normal return of function. People who seek tendon transfer surgery must tolerate several weeks of postoperative immobilization, during which time performance that had been previously gained may be diminished or lost. Family or caregiver availability is crucial during this healing phase. Several weeks of ongoing therapy follow the postoperative phase to retrain the person in the use of the returned muscle function. Successful surgery and retraining may allow the person to discontinue the use of orthotic or assistive devices used to complete specific ADL.

People with SCI at C-5 may have good shoulder control and strong elbow flexion. In this case, however, active elbow extension is absent, which makes overhead activities nearly impossible. The ability to lift the forearm and hand against gravity or reach forward more completely can greatly aid performance of certain self-care activities. Clients with SCI at C-5 may benefit from a posterior deltoid-to-triceps tendon transfer to provide for this absent muscle function (Cardenas, Burns, & Chan, 2000). Clients also may lack effective lateral pinch and therefore may benefit from a transfer of the brachioradialis to the tendon of the flexor pollicis longus (Hill, 1994). The transfer of the pronator teres to the flexor digitorum profundus may allow for active finger flexion and extension (Gansel, Waters, & Gellman, 1990).

Dental Care

A functional hand-to-mouth pattern is the first prerequisite to brushing teeth. A client with C-5 tetraplegia can use various orthoses or assistive devices to stabilize the wrist in a neutral position and a mobile arm support (MAS) to lift his or her arm against gravity. To facilitate brushing teeth and rinsing the mouth, the caregiver

- Sets up the toothbrush in a utensil holder,
- Puts toothpaste on the brush, and
- Sets up a cup of water with a straw next to a second, empty cup.

The client first brushes the teeth on one side of the mouth. He or she then turns the toothbrush around in the utensil holder by holding the brush between the teeth and rotating the head or by grasping the brush between the teeth, removing it from the holder, and then reinserting it into the holder. Then the client brushes the teeth on the other side of the mouth. The client then uses the straw to draw rinse water into the mouth, uses the lips to transfer the straw to the empty cup, and allows the rinse water to flow back out of the mouth through the straw.

Clients with adequate muscle strength to move an arm against gravity may be able to use one of the following other orthotic devices to stabilize the hand:

- Ratchet orthosis
- Long opponens splint
- Universal cuff
- Wanchik writer (Figure 9.6)
- Dorsal wrist cock-up splint
- Elastic wrist brace.

These devices usually are reasonably priced. Most people prefer a toothpaste tube with a flip-top cap because it can be easily opened by bringing it to the mouth with both hands and using the teeth to open it. As an alternative, a pump tube can be mounted on a fabricated stand to stabilize it while dispensing toothpaste.

Bathing

A client with C-5 tetraplegia requires moderate to maximum assistance from another person for task completion and safety during bathing. If a person with C-5 or C-6 tetraplegia has an accessible shower, he or she typically uses a padded, rolling shower-commode chair in a modified shower stall. Wall-mounted dispensers make accessing soap and shampoo more successful and safer during this task. Chest straps mounted to the shower-commode chair may help stabilize the upper trunk during the activity. The client also may use a D-ring wash mitt to wash the face, neck, anterior chest, and upper legs. A person with C-6 tetraplegia may use long-handled brushes to reach the feet, in-between the toes, and other hard-to-reach spots. A hand-held showerhead may be useful, but the occupational therapist may need to add an adapted handle to it. The availability of skin pro-

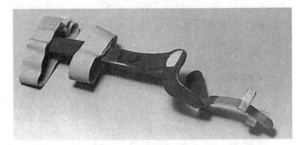

Figure 9.6. Wanchik device for daily living.

tection, postural support, and adapted handles make bathing a more independent, more private activity. Bed baths offer an alternative bathing method for people whose homes are not modified or for whom equipment is not yet available.

Washing the Face and Hands

To be totally independent in washing the face and hands, a person with C-5 or C-6 tetraplegia must be able to maneuver his or her wheelchair up to a sink. Proximity to sink and faucet handles is crucial to independent performance. Lever handles on the water faucets maximize the client's ability to turn them on and off. If the client uses a D-ring wash mitt, he or she may want to use a stabilizing wrist device under the mitt. Soap can be secured to the sink using a suction pad. Using a MAS, the person can employ a combination of head, neck, and upper extremity movements to reach all areas. Excess water is squeezed out of the wash mitt by pushing it against the side of the sink. A person with C-6 tetraplegia may use a regular washcloth, bar soap, or liquid soap dispenser.

Hair Care

Hair washing is performed most easily while showering or bathing. If a roll-in shower stall is unavailable, then hair washing is performed by leaning over a sink. Because it is necessary to stabilize the trunk while leaning forward over a sink, most people with SCI at this level choose to have someone else wash their hair. A commercially available shampoo basin can be used for hair washing when bathing in bed. This type of basin has a drain tube that can be placed in a bucket to collect the used water.

A person with C-5 tetraplegia will have difficulty holding a blow-dryer up against gravity, so drying hair is most easily achieved by mounting the blow-

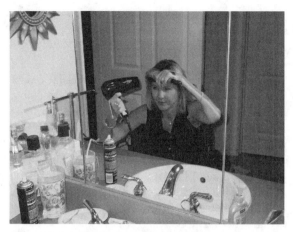
Figure 9.8. Tenodesis grasp for holding a hairbrush.

dryer on a gooseneck stand or the wall. Rather than move the blow-dryer, the person moves his or her head to catch the warm air generated by the dryer. A person with a C-6 SCI may use a modified cuff on a blow-dryer (Figure 9.7). If the person is able to prop his or her elbow on a countertop, this can enhance stability and endurance during this task.

For a person without innervated triceps, brushing and styling the hair requires creativity and skill in using substitute muscle function. A client with C-5 tetraplegia who uses a MAS will not be able to perform this task without maximal assistance. Long-handled brushes are useful, as are the small, octopus-type scrubbers with ring handles often found in drugstores. Using a curling iron or hair curlers also requires maximum assistance. The client may consider adapting by using a permanent wave or a low-maintenance hairstyle.

A client with this level of injury who can move his or her arm against gravity needs to stabilize the wrist. Brushes and combs with extended handles can be stabilized using the previously mentioned orthoses or assistive devices. People with SCI at the C-6 level can use their tenodesis grasp or a wrist-driven, wrist-hand orthosis (WDWHO) to hold a brush or comb (Figures 9.8 and 9.9). A universal cuff

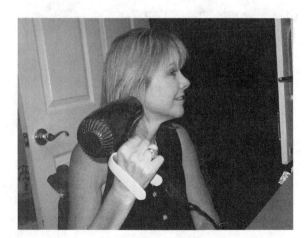
Figure 9.7. Modified cuff on blow-dryer.

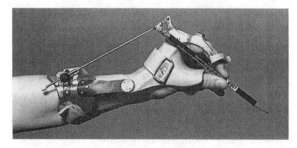
Figure 9.9. Flexor hinge/reciprocal orthosis.

and a phone holder (used as a brush holder) also can help the client perform this task.

Shaving

Shaving can be performed with either an electric razor or a safety razor, depending on the client's personal preference. Some clients prefer electric razors to avoid the cuts and nicks from blades. The therapist should work to support the client in achieving safety and independence in shaving using the selected method. A person using a MAS will need assistance setting up the razor and shaving cream. Some clients also will need assistance with shaving difficult-to-reach contours of the face, neck, and body.

Using a WDWHO, a ratchet orthosis, or a specially adapted cuff enables the client with C-5–C-6 tetraplegia to hold an electric razor. The razor's weight is a major consideration, because it may give more resistance than the limb can support. Safety razors can be adapted with a variety of low-temperature plastics for ease of handling. If the person can move his or her arm against gravity, a utensil holder can be used to stabilize the razor. Commercially available razor holders must be used in conjunction with a wrist-stabilizing brace for people with a C-5 SCI. Keeping the razor from falling can be a challenge, but it can be done using a two-handed technique. Commercially available shaving cream dispensers with a long lever handle can assist with this aspect of the activity.

Most women with C-5 tetraplegia require assistance in shaving their underarms and legs because of impaired trunk stability during forward leaning and the need to maintain upright balance while using both upper extremities for the task. A woman with C-6 tetraplegia may be able to use a WDWHO, universal cuff, or tenodesis action of her hands to hold the razor to shave her underarms and legs, but she may need the assistance of another person.

Makeup Application

Typically, a woman with SCI at level C-5 will need assistance to apply makeup to her face. The client may be able to clasp both hands together to hold makeup items. Components that require fine motor coordination are performed by a caregiver. A woman with injury at the C-6 level can use a WD-WHO, tenodesis, or adapted handles to grasp makeup brushes, pencils, or wands. Sanding or slightly filing the clasps on blush and eye shadow compacts makes them easier to open. Small tubes, such as those containing mascara, can be held in the mouth, while using the most dexterous hand to apply the makeup, allowing greater independence.

Bowel and Bladder Management

People with SCI at C-5 require assistance in bowel and bladder care because of the lack of hand function and inability to position themselves independently. The client should be able to verbally direct the caregiver in this task.

A client with C-5 tetraplegia may be able to empty his or her legbag using either a manual pneumatic legbag clamp or an electric legbag emptier. The switch that controls the clamp must be positioned so the client can access it easily. The legbag may be emptied into a floor basin, a cat litter box, or onto grass. The electric legbag emptier must be mounted onto the client's wheelchair. Gravity assists in draining urine from the tubing.

For the person with C-6 tetraplegia, self-catheterization may be made easier with bilateral WDWHO. The need to manage clothes and transfers every 4 hours, however, may complicate performance of this activity. People who must rely on themselves usually are more motivated to develop the fine motor skills necessary to manage bowel and bladder care. Practicing other fine motor skills, such as sewing, lacing, and writing, facilitate the problem solving necessary to successfully complete a clean, safe, self-catheterization.

People with SCI at level C-6 may need assistance managing a regular bowel program because of difficulty with body positioning and diminished fine motor hand movements. They should be knowledgeable in the task, however, and be verbally independent in directing the caretaker. Two examples of devices for bowel management are illustrated in Figure 9.10. The client may be able to manage an intermittent catheterization program if he or she is

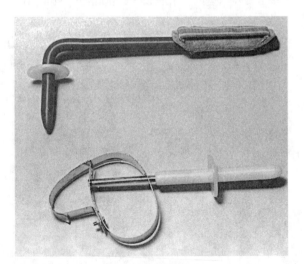

Figure 9.10. Bowel management devices.

independent with proper body positioning either in the wheelchair or in bed. The client should be able to empty the legbag with minimal adaptations. A woman with this level of injury should be able to position a sanitary napkin appropriately when dressing, but she may have difficulty inserting and removing a tampon.

A consistent, routine schedule and proper food and fluid intake help regulate waste elimination. Foods with a proper balance of fiber, nutrients, and liquids aid bladder and bowel regulation.

Occupational therapists have the unique skills required to perform an activity analysis and can be helpful in problem solving for positioning and techniques. The therapist may need to fabricate and modify equipment or provide suggestions for greater independence with bowel and bladder routines. Most important, the therapist can provide emotional support and encouragement as the client develops strategies for handling this extremely personal task (Hollar, 1995).

Eating

For clients with SCI at levels C-5–C-6, self-feeding can be achieved using a variety of techniques and adaptive devices. A person with C-5 tetraplegia may use a device to position the wrist in a neutral position, and people with SCI at C-6–C-6 may use other types of devices to hold eating utensils or for stability during the task.

The person with SCI at levels C-5–C-6 may use a universal cuff (an elastic or self-fastening strap attached to a leather pocket) that is easily donned and simply used with a regular utensil inserted into the palmar pocket. The client can pick up a modified cup or glass using a wrist-stabilizing device. A cup or glass can be given a modified handle so the hand can passively lift it to the mouth. Some clients prefer using a long straw so they do not need to lift the cup or glass from the table. For convenience and ease of reach, a straw holder can be used to keep the straw pointed toward the person's face.

If the person is using a ratchet-type orthosis, the orthosis itself can be positioned around the cup or glass for lifting. Once this is done, the client usually can drink independently. A nonbreakable, lightweight cup or glass is safer and gives less stress to arm musculature.

Eating with utensils can be accomplished with a variety of adaptations such as a hand orthosis with a utensil pocket, a long opponens orthosis, or a wrist-stabilizing splint with the ability to attach a spoon or fork. A ratchet-type orthosis can be used to hold utensils in the conventional way, allowing the client to self-feed independently once set up. A MAS or monosuspension feeder can assist clients with significantly diminished upper-extremity range of motion and strength to eat independently.

If the client has a difficult time keeping the food on the utensil because of a lack of forearm rotation, swivel utensils may be used. A plate-guard can be used as a border against which food can be scooped so that it does not fall off of the plate. Initially, a client may not have sufficient upper-extremity strength and endurance to self-feed an entire meal. Practice to gain endurance in this task should be encouraged to gain task independence. Cutting food takes much practice, and the person with tetraplegia at levels C-5–C-6 usually requires minimum to moderate assistance and adapted equipment to complete this task. A client with sufficient shoulder internal rotation may use a rocker knife. A knife with a serrated edge can be used if a sawing motion is used to cut. Some clients with C-5–C-6 lesions choose to have others cut their food because it is safer and neater. This choice should be respected.

Meal Preparation and Cleanup

Meal preparation can be difficult and time consuming for people with C-5 tetraplegia. Therefore, meals often are prepared by a caregiver. Assistance with meal preparation for clients with lesions at the C-6 level may range from no assistance to maximal assistance. Clients who use a WDWHO find it easier to accomplish more meal preparation tasks than do clients who use passive wrist-stabilizing orthoses. The performance range of clients with SCI at this level varies considerably, partly because of each person's individual functioning, but also because of varying levels of motivation to achieve the task, tolerance for problem solving, and accessibility in their kitchens.

Safely lifting pans into and out of the oven poses a major challenge for clients with SCI. A microwave or toaster oven may eliminate this problem and be adequate if the client is preparing meals for just one or two persons. Stove-top cooking is accomplished using over-the-stove mirrors, long-handled utensils, large-handled pots, shallow fry pans, and long oven mitts to prevent burns. A suction stabilizer that holds the pans stable increases safety when preparing hot food. Using adapted utensils or a palm-to-palm method to grasp utensils, the client can accomplish many mealtime tasks.

To transport food from one place to another, clients find it easiest to slide the item along the counter or use a lap-tray. Commercially available one-handed can openers with adjustable stands to support the can are difficult for a person with C-6 tetraplegia to use, but with practice the technique may be mastered. Using a blender or mixer can conserve the client's energy. Controls should be levers or push buttons.

Clients can cut food items using an adapted knife and a cutting board with a stainless or aluminum nail through it to stabilize the food. Suction cups on the bottom of the cutting board provide stability on the countertop, which allows a two-handed cutting method to be used, either palm-to-palm or allowing one hand to secure the food and the other hand to do the cutting. A table or lower counter can be used to support the client's elbows, thus bringing the objects closer and making them more easily manipulated. Because of a lack of triceps strength and the need for support to maintain trunk balance, the client is most successful when working close to the body. Jars can be opened by holding them between both hands and pushing and turning against an adaptive device that has serrated edges. In general, jar lids should be kept loosely engaged for ease of opening.

Ovens can be difficult for clients with SCI to handle because of the weight or spring action of the door. Lifting pans into and out of the oven can be unsafe. A toaster oven or a broiler used on a low tabletop offers a safer way to bake. Clients use lever action to open the door and depress buttons. Microwave ovens also are safer than conventional ovens if placed on a table at an accessible height. A button or lever often controls the door, or loops can be added to the door handle to aid in opening.

The refrigerator door also can be made easier to open by adding loops to the door handle. Frequently used items should be placed on the shelves of the refrigerator that are at eye-level or lower (Figure 9.11). Food-storage containers should be made of lightweight plastic in case they are dropped or slip from the person's grasp.

Cleanup is easier if the sink is accessible. A scrubber with soap in the handle is a useful step saver. Brushes with large open handles that the hand can fit through provide a better grasp. A rubber pad on the bottom of the sink decreases the likelihood of breakage. An adapted scrub brush and a liquid soap dispenser, a bottlebrush, a wash mitt, and levers on sink controls can help during dish washing. The dishes can be dried either in the sink or in a sink rack. Using a dishwasher is feasible but can be difficult given the weight of the door. A loop can be added to the handle to assist in opening it. Some people choose to use their dishwasher to store clean dishes in order to eliminate the step of return-

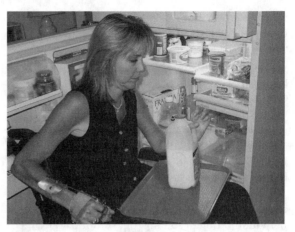

Figure 9.11. Person with C-6 tetraplegia removing items from the refrigerator.

ing them to kitchen cabinets that may be less accessible to them.

Prepared foods and microwave dishes may be relatively expensive, but they save time and energy and reduce frustration. Conventional meal preparation presents challenges that may include

- Getting the food out of the pantry, refrigerator, or freezer;
- Reaching the pots and pans;
- Opening plastic, frozen, or metal containers;
- Operating manual and small electric kitchen appliances;
- Setting the table; and
- Using large kitchen appliances.

For the client with SCI, the kitchen environment can exacerbate—or make easier—these challenges. The following elements of design and adaptation can strongly influence a client's independence in the kitchen:

- The kitchen area should have adequate room for wheelchair maneuvering to open drawers and doors.
- Cabinet doors should be easy to open, with glides and handles to assist people with limited strength and hand function (or the client may choose to remove cabinet doors altogether).
- Food and cooking items should be placed within reach at wheelchair level as much as possible, noting that clients with SCI likely will use a reacher to access items placed above head level.
- The preferred refrigerator design is a side-by-side style that makes both the freezer and the refrigerator compartments accessible.

Small manual kitchen appliances must be on a work surface at desk height to be operated with little or no adaptation. Manual appliances often require more energy to operate and often are not as effective as electric ones. Several electric appliances now are available to assist in common meal preparation tasks; electric can openers, electric peelers, food processors, and mixers are a few examples. Small electric appliances, like electric can openers, may require a supporting base and lever switches or special push buttons for efficient and safe operation (Figure 9.12).

Because of sensory deficits, the person with SCI at this level needs to be careful around sharp items and surfaces and extreme temperatures. For example, safely operating the range or oven requires that switches be within reach, eliminating the need to lean over hot burners. The therapist and client should consider where control knobs are positioned, ideally on the front or side of the stovetop, to eliminate this safety hazard.

It takes creativity to adapt the kitchen environment, appliances, and utensils to meet the needs of a person with C-5–C-6 tetraplegia. Preplanning also can help save time and increase efficiency in meal preparation.

Medication

Medications can be placed in an easy-to-open container or a shallow, open cup. A person with C-5 tetraplegia may use a ratchet orthosis and a person with C-6 tetraplegia may use a WDWHO to pick up and place medication in his or her mouth. A person with stabilized wrists will be able to raise the open cup to the mouth by clasping it between both hands. Safety issues with this method include the consequences of dropped medications and open

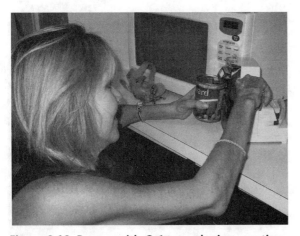

Figure 9.12. Person with C-6 tetraplegia operating an electric can opener.

containers, which could be handled by small children if they are in the home. The client should try different types of containers, requesting that the pharmacist provide containers with simple-to-open flip-top or regular screw-off caps. The most difficult containers are those with push-and-turn, or "child-proof," caps.

Dressing and Undressing

A person with C-5 SCI may require minimal to moderate assistance with upper-body dressing for pull-over or button-front clothes because of decreased upper-extremity range of motion, lack of fine motor coordination, and lack of trunk stability. The client will need assistance to fasten or unfasten buttons. Pull strings attached to zippers allow manipulation without fine motor finger movement. To put on a front-fastening shirt or jacket, the client can use the around-the-back method, which will require moderate to maximal assistance. A person with SCI at C-6 may put on pull-over or button-front shirts with little to no assistance, or may use a buttonhook–zipper pull device to fasten closures independently. Front-fastening or self-fastening bras can be modified with sewn-in loops through which the thumb can be inserted. Bras also may be put on like a T-shirt. First the caregiver fastens the bra closure, then either the client or the caregiver pulls the bra over the head and down along the upper chest into place. For men who wear ties, options include either the clip-on tie or having the caregiver preknot the tie and pull it over the client's head. Either the client or the caregiver will tighten or fasten it in place.

Because people with SCI at the C-5 level lack bed mobility, they require assistance in lower extremity dressing. Slacks and skirts cut longer and slightly larger in the hips are easier to put on and fit a person sitting in a wheelchair with flexed knees more precisely. Independent lower-body dressing begins with sitting in bed. The pants are positioned with the front facing up and pants legs over the bottom of the bed. The pants are put in position by tossing them or by using a dressing stick to move the pants legs away from the body. The client lifts one leg by using the opposite wrist or forearm placed under the knee, and tunnels the foot into the pants leg. The client may use the thumb of the other hand to hook a belt loop or pocket to hold the top of the pants open. Then the client inserts the other foot. Using the palms of the hands, the client slides the pants legs up along the calves. Some people find it helpful to wear friction gloves to provide resistance to the pants cloth for improved manipulation. Tenodesis motion or wrists hooked under the waistband inside the pants can be used to pull the pants up over the knees. These motions are continued until the waistband reaches the upper-thigh area. The person then returns to a supine position, where he or she rolls side-to-side on the bed. Lying on one side, the client hooks the thumb of the top arm in the back belt loops to pull the pants up over the buttocks. The client repeats this process on alternating sides until the pants are in place. Clients can fasten pants using a zipper pull, a loop added to the zipper, or hook-and-loop tab closures. To remove pants, the person reverses these procedures.

Socks are easiest to put on while sitting in the wheelchair. The person crosses one leg over the other and uses tenodesis grasp to put on the sock and the palms of the hands to help pull it on. A person who is unable to cross his or her legs can place one foot on a stool or chair. If trunk balance is poor, the person can hook one arm around the wheelchair upright while reaching with the other hand. Alternatively, the person can put the socks on in a sitting position in bed by crossing first one leg and then the other. Two loops may be sewn on opposite sides of the top of the sock, where the thumbs can be hooked through to manipulate the sock onto the foot, or a sock aid may used to get the sock over the toes if the person is unable to reach his or her feet. Socks are removed by pushing them off with a dressing stick, long shoehorn, or by hooking the thumb in the sock edge (Trombly, 1995a).

Modified clothing is commercially available through catalogs such as USA Jeans (www.usajeans.net), Rolli Moden (www.rolli-moden.com), Wardrobe Wagon (www.wardrobewagon.com), Adrian's Closet (www.adrianscloset.com), and Wearable (www.wearable@blvd.com) and modified sewing patterns are available through Simplicity (www.simplicity.com) to ensure a more functional fit for a person with a physical disability.

Functional Mobility

For the person with C-5–C-6 tetraplegia, transferring or moving the body from one surface to another can require a tremendous amount of effort. For this reason, many people with SCI at this level choose to rely on others to perform the total task for them. In most cases, moderate assistance from another person is needed for a person with C-5 tetraplegia to transfer to and from level surfaces. Transfers between positions of different heights require maximal to total assistance. A transfer board provides a smooth surface to slide across and decreases resistance during the task. Performance ability varies greatly among people with C-6 tetraplegia, depending on body size,

strength, motivation, and age. Some clients may need no assistance and others may need maximal assistance. A sliding board may or may not be necessary. For clients whose weight or degree of body spasticity impact on transfers may find it easier and safer to use a mechanical or electric lift.

Wheelchair Mobility

A person with C-5–C-6 tetraplegia can move independently over both level and uneven surfaces with a manual wheelchair. The wheelchair must be specifically measured to accommodate the body for proper support and occupational performance (Figure 9.13). The wheelchair's back must be high enough to support the trunk, so arm function can be maximized. Vertical–oblique or friction rims are recommended to push the wheelchair forward and reverse. The scapular stabilizing musculature must be strengthened so as not to over-stretch supporting shoulder structures. A wrist-stabilizing splint is used to enhance hand placement of the person with C-5 injury. People with SCI at the C-5–C-6 level can use a folding or rigid manual wheelchair.

A grade aid (or hill climber), a type of secondary braking device, is recommended for propelling the wheelchair up an incline or ramp. The grade aid is mounted under the wheelchair brakes. The device lies on the surface of the tire, allowing the tire to be pushed forward. The client engages the grade aid by pushing a lever handle downward. When the push stroke is completed, the device clutches the tire and prevents it from rolling backward, but continues to allow forward motion. When the incline or ramp has been climbed, the client pushes the lever up to disengage the device.

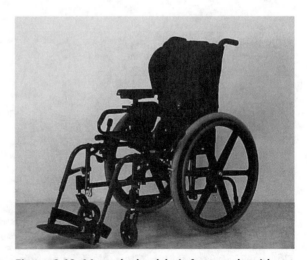

Figure 9.13. Manual wheelchair for people with C-5–C-6 tetraplegia.

Brake extensions also provide increased lever advantage in operating wheelchair brakes. On ultra-lightweight wheelchairs, anti-tip bars are a safety option, as they prevent the wheelchair from tipping backwards on an uneven surface.

For some people with SCI, propelling the weight of a manual wheelchair takes too much effort, and endurance is compromised. Sometimes the slowness of manual wheelchair propulsion limits the client's functional mobility in the community. Rough terrain, long distances, or shoulder pain can challenge the person's abilities and may necessitate a power wheelchair. Using a power wheelchair may conserve energy, allow the client greater mobility, and expand the client's opportunities for school or work. A manual wheelchair usually is purchased to serve as a backup to the power wheelchair.

A power wheelchair with a hand control usually is chosen for people with SCI at C-5 and may be selected for people with SCI at C-6 (Figure 9.14). A person who uses a MAS needs extensive practice to master driving a hand-controlled power wheelchair. It is important to look for the position of the MAS that provides the greatest mechanical advantage.

Therapists and clients must thoroughly discuss issues related to community mobility to anticipate

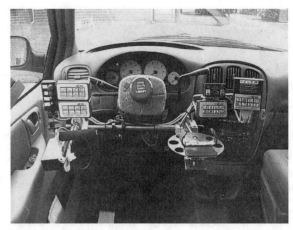

Figure 9.15. Driving controls in an adapted van for person with C-5 tetraplegia.

and solve problems. Most motorized wheelchairs do not fold easily to be loaded into a conventional vehicle. People who use motorized wheelchairs are unable to independently load the wheelchair into a car, sport-utility vehicle (SUV), or truck, which limits their independent mobility in the community. Transporting this type of wheelchair requires a modified van with an electric lift.

For safety and efficiency, some clients may need to adapt the wheelchair's hand control with an extended joystick. The wrist is supported with an orthosis or assistive device. A powered recliner or tilt system typically is considered for independent weight shifting, if the person is unable to lean side-to-side or push up independently to reduce peak sitting pressure over the pelvis.

Community Mobility

New technology in adapted driving, including modified vans with low- or zero-effort steering and electric lifts, enables some people with SCI at C-5 to be independently mobile (Figures 9.15–9.18). The person who has an injury at this level usually drives from a motorized wheelchair that is stabilized to the floor with a 4-point electric tie-down system. Evaluation and supervised driver's training are critical to ensure safety. A person who is unable to achieve this level of independence must rely on someone else to drive. The person with C-5 tetraplegia either can be transferred into the passenger seat of a van or have the wheelchair tied to the floor for transport safety. Whenever the van is in motion, both the wheelchair seat belt and the van safety restraint should be fastened.

If the person does not own a van, he or she must be transferred into a car with assistance. The

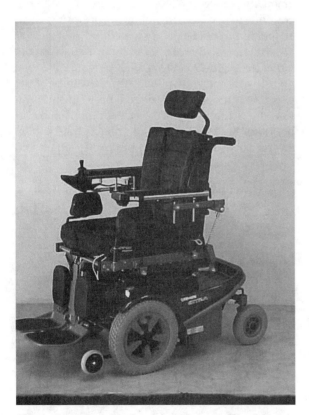

Figure 9.14. Power wheelchair for people with C-5–C-6 tetraplegia.

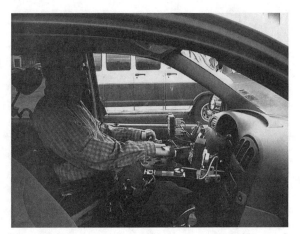

Figure 9.16. Person with C-5 tetraplegia driving adapted van.

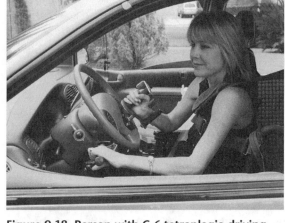

Figure 9.18. Person with C-6 tetraplegia driving adapted van.

caregiver then loads the wheelchair in the back flooring or in the trunk of the car. Loading a motorized wheelchair is a difficult and time-consuming task because of the necessary dismantling and handling of the batteries. Power wheelchairs with power-recline or -tilt systems cannot be dismantled to be loaded into a car and must be transported in an adapted van. A manual wheelchair usually is substituted, which may mean the person with SCI has less functionality once at the destination.

Some cities make available van or bus service with modified lifts. People with impaired trunk balance use a chest strap or wear lateral supports during public transportation. These supports provide stability and ensure upright sitting to counter the force of the motion. Compliance with the Americans With Disabilities Act (ADA; 1990) has resulted in more widespread use of wheelchair lifts on buses

and other public vehicles designed specifically for people with physical disabilities

Communication

Initially, assistive devices may be indicated to assist people with SCI at the C-5 level in writing. One such assistive device is a MAS in conjunction with a long opponens orthosis (Figure 9.19). Most people will gradually reduce or eliminate the use of a MAS but continue to need a wrist-stabilizing orthosis with an adaptation to hold a pen or pencil.

Other assistive devices, such as a Wanchik writer (see Figure 9.6), a WDWHO (Figure 9.20), or a dorsal wrist cock-up splint with cuff can help the client hold the wrist in a neutral position and position the writing utensil. A Dycem™ nonslip pad is useful for holding the paper in place while writing. As the client's arm control improves, letters and

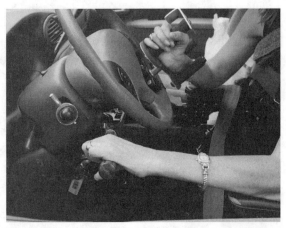

Figure 9.17. Driving controls for a person with C-6 tetraplegia.

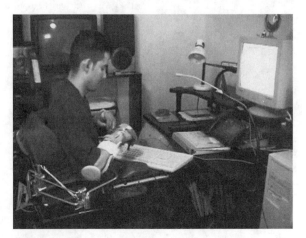

Figure 9.19. Person with C-5 tetraplegia using mobile arm orthosis.

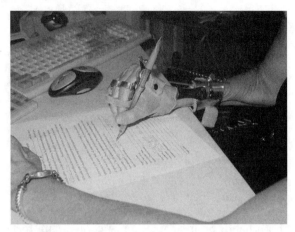

Figure 9.20. Person with C-6 tetraplegia using WDWHO for writing.

numbers may be attempted. The first attempts at writing may be difficult. Therapists should encourage clients to begin with drawing lines or circles. Asking the client to form letters or numbers early on can lead to disappointment or frustration because of the unrefined arm movement. Practice is the key to improving this skill.

Typing offers a clear visual presentation, but typing may be frustrating to the client if too much skill is called for before arm control is developed. Typing will be most efficient if done using either an electric typewriter or a computer (Figure 9.21). The client's wrists must be stabilized and a typing implement must be attached to depress the keys for typing. In most cases, another person must remove the typed text from the typewriter or computer printer to decrease the likelihood of tearing. A therapist can use typing as an exercise for a MAS because it requires fine control of the arm to select and depress exact keys. Usually the client is asked to type each row of keys individually from right to left, left to right, then up and down, before actually typing words. Once the client has achieved control of arm placement, he or she can type words.

Telephone Use

Accessing a telephone is important for people with SCI at the C-5 level. Some clients use a gooseneck stand to hold the telephone receiver to ear height and use a phone flipper (an extended lever) to depress the switch hook connector on the phone base. The lever is lifted to obtain a dial tone or to receive a call when the phone rings. Most people using a MAS use this method because they are unable to hold the receiver to the ear. People who have adequate arm strength and can hold the receiver to the ear may use a phone holder for independence with handling. Using telephones with automatic dialing, memory, or redial functions often increases efficiency. A speaker phone decreases necessary hand function but also decreases privacy. Telephones with the dialing buttons on the receiver usually are not recommended because of the increased hand function necessary to manipulate them. For people with SCI at C-6, using the phone can be made easier with an adapted handset, universal cuff, or WD-WHO used to press the buttons. Some clients at this level use tenodesis to handle a telephone without any adaptive equipment. In a vocational setting, earphones or a headset can streamline the tasks of simultaneous note writing and phone use. Cellular telephone technologies now offer more hands-free options, such as remote earpieces and speakerphone capabilities (Figure 9.22). Mainstream services like text messaging, downloading text or data, and wire-

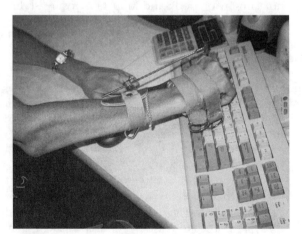

Figure 9.21. Person with C-6 tetraplegia typing on the computer.

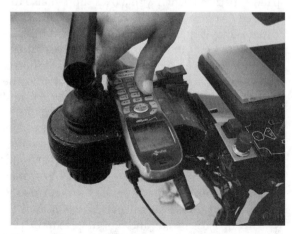

Figure 9.22. Wheelchair-mounted cellular phone.

less transmissions also can benefit people with SCI by allowing them more efficient use of their cellular telephones in ADL.

Tetraplegia: Levels C-7–C-8

People with C-7–C-8 tetraplegia have functional triceps and some finger flexor and extensor muscles innervated. They can raise their arms up against gravity and have some hand dexterity. Many such clients can live alone or without assistance with home modifications.

People with SCI at C-7–C-8 can perform upper-body grooming and hygiene independently using a sink with few or no adaptive devices. Sink accessibility is important to ensure independence while using the faucets. Lever controls are easiest for the person to use, although he or she may be able to use some twisting controls. Towels should be placed close to the sink and at a low level for greater independence.

Dental Care

People with C-7–C-8 SCI may secure the toothbrush between their fingers or use a built-up handle to enhance their grip. Some people may choose to use an electric toothbrush. Getting the toothpaste onto the brush may require using the countertop to get enough pressure to push the paste out, or the client may put the toothpaste directly in the mouth before applying the brush. Small, prethreaded dental flossing tools are also helpful.

Bathing

The person with SCI at C-7–C-8 needs some adaptations to bathe independently. A padded shower-commode chair in a roll-in shower probably provides the best level of independent functioning. A padded bathtub bench with a back support also can be used to transfer into the tub independently. Assistance may be needed for transfers when the person is wet or if he or she has a high level of spasticity that interferes with movement. A hand-held shower allows for greatest independence in showering. The person may find it difficult to reach the buttocks and lower back for cleansing; however, long-handled sponges or brushes should allow access as long as the person can maintain his or her balance. Hair washing is best done when the person is supported in the shower or tub. Towels should be placed where they can stay dry but remain within the person's reach. A towel placed on the wheelchair seat will help by soaking up excess water and moisture from the person's body while he or she completes the transfer back into the chair.

Bowel and Bladder Management

People with SCI at levels C-7–C-8 may need minimal to no assistance managing a regular bowel program. A person at this level of SCI may or may not need adaptive devices for task completion because of the amount of preserved finger dexterity. The devices previously shown for bowel management may be used, if needed (see Figure 9.10).

Eating and Meal Preparation

People with SCI at C-7–C-8 use minimal assistive devices to eat. They may intertwine utensils between their fingers for stability. To cut food, they may use both hands or an adaptation, such as a cuff, to secure the knife. These clients should be able to drink independently from a cup or glass using a tenodesis grasp or both hands.

Meal preparation is a challenge for people with SCI at C-7–C-8 primarily because of diminished trunk control, weak grasp, and poor kitchen accessibility for wheelchairs. The adaptations listed above for levels C-5–C-6, such as using toaster ovens and microwaves, may be appropriate. Adapted devices that help stabilize materials and assist in opening containers continue to be needed. Kitchens need to be modified for wheelchair accessibility, such as providing lowered work surfaces and space for wheelchair maneuverability. Other modifications are listed in the section on paraplegia.

Dressing and Undressing the Upper and Lower Body

A person with SCI at C-7–C-8 may dress the upper and lower body independently using the rolling side-to-side method on the bed; however, this technique consumes a lot of energy. Donning and doffing footwear may require assistance, if the styles are not slip-on or hook-and-loop tab closure styles. Adaptive shoelaces may help the client put on footwear independently.

Functional Mobility

Clients with SCI at C-7–C-8 can use a sliding board to transfer to and from the wheelchair. Eventually, they may be able to transfer without using the transfer board. Removable armrests and footrests are essential for safe transferring for both the person and the caregiver or assistant.

People with SCI at this level can be independent in wheelchair mobility using a manual folding or rigid wheelchair (Figure 9.23). Friction-coated hand rims may be used to assist in propulsion. Clients may still have some difficulty pushing up steep inclines or over rough terrain, but they may begin to partici-

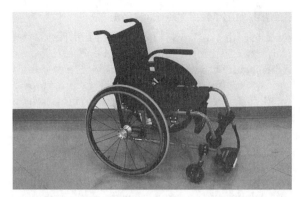

Figure 9.23. Manual wheelchair for people with C-7–C-8 tetraplegia.

pate in wheelchair sports. Clients with SCI at this level also will be independent with powered mobility using a joystick. Powered mobility conserves energy, enhancing stamina with other functional tasks, such as dressing and vocational activities.

Community Mobility

People with a C-6–C-8 injury should be able to drive a modified van or a personal vehicle (car, truck, or SUV) adapted with appropriate controls for community transportation. People with a C-7–C-8 injury should be able to transfer independently into a passenger vehicle but may need assistance with wheelchair loading, car-top loaders, or special lifts. They may choose to drive from their wheelchairs in a modified van; doing so will save energy but is more expensive (Figures 9.24 and 9.25).

Communication

Writing and typing skills are essential to independent living and handling one's own affairs. Most people with a C-7–C-8 level of SCI can use a simple writing device independently without help. The device selected for writing also can be used to type or use a computer. The wrist-driven orthosis gives dynamic grasp, which is useful for loading paper and computer disks and for picking up and moving objects. For people with SCI at C-7–C-8, using the phone can be made easier with a phone holder, universal cuff, or tenodesis motion used to press the buttons. Some people with SCI at this level need no adaptations to use a telephone, type, or write because they have well-developed tenodesis hand skills (see Figure 9.26). In a vocational setting, earphones or a headset can streamline requirements for simultaneous note writing and phone use.

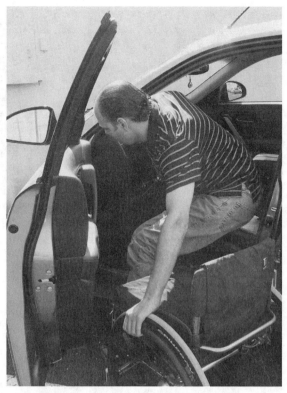

Figure 9.24. Person with C-7–C-8 tetraplegia transferring out of car.

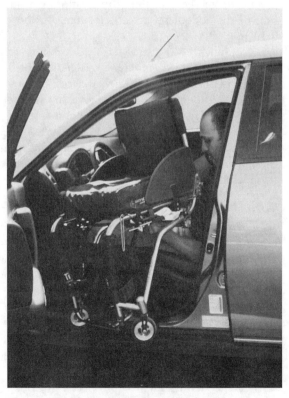

Figure 9.25. Person with C-7–C-8 tetraplegia loading wheelchair into vehicle.

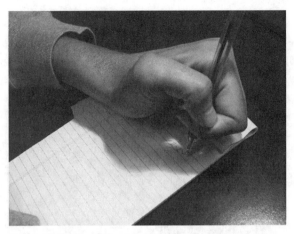

Figure 9.26. Person with C-7–C-8 tetraplegia using tenodesis for writing.

Paraplegia: Levels T-1–T-6

People with SCI at T-1–T-6 are independent with dental care, hygiene, and grooming (i.e., washing face and hands, combing hair, shaving, and applying makeup) at sink level provided the bathroom is wheelchair accessible. The muscles of the trunk and thorax have their roots from T-1 to L-4. In general, these muscles are responsible for elevation and depression of the ribs during respiration, contraction of the abdomen, and anterolateral flexion of the trunk.

People with SCI at the T-1–T-6 level have full use of their upper extremities and should be able to live independently in a wheelchair-accessible environment. Although breathing improves at this level, trunk balance remains compromised and appropriate safety precautions should be implemented. The wheelchair is the primary mode for mobility, although ambulation may be encouraged for exercise (Hoppenfeld, 1977).

Bowel and Bladder

Men with SCI at T-1–T-6 are able to apply an external catheter or independently use an intermittent catheterization program. Women with SCI at T-1–T-6 can catheterize, but they may need a mirror and an adaptive device to help position their legs during the task. Bowel management is accomplished independently by using suppositories, digital stimulation, and a consistently followed schedule. Again, positioning may be the one area requiring assistance. Women can place sanitary napkins independently, but they may need a mirror and an adaptive device to help position their legs when inserting a tampon.

Eating and Meal Preparation

People with T-1–T-6 SCI have poor trunk control but can eat and prepare meals independently from a wheelchair with use of adaptive devices or modifications, which may include lowered counter-tops or work surfaces. A mirror over a standard range is helpful for seeing inside cooking pans and avoiding touching hot areas that are not visible from the wheelchair level. The accessibility of the oven and the refrigerator from the wheelchair should be considered. Usually a side approach is best for maintaining balance and securing items from each type of appliance. Dishes, glasses, and cooking pans should be lightweight and are most accessible if located at a level no higher than the shoulders.

Dressing

People with T-1–T-6 SCI can dress without assistance. Dressing loops and oversized clothing may enhance independence in dressing the lower body. These clients do not require assistance in upper-body dressing but may have to use the bed or wheelchair for support to maintain balance. Lower-body clothing, including shoes and socks, can be put on independently if there is good hip, knee, and ankle range of motion and little interference from spasms. Applying lower-body clothing over both legs first before turning side-to-side to position the clothing helps minimize shearing over the skin of the buttocks and conserve energy.

Functional Mobility

People with T-1–T-6 paraplegia have the arm strength to transfer independently; however, body weight and height, medical problems, transfer surfaces, wheelchair position, and general endurance level may compromise transfer independence. Extremes in weight and height, in combination with poor trunk control, may complicate independent transfer enough for these people to require assistance with this task. Spasticity and muscle tone can help in some instances but compromise transfer safety in others.

People with SCI at this level usually can use a manual wheelchair independently if the wheelchair has been prescribed according to their individualized body size and activity level (Garber, Biddle, et al., 2000). The wheelchair should be lightweight, and its back height should be below the scapula for optimal propulsion. This wheelchair may be a folding or a rigid frame model (Figure 9.27). Armrests and footrests should be removable to allow for maximal independence. The occupational therapist

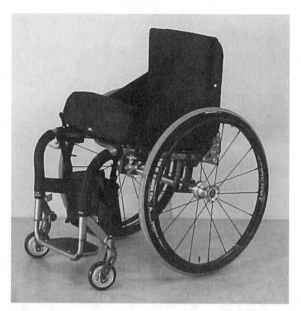

Figure 9.27. Manual wheelchair for people with paraplegia.

should consider postural stability when selecting the type of wheelchair back: Options are standard back upholstery, tension-adjustable back upholstery, or a solid contoured padded back used for the preservation of the normal spinal curves. A pressure-reducing seat cushion is recommended to reduce excessive pressure over the bony prominences of the buttocks and give pelvic stability while sitting (Garber et al., 2000; Hobson, 1992; Koo, Mak, & Lee, 1996).

Some people with SCI at T-1–T-4 may use a power wheelchair to conserve energy and time. Because many people with SCI are living longer and more active lives, musculoskeletal overuse problems are emerging. Those problems must be addressed through the use of different mobility options, which may include power wheelchairs.

Community Mobility

People with this level of injury can drive a car, SUV, or van using hand controls, a steering knob, and an emergency brake extension (Figure 9.28). The person's transfer skill and endurance will determine the decision about the type of vehicle. Transferring independently into a vehicle is an essential skill for driving, and loading the wheelchair into the vehicle requires a high level of energy, especially if performed frequently throughout the day. Some clients may choose to use a wheelchair-loading device or to drive a modified or adapted van. If the person decides to drive an adapted van, he or she should transfer from the wheelchair to the van's "captain's chair" to drive safely.

Communication

People with SCI at this level are independent in all communication skills, such as typing, writing, and use of the telephone, and they can easily access computers using either a standard keyboard or mouse. An ergonomically sound workstation will decrease musculoskeletal overuse in the upper body. Attending to the height placement and positioning of the computer monitor, keyboard, and mouse in relationship to the body minimizes effects from extended reach and abnormal postures that sometimes are seen in computer use.

Paraplegia: Levels T-7–S-5

Clients with SCI and resulting paraplegia at levels T-7 through S-5 have intact upper-extremity and thoracic function, which improves trunk stability, wheelchair sitting balance, and transfers. Functional ambulation using long leg braces and forearm crutches is possible below level T-8. People with SCI at L-4–S-2 can ambulate with short leg braces and forearm crutches; those with injuries below S-2 may only need to use a cane for safety during ambulation.

Functionally, these clients are independent in all self-care, mobility, and communication tasks. They may use some adapted equipment for energy conservation, efficiency, and maximum control. A major concern, however, is prevention of secondary SCI complications, such as urinary tract infections and pressure ulcers (Pearman, 1985; Turner, 1985). Although management of these potentially serious problems usually is addressed during the initial rehabilitation, once the client returns to the community, family, employment, or school, secondary complications often are ignored or neglected until

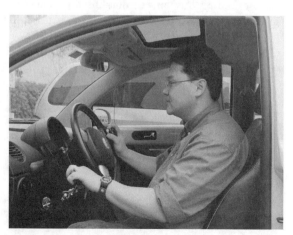

Figure 9.28. Adapted vehicle with hand controls for people with paraplegia.

the situation reaches a crisis level. People who return to outpatient clinics at facilities where they originally were rehabilitated can be reeducated or updated on advances in medical technology through their follow-up visits.

Preventing Pressure Ulcers in People With SCI

Pressure ulcers are serious, costly, and potentially lifelong complications of SCI. Clinical observations and research studies have confirmed staggering costs and human suffering, including a profoundly negative impact on the affected person's general physical health, socialization, financial status, body image, and loss of independence and control (Langemo, Melland, Hanson, Olson, & Hunter, 2000). Reported prevalence rates range from 17% to 33% among people with SCI residing in the community, and recurrence rates are high (Carlson, King, Kirk, Temple, & Heinemann, 1992; Fuhrer, Garber, Rintala, Clearman, & Hart, 1993; Schryvers, Miroslaw, & Nance, 2000; Young & Burns 1981). The financial burden of pressure ulcers ($1.335 billion in 1994 for all venues) does not begin to reflect the personal and social costs experienced by the person with the pressure ulcer and his or her family (Miller & DeLozier, 1994). Those costs include loss of independence and self-esteem; time away from work, school, or family; and reduced quality of life.

The major risk factors for pressure ulcers among people with SCI are

- Severity of SCI (e.g., immobility, completeness of SCI, urinary incontinence, and severe spasticity);
- Pre-existing conditions (e.g., advanced age, smoking, lung and cardiac disease, diabetes, renal disease, impaired cognition, and residence in a nursing home);
- Nutrition (e.g., malnutrition and anemia; Byrne & Salzberg, 1996);
- Demographic factors (e.g., age, gender, ethnicity, marital status, and education);
- Physical, medical, and SCI-related factors (e.g., level and completeness of SCI; activity and mobility; bladder, bowel, and moisture control; and comorbidities such as diabetes and spasticity); and
- Psychological and social factors (e.g., psychological distress, financial problems, cognition, substance abuse, adherence, and health beliefs and practices; Garber, Rintala, Hart, & Fuhrer, 2000).

Additional psychological factors have been associated with the development of pressure ulcers, including a person's unwillingness to take responsibility in skin care, low self-esteem, dissatisfaction with life activities (Anderson & Andberg, 1979), and poor social adjustment (Gordon, Harasymiw, Bellile, Lehman, & Sherman, 1982).

Resolving problems related to pressure ulcers requires a comprehensive evaluation and examination of the client, including

- Medical, SCI, and pressure ulcer history;
- Physical examination, including laboratory tests;
- Psychological health, behavior, and cognitive status;
- Social and financial resources, including availability and use of personal care assistance; and
- Use of equipment, including positioning and posture (Garber et al., 2000).

The examination typically is followed by a detailed description of the pressure ulcer itself.

Strategies to prevent pressure ulcers are taught to clients and their families both formally and informally during the comprehensive rehabilitation program (Garber et al., 2002). The occupational therapist also may instruct clients on turning and repositioning in bed and on shifting weight while sitting in the wheelchair. Additionally, the therapist may be directly involved in measuring the client for a wheelchair and evaluating the person for pressure-reducing seating systems. The therapist may teach the person to inspect his or her skin with an adapted mirror and practice other techniques in hygiene and positioning to help maintain the integrity of the skin.

Support surfaces are devices or systems that are intended to reduce the interface pressure between a person and his or her bed or wheelchair (Bergstrom et al., 1994). Support surfaces do not heal pressure ulcers; rather, they are prescribed by a clinician, frequently an occupational therapist, and incorporated into a comprehensive pressure-ulcer prevention and management program. Static and dynamic mattresses, mattress overlays, and specialty beds may be used at various times to reduce the risk of developing pressure ulcers or following medical or surgical treatment. Materials such as foams and gels, alone or in combination, and elements such as air and water, also alone or in combination, are used in patient care and home environments. Wheelchair cushions and seating systems of various materials and designs reduce pressure and maximize balance and stability when a person uses a wheelchair (Table 9.4). *Note:* No one product meets all patient needs.

Table 9.4. Four Seat Cushion Types: Some Benefits and Limitations

Cushion Category	Benefits	Limitations
Foams	• Can be shaped to fit the user, for lower pressures and more stable support while sitting • Lightweight • Lower in cost • Available in many forms • Can be flat or contoured	• Wear out relatively fast • Retain heat • Hard to clean • Support features change quickly when exposed to heat or moisture • Become hard in cold weather
Fluid-filled Cushions (e.g., water, gel)	• Covered with easy-to-clean material • Effective for many different users • Distribute pressure more evenly • Control skin temperatures better • Gel-filled cushions may reduce shear	• Gel-filled cushions may be better shock absorbers than pressure reducers • May be expensive • Heavier weight
Air	• Lightweight • Easy to clean • Effective for many people • Reduce shear and peak pressures	• Tendency to puncture • Must be checked frequently for proper air pressure and maintenance • Hard to repair • May interfere with balance and posture
Combination*	• Tailored to each person by combining a variety of materials	• Additional individual devices are created by using removable and adjustable parts from cushions with a variety of components such as hip guides, wedges, etc. • May be expensive

*May use foams of different densities or combinations of gel, air, and foam.
Reprinted with permission from the Paralyzed Veterans of America (PVA), *Pressure Ulcers: What You Should Know.*
© Copyright 2002, Paralyzed Veterans of America.

The client will be most effectively served by the judgment of an experienced clinician in concert with a selection of products.

Although mostly preventable, pressure ulcers deter the achievement of rehabilitation goals; can contribute to loss of independence; and interfere with the pursuit of educational, vocational, and leisure activities after SCI. Rehabilitation professionals today are challenged to implement high-quality rehabilitation services within the context of limited resources. Fortunately, it is now possible to identify people at highest risk for pressure ulcers so that effective prevention strategies can be incorporated into their lifestyles (Garber, Rintala, et al., 2000).

Leisure

The Rehabilitation Act of 1973 (Public Law 93-112), its amendments of 1986 (Public Law 99-506), and the ADA (1990; Public Law 101-336) created many opportunities for people with physical disabilities to participate in leisure activities in their communities. Engaging in leisure or recreational activities is "viewed as a means of balancing one's lifestyle in order to promote health and life satisfaction through the physical, psychosocial, and emotional benefits"

(Christiansen, 1991, p. 391). Often so much energy is exerted in retraining people with SCI to perform the basics of daily living activities that leisure and recreation may be overlooked altogether. Achieving balance in life is a key goal for all people to strive for in everyday performance. Whether a client chooses to engage in tabletop games with family, participate in an adaptive sport, or enjoy community activities, engaging in occupations that are relaxing and fun is an important aspect of the person's psychological well-being. Being involved with a leisure pursuit or being a part of the community gives people an emotional lift, a sense of belonging, and a feeling of accomplishment.

People with SCI experience a dramatic shift in the way they spend their time. Typically, immediately after an injury or returning home after rehabilitation, they learn to redefine what is meaningful to them regarding leisure time or recreation. Many of these people have lived an active lifestyle before their injury. Returning to their previous activities or identifying new activities that are enjoyable to them is crucial for life satisfaction (Dolhi, 1996). By participating in leisure or recreational activities, people with SCI can find enjoyment in engaging with others in meaningful occupations, can prevent physical

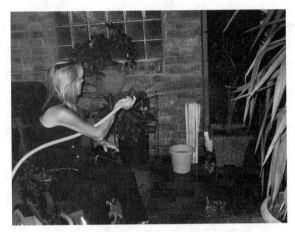

Figure 9.29. Recreational activities.

deterioration of muscle strength and endurance, and offer opportunities to experience a sense of success through a task. Occupational therapists can help clients adapt or learn new leisure or recreational activities (Figures 9.29 and 9.30). Doing so may mean adapting game pieces, using an orthosis or assistive device to manipulate objects, or exploring new activities that may interest the client.

Wheelchair sports have become a popular leisure activity for people with disabilities. These activities can offer physical, psychological, and social benefits to people with SCI (Hanson, Nabavi, & Yuen, 2001). Specialized sports wheelchairs are available with adaptations such as angled wheels for stability and ease of turning, specialized footrests for optimal positioning, ultra-lightweight frames, and low backs for maximal upper-body movement. Belonging to a team fosters a sense of companionship and gives people with SCI an outlet to be competitive. Wheelchair sports also pro-

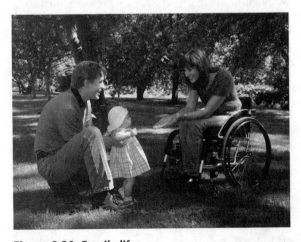

Figure 9.30. Family life.

vide physical exercise and can prevent effects of deconditioning or disuse of active musculature. Adaptive sports may lead to higher social competence and better self-esteem. Sporting activities used in the rehabilitation process can help to teach discipline and sportsmanship and assist in accomplishing necessary ADL.

Work

Once a person gains skill and proficiency in ADL and IADL, focus can be turned to returning to productive living in the community. Because people who sustain SCI tend to be relatively young at the time of injury, returning to paid employment, volunteering, or educational pursuits are common and critical for quality of life.

Factors Affecting Return to Work

It is not unusual for people who have sustained SCI to need to alter their career or life goals significantly. In general, three variables affect a client's return to work: degree of impairment, age, and rehabilitation experiences. People with paraplegia are more likely to return to work than people with tetraplegia. Within each group, people with incomplete injuries are more likely to work than those with complete injuries. People injured at a younger age are more likely to return to work. Completion of a vocational rehabilitation program also increases the likelihood of returning to work (DeVivo, Rutt, Stover, & Fine, 1987).

In looking at vocational and other life roles, researchers have found that access to equipment resources can affect role functioning. Having access to some electronic control devices is associated with increased frequency of participation in educational activities, improved performance in ADL, and increased activity by people with tetraplegia (Efthimiou, Gordon, Sell, & Stratford, 1981). Brown (1983) found that access to a private vehicle increased the probability of being employed up to 50%.

A critical step in returning to paid or volunteer work is independence in community mobility. This step could entail the client learning to drive with vehicle modifications or learning how to use accessible public transportation systems. Occupational therapists can take the lead to give clients the necessary information and training.

In addition to limited body movement, decreased mobility, and decreased independence in daily living skills, people with SCI may face environmental barriers that physically restrict their ability to access places, things, and services. Return to work appears to be related to accessing resources (e.g., through personal care assistance, electronic control units, and accessible transportation).

Examination of the SCI National Model Systems database (Dijkers, Abela, Gans, & Gordon, 1995) indicates that of people with SCI who were working at the time of injury, by the first year following the injury, 16% have returned to work, 8% have entered school, and more than 70% list themselves as unemployed. Employment following SCI increases slowly but steadily over time. At 10 to 11 years postinjury, one third of people with SCI listed in the model systems database were working. This pattern indicates that re-entry (or initial entry) into the workplace after SCI is a slow process that may span a decade or more. Significantly, two thirds of this population appears not to return to a work environment at all.

Although clearly people with SCI cannot work at jobs that require manual labor or extensive physical body mobility, many opportunities exist for them to return to work (Figure 9.31). Many psychological and societal factors, however, discourage people with physical disabilities from returning to work. At the psychological level, some people with SCI cannot envision themselves being productive at a job ever again. At the societal level, factors such as Social Security disincentives, cultural attitudes, and environmental barriers may be barriers to access to the workplace. Disincentives weigh heavily against return to work, because many people with SCI who return to work may not be able to afford essential services and products that are available through publicly funded programs only to the unemployed.

The role of the occupational therapist is to help develop a new set of goals and hopes for the person with SCI, including goals for a return to paid or volunteer work. If the client was previously employed, the therapist should discuss whether returning to that employment arena is possible. If the client is entering the workforce for the first time, the therapist should discuss his or her interests and abilities. An occupational therapist can analyze specific job performance areas that would be practical and how they can be adapted. People with SCI who have already re-entered the workplace may be considered "SCI peers" and may be asked to share their personal experiences with a newly injured client to help his or her "vision" of possibilities begin to take shape. People with SCI who have returned to work or school also may serve as role models in the community, inspiring hopes for a brighter future and a return to a normal life course that was only interrupted—not stopped—by the injury. An occupational therapist also may have clients with SCI attempt to perform typical work components to anticipate, evaluate, and solve problems. Therapists may establish a simulated work environment so that clients can practice typical work activities.

Volunteer Work

Volunteer work can serve as a "proving ground" to a client with SCI who is re-entering or entering a work setting for the first time following the injury. Volunteer work can enable the client to practice necessary skills, such as completing ADL in time to meet a work schedule, interacting with coworkers and the public, and accessing transportation. It allows testing of physical endurance and work tolerance in a noncompetitive work environment. Volunteer work frequently can be a springboard to paid employment positions; even if the client is not seeking to gain paid employment, volunteer work serves the purpose of participating and contributing to society. The meaning of volunteer work is more purposeful than monetary rewards. Volunteer work can be the initial steps to proving to oneself that paid employment might be a feasible goal. It also can prove to reluctant employers that a person with SCI can meet the demands of a job.

Paid Employment

Job seekers with SCI must think through and test specific aspects of their goals:

- Do they have reliable private transportation or convenient access to public transportation?
- Can they drive themselves to work, or can family or friends drive them to and from work?

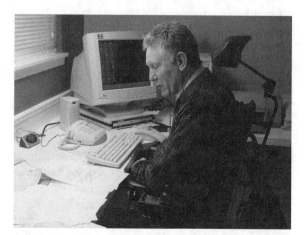

Figure 9.31. Person with C-6 tetraplegia working at home.

- Do they need further education to be successful in procuring a particular job?
- Does a potential employer have appropriate equipment that will enable the client to efficiently perform the components of the job?
- Are they knowledgeable and comfortable discussing with the employer any necessary job accommodations?
- Have they anticipated issues that may arise while on the job, and are they prepared to discuss them and offer possible solutions?

Issues that may arise on the job include situations involving bowel or bladder management or the inability to reach items or access areas of the workplace. Ideally, job seekers will be able to communicate about such issues—including suggesting ideas for possible solutions—in a manner that does not overwhelm the potential employer. Occupational therapists can help clients anticipate potential problems, generate possible solutions, and practice the communication skills necessary for applying for a job.

People with SCI need to establish what their ability will be to sustain part-time or full-time employment. Beginning conservatively with a part-time position may allow the person to prove his or her ability in the workplace and then advance to a full-time workload. Realistic expectations about energy expenditure are crucial, and they are best assessed by planning and organizing the workday. Besides the energy necessary to complete work assignments, people with SCI typically expend more energy than those without disabilities in completing the ADL necessary to prepare for and arrive at work. The client's employer must have a good understanding of his or her abilities and limitations so that work expectations can be set realistically. Depending on the worker's level of SCI, job tasks must be broken down into steps that can be analyzed to determine the most efficient and effective way for them to be performed. The better the communication between employer and employee, the more successful the work situation will be for both parties. It is incumbent on the person with SCI to ask for feedback on job performance and to present questions and concerns to the employer in a professional manner so that problem resolution can be a collaborative effort.

The Americans with Disabilities Act of 1990 provided people with SCI and many other neurological or musculoskeletal conditions opportunities to return to the workplace and gain financial success and a sense of well-being. Many of the same adaptive methods used to perform ADL can be used to accomplish work tasks on the job. No prescriptive list exists of jobs that can be performed by people with each level of SCI. People with high-level tetraplegia, such as C-2, are lawyers and office receptionists. People with C-5 tetraplegia are stockbrokers and social workers. People with C-6 tetraplegia are secretaries, teachers, or dispatchers. People with C-7–C-8 tetraplegia are computer system administrators, college professors, and school principals. People with SCI are medical supply sales representatives, theater ticket salespeople, bankers, accountants, actors, business owners, and doctors. Achieving independence and success in the workplace depends on seeking a job that best matches the person's physical and intellectual attributes, personal motivation, and problem-solving creativity.

Sexual Activity and Fertility

Since the 1970s, clinicians and researchers have advocated for sexual counseling as a mandatory part of any rehabilitation program (Cole, Chilgren, & Rosenberg, 1973; Eisenberg & Rustad, 1976; Melnyk, Montgomery, & Over, 1979). Advances in medicine and technology have enhanced sexual functioning and fertility among people with SCI. Although sexuality following SCI has been studied for at least 40 years, it is only within the past 20 years that sexual adjustment and function have become part of the occupational therapy intervention process (McAlonan, 1996).

Although sexual desire may not change after SCI, some people experience diminished sexual satisfaction (Cardenas et al., 2000). Erection and ejaculation can be improved with new devices and medical and surgical interventions. Vacuum constriction devices, intracorporeal injection of vasoactive agents, or penile prostheses can enhance erection. Vibrators or electrical stimulation may be used to induce ejaculation, and retrieval of sperm can be accomplished through microsurgical techniques if other techniques fail.

Fertility in women does not seem to be affected by SCI, although the menstrual cycle will be interrupted temporarily for weeks or months after the injury. Women with SCI may experience inadequate vaginal lubrication or problems achieving orgasm. Potential complications of pregnancy among women with SCI include inadequate vaginal lubrication; increased medical problems, such as urinary tract infections and pressure ulcers; increased spasticity; and autonomic dysreflexia.

Autonomic dysreflexia is considered the most significant potential medical complication that might occur during any stage of pregnancy, labor, delivery, or postpartum.

The role of the occupational therapist in helping clients address limitations in sexual activity has not been well studied. Neistadt (1986) described a model for occupational therapists to use in sexuality counseling. Neistadt's model involves permission, limited information, specific suggestions, and intensive therapy. According to Neistadt, the first three elements are appropriate for counseling by occupational therapists. Another consideration is the therapist's comfort level in discussing sexuality with people with SCI. Therapists should not hesitate to refer a client to a counselor trained in providing sexuality counseling to people with SCI. Therapists need to anticipate a client's concerns and questions about sexual functioning in view of the intimate personal care tasks in which they are involved. Clients may consult with the occupational therapist regarding specific performance areas, such as positioning, hand functioning, and equipment adaptation.

The psychosocial elements of building relationships, communicating needs and concerns, and satisfaction are as important as physical functioning (Adler, 1996; Versluys, 1995). Educational and emotional support provided by the occupational therapist can supplement the information people with SCI may receive from other rehabilitation or health care professionals. Sexuality is a sensitive area, however, and the topic should be broached with caution. Many times, the therapist is the person with whom the patient feels the most comfortable discussing intimate details. Therefore, it is incumbent on each therapist to develop a level of basic knowledge, develop a comfort level with imparting that basic knowledge to people who are ready to receive it, and make appropriate referrals as necessary.

High-Tech Equipment

Advances in technology influence every aspect of daily life and thus the quality of life for people with SCI. From the automated teller machines in banks to voice-activated telephone systems, technology often provides unique and dynamic solutions to otherwise insoluble problems. For people with SCI, technology expands opportunities for independence and productivity.

In the early 1970s, the U.S. government demonstrated its commitment to improving the vocational and self-care goals of people with severe physical impairments through the establishment of rehabilitation engineering centers. The centers combined the efforts of medicine, engineering, and related sciences to identify practical solutions to problems that limited the integration of people with physical impairments into productive community life (Traub & LeClair, 1975). In 1988, with the passage of the Technology-Related Assistance for Individuals With Disabilities Act (Public Law 100-407), the U.S. government further demonstrated its support for the development and use of technology to enhance rehabilitation outcomes for people with severe physical disabilities. *Assistive technology*—defined as "any item, piece of equipment, or product system, off-the-shelf, modified, or customized, that is used to increase, maintain, or improve function"—became the byword of the 1990s for consumers and health care providers alike (Technology-Related Assistance for Individuals With Disabilities Act, 1988). Assistive technology includes both high and low technology in devices that include

- Electronic aids to daily living,
- Computer access systems,
- Augmentative communication devices,
- Cellular phone technologies, and
- Mobility and seating systems.

Some mainstream technologies that are marketed as time saving or convenience items to the general public also may fit the needs of a person with SCI. These devices, such as a device to turn on lamps by clapping or an inexpensive craft tray to transport items, may be found in gift magazines, thrift stores, or home goods stores. Creative application of such devices may provide for more independent performance of a task, and they typically are available at lower cost than technologies marketed specifically as "medical" devices (Coppola-Passariello, 2003).

The appropriate prescription of upper-extremity assistive devices is a major focus of occupational therapy intervention during the rehabilitation of people with SCI. Occupational therapists have prominent roles in the assistive-technology clinics of public and private rehabilitation facilities. Therapists evaluate each client with SCI and other neuromuscular and musculoskeletal dysfunction for his or her potential to use technology to enhance and expand the skills needed to be more independent in self-care, return to school, or become more socially involved. Working with the assistive-technology team, the occupational therapist makes recommendations and trains clients to use technology to achieve their maximum potential (Mann & Lane, 1991). For people with SCI who are being assessed for assistive-technology systems for the first time, relying on knowledgeable, credentialed professionals (i.e., assistive-technology suppliers or practitioners) may ensure a more successful fit of equipment with their lifestyle and goals (Minkel, 2002).

Occupational therapists have played a leading role in evaluating and recommending environmental control units (ECUs) for people with significant disability. These electronic aids to daily living enable a person to access and manipulate objects and devices such as lamps, televisions, thermostats, blinds, and stereo systems. People without disabilities frequently use ECUs to automate and facilitate routine household tasks. A familiar ECU is the remote control device for the television or stereo. Specialized units, which can be voice-activated, also are available. The latter are especially useful for people who have impaired motor function or high-level SCI (Swenson, Barnett, Pond, & Schoenberg, 1998). Surveys have shown that the specialized ECUs used in hospitals and rehabilitation facilities have not been widely recommended for use in home settings, primarily because of their high cost and limitations on reimbursement (Holme, Kanny, Guthrie, & Johnson, 1997).

Computers

Computers have become essential tools in everyday life for education, employment, and recreation. Computers certainly have opened the door for education and job opportunities for people with SCI. It is important that people with cervical-level SCI gain access to conventional computer systems through alternative methods if the standard way is not feasible or time efficient. Occupational therapists can assess clients for the most appropriate keyboard control. To use a standard computer keyboard, the user must have sufficient upper-extremity range of motion, coordination, and strength to accurately hit target keys, depress the keys, hold down several keys at once, and release keys fast enough to avoid inadvertent repetition of keystrokes.

Keyboard adaptations eliminate the need to hold multiple keys at the same time, provide stability, isolate keys to prevent activation of incorrect keys, and slow the repeat rate to avoid unwanted repeats. Alternative keyboards can provide variety in the spacing, size, layout, and activation force of keys. They also can allow for inputting data in ways other than with the hands, such as using a head pointer or mouth stick. Voice-recognition systems allow input using consistent speech. Mouse alternatives can eliminate the need to hold the mouse, vary the movements required to point the mouse pointer, replace the button with switches that can

be activated with alternative actions, and enable pointing with alternative body parts. Trackballs and joysticks are frequently easier to control than a mouse. The mouse pointer also may be controlled using head movements, which can be tracked with infrared or ultrasound technology. Buttons on many alternative-pointing devices can be programmed to perform a double click or to lock down the mouse button for a drag function. Mouse buttons can be replaced with sip-and-puff switches or with software that performs the mouse click, double click, and drag by lingering on a target for a predetermined time and then moving the mouse cursor in one of the four directions. Free software or operating system modifications allow changes to be made to keyboard response, slowing response time, eliminating or slowing key repeat rate, and holding keys used in multiple key depressions when selected sequentially. Miniaturized keyboards can accommodate users with limited range of movement or strength (Barker, 2002; Treviranus & Petty, 2002).

Robotic Systems

Several robotic devices have been developed and evaluated at rehabilitation centers in the United States, Canada, and England (Glass & Hall, 1987). Their primary purpose is to help people with limited upper-extremity function perform daily living and vocational activities. Robotic technology has the potential to reduce dependency on full-time attendant care and provide people with severe physical impairment with a mechanism of control. Most of the robotic systems are voice activated and based on microprocessors. They usually are mounted either on a workstation or on the wheelchair. Therapists and clients have reported positive experiences with robotic systems, and several systems are being modified to become more practical, functional, and affordable.

Future acceptance and use of robotic systems will depend on several factors. Robotic systems can be expensive, so cost–benefit analyses must be done. A system's reliability and durability must be determined to assess how many hours the physically disabled person can depend on it rather than on attendant care. Another factor is acceptance of robotic systems by health care professionals, who must learn the systems and transmit the crucial information about them to the consumer. Advances in robotic technology can provide opportunities for new levels of self-care, independence, and employment. More important, robotic technology can restore a measure of personal autonomy to clients that until recently could only be imagined.

A clinical model has been developed using standard occupational therapy assessments to evaluate robotic systems' ability to augment function of an impaired extremity and compare task performance against that of an unimpaired human upper extremity (Garber, Williams, Cook, & Koontz, 2003, in press). The clinical model was applied in a two-site study funded by the Department of Veterans Affairs. The model was subsequently modified by reducing the protocol from 8 to 2 weeks of use. Overall, study participants found the robotic arm helpful in performing tasks that otherwise would have been impossible for the person with a cervical SCI. However, the robotic arm added a minimum of 2 in. to the width of the wheelchair, limiting accessibility to rooms in the participant's house and vehicles.

Service Dogs

Another alternative that could be considered a form of assistive technology is the use of service dogs (Figure 9.32) to provide compensatory functions at home and in the community (Hanebrink & Dillon, 2000). Service dogs can help people with SCI achieve greater independence in a variety of performance areas, including ADL, home management, functional mobility, socialization, emergency alerting, and environmental control (Delta Society, 2000). In addition to increasing independence in these occupational performance areas, service dog ownership has also been shown to have significant psychosocial benefits, such as improved self-esteem, increased social interaction, decreased stress, and greater internal locus of control (Valentine, Kiddoo, & LaFleur, 1993). Service dog training is tailored to meet the specific needs of each client with SCI; therefore, the particular tasks performed by the service dog vary by circumstance and master. Service dogs can perform tasks such as

- Picking up a dropped writing pen,
- Moving an obstacle out of the way of the wheelchair,
- Giving money or a credit card to a cashier,
- Dialing 911 or alerting passersby of an emergency,
- Retrieving a ringing telephone, and
- Opening the door for a delivery person (Allen & Blascovich, 1996; Delta Society, 2000; Sunderlin, 1999).

Summary

Advances in research and clinical care have provided interventions and technology for treating SCI that were unheard of a decade ago. Systems of care and assistive and adaptive devices that maximize the occupational performance potential of clients with SCI will continue to be developed, evaluated, and prescribed. With the explosive expansion of electronic technology, microprocessor-controlled, preprogrammed, "smart" devices are forthcoming in the areas of wheelchair mobility, environmental control and robotics, adapted driving, and vocational training (Swenson et al., 1998). Technological innovations present new challenges to occupational therapists, who must continue to balance the promise of technology with the practicalities of everyday life and the preferences and lifestyles of the people they serve.

Study Questions

1. Discuss how paraplegia and tetraplegia differ with respect to social participation. What aspects of social participation will likely be more difficult for people with tetraplegia? Why?
2. Describe autonomic dysreflexia and the circumstances that can cause it. What can an occupational therapist recommend to a client to help prevent autonomic dysreflexia?
3. What aspects of basic ADL are likely to be most problematic for a person with tetraplegia? Describe an adaptive strategy for one or more areas of ADL.
4. What types of orthoses might be appropriate for someone with a C-5 level SCI? Why?
5. What level of lesion would preclude someone from being able to use an adapted van? A manual wheelchair? A power wheelchair?
6. Describe the trade-off between self-reliance and independence and the cost of task completion in terms of energy and time. When should a caregiver be used for ADL? Why?

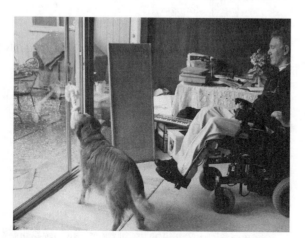

Figure 9.32. Service dog assisting person with C-6 tetraplegia

References

Adler, C. (1996). Spinal cord injury. In L. W. Pedretti (Ed.), *Occupational therapy practice skills for physical dysfunction* (4th ed., pp. 765–784). St. Louis: Mosby.

Allen, K., & Blascovich, J. (1996). The value of service dogs for people with severe ambulatory disabilities. *JAMA, 275,* 1001–1006.

American Spinal Injury Association. (2000). *International standards for neurological classification of spinal cord injury.* Chicago: Author.

Americans With Disabilities Act of 1990, Pub. L. 101–336, 42 U.S.C.A. § 12101.

Anderson, T. P., & Andberg, M. M. (1979). Psychosocial factors associated with pressure sores. *Archives of Physical Medicine and Rehabilitation, 60,* 341–346.

Barker, P. (2002). Technologies for information, communication, and access. In D. A. Olson & F. DeRuyter (Eds.), *Clinician's guide to assistive technology* (pp. 89–90). St. Louis: Mosby.

Bergstrom, N., Allman, R. M., Alvarez, O. M., Bennett, M. A., Carlson, C. E., Frantz, R. A., et al. (1994). *Treatment of pressure ulcers* (Clinical Practice Guideline No. 15, AHCPR Publication No. 96-N014). Rockville, MD: U.S. Department of Health and Human Services, Public Health Service, Agency for Health Care Policy and Research.

Brown, M. M. (1983). Actual and perceived differences in activity patterns of able-bodied and disabled men. *Dissertation Abstracts International, 43,* 2314B.

Byrne, D. W., & Salzberg, C. A. (1996). Major risk factors for pressure ulcers in the spinal cord disabled: A literature review. *Spinal Cord, 34,* 255–263.

Cardenas, D. D., Burns, S. P., & Chan, L. (2000). Rehabilitation of spinal cord injury. In M. Grabois, S. J. Garrison, K. A. Hart, & L. D. Lehmkuhl (Eds.), *Physical medicine and rehabilitation: The complete approach* (pp. 1305–1324). Malden, MA: Blackwell Science.

Carlson, C. E., King, R. B., Kirk, P. M., Temple, R., & Heinemann, A. (1992). Incidence and correlates of pressure ulcer development after spinal cord injury. *Journal of Rehabilitation Nursing Research, 1,* 34–40.

Christiansen, C. (1991). Occupational performance assessment. In C. Christiansen & C. Baum (Eds.), *Occupational therapy: Overcoming human performance deficits* (pp. 376–424). Thorofare, NJ: Slack.

Clifton, G. L., Donovan, W. H., & Frankowski, R. F. (1985). Patterns of care for the patient with spinal cord injury. *Current Concepts in Rehabilitation Medicine, 2,* 14–17.

Cohen, M. E., Sheehan, T. P., & Herbison, G. J. (1996). Content validity and reliability of the International Standards for Neurological Classification of Spinal Cord Injury. *Topics in Spinal Cord Injury Rehabilitation, 1,* 15–31.

Cole, T. M., Chilgren, R., & Rosenberg, P. (1973). A new programme of sex education and counseling for spinal cord injured adults and health care professionals. *Paraplegia, 11,* 111–124.

Coppola-Passariello, T. (2003). Creative (and cheap!) alternatives for assistive technology. *OT Practice, 8,* 21.

Delta Society. (2000). *Benefits of a service animal/service dog.* Retrieved November 18, 2003, from http://www.deltasociety.org.

DeVivo, M. J., Rutt, R. D., Stover, S. L., & Fine, P. R. (1987). Employment after spinal cord injury. *Archives of Physical Medicine and Rehabilitation, 68,* 494–498.

Dijkers, M. P., Abela, M. B., Gans, B. M., & Gordon, W. A. (1995). The aftermath of spinal cord injury. In S. L. Stover, J. A. DeLisa, & G. G. Whiteneck (Eds.), *Spinal cord injury: Clinical outcomes from the model systems* (pp. 185–212). Gaithersburg, MD: Aspen.

Dolhi, C. D. (1996). *Occupational therapy practice guidelines for adults with spinal cord injury.* Bethesda, MD: American Occupational Therapy Association.

Efthimiou, J., Gordon, W. A., Sell, G. H., & Stratford, C. (1981). Electronic assistive devices: Their impact on quality of life of high-quadriplegic persons. *Archives of Physical Medicine and Rehabilitation, 62,* 131–134.

Eisenberg, M. G., & Rustad, L. C. (1976). Sex education and counseling program on a spinal cord injury service. *Archives of Physical Medicine and Rehabilitation, 57,* 135–140.

Farmer, A. R. (1986). Dressing. In J. P. Hill (Ed.), *Spinal cord injury: A guide to functional outcomes in occupational therapy* (pp. 125–143). Rockville, MD: Aspen.

Fuhrer, M. J., Garber, S. L., Rintala, D. H., Clearman, R., & Hart, K. (1993). Pressure ulcers in community-resident persons with spinal cord injury: Prevalence and risk factors. *Archives of Physical Medicine and Rehabilitation, 74,* 1172–1177.

Gansel, J., Waters, R., & Gellman, H. (1990). Transfer of the pronator teres tendon to the tendons of the flexor digitorum profundus in tetraplegia. *Journal of Bone and Joint Surgery, 72,* 427–432.

Garber, S. L. (1985). New perspectives for the occupational therapist in the treatment of spinal cord-injury individuals. *American Journal of Occupational Therapy, 39,* 703–704.

Garber, S. L., Biddle, A. K., Click, C. N., Cowell, J. R., Gregorio-Torres, T. L., Hansen, N. K., et al. (2000). *Pressure ulcer prevention and treatment following spinal cord injury: A clinical practice guideline for health care professionals.* Washington, DC: Paralyzed Veterans of America.

Garber, S. L., Click, C. N., Cowell, J. F., Gregorio-Torres, T. L., Kloth, L. C., & Lammertse, D. P. (2002). *Pressure ulcers: What you should know—a guide for people with spinal cord injury.* Consortium for Spinal Cord Medicine Clinical Practice Guidelines. Washington, DC: Paralyzed Veterans of America.

Garber, S. L., Lathem, P., & Gregorio, T. L. (1988). *Specialized occupational therapy for persons with high-level quadriplegia.* Monograph funded in part by Grant No. G009300044 from the National Institute on Disability and Rehabilitation Research, (NIDRR), U. S. Department of Education, awarded to the Research and Training Center for the Rehabilitation of Persons with Spinal Cord Dysfunction at Baylor College of Medicine and The Institute for Rehabilitation and Research (TIRR).

Garber, S. L., Rintala, D. H., Hart, K. A., & Fuhrer, M. J. (2000). Pressure ulcer risk in spinal cord injury: Predictors of ulcer status over 3 years. *Archives of Physical Medicine and Rehabilitation, 81,* 465–471.

Garber, S. L., Williams, A. L., Cook, K. F., & Koontz, A. M. (in press). A model for evaluating wheelchair mounted robotic arm. *Journal of Rehabilitation Research and Development.*

Glass, K., & Hall, K. (1987). Occupational therapy practitioners' views about the use of robotic aids for people with disabilities. *American Journal of Occupational Therapy, 41,* 745–747.

Go, B. K., DeVivo, M. J., & Richards, J. S. (1995). The epidemiology of spinal cord injury. In S. L. Stover, J. A. DeLisa, & G. G. Whiteneck (Eds.), *Spinal cord injury: Clinical outcomes from the model systems* (pp. 21–55). Gaithersburg, MD: Aspen.

Goossens, R. H., Snijders, C. J., Holscher, T. G., Heerens, W. C., & Holman, A. E. (1997). Shear stress measured on beds and wheelchairs. *Scandinavian Journal of Rehabilitation Medicine, 29,* 131–136.

Gordon, W. A., Harasymiw, S., Bellile, S., Lehman, L., & Sherman, B. (1982). The relationship between pressure sores and psychosocial adjustment in persons with spinal cord injury. *Rehabilitation Psychology, 27,* 185–191.

Hanebrink, S., & Dillon, D. (2000). Service dogs: The ultimate assistive technology. *OT Practice, 5,* 16–19.

Hanson, C. S., Nabavi, D., & Yuen, H. K. (2001). The effects of sports on level of community integration as reported by persons with spinal cord injury. *American Journal of Occupational Therapy, 55,* 332–338.

Hill, J. (1994). Surgical options after spinal cord injury. In G. M. Yarkony (Ed.), *Spinal cord injury: Medical management and rehabilitation* (pp. 137–140). Gaithersburg, MD: Aspen.

Hobson, D. A. (1992). Comparative effects of posture on pressure and shear at the body–seat interface. *Journal of Rehabilitation Research and Development, 15,* 21–31.

Hollar, L. D. (1995). Spinal cord injury. In C. A. Trombly (Ed.), *Occupational therapy for physical dysfunction* (4th ed., pp. 795–813). Baltimore: Williams & Wilkins.

Holme, S. A., Kanny, E. M., Guthrie, M. R., & Johnson, K. L. (1997). The use of environmental control units by occupational therapy practitioners in spinal cord injury and disease services. *American Journal of Occupational Therapy, 51,* 42–48.

Hoppenfeld, S. (1977). *Orthopaedic neurology: A diagnostic guide to neurological levels.* Philadelphia: Lippincott.

James, J. J., & Cardenas, D. D. (2003). Spinal cord injury. In S. J. Garrison (Ed.), *Handbook of physical medicine* (2nd ed., pp. 270–295). Philadelphia: Lippincott Williams & Wilkins.

Koo, T. D. D., Mak, A. F. T., & Lee, Y. L. (1996). Posture effect on seating interface biomechanics: Comparison between two seating systems. *Archives of Physical Medicine and Rehabilitation, 77,* 40–47.

Langemo, D. K., Melland, H., Hanson, D., Olson, B., & Hunter, S. (2000). The lived experience of having a pressure ulcer: A qualitative analysis. *Advances in Skin and Wound Care, 13,* 225–235.

Lasfargues, J. E., Custis, D., Morrone, F., Carswell, J., & Nguyen, T. (1995). A model for estimating spinal cord injury prevalence in the United States. *Paraplegia, 33,* 62–68.

Lathem, P., Gregorio, T. L., & Garber, S. L. (1985). High-level quadriplegia: An occupational therapy challenge. *American Journal of Occupational Therapy, 39,* 705–714.

Linsenmeyer, T., Biddle, A. K., Cardenas, D., Kuric, J., Mobley, T., et al.; Consortium for Spinal Cord Medicine. (1997). *Acute management of autonomic dysreflexia: Adults with spinal cord injury presenting to health-care facilities.* Washington, DC: Paralyzed Veterans of America.

Mann, W. C., & Lane, J. P. (1991). *Assistive technology for persons with disabilities: The role of occupational therapy.*

Rockville, MD: American Occupational Therapy Association.

McAlonan, S. (1996). Improving sexual rehabilitation services: The patient's perspective. *American Journal of Occupational Therapy, 50,* 826–834.

Melnyk, R., Montgomery, R., & Over, R. (1979). Attitude changes following a sexual counseling program for spinal cord injured persons. *Archives of Physical Medicine and Rehabilitation, 60,* 601–605.

Miller, H., & DeLozier, J. (1994). Cost implications. In N. Bergstrom & J. Cuddigan (Eds.), *Treating pressure ulcers* (Guideline Technical Report No. 15, Vol. II; AHCPR Publication No. 96-N015). Rockville, MD: U.S. Department of Health and Human Services, Public Health Service, Agency for Health Care Policy and Research.

Minkel, J. L. (2002). Service delivery in assistive technology. In D. A. Olson & F. DeRuyter (Eds.), *Clinician's guide to assistive technology* (pp. 55–65). St. Louis, MO: Mosby.

National Spinal Cord Injury Statistical Center. (2002). Spinal cord injury: Facts and figures at a glance. *Journal of Spinal Cord Medicine, 25,* 139–140.

Neistadt, M. E. (1986). Sexuality counseling for adults with disabilities: A module for an occupational therapy curriculum. *American Journal of Occupational Therapy, 40,* 542–545.

Pearman, J. W. (1985). Prevention and management of infection: The urinary tract. In G. M. Bedbrook (Ed.), *Lifetime care of the paraplegic patient* (pp. 54–65). Edinburgh: Churchill Livingstone.

Ragnarsson, K. T., Hall, K. M., Wilmot, C. B., & Carter, R. E. (1995). Management of pulmonary, cardiovascular, and metabolic conditions after spinal cord injury. In S. L. Stover, J. A. DeLisa, & G. G. Whiteneck (Eds.), *Spinal cord injury: Clinical outcomes from the model systems* (pp. 79–99). Gaithersburg, MD: Aspen.

Rehabilitation Act of 1973, Publ. L. 93-112, and its amendments of 1986 (Publ. L. 99-506), 29 USC § 701.

Schryvers, O. I., Miroslaw, M. F., & Nance, P. W. (2000). Surgical treatment of pressure ulcers: A 20-year experience. *Archives of Physical Medicine and Rehabilitation, 81,* 1556–1562.

Sunderlin, A. (1999). Dog days. *Paraplegia News, 53,* 13–20.

Swenson, J. R., Barnett, L. L., Pond, B., & Schoenberg, A. A. (1998). Assistive technology for rehabilitation and reduction of disability. In J. A. DeLisa et al. (Eds.), *Rehabilitation medicine: Principles and practice* (3rd ed., pp. 745–762). Philadelphia: J. B. Lippincott Company.

Tate, D. G., Henrich, R. K., Pasuke, L., & Anderson, D. (1998). Vocational rehabilitation, independent living, and consumerism. In J. A. DeLisa et al. (Eds.), *Rehabilitation medicine: Principles and practice* (3rd ed., pp. 1151–1162). Philadelphia: J. B. Lippincott Company.

Technology-Related Assistance for Individuals With Disabilities Act, Publ. L. 100-407, 20 USC §2201.

Traub, J. E., & LeClair, R. R. (1975). The rehabilitation engineering program. *American Rehabilitation, 1,* 3–7.

Treviranus, J., & Petty, L. (2002). Computer access. In D. A. Olson & F. DeRuyter (Eds.), *Clinician's guide to assistive technology* (pp. 91–113). St. Louis: Mosby.

Trombly, C. A. (1995a). Retraining basic instrumental activities of daily living. In C. A. Trombly (Ed.), *Occupational therapy for physical dysfunction* (4th ed., pp. 289–318). Baltimore: Williams & Wilkins.

Trombly, C. A. (1995b). Spinal cord injury. In C. A. Trombly (Ed.), *Occupational therapy for physical dysfunction* (4th ed., pp. 795–814). Baltimore: Williams & Wilkins.

Turner, A. N. (1985). Prevention of tertiary complications and management: Decubiti. In G. M. Bedbrook (Ed.), *Lifetime care of the paraplegic patient* (pp. 54–65). Edinburgh: Churchill Livingstone.

Valentine, D., Kiddoo, M., & LaFleur, B. (1993). Psychosocial implications of service dog ownership for people who have mobility or hearing impairments. *Social Work in Health Care, 19,* 109–124.

Versluys, H. P. (1995). Facilitating psychosocial adjustment to disability. In C. A. Trombly (Ed.), *Occupational therapy for physical dysfunction* (4th ed., pp. 377–390). Baltimore: Williams & Wilkins.

Watson, A. H., Kanny, E. M., White, D. M., & Anson, D. K. (1995). Use of standardized activities of daily living rating scales in spinal cord injury and disease services. *American Journal of Occupational Therapy, 49,* 229–234.

Whiteneck, G., Adler, C., Biddle, A. K., Blackburn, S., DeVivo, M. J., Haley, S. M., et al. (1999). *Outcomes following traumatic spinal cord injury: A clinical practical guideline for health care professionals* (p. 13). Washington, DC: Paralyzed Veterans of America.

Wuolle, K. S., Bryden, A. M., Peckham, P. H., Murray, P. K., & Keith, M. (2003). Satisfaction with upper-extremity surgery in individuals with tetraplegia. *Archives of Physical Medicine and Rehabilitation, 84,* 1145–1149.

Young, J. S., & Burns, P. E. (1981). Pressure sores and the spinal cord injured: Part II. *SCI Digest 3,* 11–26, 48.

Chapter 10

Adaptive Strategies Following Stroke

JUDITH A. JENKINS, MA, OTR

KEY TERMS

aphasia

apraxia

ataxia

dysarthria

dysphagia

hemianopsia

hemiparesis

hemiplegia

homonymous

unilateral neglect

OBJECTIVES

Upon completion of this chapter, the reader will be able to

- Describe the three major types of stroke;

- Identify performance components and performance areas to observe during the evaluation of a person who has experienced stroke;

- Describe the challenges to occupational performance experienced by people who have experienced stroke;

- Define and compare the difference between remediation and compensatory treatment approaches; and

- Describe techniques and assistive devices that people who have one-sided weakness or paralysis from stroke commonly use for daily living activities.

Approximately 700,000 people suffer a new or recurrent stoke each year in the United States, and more than 3 million Americans currently are living with various degrees of disability resulting from strokes (American Heart Association, 2001). Stroke is the leading cause of disability in adults and is the third leading cause of death; it killed 167,661 people in 2000. Risk factors associated with onset of stroke include high blood pressure, high cholesterol levels leading to arteriosclerosis, cigarette smoking, obesity, cocaine use, coronary heart disease, and diabetes. The frequency of stroke increases with advancing age and doubles with every decade after age 55 (Post-Stroke Rehabilitation Guideline Panel, 1995).

A stroke has the potential to affect every aspect of a person's life. Loss of function or weakness on one side (i.e., *hemiparesis*) occurs in approximately 75% of clients with strokes. Persisting neurological impairments lead to partial or total dependence in basic activities of daily living (BADL) in 25% to 50% of stroke survivors (Wojner, 1996). It is common for stroke survivors to experience an initial spurt of recovery in the first few weeks after the stroke. Generally, most recovery takes place during the first year to 18 months, and many people continue to improve over a much longer period (The Stroke Association, 2003). Limitations of motor coordination after stroke may result in a failure to return to occupations important to a person's quality of life (Trombly & Wu, 1999). Stroke-related disability is a major social and economic burden (Patel, 2001).

In 1996, the American Occupational Therapy Association (AOTA) reported that people who have experienced stroke constitute the largest single population of clients seen by occupational therapists. Occupational therapy intervention is a vital part of the rehabilitation process. The primary aim of occupational therapy is to facilitate task performance by improving skills or developing and teaching compensatory strategies to overcome lost performance skills (Weimar et al., 2002). In addition to restoring functional independence, occupational therapy works to assist with psychosocial adjustment to residual disability. Baum and Christiansen (1997) stated that "the unique contribution of occupational therapy is to maximize the fit between what it is the individual wants and needs to do and his or her capability to do it" (p. 40).

What Is a Stroke?

A stroke is the result of disruption in blood supply to the brain from a blockage or bleeding in the brain. Most strokes fall into one of two categories. An *ischemic* stroke is caused when a plaque fragment or blood clot lodges in an artery and restricts blood flow to the brain. A *thrombus* is a blood clot that forms within an artery that supplies the brain. An *embolus* is a plaque fragment or blood clot that travels to the brain from the heart or an artery supplying the brain. Thrombi and emboli together account for approximately 60% of all cases of stroke (Brandstater, 1998).

The second major type of stroke, *hemorrhagic* stroke, occurs when a blood vessel ruptures from a head injury or a weak, bulging portion of an arterial wall (i.e., an *aneurysm*). Long-term high blood pressure can weaken blood vessels in the brain and cause them to bulge and eventually burst. When the blood vessel ruptures, blood spills into the brain and damages brain cells, that is, neurons and glial cells.

A third type of stroke—*lacunar* stroke—occurs as the result of an occlusion in small vessels near the end of the arterial course. Lacunar strokes affect a relatively small segment of the brain. Twenty percent of cerebral infarctions can be characterized as lacunar strokes (Brandstater, 1998).

A *transient ischemic attack* (TIA), sometimes called a "mini-stroke," occurs when blood flow to an artery inside the brain or leading to the brain is temporarily blocked. TIA symptoms are generally temporary and last less than 24 hours (The Stroke Association, 2003).

Prognosis

Several studies have concluded that most stroke recovery occurs in the first 30 days. Improvement may continue as long as 6 to 12 months after stroke (Kelly-Hayes et al., 1989; Skilbeck, Wade, Langton-Hewer, & Wood, 1983). The longer the delay in onset of recovery, the poorer the prognosis. If recovery does not begin in 1 to 2 weeks, the potential for motor and language return becomes unfavorable. Deficits such as constructional apraxia, uninhibited anger, and unilateral neglect tend to diminish and may disappear in a few weeks. D'Esposito (1997) reported that most clients who present with neglect shortly after a stroke will have little or no evidence of neglect at 3 months poststroke. Visual field loss on one side (i.e., *hemianopia*) that has not resolved in a few weeks usually will be permanent, although reading and color discrimination may continue to improve. In lateral medullary infarction, difficulty in swallowing may be persistent (lasting 4 to 8 weeks or longer); relatively normal function is restored in most cases. Aphasia, dysarthria, cerebellar ataxia, and walking may not improve for a year or longer, although it is generally accepted that whatever motor and language deficits remain after 5 to 6 months will be permanent (Adams & Victor, 1993). Clients with a lacunar infarct and pure motor hemiparesis have a good chance for full recovery, which may start within 1 to 2 days and reach almost complete restoration in a week (Adams & Victor, 1993).

Predictors of Successful Outcome

Studies that attempted to determine the factors associated with favorable functional outcomes following stroke (Granger, Hamilton, & Gresham, 1988; Granger, Hamilton, Gresham, & Kramer, 1989) found that 80% of stroke survivors will be able to attain independence in mobility and that 67% will attain independence in activities of daily living (ADL). Mauthe, Haaf, Hayn, and Krall (1996) showed that more than 70% of the variance in discharge decisions after stroke rehabilitation is determined by the ability to function independently in the performance of self-care tasks necessary for bathing, toileting, social interaction, dressing, and eating. Independence in bowel and bladder control, eating, and grooming have a cumulative influence on predicting the ability of a survivor to live independently in the community following discharge.

Davidoff, Keren, Ring, and Solzi (1991) found that patients receiving inpatient rehabilitation services were able to maintain the gains in functional independence a year following discharge. Outpatient therapy services permitted further gains, particularly in clients with unilateral neglect, impaired joint position sense, urinary incontinence, or complete upper- or lower-extremity hemiplegia.

Bernspang, Viitanen, and Eriksson (1989) found that even several years after a stroke, visual and visual-perceptual deficits were more significant than motor impairment in determining the extent to which survivors could manage self-care requirements. The authors speculated that it may be easier for people to compensate for motor impairment than for perceptual limitations. Depression often is observed in the months after a stroke and is the most common affective disorder among people experiencing stroke; it occurs in mild or more severe forms in nearly 50% of stroke survivors (Gordon & Hibbard, 1997; Hermann, Black, Lawrence, Szekely, & Szalai, 1998). Depression also has been proposed as an independent predictor of poor functional outcome after stroke (Hermann et al., 1998). Spencer et al. (2002) found that clients, including those with a history of depression, who did not return to valued activities, tended to have more serious medical conditions.

Evaluation

The occupational therapy evaluation begins with gathering information about what the client needs and wants to do and the context in which those activities take place (Coster, 1998). *The Guide to Occupational Therapy Practice* (Moyers, 1999) provides occupational therapists with a detailed description of how to conduct an evaluation. When evaluating a stroke client, knowledge of common symptoms associated with various lesion sites can help the therapist anticipate possible performance deficits and identify what may be contributing to observed activity limitations (Table 10.1). Individual variations in the size and location of the lesion will result in a unique presentation of symptoms. The therapist's evaluation can be adapted to detect the most common symptoms associated with the location of brain injury.

The occupational therapist may select a specific assessment tool to facilitate observation and focus the evaluation (Moyers, 1999). The Barthel Index (Mahoney & Barthel, 1965) and the Functional Independence Measure (FIM™) have been tested extensively in rehabilitation for reliability, validity, and sensitivity and are the most commonly used measures (Post-Stroke Rehabilitation Guideline Panel, 1995). The FIM is a measure of disability (measured in terms of burden of care) for clients regardless of impairments or limitations (Table 10.2; Uniform Data System for Medical Rehabilitation, 1993). It assesses self-care, sphincter control, transfers, locomotion, communication, and social cognition on a seven-level scale. The FIM has been incorporated into the Inpatient Rehabilitation Facility Patient Assessment Instrument, which is used to collect data to determine payment for Medicare Part A fee-for-service patients in inpatient rehabilitation facilities (*Federal Register*, 2001).

Other common assessment tools include The Katz Index of Independence in ADL (Katz, Ford, Moskowitz, Jackson, & Jaffe, 1963), the Assessment of Motor and Process Skills (AMPS; Fisher, 1994), and the Canadian Occupational Performance Measure (COPM; Law et al., 1990). The Katz Index of Independence in ADL is based on an evaluation of the functional independence of clients in bathing, dressing, toileting, transfers, continence, and feeding (Christiansen, in press). The AMPS is an assessment system that requires observation of a person performing instrumental activities of daily living (IADL) as he or she would normally perform them. The COPM measures areas of self-care, productivity,

Table 10.1. Summary of Lesion Sites and Associated Impairments

Site of Lesion	Clinical Picture
Middle cerebral artery	Contralateral hemiplegia, more upper-extremity involvement, hemisensory loss, and hemianopsia
Dominant hemisphere	Expressive and/or receptive aphasia, apraxia, and astereognosis (Chusid, 1973)
Nondominant hemisphere	Visual-spatial deficits, impaired body awareness, and visual construction deficits (Easton, 1981)
Internal carotid artery	Hemiplegia, unilateral sensory loss, and aphasia (Chusid, 1973)
Anterior cerebral artery	Diminished behavioral control, arousal, and attention Contralateral hemiplegia with the lower extremity more involved than the upper extremity, urinary incontinence, and gait apraxia
Posterior cerebral artery	Contralateral hemiplegia, hemianesthesia, and homonymous hemianopsia
Dominant hemisphere	Aphasia
Nondominant hemisphere	Visual-spatial deficits
Bilateral hemisphere	Bilateral hemianopsia, cortical blindness with denial of visual disturbance, and amnesia (Easton, 1981)
Brain stem	Lateral medullary or Wallenberg syndrome, including loss of pain and temperature sensation on the ipsilateral face and contralateral body, dysarthria, dysphagia, ipsilateral limb ataxia, vertigo, nystagmus Contralateral hemiplegia, contralateral ataxia, and a contralateral increase in the pain and temperature threshold
Vertebrobasilar artery	Cranial nerve palsy; unilateral or bilateral motor, sensory, or cerebellar signs; nystagmus; or coma
Lacunar infarct	Four lacunar syndromes: (1) Pure motor stroke (resulting in hemiplegia) (2) Pure sensory stroke (leading to paresthesia) (3) Ataxic hemiparesis (leading to hemiparesis and ipsilateral ataxia) (4) Dysarthria and clumsy hand syndrome, resulting in difficulty with speech and fine motor incoordination of the involved upper extremity

and leisure and can include an assessment of performance components (Christiansen, in press).

Phillips and Wolters (1996) noted that during the self-care assessment, the following performance components should be observed:

- Ability to sustain antigravity posture
- Ability to maintain head and trunk control
- Ability to maintain midline orientation during dynamic activity
- Functional use and quality of movement of the involved upper extremity
- Ability to perform bilateral movement
- Ability to use objects appropriately
- Endurance for self-care tasks
- Level of cognitive functioning in the areas of initiation, attention, organizational skills, and sequencing abilities
- Ability to visually attend to self-care tasks
- Presence of perceptual difficulties interfering with task performance.

Hsieh, Sheu, Hsueh, and Wang (2002) recommended assessment and management of trunk control at an early stage poststroke because it is a necessary component of occupational performance. In their study using the Postural Assessment Scale, they demonstrated the predictive value of trunk control 14 days poststroke.

Case Descriptions

The following case histories provide information on the type of stroke, resulting impairments, and occupational therapy intervention. Information from the results of an occupational therapy evaluation and a measure of the client's disability based on the FIM scale are provided.

Case Study 1

Joyce is a 58-year-old woman who experienced multiple ischemic strokes affecting multiple vascular distributions, primarily the left anterior cerebral

Table 10.2. Levels of Function and Scores: Functional Independence Measure

7 (complete independence): All of the tasks described as making up the activity are typically performed safely; without modification, assistive devices, or aids; and within reasonable time.

6 (modified independence): Activity requires any one or more than one of the following: an assistive device, more than reasonable time, or there are safety (risk) considerations.

5 (supervision or set up): Subject requires no more help than standby, cueing, or coaxing, without physical contact. Or, helper sets up needed items or applies orthoses.

4 (minimal assistance): Subject requires no more help than touching, and subject expends 75% or more of the effort.

3 (moderate assistance): Subject requires more help than touching or expends half (50%) or more (up to 75%) of the effort.

2 (maximal assistance): Subject expends less than 50% of the effort, but at least 25%.

1 (total assistance): Subject expends less than 25% of the effort.

Note. From *Guide for the Uniform Data Set for Medical Rehabilitation (Adult FIM), Version 4.0,* by Uniform Data System for Medical Rehabilitation, 1993, Buffalo, NY: Author. Used with permission.

and right occipital. She presented with a highly divergent array of deficits: right-side weakness, ataxia, impaired sensation to the right side, left unilateral neglect, and left homonymous hemianopsia.

Prior to hospitalization Joyce was employed as a nurse and lived alone in a single-story house. She was independent in all BADL and IADL. The occupational therapy evaluation revealed that active range of motion was within normal limits in both upper extremities. Her sitting balance was graded as good, but standing balance was graded as poor. She was considered to be at a high risk for falls because of her impulsivity, impaired balance, and visual perceptual deficits. Joyce required minimal assistance for most

Table 10.3. Case Assessment 1 Self-Care FIM Scores

Self-Care	Admission	Discharge
Eating	4	6
Grooming	4	6
Bathing	4	6
Dressing—upper	4	5
Dressing—lower	4	5
Bladder control	4	7
Bowel control	4	6
Bed, chair transfers	4	5
Toilet transfers	4	5
Tub, shower transfers	3	5

self-care tasks. Her rehabilitation stay was 3 1/2 weeks. Table 10.3 summarizes Joyce's FIM scores.

Intervention Strategies

Occupational therapy intervention consisted of scheduled BADL training sessions in Joyce's room. The occupational therapist coordinated with the nursing staff to ensure a consistent arrangement of Joyce's meal trays to improve her ability to locate food items. It was recommended that Joyce be placed in a private room because she was severely distracted by environmental stimuli such as conversations between other people, the television, the ringing telephone, and minor changes in the physical arrangement of her room. The structure of Joyce's rehabilitation program allowed her to improve her level of independence in feeding, grooming, and toileting from minimal assistance to modified independence.

The following activities were incorporated into the ADL training program:

- *Feeding.* After the meal tray was placed in front of her, Joyce was told what food items were being served. She was then asked to locate all items on the tray. A plate guard and an independence mug with antisplash lid were used to minimize spilling. The plate guard was also used as a guide to help Joyce locate the left side of her plate.
- *Grooming.* Joyce and her caregiver were instructed to eliminate clutter on the bathroom sink and to keep grooming tools in the same location.

- *Bathing.* Because of Joyce's impaired balance and low endurance, she used a tub transfer bench, grab bars, and hand-held shower. Because she had difficulty holding onto the bar of soap and wringing out the washcloth, liquid soap and a bathing puff improved her independence.

- *Upper-body dressing.* Joyce had difficulty manipulating small buttons and fasteners; she found hooking her bra especially frustrating. By turning the bra with the hook side up and clipping the left side to her panties with a clothes pin, she was able to fasten her bra.

- *Lower-body dressing.* Joyce had difficulty putting on her right sock and shoe. She was unable to maintain the position of crossing her right leg over her left, and when she would reach down, she would lose her balance. In addition to having Joyce routinely practice and train in donning and doffing her socks and shoes, the occupational therapist had her sit on the edge of the treatment mat and reach for items just below her knees and, eventually, from the floor. This activity helped to improve Joyce's sitting balance; by discharge, she was able to don and doff both shoes and socks with setup.

- *Leisure.* Prior to the onset of her illness, Joyce was an avid reader. Although she continued to work on reading during sessions with the speech–language pathologist, she was not proficient. She experienced some satisfaction with books on tape. The recreation therapist worked with her on obtaining access to the local library as well as to the state commission for the blind.

Because Joyce sometimes would be unsupervised after discharge from the hospital, the occupational therapist worked with Joyce and her caregiver on strategies for storing food items so that she would be able to retrieve a cold snack from the refrigerator. Due to her impairments, unsupervised cooking was not recommended. Joyce practiced making a sandwich and arranging snacks in a familiar container that she could easily locate. The caregiver participated in several training sessions with the therapist prior to Joyce's discharge from the hospital to ensure follow-through with learned compensatory strategies.

Case Study 2

Benjamin is a 55-year-old man who suffered a right middle cerebral artery distribution stroke with asso-

ciated left-side weakness, slurred speech, and decreased alertness. His hospital course was complicated by a left atrial myxoma (a tumor composed of mucous connective tissue in the atrium) excision with cardiopulmonary bypass. He also had decreased vision in the left eye, a left visual field cut, and left-side neglect. His sensation was impaired on the left side. During his acute care hospitalization, a modified barium swallow revealed paralysis of the left side of his tongue and vocal cords. A gastrostomy tube was placed due to his inability to be orally fed and his risk for aspiration. While in acute care, Benjamin had two falls while attempting to walk to the bathroom unassisted. Table 10.4 summarizes Benjamin's FIM scores.

Prior to hospitalization, Benjamin was self-employed as a handyman. He lived with his daughter in a single-story house. Prior to the stroke, he was independent in all ADL and IADL. He planned to move into an apartment for senior citizens upon discharge. The occupational therapy evaluation revealed that although Benjamin's left upper extremity had normal range of motion, his movement patterns were athetoid; in addition, edema was present in his left forearm, wrist, and hand. He complained of shoulder pain at the end of passive range. Benjamin was oriented to his name only and was able to follow one-step directions. He was impulsive and easily distracted by environmental stimuli. His sitting balance was fair, and his standing balance was poor. He needed total assistance with feeding because he was not being fed orally and was dependent on the nursing staff for his gastrostomy tube feedings. Benjamin required moderate assistance with most of his basic self-care tasks. His rehabilita-

Table 10.4. Case Assessment 2 Self-Care FIM Scores

Self-Care	Admission	Discharge
Eating	1	1
Grooming	4	5
Bathing	3	5
Dressing—upper	3	5
Dressing—lower	3	4
Bladder control	2	5
Bowel control	3	4
Bed, chair transfers	3	5
Toilet transfers	3	5
Tub, shower transfers	1	5

tion stay was 3 1/2 weeks, and he continued with therapy on an outpatient basis.

Intervention Strategies

Occupational therapy intervention consisted of daily scheduled ADL training sessions in Benjamin's room. Treatment activities focused on improving motor control in his left upper extremity, improving trunk control, developing compensatory strategies for his left field cut and unilateral neglect, and improving his safety during transfers. Because of the presence of unilateral neglect and impaired sensation, Benjamin did not use his left hand spontaneously. He also became very frustrated during remedial ADL training because he could not control his left hand. Thus, he avoided using it altogether.

Benjamin was initially taught one-handed dressing techniques by approaching his rehabilitation from a compensatory perspective (see Figure 10.1). He improved his level of independence and became more receptive to occupational therapy intervention. The occupational therapist encouraged functional use of the left arm by teaching Benjamin to use it as a gross assist to stabilize fabric while zipping his pants, bathing his right arm, and assisting with pulling up his pants. He eventually progressed to using his left arm as a fair assist and performed activities such as donning and doffing socks, putting his belt through the loops, and propelling his wheelchair.

Treatment activities to improve trunk control were similar to those used with Joyce (Case Study 1). He performed grooming activities while standing in front of the mirror to help improve dynamic standing balance. Benjamin was able to return home with his daughter, who would provide intermittent supervision. It was recommended that occupational therapy services continue through home health to

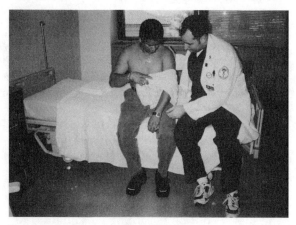

Figure 10.1. One-handed dressing.

give Benjamin the opportunity to focus on improving independence and safety in BADL as well as advance to independence in IADL. The ultimate long-term goal was to eliminate the need for supervision and allow him to live independently in a senior apartment, which was his primary goal.

Because Benjamin enjoyed playing dominoes and card games, those activities were incorporated into his home program. Shuffling cards and picking up dominoes helped facilitate spontaneous use of his left upper extremity (including pincer grasp, wrist pronation and supination, and elbow flexion and extension). Participation in those activities could also enhance his attention and concentration skills.

Setting Goals

Setting treatment goals involves estimating the amount of time it will take for the client to achieve a specific level of independence. The following factors may determine the length of stay and assist in establishing realistic and attainable goals with the client and his or her family:

- Funding sources
- Personal financial resources
- Prior level of functioning
- Age
- Lifestyle and role responsibilities
- Family support
- Presence of cognitive and perceptual deficits
- Degree of physical dysfunction
- Discharge disposition.

Goals are written to show changes in baseline performance in areas of occupation or performance skills or patterns that are expected to occur as a result of planned intervention (Moyers, 1999). A well-written goal should suggest a performance outcome and describe what improvements in performance the occupational therapist expects to achieve through the treatment intervention (Daniel & Strickland, 1992). AOTA's guidelines for documentation suggest that short- and long-term goals should be measurable and related to the occupational therapy problem list (Kron et al., 1988). For example, improvements in performance may be demonstrated by a change in the level of assistance required to perform an activity. The FIM and other ADL assessments provide baseline information that can be used to measure progress. Other improvements in performance may involve increased speed, accuracy, or frequency of the skill required; thus, baseline measurements of those skill components is useful. A goal also must include a time frame for when the goal will be attained.

It is most important for the occupational therapist to consider performance measures in motor recovery when writing goals. For example, when writing a goal to improve grip strength, the therapist should focus on skills such as the ability to hold and drink from a glass instead of the number of pounds in grip strength measured by a dynamometer. Consider what specific activity will be affected by improvement in range of motion, coordination, endurance, balance, or strength. Other examples include improving active range of motion so that the client can retrieve items from a cabinet or groom his or her hair, improving fine motor control to enable the client to button a front-closure shirt or hook a bra, and improving dynamic standing balance to enable the client to adjust his or her clothing after toileting. This focus on functional, measurable goals reflects the "uniqueness" of occupational therapy.

Ponte-Allan and Giles (1999) found that clients who made a functional, independence-focused goal statement when they were admitted to the hospital had significantly higher functional outcomes and shorter lengths of stay at the hospital than those who did not. The researchers defined a functional, independence-focused goal statement as a statement of the desire to perform a specific activity or to be able to resume a specific activity.

Remedial Treatment Approaches

Once the evaluation is complete and performance goals have been established, treatment begins. A variety of treatment approaches can be used and are generally combined to maximize both the level and the quality of independence. Note that training activities for component skills should be related to improving the client's ability to perform daily living tasks. Motor-skills teaching should not focus on how well a skill can be performed during a single treatment session but on how well the client performs the skill in context of ADL and on how well the skill is retained or remembered (Wishart, Lee, Janzen-Ezekiel, Marley, & Lehto 2000).

Learned Nonuse

Most stroke survivors are acutely affected by hemiparesis (DeBow, Davies, Clarke, & Colbourne, 2003). Spontaneous recovery occurs to some degree, but many survivors remain chronically impaired, in part because of learned nonuse of the impaired extremity (Miltner, Bauder, Sommer, Dettmers, & Taube, 1999). Learned nonuse results from repeated failed attempts to use the impaired limb soon after injury combined with successful use of the unaffected limb. Constraint-induced movement therapy (CIMT) is a treatment approach that is based on the learned nonuse theory. In CIMT the unimpaired limb is restrained in a sling for 6 hours per day for a period of 2 weeks to counteract learned nonuse and force the use of an impaired limb during normal daily activities and rehabilitative exercises (Wolf, Lecraw, Barton, & Jann, 1989). CIMT has some implications for the treatment of neglect and may assist in reducing neglect and increasing independence in ADL (Freeman, 2001). A similar principle guides the following approach used for visual field cut. Techniques such as partial visual occlusion (i.e., either patching the non-neglected half field or using hemispatial sunglasses) are thought to force the client to use head turning and eye movements to scan the neglected visual field (Freeman, 2001).

Motor-Learning Theory

Motor-learning theory, as described by Carr and Shepherd (1987), uses a sequential clinical reasoning process. A functional performance problem is identified; the limiting motor components are analyzed; the impaired components are practiced in isolation through visual, verbal, and manual guidance; and, finally, the motion is practiced in the context of the functional task with the intent of integrating the components.

Motor-Control Theory

Treatment approaches using contemporary motor-control theory emphasize practice of functional tasks as a way to organize motor behavior (Bass-Haugen, Mathiowetz, & Flinn, 2001). In this approach, the therapist determines and modifies the demands of the activity or the environment to allow maximal motor performance, given the attributes of the person. Therapy focuses on practicing the activity in a natural context. For example, if a person has residual weakness on one side and has some difficulty with dressing as a result, the most effective treatment is to actually practice the whole task of dressing with various task and environmental demands rather than practice components of the activity.

The Post-Stroke Rehabilitation Guideline Panel (1995) recommends that clients who have functional deficits and some voluntary movements of the involved arm or leg be encouraged to use the limb in functional tasks. Exercise and functional training should be directed at improving strength and motor control, relearning sensorimotor relationships, and improving functional performance.

Motor-Facilitation and -Retraining Techniques

Motor-facilitation and -retraining techniques are useful to improve upper-extremity function and the trunk control that is necessary for optimal performance of self-care skills. The techniques are directed at correcting impaired motor activity of the affected extremity, preventing overuse of the unaffected side, and preventing the development of abnormal movement patterns of the affected side. The techniques can be used in the clinic to build prerequisite skills needed for ADL. Specific techniques can enhance functional mobility while rolling, sitting, standing, or kneeling. Working on various surfaces, such as a table mat, bench, chair without arms, bed, ball, or rocker board, can provide graded challenges to balance. Reaching activities and eye–hand coordination games can improve speed and control.

Evidence suggests that internally focused instructions such as "open your hand" and "straighten your elbow" actually may slow motor performance (Fasoli, Trombly, Tickle-Degnen, & Verfaellie, 2002). Ma and Trombly (2002) recommended using actual objects within a functional goal to help the client organize movement. They reported that the presence of the object toward which movement was directed produced a significantly quicker, smoother, and more direct reaching.

The following examples of functional activities can be incorporated into one-on-one treatment sessions and were used with Joyce in Case Study 1:

- Picking up, holding, and drinking from various-sized cups and glasses with the stroke-affected hand
- Combing and brushing hair
- Opening jars, packets, and toothpaste tubes using the stroke-affected hand as a stabilizer
- Stirring liquids in a pot with the noninvolved hand while holding the handle with the stroke-affected hand
- Folding towels to encourage bilateral use of upper extremities and using a rolling pin to roll out cookie dough
- Placing the rolled-out cookies onto a cookie sheet from left to right to encourage left-side orientation.

Compensation Techniques and Contextual Training

The compensatory model emphasizes achieving independence in daily living; the focus is on improving function rather than enhancing motor recovery or minimizing impairments. Clients with persistent activity limitations should be taught compensatory techniques for performing BADL/IADL (Post-Stroke Rehabilitation Guideline Panel, 1995). Therapists should encourage use of the affected extremity when possible, but when that is not possible, clients should be taught compensatory strategies with the remaining unaffected limb. Many one-handed techniques and types of assistive devices enable someone who has experienced stroke to continue to do the things that are important to him or her. When prognosis for the return of dexterity is poor, teaching the client to deal with existing deficits and allow for the use of compensating strategies may be the most realistic approach (Kwakkel, Kollen, Vander-Grond, & Prevo, 2003).

Contextual training involves practicing a task in a specific environment until it becomes learned or habitual. This repetition of specific task sequences has been found to be effective in improving independence in people with brain injury (Soderback, 1988). Practice is most effective when it is specific to the context in which the task occurs and when it is performed in a consistent sequence (Bukowski, Bonavolonta, Keehn, & Morgan, 1996). In addition to the benefit of practicing a familiar activity, contextual training requires the client to integrate various motor, cognitive, and perceptual skills. The activity should initially begin with a low level of challenge and gradually increase in complexity as the client masters each step. Ma and Trombly (2002) recommended using task-specific practice that incorporates strategies of gradual complexity and breaks tasks into simpler steps. For example, in Case Study 2 (Benjamin), the occupational therapist first allowed the client to perform dressing activities with one hand and progressed to incorporating the use of his involved extremity. In another example, occupational therapists help clients progress from having their clothing articles placed within the area of reach or field of vision (setup) to having them search a cluttered drawer or a closet for specific articles.

Assistive Devices and Adaptive Equipment

Training in the use of assistive devices and adaptive equipment is one method occupational therapists use to improve and maintain occupational performance (Kraskowsky & Finlayson, 2001). Activities can be accomplished in more than one way, and sometimes simply using equipment that substitutes for a missing skill is all that is required (Moyers, 1999). Lysack and Neufeld (2003) found that recommendations for equipment were somewhat more common than recommendations for home modifications and that cerebrovascular accident clients tended to have more equipment recommended to them than did clients in other diagnostic groups. They also found that commode chairs, wheelchairs, and bathtub benches or chairs were prescribed for more than 50% of clients. No simple recipe exists for recommending equipment on the basis of diagnosis or performance-component deficits. The therapist must consider some of the following issues:

- Cognitive deficits
- Willingness of the client to use recommended equipment

- The physical environment in which the equipment will be used
- Whether the client can use the equipment independently or will require the assistance of another person
- The financial feasibility of obtaining the equipment.

Lysack and Neufeld (2003) reported that many small, inexpensive items, such as long-handled bath sponges, combs and shoehorns, and elastic shoelaces, were beyond the financial reach of many clients.

Table 10.5 lists some common performance-skill problems associated with stroke along with

Table 10.5. Commonly Used Assistive Devices and Techniques for Clients With Limited Use of One Extremity Following Stroke

Activity	Common Performance Skill Problems	Assistive Device and Equipment	Adaptive Techniques
Feeding, grooming	Holding utensils firmly Stabilizing objects Opening containers Two-handed tasks Reaching areas on uninvolved side	Universal cuff and built-up utensils or handles Rocker knife Lip plates, plate guard, scoop dish Extended handle utensils Dycem Wash mitt Velcro closures Suction-cup equipment stabilizers	Use teeth to open small packages and containers. Stabilize containers between knees to open.
Bathing	Reaching areas on uninvolved side Reaching lower body Getting in and out of the tub or shower Impaired sitting or standing balance	Tub bench or shower chair Handheld shower Grab bars Nonskid surface	Sit for bathing for stability. Dry off before exiting tub or shower. Keep all needed items close by.
Toileting	Getting up and down from the toilet seat Adjusting clothing Reaching perineal area for cleaning Washing both hands	Raised commode chair (drop arm) Toilet safety frame Grab bars Toilet tissue aid Velcro closures on pants or elastic waist pant Pump soap dispenser	Pull pants up or down while sitting by shifting weight. Lean against stable structures for balance. Keep floor surface nonskid.
Dressing	Adjusting clothing closures Reaching lower body	Button aid and zipper pull Velcro closures Reacher Elastic shoelaces, long-handled shoehorn	Dress the involved side first. Undress the uninvolved side first.
Cooking and cleaning	Stabilizing pans and dishes Draining liquids Opening jars and cans Washing dishes Carrying items	Dycem One-handed strainers Pan handle stabilizers Zim jar opener Electric can openers Wheeled cart Apron with front pocket	Stabilize bowls or open containers by securing them between both knees. Use teeth or mouth for light package opening. Take fewer trips by gathering supplies at the beginning (on cart or basket).

some frequently used assistive devices. Equipment can help clients who have experienced stroke solve specific skill-deficit problems related to participating in important activities. Many items are available in local department stores, supermarkets, and hardware stores. Even though many items today are available for purchase, some can be fabricated using common materials (e.g., pipe insulation can be placed on eating and grooming utensils to build up handles, or a paper clip attached to the hole in the zipper can function as a zipper pull).

IADL, such as home care, child care, community living skills, and work, provide cognitive, perceptual, and motor challenges. These activities are best performed in the actual environment in which they will take place. Because that often is not possible for hospital-based clients, occupational therapists should attempt to simulate actual environments in order to identify problem areas and help clients improve performance. Teaching clients, when appropriate, to imagine themselves performing specific functional actions is recommended (Ma & Trombly, 2002). With guidance, clients frequently are able to apply principles learned in simulated settings to their own situation.

Driving

Driving is important in maintaining the independence of older people in their daily living activities and social networking (Lee, Lee, & Cameron, 2003), and occupational therapists have an important role in addressing issues related to older drivers (Hunt et al., 1997). Readiness to return to driving following stroke is a common issue in clinical practice; a need exists for instruments that can be used to screen for cognitive functions as a way to assess driving competence (Lundqvist, Gerdle, & Ronnberg, 2000). As stated previously, stroke may affect a person's ability to see, control movement, remember, or concentrate. All of these abilities are necessary for safe driving and must be assessed (The Stroke Association, 2003). Limited research has been done to identify reliable driving evaluation criteria (Lee et al., 2003). The most common method of evaluation has been to observe the client's driving in real traffic; another method is the use of a driving simulator (Lundqvist et al., 2000).

To compensate for hemiplegia, a spinner knob may be attached to the steering wheel. A left-foot accelerator can be used for clients who have right-sided weakness or paralysis. The Association for Driver Educators for the Disabled is a useful resource for information on vehicle modifications and training. (Occupational therapists should check with the local department of public safety or department of transportation for legal implications before recommending modifications to a vehicle.) For safety reasons, it is generally illegal to drive after a stroke. Clients must inform their local driver licensing agency and insurance company, and they are not allowed to drive for at least a month (The Stroke Association, 2003). It is recommended that clients seek the advice of their physician before returning to driving.

Caregiver Training

A caregiver should be trained when a client is unable to carry out all daily activities independently. Approximately 70% to 90% of people who experience stroke are cared for in the home (Ozer, Materson, & Caplan, 1994). It may be difficult for one person to be responsible for all aspects of the client's care at home, especially if he or she is caring for other family members. Hasselkus (1991) reported that caregivers often experience ethical dilemmas when faced with conflicts between taking good care of the client and meeting other family and personal responsibilities. Evans, Bishop, and Haselkorn (1991) found that clients at risk for less-than-optimal home care had caregivers who were more likely to be depressed, had a below-average knowledge of stroke care principles, and had greater incidence of family dysfunction.

The occupational therapist should collaborate with the caregiver to develop a home program that meets the client's needs and is realistic for the caregiver. Before discharge, the home program should be demonstrated, and plenty of opportunity should be provided for practice. Picture diagrams or photographs of each activity may be helpful.

Other Intervention Considerations

In developing a treatment plan, occupational therapists must take into account a variety of stroke-associated client health issues, including heart disease, shoulder pain, dysphagia, gastrostomy, and fall risk. The following sections describe some of the health issues that may arise in the course of occupational therapy practice with stroke survivors.

Cardiac Precautions

Occupational therapists must be aware of specific precautions and secondary diagnoses, such as hypertension, coronary artery disease, and congestive heart failure, which frequently are associated with stroke (Roth, 1988). A careful review of the client's medical chart should be conducted prior to initiating therapy. Physicians may provide parameters for heart rate, oxygen saturation, and blood pressure for clients whose condition may be unstable. Such clients must be monitored before, during, and after activity to determine whether the activity is too strenuous. Isometric, resistive, and overhead activities increase cardiac stress and should be carefully monitored or avoided, depending on cardiac status. In addition, community activities in extremely cold or hot weather should be postponed.

Shoulder Pain

Elderly people frequently have some degree of joint damage due to pre-existing conditions such as osteoarthritis. Proper alignment of all joints must be maintained during self-care and passive range of motion to avoid impingement and injury to soft tissues. The affected shoulder is particularly vulnerable to injury following stroke. When the limb is too weak to resist gravity, placing the limb in a functional position is essential to avoid deformities, minimize edema, and maintain range of motion (Trombly & Radomski, 2002). The client and caregiver should be taught to position the affected arm correctly during all tasks. All caregivers must be careful to avoid pulling on the affected arm and should mobilize the scapula before attempting overhead movement of a spastic arm. The therapist should be alert for signs of *reflex sympathetic dystrophy* (also called "shoulder–hand syndrome"), which include swelling of the hand; trophic changes, including altered skin color, nail appearance, sweating, or hair growth; and pain at rest or upon motion, especially during finger and shoulder flexion, abduction, or external rotation (Eto, Yoshikaw, Ueda, & Hirai, 1980).

Dysphagia

Dysphagia, or difficulty swallowing, may affect as many as one-third of people experiencing stroke (Roth, 1988). The speech pathologist may conduct a videofluoroscopic or modified barium-swallow exam, which is the best tool for detecting deficits in oral control and swallowing. In some facilities, the occupational therapist may conduct the exam or assist with the proper positioning of the client during the exam. Foods and liquids of various consistencies are mixed with barium, which makes it visible on the video monitor. The mixture is given in small quantities. The movement of the food is observed in the mouth, through the pharynx, and into the esophagus. Any abnormality that suggests risk of aspiration (i.e., getting food in the trachea) can readily be detected, and specific recommendations about the types of food that are safe can be made.

In clients who have swallowing dysfunction, specific guidelines may include avoid drinking with a straw, taking one or two sips of liquid followed by eating solid foods, tilting the head forward while swallowing, and limiting environmental distractions during eating. During feeding training, the occupational therapist should be aware of possible restrictions, such as no oral intake, as well as specifications for texture or consistency of food and beverages. A dietitian also will be consulted to ensure that protein and caloric needs are met and dehydration is prevented.

Gastrostomy Tube

If the client has severe dysphasia, he or she may have a gastrostomy tube. The tube must be monitored to avoid disruption during activity. When gastrostomy feedings are given, the client must be maintained in an upright position (at least 45 degrees) for generally 1 hour following meals. This prevents food from flowing back into the trachea, which can lead to aspiration pneumonia. Therapists also should be aware of the location of the tube to avoid pressure from clothing or a gait belt.

Fall Risk

Stroke survivors are more likely to fall than any other population (Vlahov, Myers, & Al-Ibrahim, 1990). Studies report that from 41% to as much as 83.3% of patients who fell had a diagnosis of stroke (DeVincenzo & Watkins, 1987; Grant & Hamilton, 1987; Mion et al., 1989; Vlahov et al.,1990). Clients with impaired balance, impaired vision, lower extremity weakness, impulsivity, confusion, gait disturbances, and perceptual deficits such as depth perception and unilateral neglect are at an increased risk for falls. They may require constant or intermittent supervision. If sitting balance or judgment is impaired, safety belts should be used in wheelchairs and on the toilet. A gait belt is recommended when transferring, standing, or walking with a client. Brakes on the wheelchair, bed, or other unstable items should be locked prior to a transfer.

Discharge Planning

When a reasonable number of goals have been met or changes in performance no longer occur, it may be time for discharge from the rehabilitation unit. The Post-Stroke Rehabilitation Guideline Panel (1995) recommended that absence of progress on two consecutive evaluations should lead to reconsideration of the intensive rehabilitation setting. It is generally understood that discharge planning should begin on the day of admission to the unit. The occupational therapist, working with the rehabilitation team, the client, and his or her caregivers, must determine whether the client will be safe in his or her discharge environment.

Therapeutic Day Pass

If the client is in an inpatient rehabilitation facility, a therapeutic day pass can be arranged. The pass permits the client to go home for a period of 4 to 6 hours with a caregiver. This opportunity can help identify problems that may require specific environmental adaptations or further training. An assessment of actual behavior must take place in the daily living environment in which the person performs the tasks (Christiansen, in press). Reliable friends or family may report performance during a home pass. The report should include information on what kinds of activities were done; any problems the client may have encountered, such as household ambulation, wheelchair mobility, kitchen and bathroom mobility; and general accessibility in and around the home. The client's companion or caregiver should note any problems that would prevent him or her from using any of the recommended equipment.

Home Safety Assessment

Another valuable assessment for discharge planning is the home safety assessment. This generally involves a visit by the occupational therapist, physical therapist, the client and, if necessary, the caregiver visiting the home. The main purpose of the home safety assessment is to ensure safety in the home and determine whether the client has received sufficient training to safely move around the home and participate in his or her important everyday activities. Careful assessment of the client's abilities within his or her home is critical to identifying barriers that can be eliminated or modified in preparation for a successful return home (Lysack & Neufeld, 2003).

The therapist observes whether the client is able to generalize to the home setting some of the basic skills learned in the rehabilitation or skilled nursing facility setting, such as stair climbing, tub and toilet transfers, kitchen mobility, and household ambulation. The advantage of the home safety assessment is that it allows the therapist to see the physical structure of the home and determine whether space is adequate to use recommended equipment, such as a tub transfer bench. Another added benefit of the home evaluation is prevention of secondary injuries (Lysack & Neufeld, 2003). During the home safety visit, the therapist can make recommendations specific to the client's home environment.

Continuity of Care

The final concern in discharge planning relates to continuity of care. If therapy is to continue through home health services, on an outpatient basis, or at a skilled nursing facility, arrangements should be made. The occupational therapist should establish a plan for follow-up care, which may be done by the client's primary care physician or the rehabilitation physician.

Summary

Current trends in health care continue toward shorter lengths of hospital stay. One-third of all stroke patients are moved from an acute care setting to rehabilitation units within 14 days of onset, and length of stay has been declining since 1989 (Joe, 1995). The challenge for occupational therapists is to provide the treatment approach that will best enable their clients to achieve maximal benefits and functional gains within shortened time frames. Ma and Trombly (2002) concluded that treatments occupational therapists use to improve impairments after stroke generally are effective, especially those involving activity or occupation to effect change. They challenged the occupational therapy profession to research those and other treatments used in occupational therapy.

Study Questions

1. Discuss how hemiplegia, the most common performance-component deficit associated with stroke, affects a client's ability to perform ADL.
2. What are some important secondary factors that affect full recovery from a stroke?
3. What should be observed during the self-care evaluation?
4. What are some ways to ensure the best outcome when a client returns home from the hospital?
5. What are the most effective ways to improve motor performance during ADL for a person who has hemiparesis?
6. What are some techniques or equipment that may be useful for cooking, cleaning, and driving for someone who has hemiparesis?

References

Adams, R. D., & Victor, M. (1993). Cerebral vascular diseases. In W. J. Lamsback & M. Navrozov (Eds.), *Principles of neurology* (5th ed., pp. 669–748). New York: McGraw-Hill.

American Heart Association. (2001, February). *American Heart Association 2001 heart and stroke statistical update*. Retrieved September 2003 from *www.ameri-canheart.org/statistics/stroke.html*.

American Occupational Therapy Association. (1996). *Member data survey*. Bethesda, MD: Author.

Bass-Haugen, J., Mathiowetz, V., & Flinn, N. (2001). Optimizing motor behavior using the occupational therapy task-oriented approach. In C. A. Trombly & M. V. Radomski (Eds.), *Occupational therapy for physical dysfunction* (5th ed., pp. 481–499). Philadelphia: Lippincott Williams & Wilkins.

Baum, C., & Christiansen, C. (1997). The occupational therapy context: Philosophy-principles-practice. In C. Christiansen & C. Baum (Eds.), *Occupational therapy: Enabling function and well-being* (2nd ed., pp. 26–45). Thorofare, NJ: Slack.

Bernspang, B., Viitanen, M., & Eriksson, S. (1989). Impairments of perceptual and motor functions: Their influence on self-care ability 4–6 years after a stroke. *Occupational Therapy Journal of Research, 9*(1), 38–52.

Brandstater, M. (1998). Stroke rehabilitation. In J. DeLisa et al. (Eds.), *Rehabilitation medicine: Principles and practice* (3rd ed., pp. 1165–1189). Philadelphia: Lippincott Williams & Wilkins.

Bukowski, L., Bonavolonta, M., Keehn, M. T., & Morgan, K. A. (1996). Interdisciplinary roles in stroke care. *Nursing Clinics of North America, 21*, 359–374.

Carr, J. H., & Shepherd, R. B. (1987). *A motor relearning programme for stroke* (2nd ed.). Rockville, MD: Aspen.

Christiansen, C. H. (in press). Assessment and management of basic and extended daily living skills. In J. Delisa et al. (Eds.), *Rehabilitation medicine: Principles and practice* (4th ed.). Philadelphia: Lippincott, Williams & Wilkins.

Coster, W. (1998). Occupation centered assessment of children. *American Journal of Occupational Therapy, 52*, 337–344.

Daniel, M. S., & Strickland, L. R. (1992). Writing goals for documentation. In *Occupational therapy protocol management in adult physical dysfunction* (pp. 389–407). Gaithersburg, MD: Aspen.

Davidoff, G. N., Keren, O., Ring, H., & Solzi, P. (1991). Acute stroke patients: Long term effects of rehabilitation and maintenance of gains. *Archives of Physical Medicine and Rehabilitation, 72*, 869–873.

DeBow, S. B., Davies, M. L., Clarke, H. L., & Colbourne, F. (2003) Constraint-induced movement therapy and rehabilitation exercises lessen motor deficits and volume of brain injury after striatal hemorrhagic stroke in rats. *Stroke, 34*, 1021–1026

D'Esposito, M. (1997). Specific stroke syndromes. In V. M. Mills, W. Cassidy, & D. I. Katz (Eds.), *Neurologic rehabilitation: A guide to diagnosis, prognosis, and treatment planning* (pp. 59–103). Malden, MA: Blackwell Science.

DeVincenzo, D. K., & Watkins, S. (1987). Accidental falls in a rehabilitation setting. *Rehabilitation Nursing, 12*, 248–252.

Eto, F., Yoshikawa, M., Ueda, S., & Hirai, S. (1980). Posthemiplegic shoulder-hand syndrome, with special reference to related cerebral localization. *Journal of the American Geriatrics Society, 28*(1), 13–17.

Evans, R. L., Bishop, D. S., & Haselkorn, J. K. (1991). Factors predicting satisfactory home care after stroke. *Archives of Physical Medicine and Rehabilitation, 72*, 144–147.

Fasoli, S. E., Trombly, C. A., Tickle-Degnen, L., & Verfaellie, M. H. (2002). Effect of instructions on functional reach in persons with and without cerebrovascular accident. *American Journal of Occupational Therapy, 56*(4), 380–390.

Fisher, A. (1994). *Assessment of motor and process skills (Research edition 7.0)*. Fort Collins: Colorado State University.

Freeman, E. (2001). Unilateral spatial neglect: New treatment approaches with potential application to occupational therapy. *American Journal of Occupational Therapy, 55*, 401–408.

Gordon, W. A., & Hibbard, M. R. (1997). Poststroke depression: An examination of the literature. *Archives of Physical Medicine and Rehabilitation, 78*, 658–663.

Granger, C. V., Hamilton, B. B., & Gresham, G. E. (1988). The stroke rehabilitation outcome study: Part I. General description. *Archives of Physical Medicine and Rehabilitation, 69*, 506–509.

Granger, C. V., Hamilton, B. B., Gresham, G. E., & Kramer, A. A. (1989). The stroke rehabilitation outcome study: Part II. Relative merits of the total Barthel Index score and a four-item subscore in predicting patient outcomes. *Archives of Physical Medicine and Rehabilitation, 70*, 100–103.

Grant, J., & Hamilton, S. (1987). Falls in a rehabilitation center: A retrospective and comparative analysis. *Rehabilitation Nursing, 12*, 74–76.

Hasselkus, B. (1991). Ethical dilemmas in family caregiving for the elderly: Implications for occupational therapy. *American Journal of Occupational Therapy, 45*, 206–212.

Herrmann, N., Black, S. E., Lawrence, J., Szekely, C., & Szalai, J. P. (1998). The Sunnybrook stroke study. A prospective study of depressive symptoms and functional outcome. *Stroke, 29*, 618–624.

Hsieh, C., Sheu, C., Hsueh, I., & Wang, C. (2002). Trunk control as an early predictor of comprehensive activities of daily living function in stroke patients. *Stroke, 33*, 2626–2630.

Hunt, L. A., Murphy, G. F., Carr, D., Duchek, J. M., Buckles, V., & Morris, J. C. (1997). Reliability of the Washington University Road Test. A performance based assessment for drivers with dementia of the Alzheimer's type. *Archives of Neurology, 54*, 707–712.

Joe, B. E. (1995, October 19). Accelerating stroke rehab. *OT Week*, 14–15.

Katz, S., Ford, A. B., Moskowitz, M., Jackson, B. A., & Jaffe, M. W. (1963). Studies of illness in the aged. The index of ADL: A standardized measure of biological and psychosocial function. *Journal of the American Medical Association, 185*, 914–919.

Kelly-Hayes, M., Wolf, P. A., Kase, C. S., Gresham, G. E., Kannel, W. B., & D'Agostino, R. B. (1989). Time course of functional recovery after stroke: The Framingham study. *Journal of Neurologic Rehabilitation, 3*, 65–70.

Kraskowsky, L. H., & Finlayson, M. (2001). Factors affecting older adults' use of adaptive equipment: Review of the literature. *American Journal of Occupational Therapy, 55*, 303–310.

Kron, L., McGourty, L., Foto, M., Kronsnoble, S., Lossing, C., Rask, S., et al. (1988). Guidelines for occupational therapy documentation. In E. Hopkins & H. Smith

(Eds.), *Willard and Spackman's occupational therapy* (7th ed., pp. 811–813). Philadelphia: Lippincott.

Kwakkel, G., Kollen, B. J., VanderGrond, J., & Prevo, A. J. (2003). Probability of regaining dexterity in the flaccid upper limb. *Stroke, 34*, 2181–2186.

Law, M., Baptiste, S., McColl, M., Opzoomer, A., Polatajko, H., & Pollock, N. (1990). The Canadian Occupational Performance Measure: An outcome measure for occupational therapy. *Canadian Journal of Occupational Therapy, 57*(2), 82–87.

Lee, H. C., Lee, A. H., & Cameron, D. (2003). Validation of a driving simulator by measuring the visual attention skill of older adult drivers. *American Journal of Occupational Therapy, 57*, 324–328.

Lundqvist, A., Gerdle, B., & Ronnberg, J. (2000). Neuropsychological aspects of driving after a stroke—in the simulator and on the road. *Applied Cognitive Psychology, 14*, 135–150.

Lysack, C. L., & Neufeld, S. (2003). Occupational therapist home evaluations: Inequalities, but doing the best we can? *American Journal of Occupational Therapy, 57*, 369–379.

Ma, H., & Trombly, C. A. (2002). A synthesis of the effects of occupational therapy for persons with stroke, part II: Remediation of impairments. *American Journal of Occupational Therapy, 56*, 260–274.

Mahoney, F., & Barthel, D. (1965). Functional evaluation: The Barthel Index. *Maryland State Medical Journal, 14*, 56–61.

Mauthe, R., Haaf, D., Hayn, P., & Krall, J. (1996). Predicting discharge destination of stroke patients using a mathematical model based on six items from the Functional Independence Measure. *Archives of Physical Medicine and Rehabilitation, 77*, 10–30.

Miltner, W. H. R., Bauder, H., Sommer, M., Dettmers, C., & Taub, E. (1999). Effects of constraint-induced movement therapy on patients with chronic motor deficits after stroke: A replication. *Stroke, 30*, 586–592.

Mion, L. C., Gregor, S., Buettner, M., Chwurchak, D., Lee, O., & Paras, W. (1989). Falls in the rehabilitation setting: Incidence and characteristics. *Rehabilitation Nursing, 14*, 17–21.

Moyers, P. A. (1999). The guide to occupational therapy practice. *American Journal of Occupational Therapy, 53*, 247–322.

Ozer, M. N., Materson, R. S., & Caplan, L. R. (1994). *Management of persons with stroke*. St. Louis: Mosby.

Patel, A. T. (2001). Disability evaluation following stroke. *Physical Medicine and Rehabilitation Clinics of North America, 12*, 613–619.

Phillips, M. E., & Wolters, S. (1996). Assessment in practice: Common tools and methods. In C. B. Royeen (Ed.), *Stroke: Strategies, treatment, rehabilitation, outcomes, knowledge, and evaluation* (pp. 1–47). Bethesda, MD: American Occupational Therapy Association.

Ponte-Allan, M., & Giles, G. (1999). Goal setting and functional outcomes in rehabilitation. *American Journal of Occupational Therapy, 53*, 646–649.

Post-Stroke Rehabilitation Guideline Panel. (1995). *Post-stroke rehabilitation* (Clinical Practice Guideline No. 16; AHCPR Publication No. 95-0662). Rockville, MD: U.S. Department of Health and Human Services, Public Health Service, Agency for Health Care Policy and Research.

Roth, E. J. (1988). The elderly stroke patient: Principles and practices of rehabilitation management. *Topics in Geriatric Rehabilitation, 3*(4), 27–61.

Skilbeck, C., Wade, D., Langton-Hewer, R., & Wood, V. (1983). Recovery after stroke. *Journal of Neurology, Neurosurgery, and Psychiatry, 46*, 5–8.

Soderback, I. (1988). The effectiveness of training intellectual functions in adults with acquired brain damage. *Scandinavian Journal of Rehabilitation Medicine, 20*, 47–56.

Spencer, J., Hersch, G., Shelton, M., Ripple, J., Spencer, C., Dyer, C., et al. (2002). Functional outcomes and daily life activities of African-American elders after hospitalization. *American Journal of Occupational Therapy, 56*, 149–159.

The Stroke Association. (2003). *Driving after a stroke*. Retrieved October 21, 2003, from *http://stroke.org.uk/noticeboard/Driving.htm*.

Trombly, C. A., & Wu, C. (1999). Effect of rehabilitation tasks on organization of movement after stroke. *American Journal of Occupational Therapy, 53*, 333–344.

Uniform Data System for Medical Rehabilitation. (1993). *Guide for the Uniform Data Set for Medical Rehabilitation (Adult FIM), Version 4.0*. Buffalo, NY: Author.

Unsworth, C. A., & Cunningham, D. T. (2002). Examining the evidence base for occupational therapy with clients following stroke. *British Journal of Occupational Therapy, 65*, 21–29.

Vlahov, D., Myers, A. H., & Al-Ibrahim, M. S. (1990). Epidemiology of falls among patients in a rehabilitation hospital. *Archives of Physical Medicine and Rehabilitation, 71*, 8–12.

Walker, C. M., & Walker, M. F. (2001). Dressing ability after stroke: A review of the literature. *British Journal of Occupational Therapy, 64*, 449–454.

Weimar, C., Kurth, T., Kraywinkel, K., Wagner, M., Busse, O., Haberl, R. L., et al. (2002). Assessment of functioning and disability after ischemic stroke. *Stroke, 33*, 2053–2059.

Wishart, L. R., Lee, T. D., Janzen-Ezekiel, H., Marley, T. L., & Lehto, N. K. (2000). Application of motor learning principles: The physiotherapy client as a problem-solver. I: Concepts. *Physiotherapy Canada, 52*, 229–232.

Wojner, A. (1996). Optimizing ischemic stroke outcomes: An interdisciplinary approach to poststroke rehabilitation in acute care. *Critical Care Nursing Quarterly, 19*(2), 47–61.

Wolf, S. L., Lecraw, D. E., Barton, L. A., & Jann, B. B. (1989). Forced use of hemiplegic upper extremities to reverse the effect of learned nonuse among chronic stroke and head-injured patients. *Experimental Neurology, 104*(2), 125–132.

Chapter 11

Self-Care Strategies for People With Movement Disorders

JANET L. POOLE, PHD, OTR/L, FAOTA

KEY TERMS

adaptive strategies

assistive devices

augmentative communication

dysphagia

energy conservation

independent living movement

routines

OBJECTIVES

Upon completion of this chapter, the reader will be able to

- Identify the difference between occupational therapy aimed at remediation of performance skills and occupational therapy aimed at independent living;
- Describe factors to consider when recommending adaptive strategies;
- Describe adaptive strategies that involve equipment and techniques for feeding, meal management and shopping, community mobility, and communication for people with movement disorders;
- Describe adaptive strategies that involve routines and social support for communication, feeding, and meal management for people with movement disorders; and
- Identify ways in which routines and social supports can be facilitated.

This chapter presents anecdotal accounts of how adults with movement disorders view and manage daily occupations. Drawing from case examples, it suggests principles for problem solving from the perspectives of the client and the occupational therapist. This approach differs from the traditional presentation of problems according to disability and of solutions in terms of physical performance. The emphasis is on the client's perspective and experience of self, within the context of his or her social and physical environments, as they re-late to occupational performance. The chapter also describes the therapist's role in helping the client develop adaptive strategies. The chapter uses a framework that considers techniques, equipment, routines, and social supports as categories of adaptive strategies that help people with movement disorders compensate for the lack of or excess movement with which they must contend.

The material in this chapter is designed to help occupational therapists work with people who have movement disorders such as amyotrophic lateral

Table 11.1. Movement Disorder Terms and Examples of Associated Conditions

Term	Description	Example
Ataxia	Movement, usually of the extremities, that is reduced in speed and distorted in terms of timing and direction	Multiple sclerosis; Charcot–Marie–Tooth
Athetosis	Slow sinuous movement with fluctuations in tone and most commonly found in the distal extremities; more rhythmic and slower than choreiform movements; exacerbated by anxiety and attempted voluntary movements	Cerebral palsy; tardive dyskinesia
Bradykinesia	Slowness of movement resulting in a person "freezing"; often misinterpreted as depression and withdrawal; presents as a loss of spontaneity	Parkinson's disease
Chorea	Usually describes a random pattern of rapid, irregular, unpredictable, and involuntary contractions of a group of muscles; resulting clinical picture may be one of a "dancing" or "clownish" gait with the distal extremities more involved than the proximal ones; movements attenuated during sleep, exacerbated with stress and attempts at action	Huntington's chorea; tardive dyskinesia
Dystonia	Although often found as a clinical descriptor, is in fact used to describe a neurological syndrome in which there is an abnormality of tone; affects muscle groups in the trunk, neck, face, and proximal limbs; presents with slow, sustained, involuntary twisting movement patterns that may be generalized, segmental, or focal; confused with athetosis when slow, and chorea when rapid	
Hyperkinesia and hypokinesia	An excess and a paucity of movement, respectively; difficulty with initiation and enactment of a normal speed of movement	All movement disorders, with exception of amyotrophic lateral sclerosis
Spasticity	Extreme or excessive muscle tone; presents as resistance to passive movement; a constant cocontraction of muscle groups inhibiting relaxation pulls the body into abnormal patterns, rendering it vulnerable to deformities; exacerbated by effort	Cerebral palsy; multiple sclerosis
Rigidity	Resistance of proximal and axial muscles to passive movement; frequently experienced as stiffness and associated with pain	Parkinson's disease
Tremor	Simple, involuntary, rhythmic movement, frequently starting in the hands; difficult to differentiate from generalized shivering or shaking; frequently found at rest, but disappears in sleep; most pronounced under stress	Parkinson's disease; multiple sclerosis

Table 11.2. Summary Data of Major Motor Control Disorders: Manifestations and Presenting Problems

Condition	Features	Movement Problems
Amyotrophic lateral sclerosis	Motor neuron disease of rapid onset; more prevalent in men over 30; affects central and peripheral motor neurons	Progressive muscle weakness and atrophy distally, then proximally; fatigue
Cerebral palsy	Motor disorder resulting from a nonprogressive lesion in the developing brain, resulting in abnormal and fluctuating muscle tone and reflexes	Ataxia; athetosis; flaccidity; spasticity; or mixed pattern of movement affecting the limbs, trunk, head, and neck
Charcot–Marie–Tooth	Inherited, progressive, sensorimotor disorder of nervous system; included mild loss of sensation	Progressive muscle weakness starting in extremities, resulting in loss of balance and tripping
Duchenne muscular dystrophy	Hereditary and progressive disease of the muscles; onset in males ages 2 to 6 years; marked wasting of proximal muscle groups; moves distally	Rapidly progressive muscle weakness, initially affecting pelvic and pectoral groups; fatigue
Huntington's chorea	Hereditary, progressive disorder of the basal ganglia; characterized by abnormal, involuntary choreiform movements; amplified by progressive cognitive impairment	Abrupt, involuntary choreiform movements; exacerbated by stress and effort
Multiple sclerosis	Lesions in the central nervous system; demyelination results in a series of exacerbations and remissions; progressive weakness; sensory disturbances; cognitive damage	Progressive muscle weakness and spasticity; tremors, ataxia, and fatigue
Parkinson's disease	Degeneration of the basal ganglia; progressive; found most frequently in men and women more than 50 years of age; results in muscle rigidity, postural changes, dementia, loss of autonomic reflexes	Slowness in motor planning; difficulty initiating movement; tremors at rest and with intention; shuffling gait; slurred speech; symptoms exacerbated by fatigue and stress
Tourette's syndrome	Involuntary movement disorder; onset 2 to 5 years of age, primarily males; includes sensory disturbances, impulsivity, compulsive and ritualistic behaviors, with possible attention deficits	Recurrent involuntary, repetitive, rapid movements; hyperactivity; symptoms increase with stress

sclerosis, cerebral palsy, dystonia, Huntington's chorea, multiple sclerosis, muscular dystrophy, Parkinson's disease, tardive dyskinesia, and Tourette's syndrome. This list includes both hyper- and hypokinetic movement disorders, but it is not exhaustive (Jain & Francisco, 1998). Table 11.1 provides common definitions of frequently used terms, and Table 11.2 describes features and problems of selected movement disorders.

Framework for Identifying Problems in Occupational Performance

People with movement disorders face the challenge of living with too much or too little movement, which is associated with some degree of paralysis or weakness. Their actions are frequently difficult to start, stop, or control. Many conditions have a progressive component—which often is rapid. Some disorders create a disturbance in mental functioning that may affect memory, concentration, and the ability to organize and sequence events. Sensory abilities, including awareness of the body's posture, movement, and position in space (i.e., *proprioception*) may be impaired. Problems performing daily occupations often are intensified by stress and the aging process, even if the medical condition itself is stable (Finlayson, Impey, Nicolle, & Edwards, 1998; Watts & Koller, 1997). Many people with movement disorders experience pain and have constant fatigue; poor balance; and difficulties with most occupations, including communication, mobility, eating, dressing, toileting, bathing, and grooming (Finlayson et al., 1998).

A client's environment can support or inhibit independence. Social supports, cultural beliefs and values, environmental designs and furnishings, and the availability of structures and tools are all significant factors in a person's engagement in daily occupations. For that reason, when addressing problems with the performance of everyday occupations, it is important to evaluate and intervene within the context of the client's social, cultural, and physical environments (Christiansen, 2004).

Traditionally, medical rehabilitation focused on elimination of impairments (Christiansen, 2004). Problems related to daily occupations, however, often are addressed through adaptive strategies within the domains of techniques and equipment, routines, and social supports. Occupation-related needs can be met despite the presence of movement disorders and without emphasizing remediation of physical performance skills.

Occupational therapists who work with adults who have movement disorders need to be knowledgeable about the context of the client's life, committed to supporting the client's perspective, and willing to use approaches reflecting principles of the independent living movement. This framework requires occupational therapists to support clients' acquisition of skills and capabilities for self-direction and to acknowledge their ability to be managers who can communicate effectively, identify and use resources, make choices and decisions, set priorities, and make sound judgments (American Occupational Therapy Association, 2002).

Principles of Adaptations in Daily Living Activities

Adaptive strategies can be categorized in two domains: (1) techniques and equipment and (2) routines and social supports. *Techniques and equipment* are the actions or assistive devices a client uses to accomplish activities of daily living (ADL), which serve to organize life. *Routines* are the established sequences and patterns clients use to perform occupations, and *social supports* include the availability and expectations of significant people. Within these domains of adaptive strategies are areas of occupation, such as eating, communicating, mobility, and preparing a meal.

A client's choice of a specific adaptive strategy is not based on performance alone (Lyons & Tickle-Degnen, 2003; McCuaig & Frank, 1991). Deciding how to accomplish a task is highly dependent on values that determine the importance and order of potential actions. Such decisions also are based on

the client's occupational profile (including his or her history, values, and interests), the context of an activity, and the requirements of the situation.

All too often, the clinical focus in occupational therapy intervention has been to increase function without consideration of the context in which it is performed. Living with a movement disorder involves more than learning a number of techniques in a clinical setting or choosing a particular piece of equipment. Physical and social supports and limitations, as well as individual constraints and beliefs, strongly influence behavior and adaptation (Lyons & Tickle-Degnen, 2003). The choice of action or adaptive strategy will be shaped by temporal factors; client values; and client beliefs about the activity, self, and environment, as illustrated in the case example below (Law, 2002; Lyons & Tickle-Degnen, 2003).

Meghan, who has athetoid cerebral palsy, has personal criteria for choosing her adaptive strategies in self-care activities. Her criteria include being viewed as mentally competent, physically able, and socially acceptable (McCuaig & Frank, 1991). To carry out her activities, she chooses from a variety of strategies that include techniques and equipment, routines, and social resources. As might be expected, Meghan's choice of strategy is frequently based not on functional efficiency but on self-presentation (i.e., how she wishes to appear to others). She prefers techniques, equipment, routines, and people that support her appearance as a competent and socially and physically able person.

Meghan's athetosis, physical deformities, and inability to speak affect her ability to function. Therefore, if she makes tea for her sister, whom she believes views her as incompetent and dependent, she completes every step herself, from boiling the water to pouring the cream in the cups and serving the food. When she is with those whom she feels acknowledge her as a competent person, her desire to present a social self and to communicate are more important than her physical abilities. Under such circumstances, she will ask her guests to fix and serve the tea. This leaves her free to use her hands for pointing to her communication system to "chat" with her visitors. However, Meghan directs the activity: She indicates which dishes to use, notes where the items are located, and decides where tea will be served. Who is present and how she is perceived are more important considerations than simply getting the tea from the kettle into the cups.

In the preceding case example, Meghan has a repertoire of strategies for making tea and chooses one according to the context of the event. The case illustrates the point that the client's desired identity is a key factor in choosing an adaptive strategy (Christiansen, 1999).

Adaptive Strategies Using Equipment and Techniques

Adaptive strategies to address engagement in occupations for people with movement disorders often include methods or techniques involving either specialized or ordinary equipment. See Table 11.3 for factors to consider when making recommendations.

Equipment

Highly specialized equipment used by people with movement disorders might include power wheelchairs (which are discussed later in the chapter) and environmental control systems. Environmental control units are electronic switching devices that govern stereo sound systems, telephones, apartment intercoms, lights, fans, and televisions. They provide easy access to many functions within living environments for people lacking the dexterity, coordination, or strength to turn knobs or push buttons directly (Bain, 1996; Cook & Hussey, 2002). Computers with an Internet connection are not just a source of leisure for people with movement disorders but also are a means to completing instrumental tasks of daily living such as banking, bill paying, shopping, and socialization (Angelo & Buning, 2001; Cook & Hussey, 2002).

Table 11.3. Factors to Consider When Recommending Adaptive Strategies

What is important to the individual about the task?

Is the strategy viewed as compatible with the particular social context?

Does the strategy enhance the person's sense of personal control?

Does the strategy minimize effort?

Does the strategy interfere with social opportunities or diminish the presentation of self?

Is the recommended strategy temporally realistic, given the context?

Does the strategy provide for safety?

Some equipment may be "transparent"—that is, not readily identifiable as an adaptive device. Examples of transparent adaptive equipment include keyboards with widely spaced keys for people who lack the coordination and dexterity to type; felt-tipped pens for people too weak to exert pressure to write; and front-opening, lightweight clothing to make dressing easier for people with excess movement. Wall-mounted grab bars, which provide stability for transferring to the toilet, are becoming common in many apartment dwellings. Many people with movement disorders use commercially available nonskid mats and adhesive strips for bathtubs and showers. Several models of pagers and cellular phones have features that meet the needs of people with movement disorders (Barker, 2002). Commercially available equipment has several important advantages, including lower cost, availability, and service and maintenance warranties that frequently accompany major items. Manufacturers should be contacted before making modifications to ensure that adaptations will not jeopardize the item's warranty.

Assessment, prescription, and adaptation of equipment are familiar activities for occupational therapists. Batavia and Hammer (1990) noted the general absence of consumer-based criteria for the evaluation of equipment. Such criteria could benefit designers, manufacturers, funding agencies, occupational therapists and, ultimately, the consumers themselves. Batavia and Hammer cited research showing that important criteria for consumers include effectiveness, affordability, operability, acceptability, and dependability. Criteria ranking changed according to the equipment function. For example, acceptability (i.e., the aesthetics, or psychological "fit") was a high priority for something as personal as a power wheelchair but of little consequence in an environmental control unit to operate the stereo.

Criteria for equipment specifically to be used by people with movement disorders include an ability to undergo unusual physical force or stress, which includes falling and inadvertent, uncoordinated hitting. Equipment often needs to be lightweight (to compensate for weakness) as well as durable (to withstand being dropped or struck through excess movement). If a client has involuntary movement, safety factors such as stability, absence of sharp edges, and flexibility must be considered. Equipment may need extra padding, bolts may need to be covered, and raw edges may need to be smoothed or sanded. If the client has difficulty initiating and sustaining movement, then sensitivity to touch and the use of lightweight materials are important features of equipment. If the client's condition is deteriorating, the equipment must be flexible and easily, inexpensively, adaptable to meet changing requirements.

Techniques

Techniques are the methods a person uses in order to accomplish a task. Techniques often involve equipment. Adults with movement disabilities frequently use methods that have evolved over the years, often by trial and error, through family intervention, persistence, and experimentation. Techniques that appear to be awkward, uncoordinated, and precarious in fact may be finely honed and efficacious elements of a highly integrated system (see the example of Meghan).

The occupational therapist's role in teaching adaptive techniques to clients with movement disorders is to observe clients closely, assess them in their normal environments, and give attention to the larger and potentially fragile system of movement. Techniques designed for people with movement disorders require observation of timing and an understanding of peoples' adaptive use of their physical abilities and limitations. Body postures that decrease excessive movements and provide trunk support and proximal stability need to be taught and developed (see, e.g., Gillen, 2002). For people with decreased movement, as seen in Parkinson's disease, it is important for the occupational therapist to locate body parts that provide consistent, voluntarily controlled movement and do not fatigue easily. Auditory and visual cues may be necessary to facilitate initiation and speed of movement in clients with movement disorders. Several studies have shown that visual cues (e.g., lines on the floor) and auditory cues (e.g., the sound of a metronome) can increase functional ambulation speed in people with Parkinson's disease (Morris, Iansek, Matyas, & Summers, 1994; Thaut et al., 1996).

Energy-Conservation Strategies

Teaching strategies that minimize fatigue, conserve energy, enhance safety, and foster adequate stability (particularly postural stability) are essential for managing ADL for people with movement disorders (Baker & Tickle-Degnen, 2001; Gauthier, Dalziel, & Gauthier, 1987; Gillen, 2002; Mathiowetz, Matuska, & Murphy, 2001). A client who fatigues easily through the course of the day may need to have at least three different strategies for getting to the toilet: one using bars on the wall, one using a sliding transfer board, and one requiring the presence of another person for physical support. The choice of strategy will depend on the client's energy level, resources available, urgency, and timing. To save energy, people with movement disorders plan and prioritize their occupations and pace themselves. Energy-conservation education courses have been shown to be beneficial for people with multiple sclerosis (Mathiowetz et al., 2001; Vanage, Gilbertson, & Mathiowetz, 2003). Providing postural stability using lateral supports and a tilt-in-space wheelchair resulted in increased upper-extremity control in a man with multiple sclerosis, which allowed him to propel his wheelchair independently using a joystick (Gillen, 2002).

Adaptations for Specific Performance Areas

Feeding

Occupational therapists have paid considerable attention to the development of equipment and specialized techniques for self-feeding. Sophisticated feeding apparatus, such as the Winsford Feeder and the Beeson Automaddak Feeder (Cook & Hussey, 2002), move food from the plate to the mouth by means of a spoon set in motion with an electronic switch (Figure 11.1). In other instances, highly individualized devices are fabricated; for example, a feeding harness was developed for a man with amyotrophic lateral sclerosis (Takai, 1986). Nonskid mats, plate guards, weighted utensils, and utensil holders, such as the universal cuff, can enhance stability for people with movement disorders (Foti, 2001). People with poor coordination may use ordinary equipment, such as straws and heavy mugs. Although weights have been shown to decrease the amplitude of tremors in people with cerebellar tremors (McGruder, Cors, Tiernan, & Tomlin, 2003), one study reported that using weighted utensils or weight cuffs did not reduce tremors in people with Parkinson's disease (Meshack & Norman, 2002). Cold temperature also has been shown to decrease essential tremor, but not tremors from Parkinson's disease (Cooper et.al., 2000).

Difficulty swallowing, or *dysphagia*, frequently occurs in people with movement disorders, particularly those with amyotrophic lateral sclerosis, cerebral palsy, multiple sclerosis, and Parkinson's disease. This condition is potentially life threatening because of the possibility of aspiration and inadequate nutrition. Weakness of the tongue and palate leads to food retention in the mouth and throat and difficulty maneuvering food in the mouth, such that food may slip into the airway. Poor lip closure may

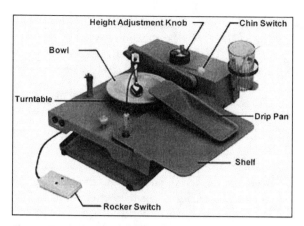

Figure 11.1. Model 5 Winsford Feeder; can be operated by chin or rocker switch.

Note. Available from Winsford Products, Inc. 179 Pennington-Harbourton Road, Pennington, NJ 08534; (609) 737-3311.

result in drooling. Often, correct evaluation and diagnosis, coupled with simple intervention, helps normalize oral food intake. Occupational therapy intervention for clients with dysphagia has been well-documented (Avery-Smith, 2001; Jenks, 2001).

We return to the example of Meghan, a woman with athetoid cerebral palsy, for examples of how techniques and equipment can be part of an adaptive strategy for meal management:

Meghan has deformities in her trunk and limbs and an inability to communicate verbally, so she uses her body as a tool to compensate for the changes in tone that make her movements difficult to predict and control (McCuaig & Frank, 1991). She holds a fork woven unconventionally in and out of the fingers of her right hand. She spears the food with her fork and, balancing on her forearm and elbow, brings the food to her mouth. Her chin rests on her chest with her neck rotated so that her left ear is almost touching her shoulder. This seemingly contorted body position provides the balance she lacks when sitting erect and decreases the effects of the excess movements in her arms when her elbow is not stabilized. A colorful, plastic-coated mat stabilizes her dishes, countering the excess movement in her hands. Meghan is not set apart as different from her mealtime partners by her use of "adapted" equipment. She uses ordinary utensils in extraordinary ways.

Equipment and techniques address only the functional aspect of moving food from the plate to the mouth. Of equal or greater importance for Meghan is the social context of meal management and eating. Although

Meghan often invites people for tea or lunch, she rarely eats at those functions. The physical stress of eating, the ensuing fatigue, and her inability to use her hands to access her communication systems when eating led to her decision not to eat with others. She explained her decision in the following comment: "The reason I very often don't eat with people is I feel I can eat after they go, but I won't be able to talk [after they are gone]."

Like most of us, Meghan uses the occasion of tea or meals for social purposes. Occupational therapists who emphasize the functional and nutritional aspects of mealtime management have sometimes overlooked this social aspect. Thus, important considerations for therapists in recommending equipment and techniques may be the extent to which they permit social interaction and whether independence in meal management is important to the client. Some of the questions that occupational therapists may need to answer in determining appropriate adaptive strategies for mealtimes are as follows:

- Is eating viewed as a social occasion?
- Is eating "independently" with equipment more important than the length of time or the physical effort it takes to finish a meal?
- Is appearance important and, if so, are the utensils attractive and pleasant to hold to the tongue and lips?
- Does the plate guard blend with the plate? Does the color of the nonskid mat clash with that of the table?
- Do the techniques, such as sliding rather than lifting, minimize effort?
- Does the independent use of the equipment detract from the potential social opportunities that arise when one person is fed by another (Einset, Deitz, Billingsley, & Harris, 1989)?
- What are the time considerations and the fatigue factors? Would several smaller meals per day be more manageable than the traditional three main meals?

Additional suggestions for adaptive strategies for feeding are described in the section "Adaptive Strategies Using Routines and Social Supports."

Mobility

Another factor identified as central for adults with movement disorders is independent mobility, both within and outside the person's dwelling (Reid, Laliberte-Rudman, & Hebert, 2002). The physical control a person has over the environment and the ease with which he or she can move within it influence feelings of independence, dignity, and competence. Physical control also helps conserve energy. Equipment recommended for mobility must be considered from perspectives other than function (Reid et al., 2002). Stronger than the desire to be mobile may be the need to maintain the view of an able self, which may not include using a wheelchair or power chair.

Clients with movement disorders may have substantial changes in ability and endurance over time, even during the course of a day. Accordingly, they may require highly flexible mobility systems. For example, a client with multiple sclerosis may wish to use a manual wheelchair for exercise in the morning and a power chair for transportation as the day and ensuing fatigue progress.

Particular concerns for occupational therapists in addressing powered mobility for people with movement disorders are physical and cognitive control, flexibility, and safety. Positioning for maximum stability is critical and may require special seating that provides trunk and head support. Proximal joints and limbs must be stabilized, and extraneous movements must be controlled in order to enhance distal control. In general, clients with severe movement disorders involving abnormal or fluctuating muscle tone require customized seating systems, which typically include carefully fabricated seating surfaces. Recently, Cook and Hussey (2002) provided a useful overview of the issues of seating and positioning for clients with different levels of need.

Once the most reliable, consistent, voluntarily controlled body movement and location have been determined, the mobility system's control mechanism (often a joystick) can be adapted to compensate for almost any degree of excess or lack of movement. Wheelchair control mechanisms can be mounted easily in various places on the chair: on the right, the left, centrally, under the chin, or at the back or side of the head. *Latching*, or "cruise control," is an option for clients who fatigue easily. Tremor dampening is a mechanical means for adjusting the sensitivity of switches so unintentional movement does not activate them. With this feature, switches can be adjusted to work appropriately with almost any degree of excess movement. The speed at which the braking system engages also can be adjusted for clients with a startle reflex. Particular safety points for powered mobility systems include replacing square-headed bolts with round ones, padding sharp edges, removing heel loops if necessary, and using safety belts and antitipping devices.

Meghan uses a conventional power wheelchair with a joystick; the footrests have been removed. This chair, along with ramped sidewalks, paved roads, and an accessible apartment, gives her the independence she requires to get about in her home environment, go to her appointments, do her shopping, and visit friends who are within commuting distance. She can approach and leave clerks, friends, store displays, and buildings with the same timing, speed, and grace as the general public. She moves across busy streets during the prescribed "walk" interval.

Meghan's ability to extend her body image to include the wheelchair is an important adaptation in her mastery of techniques and the use of equipment. A cloth sack made by a friend hangs over her wheelchair handles, allowing Meghan to carry items in the same manner in which a person might use a backpack or a tote bag over a shoulder. Meghan hangs her purse on the right side of the chair. She has personalized the chair with a sticker saying, "Writers have the last word." When looking at Meghan, one had the sense not of a person confined in a wheelchair, but of an individual unit, a "goodness of fit."

Community Mobility

Occupational therapists must carefully assess the driving potential of clients with movement disorders. Possible perceptual and cognitive involvement may make it difficult for clients to compensate for the changes in speed and direction needed to safely operate motor vehicles. Decisions must be made regarding vehicle selection and access. In addition, seating and positioning must be considered if the client is going to sit in the wheelchair when driving. Numerous options are available for hand controls for braking, accelerating, steering, and gripping. If an evaluation determines that driving is not an option, transportation by personal and public transportation is becoming more accessible to people with movement disorders. Cook and Hussey (2002) stated that users of personal and public transportation need to be concerned with wheelchair tie-downs, occupant restraint systems, and the seating system of the wheelchair. Cook and Hussey (2002) and Babirad (2002) discussed how to make decisions about driving assessment and transportation technology.

Communication

People engage in different modes of communication, but the main forms are conversation and messaging. *Conversation* is commonly thought of as a brief, temporal, and spontaneous verbal exchange. Conversation includes changes in intonation and timing and is accompanied by facial expressions, gestures, and body language. It can take place face-to-face, over the telephone, or simultaneously with an activity. *Messaging* is the delayed presentation of previously prepared information. Common tools for messaging include pens or pencils, typewriters, fax machines, telephone answering devices, and computers. When someone is unable to use conventional modes and tools of communication for conversation or sending messages, the dynamics and quality of the interaction are affected.

Augmentative communication includes any personal or technical system that enhances a person's present communication abilities. Devices may produce speech, a visual display, or a written message. Clients use body parts, such as a hand, the head, or eyes, to access devices directly or indirectly (Cook & Hussey, 2002).

Meghan has a wide variety of universal or ordinary communication devices, including felt-tipped pens, an electric typewriter with widely spaced keys, a computer, and a telephone. She also uses specialized equipment, including an 8.5" × 11" letter board indicating the letters of the alphabet, to which she points to spell her message; a small, portable, battery-operated communication device with keys that she presses to produce a ticker-tape printed message; and a device attached to her telephone that produces synthesized sounds in the form of letters and enables her to spell messages to callers. Meghan also uses her voice, facial expressions, and gestures to convey messages. She has a repertoire of equipment and techniques from which to choose according to the context of the communication that is taking place. Meghan's choice of equipment is based on her desire to present an able self, her need to accommodate the demands of the situation, and her expectations of the exchange. If Meghan is having a conversation with a friend, she likes to sit close to him or her and use the letter board; she points to the letters as she spells out her message, and her friend repeats the letters and says the resulting words. Although this method is slow (approximately 12 words per minute), it allows Meghan to make frequent eye contact and stay engaged with her conversation partner. She can use her other hand to gesture, and she can use her face and body to express feelings. The "voice" is personal and not synthesized.

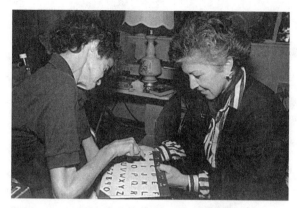

Figure 11.2. Meghan communicating through her letter board.

When Meghan is in a public place, such as the drug store, a situation that has fewer personal communication expectations, she uses her electronic communicator. The attractive device resembles a small pocket calculator and produces a written message that is easy to see and is understood by anyone who can read. Meghan has attempted to use her letter board in public, but people reacted as though she were mentally impaired. She has found that people are interested in her communication device, and it serves as a conversational icebreaker for people who are not familiar with her methods. When interacting with a store clerk, Meghan needs only to deliver a message to obtain the items she requires.

Meghan's desire to present a sophisticated and capable image is supported by her use of her communication device in public. In evaluating and designing interventions for communication needs, occupational therapists work closely with speech and language pathologists to determine access to the equipment and the requirements of the social and physical environment. For people who have movement disorders, specific recommendations for communication needs include enlarged pencils, writing aids that hold a pen or pencil, and felt-tipped pens. People who can use typewriters, computers, or electronic communicators might also need key guards, which prevent more than one key from being pressed at the same time and help compensate for poor coordination. Enlarged computer keyboards are useful for people who lack the fine motor skills to access a standard size keyboard. Mini-keyboards are available for people who lack range and muscle strength in their upper extremities (Cook & Hussey, 2002).

Often a client has sufficient control of the head and neck to permit the use of mouth sticks or head wands for operating augmentative communication devices (see Jasch, 2002, for a review of mouth stick types and uses). Mouth sticks made of lightweight doweling or arrow shafts with rubber tubing on the end may be useful for people with adequate neck and jaw control and movement. Smith (1989) noted that inadequate attention has been given to the potential problems from improperly fitted mouth sticks, which include, in addition to dental problems, fatigue, gagging, and temporal mandibular joint dysfunction. Therapists are urged to consider the techniques described by Duncan and Puckett (1993) when prescribing or fabricating mouth sticks. Head pointers, which can be custom made or obtained commercially, offer another option for using augmentative communication devices.

Several other considerations are important when determining appropriate equipment and techniques for communication:

- The speed of message transmission
- The portability of the system
- The device's reliability and flexibility
- Whether the device can be used spontaneously
- The system's potential for communicating the message completely (i.e., not just the words, but the intended meaning and tone).

An augmentative communication system should require as little expenditure of energy as possible for both the sender and receiver of the message. It must enhance the user's personal abilities and, whenever possible, encourage physical gestures and expressions of sound. The equipment also must meet the requirements of the physical and social environment.

Adaptive Strategies Using Routines and Social Supports

Behaviors that are repeated over time and organized into patterns and habits form routines. Routines and the use of social supports are adaptive strategies for people with movement disorders because they compensate for the inability to perform certain activities, the additional time and energy required to accomplish tasks, and limited coordination and strength. Social supports include family and friends, casual acquaintances, formal and informal organizations, and health care workers. Frequently, a client's strategy for accomplishing a task uses a unique combination of equipment, techniques, routines, and social supports.

The use of routines and social supports often depends on specific factors. The person engaging in

the routine needs to know that a certain activity or interaction is going to take place and what the requirements of the situation will be. He or she also must have time to plan, a well-developed ability to organize personal and environmental resources, a sense of how long an activity will take, and an understanding of the specific steps involved and the amount of energy required. Routines generally are predictable and familiar; clients generally have used a given routine successfully in the past under similar, if not exact, conditions. Social supports must be initiated, nurtured, and developed and are not as predictable as routine.

Communication Routines

For an illustration of how a client might use a communication routine, consider the following case example.

Emma has amyotrophic lateral sclerosis and lives in a long-term-care unit. She uses a variety of techniques and equipment for communication to adapt to her inability to speak and her lack of movement in her limbs. She has a letter board to which she can point with hand movements that are slow and difficult. She also has a computerized message system, which she operates with a microswitch in her palm, and a system of blinking, which she uses along with her communication partner's verbal spelling. In addition, Emma has established routines for communication that are considered adaptive because of their premeditated, compensatory nature.

Like Meghan, Emma determines which strategy to use after considering outcome, context, and values. She decides in advance the purpose of the communication, the intended recipient of the message, what she expects from the exchange, and what is important for her to achieve. Emma decides ahead of time whether it is more important to save the other person time by having information ready, or whether the conversation process and the elements of the interaction are of greater significance than the message itself. One of Emma's routines for communicating is to provide her communication partner with information that she writes using and prints out from her computer. This routine requires Emma's knowledge of the visit before it occurs, adequate time to compose her thoughts and messages at the computer, and the ability of her communication partner to read.

Emma is highly aware of the importance of her social support system and consciously works at sustaining those networks. It requires much more of Emma's time, but significantly less of her partner's, if she puts her thoughts on paper before the interaction. The printouts also provide the partner with something to read and on which to focus. Emma can work at her own pace at her computer when she has the energy, and she can take rest periods; in conversation, such rest periods would be awkward and possibly stressful for the partner.

Many people with movement disorders that include loss of speech struggle with other people assuming one disability based on the presence of another (Pentland, Gray, Riddle, & Pitcairn, 1988). An inability to speak is frequently equated with an inability to think. Emma's strategy of communicating with people through a prepared note helps dispel any misconceptions the conversation partner might have of her cognitive abilities. The notes contain witticisms, inquiries about the partner's well-being, social comments about the news or weather, descriptions of Emma's sons' activities, and her feelings about events on the ward. Emma presents herself as a socially competent woman who is full of ideas and feelings and actively engaged in life.

Meal-Preparation and Shopping Routines

The following incident demonstrates the use of routines and social supports as an adaptive strategy for meal preparation and shopping:

> Lee is a woman who has Parkinson's disease, which has resulted in intention tremor in her upper extremities, head, and neck; a slow and shuffling gait; rigidity in her trunk; and slurred speech. She shares a home with her elderly husband. Having friends in for tea once a week is an important social event for her. When her guests arrive, the cups and saucers, along with the cream and sugar, napkins, and a cake, are set out on a cart. During the tea, Lee plays the host, directing the event. She manages everything: She decides when to hold the tea, what to serve, and who will pour. She has a keen sense of timing, is extremely gracious and social in her requests, is well-organized, and gives clear directions.
>
> For Lee to execute this ordinary but important occasion, she must invest considerable planning time and effort. She needs to travel in her scooter to the local mall to buy the cake and other grocery items and transport them safely home. She has to have her cups clean and arranged on the tray ahead of time. Her problems with strength, balance, manipulation, and coordination make an apparently easy task one that requires considerable orchestration.

Eating Routines

For many people with movement disorders, eating can be an exhausting and undignified experience, whether managing food independently or being fed. Getting the food on the utensil, bringing it safely to the lips, keeping it in the mouth, chewing adequately, swallowing smoothly, and maintaining a comfortable posture can involve great physical and emotional strain. Weighted handles, nonskid mats, plate guards, and even automatic feeding devices often are inadequate to support a client's nutritional, social, and personal needs related to eating. As with other ADL, function alone is not sufficient for a satisfying experience at mealtime. Although being fed brings its own set of problems, it is often the strategy of choice for people unable to manage a meal in a reasonable amount of time and with a minimum of effort. Consider the following case example:

> Catherine, a young woman with cerebral palsy living in an extended-care facility, prefers to be fed rather than to feed herself. She has spent countless hours practicing and has tried different pieces of equipment and physical positions. The combination of her severe athetoid movements, poor head control, and general weakness makes eating independently an unpleasant chore. She now prefers to spend her energy writing at her computer, visiting with friends, and going to school. To make her mealtime pleasant, she has asked to be fed in her room and to invite one other person who also needs to be fed to join her and the aide who is feeding her. When she orders her meal, she includes an extra tea and biscuit for the aide. This is a treat for the aide, and it adds to the feeling of the meal being more of a shared and social experience. Catherine also has the television turned on to her favorite soap opera at noon and to the news in the evening. This, too, is a treat for the aide, and it gives them something on which to focus and to discuss. The conversation, the tea, and the company promote a relaxed atmosphere and help minimize the aide's potential boredom and, therefore, his or her stress.

When occupational therapists plan mealtime interventions, they always should consider how to create an environment that promotes eating as an enjoyable social event rather than as simply a nutritional exercise. At its best, eating is an intimate affair; at its worst, it is traumatic. Whenever possible, the physical environment should promote relaxation and comfort. Attention should be given to room temperature, noise level, and visual stimulation, particularly if the client has a sensitive startle reaction. A quiet room may suit one client, whereas other clients might prefer company. Clients who need to be fed can be taught how to engage the interest and attention of the person feeding them. They can be encouraged to take control of choices by determining what foods to eat, when to eat them and how quickly, and the order in which they are presented. Clients also can help identify which elements of the mealtime event are stressful and collaborate with practitioners to address them.

Sexuality

Sexuality is another important concern of people with movement disorders. Physical impairments such as tone, contractures, loss of mobility, fatigue, medications and, in some cases, actual sexual dysfunction may affect sexuality (Burton, 2001). Primary dysfunction, such as erectile dysfunction and decreased vaginal lubrication, can be managed with medications. Tone, contractures, and loss of mobility can be managed by using pillows to support body parts, experimenting with different positions, and creative problem solving by the client and his or her partner. Energy-conservation techniques, such as engaging in sexual relations when the person with the movement disorder has the most energy and assuming positions that use less energy, are helpful in managing fatigue (Burton, 2001; Sipski & Alexander, 1997).

Facilitating the Development of Routines and Social Supports

Research on several movement disorders, including multiple sclerosis (Somerset, Peters, Sharp, & Campbell, 2003), Parkinson's disease (Karlsen, Tandberg, Arsland, & Larsen, 2000), and amyotrophic lateral sclerosis (Young & McNicoll, 1998), suggests that social psychological variables play the most important role in adjustment to such diseases. In particular, integrating the realities of a disease into one's lifestyle and creating strong social support networks have been identified as important variables for people with progressive, episodic, and debilitating neuromotor conditions. Thus, the development of adaptive routines and social supports is an effective therapeutic strategy.

Therapists can help clients who have all types of movement disorders develop strategies that use routines and social supports by facilitating their repeated action beyond basic problem solving until a routine is established and acceptable to the client and those in his or her environment. During this process, therapists should help develop routines that minimize stress and conserve energy. Routines require planning and organization to allow people to do their most important activities when they have the most energy, maximizing both safety and enjoyment.

Therapy sessions can be planned to support the shift in the client's focus from the physical to the cognitive domain. A client who is no longer able to execute an activity physically may need to learn to organize and plan in order to direct care. Overvaluing the concept of independence may lead to goals that seek to achieve levels of function that are too costly in terms of expended energy. Assistance with personal care may be preferable to independence in ADL if the physical and mental costs of attaining independence interfere with social interaction or life satisfaction (Gillette, 1991). Social supports must be sought out, developed, nurtured, and maintained. Attention must be given to ways in which the distress, enormous effort, and tedium of living with and supporting someone with a physical disability can be managed so that important social supports can be maintained as integral components of a client's adaptive strategies.

Summary

It is important for occupational therapists to focus on strategies that minimize fatigue, enhance safety, and reduce stress. To manage self-care, people with movement disorders must attend to issues involving organization, pacing, timing, and energy conservation (Mathiowetz et al., 2001). A philosophy of independent living that emphasizes the importance of a person's acquisition of skills and capabilities for self-direction in managing physical and social resources has been embraced in this chapter. This philosophy, however, also acknowledges that a person can exhibit an independent spirit while accepting assistance from others and that all adaptive strategies must be considered in terms of their contribution to well-being and life satisfaction. In working with clients with movement disorders, the role of the therapist is to help the client identify an array of adaptive strategies that can be used comfortably within the context of the client's daily life.

Acknowledgment

The research and contributions of Margaret McCuaig to earlier versions of this chapter are appreciated.

Study Questions

1. What is energy conservation, and how is it used for people with movement disorders?
2. What types of adaptive strategies or equipment are useful for communication, mobility, meal preparation, and feeding?
3. List two examples of adaptive strategies for communication, mobility, meal preparation, and feeding.
4. What are important factors to consider when recommending equipment for people with movement disorders?
5. How can routines and social supports be facilitated?

References

American Occupational Therapy Association. (2002). Occupational therapy practice framework: Domain and process. *American Journal of Occupational Therapy, 56,* 609–639.

Angelo, J., & Buning, M. E. (2001). High-technology adaptations to compensate for disability. In C. A. Trombly & M. V. Radomski (Eds.), *Occupational therapy for physical dysfunction* (5th ed., pp. 389–419). Philadelphia: Lippincott Williams & Wilkins.

Avery-Smith, W. (2001). Dysphagia. In C. A. Trombly & M. V. Radomski (Eds.), *Occupational therapy for physical dysfunction* (5th ed., pp. 1091–1109). Philadelphia: Lippincott Williams & Wilkins.

Babirad, J. (2002). Driver evaluation and vehicle modification. In D. A. Olson & F. DeRuyter (Eds.), *Clinician's guide to assistive technology* (pp. 351–386). St. Louis: Mosby.

Bain, B. (1996). Environmental controls and robotics. In J. Hammel (Ed.), *Technology and occupational therapy: A link to function* (pp. 1–44). Bethesda, MD: American Occupational Therapy Association.

Baker, N. A., & Tickle-Degnen, L. (2001). The effectiveness of physical, psychological, and functional interventions in treating clients with multiple sclerosis: A meta-analysis. *American Journal of Occupational Therapy, 55,* 324–331.

Barker, P. (2002). Information technology. In D. A. Olson & F. DeRuyter (Eds.), *Clinician's guide to assistive technology* (pp. 115–164). St. Louis: Mosby.

Batavia, A. I., & Hammer, G. S. (1990). Toward the development of consumer-based criteria for the evaluation of assistive devices. *Journal of Rehabilitation Research, 27,* 425–436.

Burton, G. U. (2001). Sexuality and physical dysfunction. In L. W. Pedretti & M. B. Early (Eds.), *Occupational therapy: Practice skills for physical dysfunction* (5th ed., pp. 212–225). St. Louis: Mosby.

Christiansen, C. H. (1999). Defining lives: Occupation as identity: An essay on competence, coherence, and the creation of meaning. *American Journal of Occupational Therapy 53,* 547–558.

Christiansen, C. H. (2004). Functional evaluation and management of self care and other activities of daily living. In J. DeLisa, B. Gans et al. (Eds.), *Rehabilitation medicine: Principles and practice* (4th ed., pp. 137–165). Philadelphia: Lippincott Williams & Wilkins.

Cook, A. M., & Hussey, S. M. (2002). *Assistive technologies: Principles and practice* (2nd ed.). St. Louis: Mosby.

Cooper, C., Evidente, V. G. H., Hentz, J. G., Adler, C. H., Caviness, J. N., & Gwinn-Hardy, K. (2000). The effect of temperature on hand function in patients with tremor. *Journal of Hand Therapy, 13,* 276–288.

Duncan, J. D., & Puckett, A. D., Jr. (1993). A one-appointment mouthstick appliance. *Journal of Prosthodontics, 2,* 196–198.

Einset, K., Deitz, J., Billingsley, F., & Harris, S. R. (1989). The electric feeder: An efficacy study. *Occupational Therapy Journal of Research, 9,* 38–52.

Finlayson, M., Impey, M. W., Nicolle, C., & Edwards, J. (1998). Self-care, productivity, and leisure limitations of people with multiple sclerosis in Manitoba. *Canadian Journal of Occupational Therapy, 65,* 299–308.

Foti, D. (2001). Activities of daily living. In L. W. Pedretti & M. B. Early (Eds.), *Occupational therapy: Practice skills for physical dysfunction* (5th ed., pp. 124–171). St. Louis: Mosby.

Gauthier, L., Dalziel, S., & Gauthier, S. (1987). The benefits of group occupational therapy for patients with Parkinson's disease. *American Journal of Occupational Therapy, 41,* 360–365.

Gillen, G. (2002). Improving mobility and community access in an adult with ataxia. *American Journal of Occupational Therapy, 56,* 462–466.

Gillette, N. (1991). The challenge of research in occupational therapy. *American Journal of Occupational Therapy, 45,* 660–662.

Jain, S. S., & Francisco, G. E. (1998). Parkinson's disease and the movement disorders. In J. DeLisa et al. (Eds.), *Rehabilitation medicine: Principles and practice* (2nd ed., pp. 1045–1056). Philadelphia: Lippincott-Raven.

Jasch, C. R. (2002). Adaptive aids for self-care and child care at home. In D. A. Olson & F. DeRuyter (Eds.), *Clinician's guide to assistive technology* (pp. 405–423). St. Louis: Mosby.

Jenks, K. N. (2001). Dysphagia: Evaluation and treatment. In L. W. Pedretti & M. B. Early (Eds.), *Occupational therapy: Practice skills for physical dysfunction* (5th ed., pp. 730–766). St. Louis: Mosby.

Karlsen, K. H., Tandberg, E., Arsland, D., & Larsen, J. P. (2000). Health related quality of life in Parkinson's disease: A prospective longitudinal study. *Journal of Neurology, Neurosurgery, and Psychiatry, 69,* 584–589.

Law, M. (2002). Participation in the occupations of everyday life. *American Journal of Occupational Therapy, 56,* 640–649.

Lyons, K. D., & Tickle-Degnen, L. (2003). Dramaturgical challenges of Parkinson's disease. *Occupational Therapy Journal of Research, 23,* 27–34.

Mathiowetz, V., Matuska, K. M., & Murphy, M. E. (2001). Efficacy of an energy conservation course for persons with multiple sclerosis. *Archives of Physical Medicine and Rehabilitation, 82,* 449–456.

McCuaig, M., & Frank, G. (1991). The able self: Adaptive patterns and choices in independent living for a person with cerebral palsy. *American Journal of Occupational Therapy, 45,* 224–243.

McGruder, J., Cors, D., Tiernan, A. M., & Tomlin, G. (2003). Weighted wrist cuffs for tremor reduction during eating in adults with static brain lesions. *American Journal of Occupational Therapy, 57,* 507–516.

Meshack, R. P., & Norman, K. E. (2002). A randomized controlled trial of the effects of weights on amplitude and frequency of postural hand tremor in people with Parkinson's disease. *Clinical Rehabilitation, 16,* 481–492.

Morris, M. E., Iansek, R., Matyas, T. A., & Summers J. J. (1994). The pathogenesis of gait hypokinesia in Parkinson's disease. *Brain, 117,* 1169–1181.

Pentland, B., Gray, J. M., Riddle, W. J., & Pitcairn, T. K. (1988). The effects of reduced non-verbal communication in Parkinson's disease. *British Journal of Disorders of Communication, 23,* 31–34.

Reid, D., Laliberte-Rudman, D., & Hebert, D. (2002). Impact of wheeled seated mobility devices on adult users' and their caregivers' occupational performance: A critical literature review. *Canadian Journal of Occupational Therapy, 69,* 261–280.

Sipski, M., & Alexander, C. (1997). *Sexual function in people with disability and chronic illness.* Gaithersburg, MD: Aspen.

Smith, R. (1989). Mouthstick design for the client with spinal cord injury. *American Journal of Occupational Therapy, 43,* 251–255.

Somerset, M., Peters, T. J., Sharp, D. J., & Campbell, R. (2003). Factors that contribute to quality of life outcomes prioritized by people with multiple sclerosis. *Quality of Life Research, 12,* 21–29.

Takai, V. L. (1986). Case report: The development of a feeding harness for an ALS patient. *American Journal of Occupational Therapy, 40,* 359–361.

Thaut, M. H., McIntosh, G. C., Rice, R. R., Miller, R. A., Rathbun, J., & Brault, J. M. (1996). Rhythmic auditory stimulation in gait training for Parkinson's disease patients. *Movement Disorders, 11,* 193–200.

Vanage, S. M., Gilbertson, K. K., & Mathiowetz, V. (2003). Effects of an energy conservation course on fatigue impact for persons with progressive multiple sclerosis. *American Journal of Occupational Therapy, 57,* 315–323.

Watts, R. L., & Koller, W. C. (1997). *Movement disorders: Neurologic principles and practice.* New York: McGraw-Hill.

Young, J. M., & McNicoll, P. (1998). Against all odds: Positive life experiences of people with advanced amyotrophic lateral sclerosis. *Health & Social Work, 23,* 35–43.

Chapter 12

Managing Daily Activities in Adults With Upper-Extremity Amputations

SANDRA FLETCHALL, OTR, CHT, MPA

DIANE J. ATKINS, OTR, FISPO

KEY TERMS

biscapular abduction

body-power prosthesis

disarticulation

electronic prosthesis

greifer

humeral flexion

hybrid prosthesis

myoelectric prosthesis

specialized amputee clinic

specialized amputee team

terminal device

transhumeral amputation

transradial amputation

OBJECTIVES

Upon completion of this chapter, the reader will be able to

- Identify some assessments appropriate for determining whether a client is a candidate for a prosthesis;
- Identify when a preprosthetic program can begin;
- List goals of a preprosthetic program;
- Name the components of success that lead to incorporation of the prosthesis into daily life; and
- Describe the differences among a body-power, myoelectric, and electronic prosthesis.

Upper-extremity amputation presents a complex loss for the client. The hand functions in prehensile activities as a sensory organ and as a means of communication. Any loss interferes with the client's productivity and feeling of completeness and alters his or her interactions with the environment (Bennett & Alexander, 1989).

Everyone with an upper-extremity amputation is unique, and no two amputations are identical. The ability to acquire independence in performance areas such as self-care, work, and leisure is frequently attributed to performance skills in the upper extremities. Without motor, sensory, grasp, and prehension skills, a client who has sustained bilateral loss of the upper extremities may not be able to resume satisfactory performance in important occupations; this change may lead to depression or a feeling of helplessness. The occupational therapist, through evaluation of existing sensory and motor skills, preexisting process and communication skills, and environmental influences such as cultural and social contexts, develops an intervention plan unique to such clients to improve their level of independence, self-confidence, and body image.

With appropriate intervention, most clients with upper-extremity amputation can resume independence in activities of daily living (ADL) and instrumental activities of daily living (IADL) and return to work or education environments. People with amputations of bilateral short transhumeral or bilateral shoulder disarticulations may have difficulty achieving independence in all areas of daily living, although performance in selected ADL, IADL, and return to work or school environments is feasible.

When clients are provided the appropriate training and education, they often can return to independent living and regain good bilateral upper-extremity use. Sudden loss of the upper extremity as the result of an illness or trauma does not disrupt the motor cortex in the central nervous system; thus, motor control, motor learning, and coordination remain intact. Through the program developed by the occupational therapist, the prosthesis is incorporated into the body image and integrated into the client's activities and occupations. Therapy provides the client with the opportunity to use the prosthesis in everyday life; however, the client makes the final decision to wear and use a prosthesis.

This chapter focuses on the process of prosthetic and prosthetic training. It presents case studies to illustrate concepts and demonstrate the outcomes that can be achieved in occupational therapy programs.

> *We are often enriched by the personal aura and spirit of persons who manage life with disabilities, each in his individual special way.*
>
> (Marquardt, 1989, p. 242)

The Preprosthetic Therapy Program

If the occupational therapist works closely with surgeons who perform upper-extremity amputations, the preprosthetic program can began within a few hours of the surgery to within 2 to 3 weeks after surgery. Early intervention can involve wound care, edema control, residual limb shaping, and assessment of the client's desired areas of future performance in ADL, IADL, leisure, work, or school.

Educating nursing staff about potential accomplishments of patients with amputations can create an environment of hope and opportunity. Length of inpatient hospital stay following uncomplicated upper-extremity amputation currently ranges from 1 to 7 days. Patients with bilateral uncomplicated, upper-extremity amputations may have a short inpatient rehabilitation stay, with most occupational therapy occurring in an outpatient setting.

Regardless of the client's unique social, cultural, or physical contexts, the preprosthetic therapy program's general goals are as follows:

- To provide residual-limb edema control and shaping
- To promote residual-limb tolerance to sensory stimuli
- To maintain or acquire normal joint range of motion
- To increase muscle strength and endurance of the total body and residual limb
- To provide education regarding residual-limb hygiene
- To assess the client's preinjury and postinjury performance roles
- To initiate training to acquire independence in selected basic ADL
- To educate the client about appropriate prosthetic options
- To assess the client's learning style and visual-motor skills
- To assess the client's voluntary motor control of the residual limb. Voluntary motor responses are needed if myoelectric prosthetic components are to be prescribed (Atkins, 1989b; Fletchall, 1998).

Assessment of voluntary muscle control helps determine whether peripheral nerve injury has been sustained. Understanding the client's learning style (e.g., kinestic, visual, auditory) enables the occupational therapist to adapt his or her approach to the client when presenting new information and designing the intervention.

The Prosthetic Training Program

The prosthetic training program will be more successful in reaching the client's desired goals if the occupational therapist provides education on the functions and components of the prosthesis and how it can be used to accomplish valued daily activities. The training program also will be more effective if time frames for achieving identified tasks are established and if training quickly progresses to client-directed activities. The training program is considered effective or successful if it leads to the client's acceptance of the prosthesis as a tool to improve performance (Atkins, 1989a; Fletchall & Hickerson, 1991).

The client's learning is facilitated by conducting the therapy in a quiet environment. Initial sessions should familiarize the client with the prosthetic components and terminology. The design of the harness should be based on collaboration among the occupational therapist, prosthetist, and physician. The client's physical abilities, prosthetic components, and goals all influence the style of the harness.

During the initial session, training should be directed toward donning and doffing procedures for the prosthesis. Clients with bilateral high-upper-extremity amputations may require innovation and creativity in techniques to achieve independence in donning and doffing the prosthesis. Daily use of the prosthesis can be influenced by the ease of donning, comfortable fit, and cosmetic appearance (Atkins, 1994).

Training should progress to body motions appropriate for operating the terminal device, elbow, or shoulder. Even with prostheses for high-level amputations, training should begin with simple grasp and release of items before progressing to operation of the other components. Performing activities at tabletop height requires less motor response from the client compared to self-care activities (e.g., feeding self, grooming). Training activities involving bilateral upper-extremity use should be performed sitting and standing, just as the client would perform basic ADL in his or her environment.

Pre-positioning of the terminal device, elbow, or shoulder is important to incorporating the prosthesis into tasks in a time-efficient manner. Appropriate instruction in pre-positioning the prosthetic components can minimize irritation of the noninvolved extremity secondary to abnormal posturing. One method of instructing the client to pre-position the prosthesis is to have the client attempt to simulate the position of the nonamputated extremity by positioning the components of the prothesis (e.g., wrist flexion, terminal device supinated or pronated; Atkins, 1989a).

Providing activities that lead to success will further reinforce the value of the prosthesis. The occupational therapist can grade the difficulty of activities progressing from simple grasp-and-release to use of the prosthesis in self-care. The clinic provides an environment for performing bilateral upper-extremity tasks such as cutting food, opening jars, tying shoes, preparing meals, driving, and using hand and power tools. Incorporation of the prosthesis into the client's leisure activities also should be explored, taking care to identify procedures for safety. Treatment in a clinic with other clients with amputations reinforces the functional value of the prosthesis, assists with psychological acceptance of the amputation and injury, and reinforces the accomplishment of established goals (Figure 12.1; Fletchall & Torres, 1992).

Although training should be individualized, several training concepts typically apply to everyone who wears a prosthesis:

- The prosthesis functions as the nonpreferred extremity and acts to stabilize objects.
- Dress the prosthesis first, and undress it last.

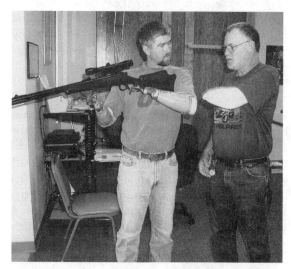

Figure 12.1. Specialized clinic provides environment for peer support and goal completion.

• In cutting meat with the prosthesis, the fork is placed between the hook fingers and behind the prosthetic thumb, and the knife is held by the noninvolved extremity.

People with amputations frequently define prosthetic success as daily wear of the device and its incorporation into most of their tasks. Inconsistent prosthetic use with high-level amputations is influenced by the amount of components needed and by the perceived "heavy feel" of the device secondary to the short residual limb. The prosthesis, which is a tool, appears to be incorporated into body image for unilateral and bilateral amputations when

• Posttraumatic intervention occurs early,
• An experienced team provides intervention,
• A client-centered approach is used in the assessment and treatment,
• The client is provided ongoing education, and
• The client is placed into structured follow-up (Atkins, 1989a; Fletchall & Torres, 1992).

Body-Power, Myoelectric, or Electronic Prosthetic Prescription

Prosthesis type—body power, myoelectric, electronic, or hybrid (i.e., a combination of two or more styles)—must be determined for each client, regardless of the length of amputation. Advantages of body-power prostheses are their relatively light weight, durability, provision of sensory feedback, and cost-effectiveness; in addition, the residual-limb shape does not need to be definitive in size. The hook terminal device of body-power prostheses allows easy visibility of objects. The disadvantages of body-power prostheses are the need for a harness, the uncomfortable feeling of the axillary loop, and the appearance of the hook terminal device. Many clients who have multiple types of prostheses and who perform rigorous or outdoor activities wear a body-power prosthesis most the time.

Whether the amputation is transradial or transhumeral, operation of the terminal device on a body-power prosthesis is through tension on a cable by biscapular abduction or humeral flexion. Without proper training, the client's use of the terminal device may be limited to an area between the chest and knees and within the frontal span of the body. Clients with transhumeral amputation who use a body-power prosthesis operate the elbow through the same cable for terminal device function. Skilled occupational therapists teach the client to activate elbow movement through shoulder abduction, depression, and extension without operating the terminal device. This approach allows the client to be proficient in using the prosthesis in a variety of positions and activities.

A myoelectric prosthesis operates the terminal device and other components through surface electrodes placed over muscles in the residual limb. In a transradial amputation, the residual forearm muscles, if under voluntary control, can be used to generate the myoelectric signal. An electronic prosthesis functions by toggle or pull switch to activate the prosthetic motor units of the terminal device, elbow, or both. To successfully operate either type of prosthesis consistently and daily, the client must have the cognitive ability to comprehend the maintenance, care, and use of the prosthesis along with the battery-charging procedure. Occupational therapists will verify this ability as part of their ongoing evaluation process. Battery cost can be high for some myoelectric and electronic prostheses. Compared with body-power prostheses, the advantages of myoelectric and electronic prostheses are as follows:

• Less body movement is required to operate the components.
• The terminal device's prehension power is greater.
• The terminal device opening is larger.

Clients with transradial amputation can operate a myoelectric prosthesis with minimal or no harness. The disadvantages of myoelectric and electronic prostheses are that the weight on the residual limb is greater than with a body-power prosthesis, the transradial or transhumeral residual-limb shape and size must be stable, and they are more expensive than other prostheses. The decision to move the client into a myoelectric prosthesis can best be assessed by the amputee team. Residual-limb shape and size, total residual-limb strength and endurance, and the client's ability to use a body-power prosthesis must be assessed when considering a myoelectric prosthesis.

A specialized amputee team can effectively progress the client into the prosthesis that has the most appropriate components. Team members may include, in addition to the client and occupational and physical therapists, a physician, prosthetist, nurse, social worker, and psychologist. The team can provide documentation that is necessary to receive reimbursement for the prosthesis from health care payers. The cost for a unilateral prosthesis, depending on the style, can range from $15,000 to $80,000. For clients with complex upper-extremity amputations or bilateral amputations, prosthetic costs will be greater. Specialized amputee team members can provide creative options for clients who have complex amputations to help them return to satisfactory performance of everyday activities.

Achieving Successful Amputee Rehabilitation

Successful *amputee rehabilitation* can be defined as the ability of the client to participate independently and satisfactorily in valued ADL and roles. Successful *prosthetic rehabilitation* can be defined as the ability of the client to wear and use the prosthesis for a minimum of 8 hours daily. Achieving successful prosthetic wear and use also requires involving the client early in the rehabilitation process. Talking about strengths and weaknesses with clients and developing a time frame for achieving their goals encourages them to regain control over their lives. Providing education about different prosthetic styles and components and relating those options to the clients' lifestyles also can foster successful goal achievement (Myers 1999). Additional success can be achieved when a specialized amputee team analyzes the client's social, physical, and emotional areas of occupation and makes appropriate recommendations regarding prosthetic type and components.

Functional training is a prolonged stage of the prosthetic training process. The most challenging parts of the training are identification of the most efficient body motion(s) and development of skills in the prosthetic pre-positioning process. The success or failure of the client's use of the prosthesis depends on the motivation of the client, the comprehensiveness and quality of the tasks and activities practiced and, most important, the experience and enthusiasm of the occupational therapist. The functional training experience is most effective if the same therapist remains with the client throughout the process (Atkins, 1989a).

The high rejection rate of upper-extremity prostheses often can be attributed to the following causes (Burrough & Brook, 1985):

- Development of one-handedness, which removes the functional need for the prosthesis
- Lack of sufficient training or skill in operating the prosthesis
- Poor comfort or quality of the prosthesis
- The unnatural look or profile of the prosthesis
- Reactions that the wearer receives from other people.

Potential Problems

Client with an amputation may develop a variety of problems, which can interfere with independent ADL performance. As the residual limb ages, atrophy occurs, which can produce bone irritation or poor socket fit. Poor socket fit frequently results in skin irritation or breakdown and an inability to operate the prosthesis. Total body weight loss or gain also can affect the socket fit. Different types of pain and abnormal sensations can interfere with ADL performance and prosthetic use.

Early intervention and education frequently can minimize phantom sensations' interference with prosthetic use. Neuroma irritation can be minimized through the use of pressure and a properly fitting socket. Additional medical problems, such as cardiac conditions or diabetes, may require consideration of alternative prosthetic components or prosthetic styles. As clients age, participation in activities may change, which in turn can influence prosthetic design or needs.

Functional Outcomes at Various Levels of Amputation

For clients with a unilateral amputation, most IADL, work tasks, and leisure activities can be accomplished independently with the use of the noninvolved extremity. Early intervention, including prosthetic fitting within 30 days of the last surgical procedure on the amputated extremity, can foster daily prosthetic wear and use (Fletchall & Torres, 1992). When the client also sustains a significant injury to the nonamputated extremity, early prosthetic fit and training can assist in resuming performance in ADL.

Unilateral Transradial Amputation

With the loss of the hand, the most desired length of the amputated limb is a medium or long transradial amputation, because the procedure preserves forearm rotation. Wrist or elbow disarticulation will lead to problems of bone irritation secondary to atrophy of the soft tissue. The shape of the residual limb with either wrist or elbow disarticulation may not be appropriate for comfortable donning of the socket. A medium or long transradial amputation ideally should be conical.

Before initiating functional prosthetic training, the prosthesis should fit well and the client should operate all components correctly. Frequent communication between the occupational therapist and prosthetist initially determines the style and type of components, and ongoing communication can quickly identify the need for prosthetic revision. The client should visit a clinic specializing in amputations and prosthetics on a routine schedule, even after completing the therapy program.

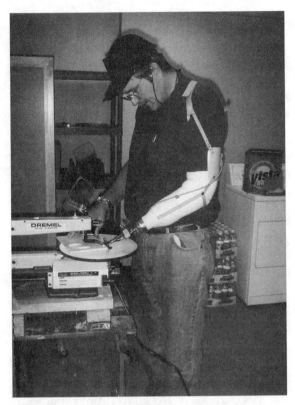

Figure 12.2. Using saw with transradial body power prothesis.

Clients with unilateral transradial amputation and a noninjured upper extremity should be able to achieve independence in all activities. The non-involved hand will provide prehension in bilateral tasks, and the prosthesis will provide stabilization. Initially, certain self-care tasks, such as buttoning, tying shoes, and cutting food, may require special adaptive equipment. With daily practice, however, clients with wrist disarticulation or transradial amputation will minimize the use of adaptive equipment as they complete their activities (Atkins, 1994).

Case Study 1

D. F. is a 46-year-old man from the Memphis, Tennessee, area. He sustained a partial hand amputation while at work stacking cargo containers for ships and trucks. D. F.'s hand became trapped in the pinlocking mechanism for stacking the containers, resulting in crush injury with partial hand amputation at the site. Following attempts to stabilize several fractures in the partial hand, D. F. requested an amputation. Because his was an elective procedure, he received education about the value of a prosthesis for his life activities and work. He was provided ongoing exposure to other people with upper-extremity amputations, where he observed the functional performance abilities of body-power prostheses.

Within 1 day of the transradial amputation, D. F. resumed outpatient occupational therapy. Initially, the program focused on edema control, residual-limb shaping, range of motion, and residual-limb and total body strengthening.

Within 30 days following the primary closure transradial amputation, D. F. was fitted with a body-power prosthesis. Functional prosthetic training focused on independence in bilateral IADL, work simulation, and leisure activities. After the shape and size of the residual limb stabilized, he was fitted with a myoelectric prosthesis that included an interchangeable terminal device consisting of a greifer and hand. D. F. returned to his former employer and was performing his previous job within 4 months after the transradial amputation. He uses both types of prosthesis, preferring the body-power prosthesis when performing outdoor activities.

Unilateral Transhumeral Amputation

Transhumeral amputation results in shorter extremity length and greater loss of movement than transradial amputation does. Without a prosthesis, the ability of the residual limb to provide stabilization for the noninvolved extremity may be limited secondary to the length of the residual limb. Attempting to perform a bilateral upper-extremity activity with the transhumeral residual limb stabilizing an item on the table frequently results in neck flexion (i.e., forward cervical posturing), which may lead to pain.

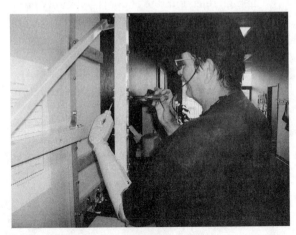

Figure 12.3. Using transradial myoelectric prosthesis to handle small hand tools.

Prosthesis selection requires thorough assessment of total body function, bilateral shoulder function, and types of occupational activities to be performed. Shaping and edema control of the residual limb remain vital to achieving an appropriate socket fit. At a minimum, mobility, endurance, and strength of the residual limb shoulder must be adequate to tolerate the weight of prosthesis as well as to reposition the prosthesis in relationship to the body, as when donning clothing.

If the client is strong or can regain good muscle strength, performance of activities can be accomplished with a body-power prosthesis. When the client has limited endurance or strength, the occupational therapist should consider a hybrid, myoelectric, or electronic prosthesis. Amputee team members will analyze all factors to make the most appropriate prosthetic recommendations. Clients with transhumeral amputation and no physical involvement of the remaining extremity should be able to achieve independence in most ADL.

Case Study 2

R. V. is a 25-year-old Latina woman who sustained a short transhumeral amputation while working for a frozen food company. During the accident, the nondominant extremity came into contact with the conveyor system, with rotary forces creating a crush and amputation injury. R. V. required circumferential skin graft to the short residual limb. Even though she began the outpatient occupational therapy within 2 weeks of the skin graft, her initial attending surgeon was not supportive of an aggressive preprosthetic program and was not familiar with the benefits of a prosthesis. Following education of the client and case manager about the benefits to the client and cost effectiveness for the insurance payer, R. V. was referred to the amputee team.

The initial therapy program included edema control, residual-limb shaping, wound care to areas where the skin graft had failed, shoulder and upper-quadrant range of motion, and scar-tissue elongation; those efforts were followed by residual-limb muscle endurance and strengthening. R. V. received training in how to independently perform self-care and selected household tasks. She is a mother of three children—one in diapers—so adaptive techniques for managing child care with the noninvolved extremity were taught. Until R. V. received training with the prosthesis, she was instructed in safe techniques for bathing the small child, changing diapers, and physically managing items needed when in the community with the infant. Once

wounds had healed and shoulder motion had improved, the occupational therapist fabricated an "extendoarm" from low-temperature thermoplastic. The extendoarm provides additional length to the residual limb, thereby facilitating use of the extremity in bilateral midline activities and reinforcing shoulder and scapular muscle skills until delivery of the prosthesis.

R. V. was given information on the type of prosthesis and components that were most appropriate for her strength, motion, and endurance and could act as an assist to accomplish several activities bilaterally. She initially was fitted with a hybrid prosthesis, which had an electronic hand, a passive counterswing elbow, and a passive humeral rotation plate. Obtaining control of the terminal device, positioning the elbow and pre-positioning the hand was achieved prior to training in functional tasks. Initial functional prosthetic training focused on cutting food and opening packets, then progressed to meal preparation and household chores. Following occupational therapy, R. V. resumed her role as mother to three small children and returned to competitive employment. R. V. returns to the Amputee Clinic for regular follow-up to assess residual-

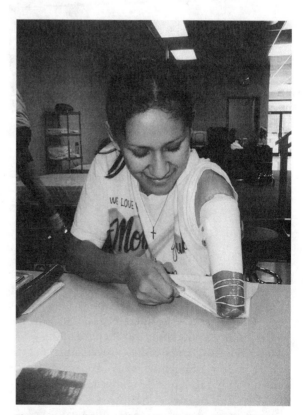

Figure 12.4. "Extendoarm" assists individual with transhumeral amputation in bilateral tasks.

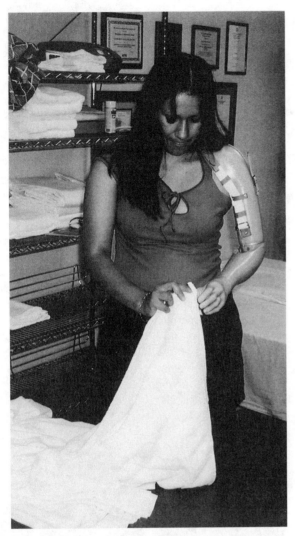

Figure 12.5. Working on folding clothes with hybrid transhumeral prosthesis.

limb change, appearance, and ADL to determine prosthetic needs.

Bilateral Transradial Amputation

Loss of both hands can significantly affect ADL performance. A client's sense of helplessness and depression can be minimized with early intervention. Depending on the type of trauma sustained, the client may require a treatment program that focuses on flexibility; endurance; and strength of the upper trunk, quadrant, and extremity. Evaluation and upgrade of lower-extremity skills can enhance the client's ability to return to complete independence in ADL. With creativity on the part of the client and therapist, many clients sustaining a bilateral transradial amputation can obtain some independence

in selected activities while undergoing a traditional physical rehabilitation program. Upper-extremity movement across the midline, above the head, and to the back can be fostered through use of adaptive techniques and equipment to perform basic self-care, such as eating, washing, and donning upper-extremity garments. Adaptive techniques for toileting must be taught for use with and without the prosthesis. The adaptive toileting techniques are individualized to each client and depend on balance, lower-extremity skills, trunk flexibility, and midline positioning of the upper extremities and/or prostheses (Leonard & Meier, 1998).

Due to the changes in the residual limb and the initial decreased endurance and strength, it is usually preferable to fit clients who have had transradial amputation with body-power prostheses. Compared with hand or greifer, the hook terminal device weighs less and provides greater visual feedback when interacting with objects. The harness and socket of a body-power prosthesis provide the client with kinesthetic feedback while he or she performs activities. Wrist-flexion units provide easier access to midline activities, such as feeding and managing clothing. Automatic wrist rotators may be added to the prosthesis to position the terminal device, but they add weight and generate stress on the residual limb.

Prosthetic training for clients with bilateral transradial amputation is similar to what has been previously described. Training focused on terminal device operation and prepositioning can influence the time it takes to perform activities. Use of the prosthesis in writing, feeding, hygiene, toileting, and dressing reinforces the daily use of the devices. Obtaining independence with the prosthesis in basic self-care facilitates preinjury leisure activities. A thorough understanding of the client, the prosthetic components, and style is necessary to help the client return to competitive employment or the educational system. For some clients, state vocational rehabilitation services may provide funding for retraining or education.

Following appropriate pre- and postprosthetic training, clients with bilateral transradial amputations who have good muscle function, mobility, and cognitive skills can achieve a high level of independence and resume many preinjury activities, including competitive employment. Once strength is obtained and appropriate prosthetic training has been completed, few clients require adaptive devices to perform everyday tasks. For many clients, the prostheses become an essential part of their life and body image (Atkins, 1994, p. 295).

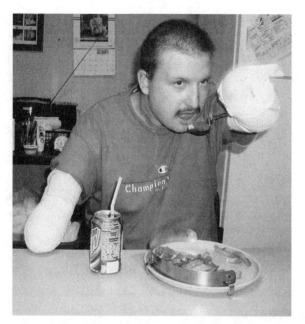

Figure 12.6. Prior to prosthesis, adaptive techniques are used to provide some independence.

Case Study 3

J. C. is a 31-year-old man who sustained 89% total body surface burns, more than 50% of which were third degree, from a thermal explosion while at work. As a result of the deep burns to both hands, he required bilateral transradial amputations. Burn injuries were sustained to all parts of the body except the ankles distally, genital area, and top of the head. Immediately following his discharge from the burn center, he began an intense, daily outpatient program, which encompassed up to 6 hours per day. His treatment program initially focused on multiple problems associated with burn injuries and amputations. Simultaneous burn and amputation rehabilitation programs minimize or prevent potential problems of contracture development, residual limb edema, and shoulder and scapular weakness (Fletchall & Hickerson, 1991, 1995).

During J. C.'s first day of treatment, adaptive equipment was used to allow him to feed himself, a task he had not performed for 8 weeks. While receiving traditional burn rehabilitation treatment, he was also involved in a preprosthetic program. Burns to the back can interfere with horizontal shoulder adduction, which can limit functional use of prostheses. Therefore, before receiving prostheses, J. C. focused on activities and tasks that fostered midline use of upper extremities to increase his performance of the prosthesis in dressing and hygiene tasks.

As a result of heterotophic ossification of the right elbow, J. C. was initially placed into a left-unilateral body-power prosthesis with hook prehensor and wrist-flexion unit. His initial prosthetic program focused on attaining independence with one prosthesis while continuing to improve the function of the remaining upper extremity. He achieved independence in donning and doffing the prosthetic socks and prosthesis, self-feeding, basic meal preparation, dressing with selected fasteners, bathing, and managing household objects such as a telephone and keys (Figure 12.8). With improvement in strength, J. C. progressed to driving, for which he used the minimal adaptation of a removable amputee driving ring (Figure 12.9).

Following surgery for removal of the heterotophic ossification in the elbow, J. C. was placed into a bilateral body-power prosthesis with hook prehensors and wrist-flexion units. Return to outpatient therapy provided for prosthetic training with the new prosthesis and an upgrade of his skills in all areas of IADL.

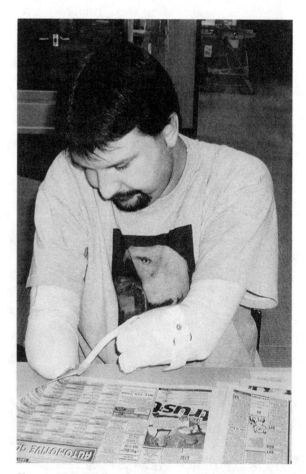

Figure 12.7. Midline activities can improve prosthetic control.

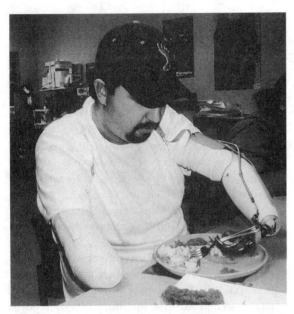

Figure 12.8. With complicated bilateral transradial amputations, prosthetic training can begin with one device.

The occupational therapist performed muscle assessment of the forearms and found peripheral nerve loss to flexors and extensors of the forearm in J. C.'s previously dominant extremity. Therefore, myoelectric forearm muscle training was initiated with the one residual limb that exhibited voluntary muscle control of the forearm muscles. Following J. C.'s request, the stronger residual limb is progressing to myoelectric prosthesis, with greifer and hand, and the other extremity is using a unilateral body-power prosthesis. He is scheduled for return to the occupational therapy clinic for training with the myoelectric prosthesis in functional activities. For clients

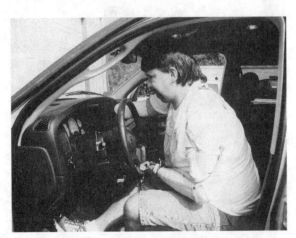

Figure 12.9. Driving with adaptations increases independence with bilateral transradial amputation.

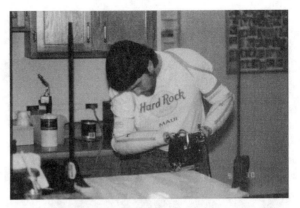

Figure 12.10. With specialized training, power tool use is possible with transradial amputations, bilaterally.

with bilateral transradial amputations, training in preinjury activities and specific job duties improves their ability to remain productive (see Figure 12.10).

Bilateral Transhumeral Amputation

In a bilateral transhumeral amputation, the loss of both elbows requires that the prosthesis provide motion at the elbow, wrist, and terminal device. In addition, the residual-limb length is shorter than with transradial amputation, thereby placing additional demands on the structures of the shoulder and on cervical and upper-torso mobility.

Prosthetic components can provide for elbow flexion and extension, but the client must use more energy to position the prosthesis and operate the terminal device. The ability to construct a lightweight elbow component that has extreme durability remains a challenge to manufacturers. Most clients with bilateral transhumeral amputations prefer body-power elbow units to electric units. Body-power units are lighter weight and more dependable, durable, and cost-efficient than electric elbows; they also require less maintenance.

Prosthetic training will be influenced by the client's tolerance for new information, "gadgets," and family support as well as emotional and physical factors. The ability to achieve independence in basic self-care will require creativity from the therapist and motivation from the client, and it should be explored with and without the use of prostheses. Staged treatment sessions, which allow the client to practice levels of skills in the clinic then within the home environment, may be appropriate.

Case Study 4

G. H. is a 44-year-old man who sustained bilateral transhumeral amputations following damage from

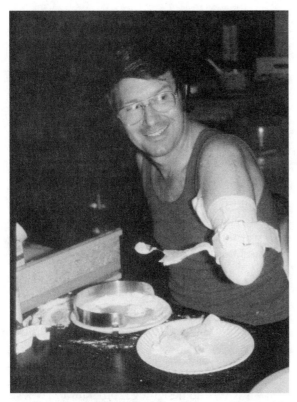

Figure 12.11. While awaiting prosthesis, client with bilateral transhumeral amputation uses adaptive techniques to feed self.

a high-voltage electrical burn. In addition to the transhumeral amputations, he sustained loss of both biceps and presented with deep burn wounds to both axillas. G. H. entered the burn–amputee program on the day of injury. The treatment program focused on both catastrophic injuries simultaneously. While achieving wound closure, the

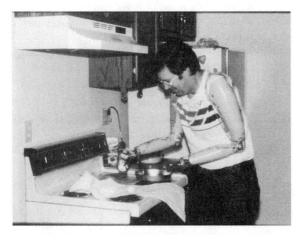

Figure 12.12. Using bilateral body power prosthesis, client works on meal preparation.

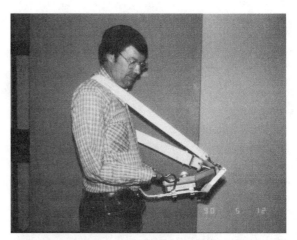

Figure 12.13. Equipment modification assisted with RTW for client with bilateral transhumeral amputations.

preprosthetic program focused on shoulder motion and strength, and training for independence in selected self-care activities such as self-feeding (Figure 12.11). Initially, G. H. was fitted with a bilateral prosthesis with electronic elbows and electronic hooks. Prosthetic training with the electronic prosthesis focused on self-care and the ability to be alone for several hours in the home environment. As total body strength and endurance improved, he returned to the clinic for additional prosthetic training with bilateral body-power elbows and hooks.

G. H. chose to use the bilateral body-power prosthesis due to the reliability of its components and the speed with which he could operate the elbow and hooks. He resumed independence in many self-care activities with and without the prostheses; he drove and participated in leisure activities with the prostheses. His return to employment required work assessment by the authors' staff, which also designed and fabricated custom adaptive equipment for stabilizing items while working outside of the office. G. H. returned to employment within 54 weeks from the date of injury, where he retired 14 years later (Figures 12.12 and 12.13).

Unilateral Shoulder Disarticulation

Loss of the upper extremity at the shoulder reduces the physical performance of the prosthesis. Prosthetic components must attempt to duplicate or replace the hand, wrist, elbow, and shoulder. No limb is available, so the prosthesis must lie on the upper quadrant and trunk. Prosthetic components for shoulder disarticulation frequently are electronic and involve pull or toggle switches to operate the elbow and terminal device. Chest-expansion movements can be used to operate a pull switch.

Self-care training should focus on achieving independence with and without the use of the prosthesis. Prosthetic training must focus on operation of the prosthesis without exaggerated trunk motions and without prosthetic activation during activities of ambulation, coming to standing, reaching with the noninvolved extremity. Portions of the training should use the prosthesis to provide stabilization to items while the noninvolved extremity performs the detail work. Providing instruction in use of the prosthesis in everyday activities, including work duties, can minimize potential of overuse of the noninvolved extremity.

Case Study 5

V. B. is a 30-year-old man who sustained high-voltage electrical injury while at work. The depth of electrical injury resulted in physical loss of several muscles in the posterior neck, loss of axillary nerve and interosseous branch of the median nerve of the nonamputated extremity, and left shoulder disarticulation.

Following V. B.'s initial burn care, he received more than 9 months of inpatient and outpatient treatment. His referral to the center occurred 13 months after the date of injury. V. B. was totally dependent in all ADL, including self-feeding. Through the rehabilitation center, he had been fitted with a prosthesis, which had body-power hook and elbow components. Efforts had not been directed towards achieving soft-tissue and scar-tissue elongation of the neck, right shoulder, or hand. Emotionally, V. B. was distraught and depressed, but he articulated goals of achieving independence in ADL, including driving and fishing.

V. B. began the conditioning program, which is geared toward improving total body endurance, motion, and strength. Selected tasks incorporated neck flexion and progressed to hand prehension and strength skills for the right upper extremity. Following a thorough assessment by the Amputee Clinic, the previous body-power prosthesis was discontinued and V. B. was placed into a hybrid electronic prosthesis with a chest expansion pull switch, which operated the elbow and terminal device. The prosthetic frame construction respected skin grafts and scar-tissue areas, especially at the shoulder disarticulation site.

Functional training began within 1 week of receiving the hybrid electronic prosthesis. V. B. achieved independence in all areas of self-care. A home assessment was completed, which provided recommendations for architectural modifications to accommodate V. B's inability to achieve right shoulder flexion secondary to loss of axillary nerve. Vehicle modifications were minimal once neck motion increased and included additional mirrors.

After 3 months in the program, V. B. achieved total independence in IADL and driving and returned to employment. He lives alone, remains employed full-time, and has participated and placed in several competitive fishing tournaments. Because of V. B.'s active lifestyle and physical limitations of the right upper extremity, he has two electronic hybrid prostheses. He returns to the Amputee Clinic yearly for reassessment of prosthetic needs in relationship to his skin, soft-tissue atrophy, and lifestyle tasks.

Summary

Clients who have sustained loss of the upper extremity can achieve success in many preinjury activities when treatment is initiated early and by professionals who specialize in amputations and prosthetics. Thorough evaluation and early intervention is vital to designing a program to achieve the client's goals and minimize costs. Return to independence and prosthetic daily use are related to the prosthetic style, components, training, and follow-up. The specialized amputee team members educate clients about the abilities of a prosthesis and emphasize that it is a tool, not a replacement for an extremity.

Study Questions

1. Describe why a preprosthetic program should begin early.
2. Describe the advantages of a body-power hook compared over a hand terminal device.
3. What is the difference between myoelectric prostheses and body-power prostheses?
4. What type of prosthesis is frequently considered for clients with shoulder disarticulation?
5. Explain how clients with bilateral transradial amputations can achieve independence in IADL.
6. What information about the client should be considered before suggesting an electronic prosthetic device?

References

Atkins, D. J. (1989a). Adult upper limb prosthetic training. In D. J. Atkins & R. H. Meier (Eds.), *Comprehensive management of the upper limb amputee* (pp. 39–59). New York: Springer-Verlag.

Atkins, D. J. (1989b). Postoperative therapy programs. In D. J. Atkins & R. H. Meier (Eds.), *Comprehensive management of the upper limb amputee* (pp. 11–15). New York: Springer-Verlag.

Atkins, D. J. (1994) Managing self-care in adults with upper extremity amputations. In C. H. Christiansen (Ed.), *Ways of living* (pp. 277–304). Rockville, MD: American Occupational Therapy Association.

Bennett, J. B., & Alexander, C. B. (1989). Amputation levels and surgical techniques. In D. J. Atkins & R. H. Meier (Eds.), *Comprehensive management of the upper limb amputee* (pp. 1–10). New York: Springer-Verlag.

Burrough, S., & Brook, J. (1985). Patterns of acceptance and rejection of upper limb prostheses. *Orthotics and Prosthetics, 39,* 40–47.

Fletchall, S. (1998, October). Sandy Fletchall ...Using professional experience to lead people with recent amputations to success. *Capabilities Quarterly Newsletter, 7*(4), 6–7.

Fletchall, S., & Hickerson, W. L. (1991, May). Early upper-extremity prosthetic fit in patients with burns. *Burn Care and Rehabilitation Journal, 12,* 234–236.

Fletchall, S., & Hickerson, W. L. (1995, September/October). Quality burn rehabilitation: Cost-effective approach. *Journal of Burn Care and Rehabilitation, 16,* 539–542.

Fletchall, S., & Torres, H. (1992, July). Benefits of early upper extremity prosthetic training. *Capabilities Quarterly Newsletter, 2*(2), 6–8.

Leonard, J. A., Jr., & Meier, R. H., III. (1998). Upper and lower extremity prosthetics. In J. A. DeLisa et al. (Eds.), *Rehabilitation medicine: Principles and practice* (pp. 669–696). Philadelphia: Lippincott-Raven.

Marquardt, E. (1989). The Heidelberg experience. In D. J. Atkins & R. H. Meier (Eds.), *Comprehensive management of the upper limb amputee* (pp. 240–252). New York: Springer-Verlag.

Myers, C. (1999, December/January). A one-woman show. *Rehab Management,* 74–77.

Chapter 13

Adaptive Strategies After Severe Burns

SANDRA UTLEY REEVES, OTR/L

KEY TERMS

autograft

boutonnière deformity

boutonnière precautions

donor site

ectropion

eschar

full-thickness burn

heterotopic ossification

hyperpigmentation

hypertrophic scar

hypopigmentation

keloid scar

microstomia

partial-thickness burn

scar maturation

split-thickness skin graft

OBJECTIVES

Upon completion of this chapter, the reader will be able to

- Recognize and understand the characteristics of the different depths of burn injury;

- Describe the phases of recovery and the focus of occupational therapy intervention for each phase;

- Identify factors that increase the potential for scar hypertrophy or contractures;

- Understand how early patient–caregiver education and the active involvement of patient and caregiver in establishing goals influence long-term compliance with the treatment program;

- Understand the rationale and benefits of early involvement of burn patients in their self-care;

- Recognize the impact that a severe burn has on a person's life roles, self-image, values, and occupational performance; and

- Describe factors to consider when recommending adaptive techniques, equipment, or environmental modifications for people recovering from burns.

The primary purpose of occupational therapy intervention with burn patients is to return them to their preinjury level of independent occupational performance. Pain, discomfort, loss of joint mobility, cosmetic disfigurement, and adverse psychological reactions, however, can limit burn patients' potential for resuming previous life roles, occupations, and interests. Because the focus of occupational therapy is on returning burn patients to their preinjury lifestyle, effective treatment planning requires ongoing evaluation of the client's physical activity level, social needs, and psychological status. Understanding and respecting clients' personal goals and priorities are essential, because clients' wishes directly affect adherence to treatment regimens, motivation, and functional outcomes.

It takes a coordinated effort by a multidisciplinary team to effectively manage the many medical, functional, and psychosocial problems encountered during burn recovery and rehabilitation. Only through continual interaction among the patient and members of the burn team can rehabilitation progress efficiently. Ideally, the burn team should consist of physicians, nurses, occupational therapists, physical therapists, respiratory therapists, a nutritionist, a social worker or case manager, a psychologist, a chaplain, a recreational therapist, and a vocational counselor.

Traditionally, a burn patient's recovery was considered successful if he or she survived the injury, returned home, and was able to perform basic self-care tasks (i.e., activities of daily living [ADL]), which include eating, dressing, grooming, toileting, and ambulating. Today, successful burn care is measured by a patient's *quality of life* once he or she is discharged from the acute care or rehabilitation setting. Functional recovery now includes the burn patient being able to perform complex activities (i.e., instrumental activities of daily living [IADL]). The ability to perform ADL and IADL allows the patient to resume self-determined roles at home, work, school, and in the community, including social and recreational activities.

Factors That Influence Burn Injury Outcomes

Burn team members consider many factors while developing goals and treatment plans for specific patients. Those factors include the depth of the burn; the mechanism of injury; the percentage of total body surface area burned (%TBSA); and the severity of the burns, including the location and subsequent quality of wound healing. A patient's age, preinjury health and emotional stability, motivation and compliance with treatment, and family support are other factors that can directly affect the recovery process.

Burn Depth

Prediction of the potential for long-term activity impairment begins with an evaluation of burn depth. In the past, it was customary to classify burns as first, second, and third degree; however, burns are now more accurately described as superficial, superficial partial-thickness, deep partial-thickness, full-thickness, and subdermal injuries (Table 13.1). The period required for healing and the risk for scarring are directly related to the depth of the burn, which is estimated from clinical evaluation of its appearance, vascularity, sensitivity, and pliability.

Superficial and deep partial-thickness burns usually heal without surgical intervention. Once healed, however, they tend to be excessively dry, itchy, and vulnerable to injury from trauma and shearing forces, which often are caused by rubbing or scratching. Shearing forces may result in separation of the newly healed skin layers and subsequent formation of blisters. With repeated injury, the skin's integrity is further compromised and potential for scarring increases. Partial-thickness and full-thickness burns usually develop uneven pigmentation as a result of combinations of hypopigmentation and hyperpigmentation of the healed skin tissue. Deep partial- and full-thickness burns also carry a high potential for thick, hypertrophic scar and contracture formation because of their prolonged healing period and resulting collagen overgrowth. This potential is even higher with partial-thickness burns that convert to full-thickness injuries due to infection or repeated trauma. To obtain prompt wound closure, large full-thickness wounds require surgical intervention, such as skin grafting. Skin-graft donor sites usually have healing time frames and end results similar to those of superficial partial-thickness burns; they result in less scarring but similarly uneven pigmentation. If healing is delayed by trauma or infection, however, a donor site will have the same scarring potential as a deep partial-thickness burn.

Mechanism of Injury

The mechanism of a burn injury and the duration and intensity of exposure to the damage-causing agents also are determinants of severity. Superficial partial-thickness burns typically occur after brief contact with hot liquids, heated surfaces, or flash flames. Deep partial-thickness burns are caused by

Table 13.1. Burn Wound Characteristics

Burn Depth	Tissue Depth	Clinical Findings	Healing Time	Common Causes	Scar Potential
Superficial (first degree)	Epidermis	Erythema, dry, no blisters Moderate pain	3–7 days	Sunburn, brief flash burns, brief exposure to hot liquids or chemicals	No potential for hypertrophic scarring or contractures
Superficial partial thickness (superficial second degree) and donor sites	Epidermis, upper dermis	Erythema, wet, blisters Significant pain	Less than 2 weeks	Severe sunburn or radiation burns, prolonged exposure to hot liquids, brief contact with hot metal surfaces	Minimal potential for hypertrophic scarring or contractures unless secondary infection or trauma delays healing for longer than 2 weeks or if the patient has a genetic predisposition for scarring
Deep partial thickness (deep second degree) and traumatized or infected donor sites	Epidermis and deeper dermis but skin appendages survive, from which skin may regenerate	Erythema; usually broken blisters (but palms and soles of feet have large, possibly intact blisters over beefy red dermis) Severe pain to touch Hypersensitivity to heat	More than 2 weeks May convert to full thickness with onset of infection or repeated trauma	Flames; firm or prolonged contact with hot metal objects; prolonged contact with hot, viscous liquids	High potential for hypertrophic scarring and contractures across joints, web spaces, skin cleavages, and facial contours; high risk for boutonnière deformities if dorsal fingers are involved
Full thickness	Epidermis and dermis; skin appendages and nerve endings are nonviable	Pale, nonblanching, dry, coagulated capillaries may be seen No sensation to light touch except at deep partial-thickness borders	Large areas require surgical intervention for wound closure; small areas may heal in from the borders over an extended period of time.	Extreme heat or prolonged exposure to heat, hot objects, or chemical agents	Very high potential for hypertrophic scarring and contractures, depending on the method used for wound closure and period required for wound healing
Subdermal	Full-thickness burn with damage to underlying tissues	Nonviable surface; may be charred or with exposed fat, tendons, muscle, or bone Electrical injuries may have small external wounds but significant subdermal tissue damage and peripheral nerve damage	Requires surgical intervention for wound closure May require amputation or significant reconstruction	Electrical burns and severe long-duration burns (e.g., house fires, motor vehicle accidents with passenger entrapment inside the burning vehicle or under the hot exhaust system, smoking in bed, or alcohol-related burns)	Similar to full-thickness burn except when amputation removes the burn site and the borders of the surgery are closed primarily without grafting

exposure to intense heat, as with hot-water immersion scalds or prolonged exposure to flaming materials and hot surfaces. Full-thickness and subdermal burns usually result from electrical current, prolonged contact with viscous liquids or adhesive melted substances (e.g., hot grease, tar, or melted plastics), caustic chemical agents such as battery acid, extended exposure to flames, and high-temperature immersion scalds.

%TBSA

The severity of a burn injury is also measured by estimating the proportion of the body's skin that has been affected. The two traditional methods for estimating the %TBSA burned are the "rule of nines" and the Lund and Browder chart (Solem, 1984). The rule-of-nines method developed by Pulaski and Tennison in 1947 is simple and quick; it is useful for fast estimates in the emergency department but is relatively inaccurate. It divides the body surface into areas of 9% (or multiples of 9%); the perineum or neck constitutes the final 1%. The head area is 9%, each upper extremity is 9%, each leg is 18%, and the front and back of the trunk are each 18%. The rule of nines applies only to adults, however; body proportions vary in children, especially in the head and legs, depending on their age (Carvajal, 1988).

The Lund and Browder chart (Lund & Browder, 1944), which is used in most burn centers, provides a more accurate estimate of the %TBSA. The chart assigns a percentage of surface area to body segments and adjusts calculations for different age groups. For low %TBSA injuries, the therapist can make a quick estimate using the size of the patient's palm (i.e., the hand excluding the fingers), which equals approximately 1% of the person's TBSA.

Severity of Injury

The %TBSA and the depth of the burn together serve as the primary determinants of burn injury severity. A deep partial- or full-thickness burn to more than 20% TBSA is often the threshold for admission to a burn intensive care unit. For most adults, a deep partial-thickness and full-thickness burn of more than 40% TBSA is considered severe. Depending on the patient's age and preinjury health, however, partial-thickness or full-thickness burns of less than 20% TBSA can still be considered severe burn injuries. Children younger than 5 years of age and adults older than 50 years of age are considered to be at greater risk of death from large burns, so a 20% burn is considered severe for these populations. The presence of associated injuries, such as inhalation injury, fractures, or other trauma, contributes to severity.

Burns to specific body areas also influence severity, even though the %TBSA may be relatively small. Deep partial- or full-thickness burns of the hands, face, or perineum usually are considered severe (Wachtel, 1985). Burns of the face, eyes, and neck often interfere with respiration, vision, and feeding and may result in long-term functional and cosmetic impairment. Bilateral hand burns initially may limit the person's self-care ability, but they also can result in permanent impairment of occupational performance if not properly managed from the onset of treatment.

Wound Care and Surgical Intervention

Most burns are treated with some form of antibacterial agent to reduce the potential for wound infection (Hartford, 1984). If the wound is relatively clean, a biological dressing may be used as a temporary wound covering. Types of biological dressings include homografts, which are processed cadaver skin; xenografts, which are processed pig skin; and synthetic products or artificial skin substitutes. The extent and depth of the burn wound determine the need for surgical treatment. When it appears that a deep partial-thickness burn will take more than 2 weeks to heal, surgery may be decided upon to accelerate wound healing, shorten hospital length of stay, and reduce the potential for hypertrophic scarring.

The most common form of surgical intervention for serious burn wounds is split-thickness skin autografting. In this procedure, the dead burned tissue, or *eschar,* is surgically debrided. Then the top layer of skin is harvested from an unburned donor site and applied over the debrided burn site. In 3 to 7 days, the transplanted split-thickness skin graft is revascularized and permanently adhered. During this period, the graft site is kept immobilized to keep the skin graft from being dislodged. The donor site has the appearance and discomfort of a severe abrasion and usually heals in 7 to 10 days. If adequate donor sites for autografting are not available, or when burn depth or infections create conditions such that the grafted tissue will not survive, temporary porcine, cadaver, or synthetic biological dressings may be used over the burns until the site is ready for autografting. Full-thickness skin grafts may be used around facial features or areas of chronic skin breakdown, which require greater flexibility, durability, and a lower potential for scar contraction than split-thickness grafts can provide. This type of autografting usually involves excising a full-thickness fold or flap of unburned skin and transplanting it to an open area created where a tight scar has been incised and released. The full-thickness donor site is then closed primarily by approximating the borders of the wound or repaired using a split-thickness skin graft to close the defect.

Scar Formation

The quality of burn healing is affected by many factors, some of which occur during early phases of care (Helm & Fisher, 1988). The most common burn injury complication that limits independence with ADL is the development of hypertrophic scars and contractures. Burn-scar formation is strongly influenced by the time needed for the initial wound to close and the subsequent amount of disorganized collagen deposited by the fibroblasts in response to this inflammatory phase of healing (Abston, 1987). The longer the scar stays inflamed, the higher the potential for excessive scarring. After initial healing, some scars rise above the original level of the skin surface, become thick and rigid, and remain erythemic in appearance. These are referred to as *hypertrophic* scars. Hypertrophic scars usually begin developing during the first few months after a deep-partial or full-thickness burn heals. Secondary trauma and infection can impede healing and prolong the inflammatory response, resulting in collagen overgrowth and the development of hypertrophic scar tissue. A hypertrophic scar that not only rises above the original skin surface but also expands horizontally beyond the original borders of the scar is referred to as a *keloid* scar.

A scar's functional or cosmetic significance depends on its anatomical location. Joint motion is limited when a scar complex develops across a joint surface and contracts, creating a restrictive band of scar tissue known as a *scar contracture*. When tight or hypertrophic scars develop on the face, they distort facial features and interfere with eating, eye closure, and facial expression.

Regardless of the wound care methods used and the time taken for wound closure, scar maturation differs with each person. Superficial, partial-thickness, nonhypertrophic scars can mature in 5 to 8 weeks. Hypertrophic scars, however, can take 18 to 24 months to mature, and keloid scars can take even longer. Surgical scars from reconstruction procedures may mature faster, depending on the length of time to heal. As a scar matures, it becomes metabolically inactive and no longer attempts to contract. The erythema fades, the texture softens, and the scar becomes more pliable and elastic. At that point compression therapy, massage, and other scar-management interventions may be discontinued, although skin care precautions will continue for the rest of the patient's life.

Although it is sometimes possible to predict outcomes on the basis of the depth and location of the wound, other factors can affect the final results. Genetic predisposition for scarring, age, and preexisting health problems, for example, influence healing and scar formation. People of Asian, African, and Native American descent and those with deep pigmentation are more likely to develop hypertrophic scarring and uneven repigmentation of burned and grafted skin. Elderly patients may heal more slowly than young patients, but they have a lower incidence of collagen overgrowth. Small children tend to heal quickly but have a much higher potential for hypertrophic scarring. Patients with diabetes, peripheral vascular disease, or other conditions that restrict circulation may heal more slowly and be at greater risk for secondary infection.

Phases of Recovery

Burn rehabilitation can be divided into three basic phases of recovery: acute care, inpatient rehabilitation, and outpatient rehabilitation. The acute phase begins immediately after injury and usually continues until extensive wound care needs are minimal. During the first few days of this phase, the primary focus of the burn team is on the survival of the patient. During this time, when a severe fluid shift into the interstitial tissues and generalized swelling takes place, the burn team must work to reduce edema while ensuring that circulatory fluid resuscitation is accomplished. Fluid loss resulting from severe burns can cause burn shock and subsequent kidney failure if not managed carefully. Smoke- and heat-inhalation injuries often accompany burns and result in the need for mechanical ventilation or a tracheostomy to protect the patient's airway. As the medical team works to stabilize the patient, the occupational therapist should be anticipating and planning for the patient's rehabilitation needs. This initial evaluation should involve the total patient, not just the burn wound, so the occupational therapist should learn as much as possible about the patient's preinjury personality, performance patterns, and life context.

As the patient becomes medically stable, prevention of deformity and preservation of function become priorities. The occupational therapist performs an extensive evaluation of range of motion (ROM), sensation, strength, cognition, and abilities. He or she then develops and initiates a customized intervention program designed to minimize or prevent long-term loss of occupational performance.

When a burn patient enters the inpatient rehabilitation phase of recovery, preserving independent function and preventing disability and deformity become the central themes of intervention. Wound care continues, and the patient and his or her family take an increasingly active role in it. This phase emphasizes general reconditioning (i.e., strength, flexibility, and endurance), scar management, improving performance with self-care activities (i.e., self-feeding, wound and skin care, personal hygiene and grooming skills, and dressing), and social reintegration.

The outpatient rehabilitation phase is an extension of the rehabilitation phase, but patients typically live at home and attend therapy sessions during the day. The focus of care continues to center on minimizing hypertrophic scar and contracture formation; improving flexibility, strength, and endurance; ensuring proper skin and scar care techniques; and promoting independence in normal daily activities, including social and recreational pursuits. Community reintegration and socialization issues become more important. A primary objective is to help the patient adjust physically and emotionally to residual effects of the injury.

Most burn patients discontinue routine outpatient rehabilitation services when they achieve the skills needed to perform ADL independently at home and can return to school or work full-time. They often reach this point before scar maturation is complete. The total time required before returning to work is related to the site and severity of the burn, age of the patient, the patient's occupation, and the location of the thermal injury (Bowden, Thomson, & Prasad, 1989; Helm, Walker, & Peyton, 1986). Before discharge from the hospital, follow-up visits to a burn outpatient clinic should be scheduled to monitor the scar-maturation process and address unanticipated problems (Petro & Salisbury, 1986).

Role of Occupational Therapy

The role of occupational therapy in intervention with patients who have severe burns is multifaceted and changes as healing progresses. It is necessary to preserve ROM, strength, and endurance so that the patient can perform ADL (Trombly, 1995). These goals are essential to preventing contractures and physical deformities (Alvarado, 1995) but do not address all aspects of burn rehabilitation.

Systems models of occupational therapy are useful in understanding the effects of a serious burn injury on the life of a patient (Christiansen & Baum, 1997; Kielhofner, 1995; Law et al., 1996). These models help the therapist identify problems and understand the relationships among various aspects of intervention. Such models suggest that restrictions in the ability to move and perform tasks reduce the patient's ability to accomplish necessary roles. This impaired ability influences the patient's view of him- or herself as a competent person. Over time, a diminished self-conception can affect interests and values and reduce motivation, resulting in adverse physical, social, and emotional consequences.

When people sustain severe burn injuries, they initially are unable to complete self-care activities for many reasons, including the severity and location of the wounds; restrictive dressings, medication, and hospital routines; and pain and anxiety. Impaired physical abilities, isolation, and dramatic changes in one's usual daily routines seriously alter the patient's previous roles. The new role of patient replaces previous roles of worker, student, parent, or spouse (Reilly, 1962).

Psychological effects are a major concern (Fleet, 1992). Changes in motivation may occur at the time of injury and could continue for many years after discharge. Values can change, and self-esteem and confidence may be adversely affected because of negative body image. Social and personal interests may diminish, particularly if the injury occurred during a specific type of social gathering or is connected to a tragedy that resulted in loss of a loved one.

Cheng and Rogers (1989) studied men who had completed rehabilitation for severe burn injuries to determine how their role performance changed in the areas of self-care, leisure, home management, and work. They found that some men experienced minimal role reduction, whereas others managed their self-care requirements but experienced role disruption in their leisure, work, and home management. A third group experienced substantial disruption of all roles. The study found that loss of roles was associated with reduced endurance, the presence of impaired grip strength and upper-extremity skill, and difficulty with walking and standing. Although most of the men studied had achieved independence in self-care within a year after discharge, this achievement did not coincide with role resumption in the areas of home management, work, and leisure.

Because occupational therapy views the patient within a dynamic conceptual framework of occupation, the rehabilitation process can focus on the relationship between the injury and the patient as a multifaceted being. Within this context, evaluation and intervention strategies should address the patient's personal, emotional, social, cultural, and spiritual priorities as well as the easily identified physical and performance-skill deficits.

Acute Care Phase: Evaluation

Whenever possible, a patient should be evaluated by an occupational therapist within the first 24 hours after admission to the hospital. A pre-assessment review of the medical record is needed to obtain information regarding the mechanism of injury; the %TBSA affected; the depth of the burn; the presence of associated injuries, such as inhalation injury or fractures; and the patient's previous medical history and living situation. This information should be confirmed and supplemented by communication with the patient and his or her family.

Ideally, at least part of the initial occupational therapy evaluation should take place during a dressing change, when the patient has had pain medications and the depth and exact location of the burns can be viewed directly and documented in detail (Figure 13.1). Using appearance and quality of sensation, the therapist should differentiate each burn wound as a superficial, deep partial-thickness, or full-thickness burn as soon as possible after the injury. Burn eschar develops quickly, and it makes accurate evaluation of burn depth difficult because it causes deep partial-thickness burns to closely resemble full-thickness burns in appearance and sensitivity. Attention also should be directed to burned joint surfaces and the presence of any circumferential burns. The extremities should be screened for possible peripheral nerve damage by checking for the presence and quality of sensation. This screening is especially important with electrical or multiple-trauma injuries. The dorsum of the hands should be checked for deep burns, especially over the proximal interphalangeal (PIP) joints, which could indicate the need to initiate special therapy precautions or hand splints. If time allows, an active range of motion (AROM) or active-assistive range of motion (AAROM) assessment should be conducted to evaluate joint mobility and general strength before restrictive dressings are applied or serious edema develops.

Once the dressings are in place and nursing care is completed, a comprehensive occupational therapy evaluation can be performed. A careful history is needed from the patient or family members to establish the patient's preburn level of occupational performance, including physical, cognitive, and social skills and prior performance patterns (i.e., habits, routines, and roles). This history should include information about the patient's home environment and responsibilities; occupational background and work skills; educational level; hand dominance; and any preexisting physical, psychological, or social conditions that would affect the patient's occupational performance. Understanding the patient's preinjury performance patterns and life context is important not only for setting realistic treatment goals but also for establishing a therapeutic relationship with the patient and his or her family. Patient and caregiver education should be initiated on this first contact and continued as an essential part of therapy throughout the stages of recovery.

During the first 24 to 72 hours after the burn injury, acute, generalized edema develops, limiting the end ranges of joints, weighing down extremities, and impairing participation with active ROM. For this reason, formal joint goniometry may not be practical. The therapist, however, should note any developing joint stiffness not explained by preexisting conditions such as old injuries, congenital abnormalities, or age-related joint disease. Acute edema in the extremities can be monitored by taking circumferential measurements over established anatomical landmarks or by the finger-impression method. The impression method measures pitting edema by documenting in millimeters (mm) the depth of the impression a fingertip will make if pressed over a bony prominence for 5 seconds. Traditional scoring is as follows: 0 for no edema, 1+ for a barely discernable impression, 2+ if the depression is less than 5 mm, 3+ if the impression is 5 to 10 mm deep, and 4+ if the impression is more than, 10 mm deep. Intervention and recommendations regarding positioning and splinting are initiated and modified in response to changes in joint mobility and edema severity.

If lost AROM is not promptly regained as acute edema decreases, then goniometric measurements should be used to formally document changes in joint mobility. When possible, goniometer measurements of involved and uninvolved joints should be compared to assist in establishing the patient's norms. The extent and causes of limitations in motion should be determined from both the physical and psychological perspectives. A comparison of AROM and AAROM is preferred, but a patient may resist assistive or passive motion because of apprehension, pain, or confusion. If the patient is unresponsive or unable to participate, the therapist should evaluate joint mobility using gentle passive ROM.

An initial screening of gross strength is performed by a manual test of major muscle groups.

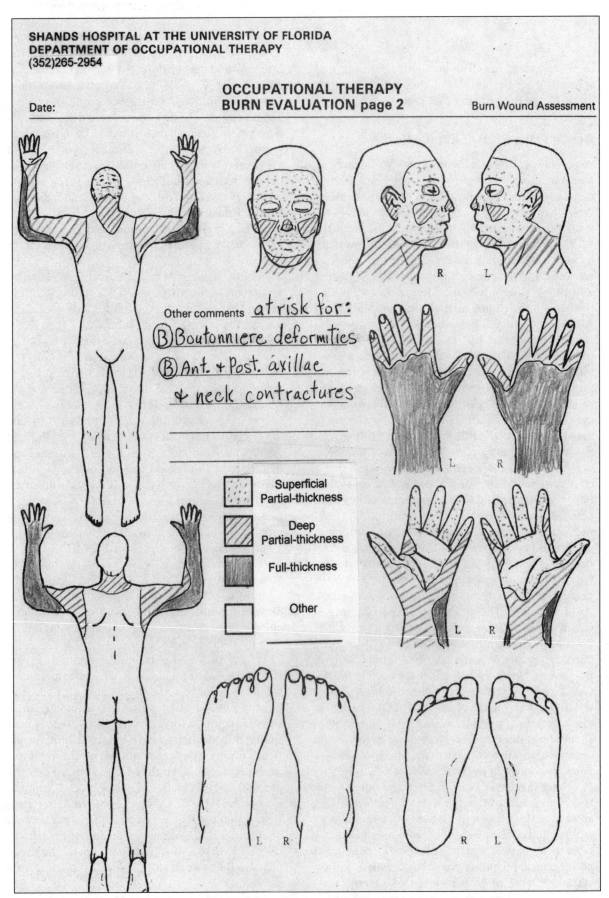

SHANDS HOSPITAL AT THE UNIVERSITY OF FLORIDA
DEPARTMENT OF OCCUPATIONAL THERAPY
(352)265-2954

Date:

OCCUPATIONAL THERAPY
BURN EVALUATION page 2

Burn Wound Assessment

Other comments *at risk for:*
(B) *Boutonniere deformities*
(B) *Ant. + Post. axillae*
+ neck contractures

Superficial
Partial-thickness

Deep
Partial-thickness

Full-thickness

Other

Figure 13.1. After direct visual assessment of the burns, the depth, exact location, and potential problem areas should be documented in detail and communicated to the team.

Because the burn does not initially affect muscle strength, this test can help identify any associated injuries, peripheral nerve damage, or preexisting conditions. Assessment of muscle strength several days postinjury can be adversely affected by pain, medications, and edema.

Actual performance of daily skills should be assessed beginning in the acute phase and should continue throughout the phases of recovery. Observation of eating, grooming, and basic self-care skills is important in determining whether appropriate or compensatory motions are being used. To overcome interference from dressings, edema, or pain, patients often demonstrate resourcefulness by initiating adaptive methods on their own. Some compensatory motions may also be associated with abnormal posturing, however, which may lead to subsequent problems and should be addressed in intervention planning.

Acute Care Phase: Intervention

During acute care, pain is a primary issue for patients. Most patients with a severe burn injury naturally respond to pain by resisting painful motions or activities. It is also normal for most children (and many adults) to regress in their behavior. When negative behaviors occur, the therapist should be supportive; he or she should continually explain beforehand what is to be done and why using terms the patient can understand (Figure 13.2). Limits need to be set on

behaviors that interfere with progression of treatment, such as intentional delaying of treatments (e.g., inappropriate requests or excessive socialization) or combative or verbally abusive behaviors. Involving the patient in setting goals and offering choices when establishing schedules give the patient some control, which can help avoid inappropriate behaviors or power struggles later during treatment.

The patient is usually more interested in whether a procedure will be painful or how long it will last than in technical information. Coordinating treatments with scheduled pain medications is often helpful and is highly recommended, especially if active participation is needed. Relaxation techniques, such as breathing exercises and guided imagery, may be helpful with motivated patients. If a patient's anxiety or pain is disproportionate to the treatment, however, antianxiety medication may be indicated both to relieve anxiety and to increase the effectiveness of pain medication. Time limits on painful treatment sessions should be predetermined with all patients who are cognizant and capable of participation. The therapist should consistently adhere to those limits to foster trust and provide a sense of control for the patient.

Depending on the presence of associated conditions or complications, the patient may be disoriented or unable to follow verbal cueing and therefore require passive ROM (PROM) exercise. In those circumstances, it is still important to continue to attempt full ROM using verbal encouragement and

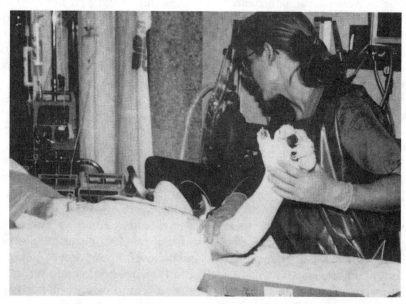

Figure 13.2. Before and during active-assistive or passive range of motion exercises, the therapist should continually reassure the patient and describe what is being done and why.

smooth, rhythmic patterns of movement with nonaggressive, sustained, end-range stretches. Individual joint ROM may be needed for problem areas, but in most cases, combined joint stretches are more effective when stretching burns that cover a large surface area. This combined joint stretching also decreases the length of time spent in painful therapy for the patient.

Positioning

Positioning and splinting recommendations should be made as needed to reduce edema, preserve joint mobility and structural integrity, and protect trauma or surgical sites. The general rules for positioning are to keep the head and extremities elevated above the heart and to keep all joints positioned in the *antideformity position,* defined as the position in which the specific body area (i.e., extremity, trunk, neck, or facial feature) is oriented with the healing skin stretched opposite to the line of pull of any anticipated contracture (Reeves, 2001). This positioning is accomplished by elevating the head of the bed, propping extremities on pillows, and using commercially or custom-fabricated positioning devices and splints. AROM, AAROM and, if necessary, PROM exercises should be initiated promptly for all joints that develop stiffness due to edema or that show evidence of skin tightness.

During the transition from dependence on others to self-reliance, patients frequently demonstrate abnormal posturing during exercise or self-care activities. This protective self-positioning usually begins as a guarding response to avoid pain and discomfort and usually involves a flexed position. For example, a patient with a burned arm may hold the extremity close to his side, giving in to the pull of tight scars. This behavior results in a progressive loss of active motion that eventually leads to difficulty performing activities such as dressing and bathing. This protective self-positioning often has been referred to as the "position of comfort." Unfortunately, this position is often the "position of deformity" as well. For this reason, preventive positioning and corrective splinting may be needed to preserve long-term joint mobility.

Splinting

Splints generally are used to maintain the extremities in the antideformity position. A splint may become constrictive, however, if applied the first day postinjury, when the patient is undergoing fluid resuscitation and the swelling is actively increasing. It may be advantageous to postpone formal splinting until after the swelling plateaus. Instead, the occupational therapist should emphasize positioning and active exercise to mobilize the edema. This approach is not appropriate, however, if the patient requires splinting to immobilize surgical sites or if subdermal structures have been compromised and immobilization is needed to prevent progressive damage. Exposed tendons can quickly become denatured and may rupture if not kept moist and splinted to prevent tension or stretching. Another situation requiring early splinting is if the patient is at risk for boutonnière deformities.

When deep burns are sustained to the dorsal PIP joints, the fingers are at risk for dorsal hood disruption and subsequent boutonnière deformities. When disruption occurs, the central slip of the extensor tendon is ruptured, allowing the head of the proximal phalanx to protrude dorsally through the extensor tendon mechanism and the lateral bonds drift volarly. All attempts to actively extend the finger will then result in flexion of the PIP joint and hyperextension of the distal interphalangeal (DIP) joint. If the PIP joints of a hand with deep dorsal burns are passively or forcefully flexed, the risk for dorsal hood disruption increases significantly. When exercising a finger under boutonnière precautions, the PIP joint is passively extended but *never* passively or forcefully flexed by either the patient or the practitioner. The adjacent DIP and metacarpophalangeal joints can be individually flexed only with the remaining two joints of the finger held in full extension. For 6 weeks, the finger should be kept in a digit extension splint to maintain full extension of the PIP and the dorsal hood on slack and removed only to exercise the DIP. This technique allows scar tissue to form over the dorsal surface of the PIP joint and reinforce or substitute for the damaged extensor hood (Pullium, 1984). The resulting stiff PIP joint will later respond to exercise, whereas a ruptured extensor hood mechanism results in permanent loss of joint mobility and hand disfigurement (Figure 13.3).

Most splinting falls into three categories: preventive, protective, and corrective. *Preventive* splints are static splints used to keep the extremities, neck, or mouth from losing functional mobility due to skin tightness or contractures. The affected area is immobilized in the antideformity position—the position that holds the skin and underlying tissues on maximum safe and tolerable stretch. They are usually worn at night or during periods of rest. Volar antideformity hand splints and elbow or knee extension conformers are examples of preventive splints.

Protective splints are static splints that immobilize an area to prevent motion that could compromise damaged subcutaneous structures or disrupt recently placed skin grafts and surgically reconstructed tissues. Positioning for these splints varies with the

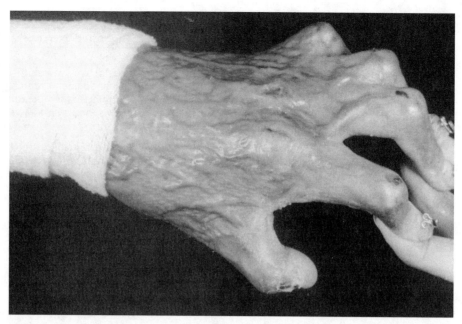

Figure 13.3. Boutonniére deformities, if not prevented in the acute phase, can result in severe deformity and loss of function.

surgical procedure performed and is not necessarily the antideformity or functional position.

Corrective splinting includes dynamic or serial static splints that exert a force to stretch tight tissues or correct a contracture. Examples of corrective splints are adjustable appliances for stretching mouth contractures (i.e., *microstomia*), serial casting of a flexion contracture, or hand splints with dynamic traction to correct MP joint hyperextension tightness (Pullium, 1984).

If the patient is able to participate, an AROM exercise program should be initiated and taught to the patient and family members. AROM exercise programs should be simple and easy to remember and should follow functional patterns of movement. Positioning recommendations, precautions, schedules for splint wear, and instructions for exercises should be documented in the medical record. They also should be posted bedside in the form of simple drawings that the staff, patient, and family members can easily see from a distance.

Managing extremity edema remains an acute care objective, and many of the positioning techniques established initially will be continued throughout recovery. Legs should be elevated in bed or when sitting. If a patient has upper extremity burns, the arm should be elevated on a pillow incline with the elbow above the heart and the hand above the elbow. For persistent edema, external compression, through use of pressure wraps, compression garments, or treatment with intermittent compression devices, may be indicated. Patients should be expected to exercise their hands independently, especially using the intrinsic muscles. They also should be encouraged to use their hands for eating, grooming, and other functional activities as much as possible, using adaptive aids as needed. The combination of active exercise, self-care activities, elevation, and external compression not only helps decrease hand edema but also promotes recovery of strength and coordination (Table 13.2).

Self-Care

Regardless of the education and emotional support provided, some patients may perceive their injury as a permanent disability. They experience decreased self-confidence and become increasingly dependent on staff and family members. When asked to perform an ADL task, their immediate response is to anticipate failure and refuse to even try. Rather than label the patient "uncooperative" or "unmotivated," the therapist should grade and carefully select tasks to promote success and increase self-confidence. Self-feeding is one of the first ADL tasks learned as a child, and the inability to do so carries much significance for a person's self-esteem. Therefore, as soon as a patient is allowed any oral intake, self-feeding should be introduced regardless of the assistance required. Early involvement in basic self-care activities, however limited, promotes a sense of efficacy by engaging the patient in goal-directed tasks that focus

Table 13.2. Antideformity Positioning and Exercises

Body Area	Position	Positioning Devices or Splints	Suggested Exercises
Face			
Mouth	Head of bed elevated to decrease facial and head edema	Microstomia prevention appliance or custom thermoplastic splint to preserve oral commissures and size of mouth opening	Early active "yawning" and passive sustained lateral stretch to mouth with fingers, temperature probe covers, or acrylic straws
Cheeks		Foley catheter placed between teeth and inner cheek and inflated to point of slight outer cheek blanching, applied no more than 10 minutes	Passive sustained stretch to cheeks and mouth using increasing number of tongue depressors stacked between uncompromised teeth
Eyes		Face mask; ectropion releases usually immobilized with cotton stint dressings sutured into place, then face mask reapplied posthealing over adjacent skin	Active eye opening with eyebrows up and mouth open Tight eye closure Frequent sustained lateral eye stretches to help prevent ectropion and eyelid tightness
Nares		Nasal trumpet to preserve opening; nasal flange added to facial conformer	Scar massage and manual stretching of nares
Ears	Avoid pressure to the burned helix when side-lying	Foam cutout instead of pillow; thermoplastic ear protectors after surgery	Posthealing scar massage Prompt use of Otoform-K® silicone putty or Silastic® elastomer conformers under elastic face mask with no ear openings in mask
Neck			
Anterior	No pillows under head; folded towels along thoracic spine to simultaneously extend neck and stretch chest; short mattress	Snug, custom-fitted, soft foam collar and elastic chin strap applied early over dressings to extend neck and compress healing scars; if scar bands or contractures develop, a rigid thermoplastic splint is used over dressings during the day	Gentle frequent AROM and sustained passive stretch with massage to stretch scar bands (Avoid neck hyperextension, especially in older adults.)
Posterior	Pillows under head	Same as anterior	Drag chin across chest from shoulder to shoulder
Shoulders and chest			
Anterior axilla and chest	Shoulders abducted to 100° and slight flexion supported on pillows; towel roll along thoracic spine to stretch chest	Figure 8 wrap around shoulders over axilla pads to protract shoulders and prevent or compress axillary web scar bands; airplane splint postgrafting worn full time for 3–5 days, then nights only	Frequent AROM and PROM of shoulders in all functional planes Sustained end-range stretch in flexion and horizontal abduction combined with massage and use of modalities to stretch axilla contractures
Posterior axilla and back	Shoulders abducted to 90° with 45° horizontal flexion supported on pillow or tray tables	Same as anterior	Frequent AROM and AAROM of shoulders in flexion and horizontal adduction using pulleys and wall-stretch exercises

Continued

Table 13.2. *Continued*

Body Area	Position	Positioning Devices or Splints	Suggested Exercises
Elbows Anterior	Position with elbows in 0°–5° flexion, avoid hyperextension	Thermoplastic anterior or posterior elbow splint in position to maintain maximum surface area of burn site; 5° flexion; dynamic splints or serial casting to stretch established flexion contractures or scar bands	Frequent AROM and self-assisted PROM with sustained stretch at end ranges (If patient has disproportionate pain, avoid rigorous PROM and evaluate for heterotopic ossification.)
Posterior	Position elbows in 45°–90° flexion with pillows	Posterior elbow splint with ≥ 90° flexion for posterior elbow burns or grafts	
Hands Dorsal and volar	Elevate UE on pillow elbow; elbow above incline with hand above palm until initial acute edema resolves heart and hand roll in	Resting hand splint in 75° flexion, IPs at 0°, thumb in antideformity position (MPs at combined radial and palmar abduction and wrist at 30° extension) secured over dressings with elastic wraps and well elevated on pillow incline	Boutonnière precautions if deep partial-thickness burns are present with *no* passive flexion of PIP joints, *no* combined MP and IP flexion and *no* fisting If no deep burns cover PIPs, combined IP, MP, and 45° wrist flexion with thumb in opposition to give maximum sustained stretch to dorsal hand and preserve palmar arch
Volar only	Elevate UE on pillow incline with hand above elbow, elbow above heart, and hand out flat with no hand roll	*Early* initiation of "banjo" hand splint in palmar stretch position (fingers extended and abducted with wrist extended 45°) worn during all periods of inactivity, off during the day for exercise and ADL	*Early* initiation of palmar stretchskin exercises with combined IP and MP extension, finger abduction, thumb radial abduction and extension, and and 45° wrist extension to give maximum sustained stretch to volar skin
Web spaces	Velfoam strips between fingers wrapped with figure 8 pattern, using Coban elastic wrap or secured with compression gloves	Splint as with volar only with conformers under promptly applied temporary or customized scar-compression glove	Massage and passive stretch of web spaces and active finger-abduction exercises Lacing fingers together and pushing distal palms tightly together
Trunk Anterior and posterior	Keep shoulders aligned with hips at all times when in bed	Keep upright when sitting with pillows or support both arms on tray table	ROM and sustained stretch in trunk flexion, extension, and rotation over bolster
Hips Anterior	Use reclining chair and minimize time spent in hip flexion; when supine, keep bed flat as possible, support lateral legs in abduction and neutral rotation; if possible, have patient rest prone on firm mattress with feet off end of bed	Posterior splint for postoperative immobilization	Supine on mat table with pillow below buttocks Sit at edge of mat table with feet on floor and lie back slowly until supine

Continued

Table 13.2. *Continued*

Body Area	Position	Positioning Devices or Splints	Suggested Exercises
Posterior	Sit upright with pillows under thighs; when supine, head and knees on bed raised to allow hip flexion, support lateral legs in abduction and neutral rotation	Splinting usually only needed for postoperative immobilization in agitated patient	"Knee hugs," squats, toe touches
Perineum	Sit or lie with legs abducted	Abduction pillow or splint to keep knees apart	"Frog sit" with soles of feet together and slowly spread knees and pull feet toward body
Knees Anterior only	Pillow under knees to allow moderate flexion	Splinting usually only needed for postoperative immobilization	"Knee hugs" and squats
Anterior or or posterior	Pillows under distal legs to minimize knee flexion; avoid hyperextension	Thermoplastic posterior knee conformer applied with elastic wrap; serial casting or dynamic splint for established knee contracture	Touch toes with knees bent, then slowly straighten knees Prone with pillow under knee, ankle weights give slow stretch
Ankles Anterior	Pillow under lower leg with heel suspended	Thermoplastic dorsal conforming resting splint to maintain combined ankle and toe plantar flexion	Kneel with dorsum of foot as flat as possible on mat surface, slowly sit on heels
Posterior	Ankle supported in dorsiflexion with footboard, blanket roll or posterior splint	Ankle foot orthosis or molded posterior conforming splint with ankle held in neutral, posterior heel of splint "bubbled out" to avoid excessive pressure to calcaneus and Achilles' tendon	Sustained stretches in dorsiflexion Ambulation Ankle pumps and toe raises with distal foot on 2 in. pad (see volar toe exercises)
Toes Dorsal	Toes supported in plantar-flexed position with dorsal padding and elastic wrap, lace-up shoe with insert or splint to maintain toe flexion	Thermoplastic dorsal conforming resting splint to maintain combined ankle and toe plantar flexion	Sit with foot on opposite knee and pull foot into combined ankle and toe plantar flexion; hold to sustain stretch
Volar	Toes supported in dorsiflexion with volar padding and elastic wrap, lace-up shoe or splint to maintain toe dorsiflexion		With knees extended, place a long, wide strap or lengthwise folded sheet under the distal foot and toes and pull foot and toes dorsally
Web spaces		Long Velfoam padding strips between toes and secured to the foot with self-adhesive elastic wrap or worn under "foot glove" customized scar-compression garment	Massage and passive stretch of web spaces Active toe-abduction exercises

Note. AAROM = active-assistive range of motion; ADL = activities of daily living; AROM = active range of motion; IP = interphalangeal; MP = metacarpophalangeal; PIP = proximal interphalangeal; PROM = passive range of motion; ROM = range of motion; UE = upper extremity.

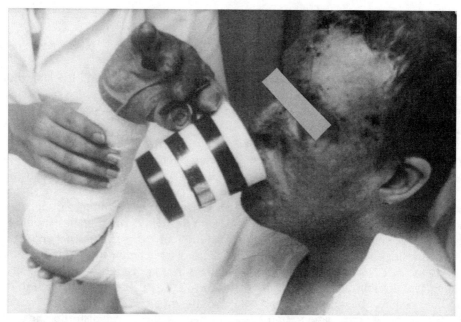

Figure 13.4. As soon as oral intake is allowed, the patient should be encouraged to begin self-feeding regardless of the assistance needed.

attention on accomplishment instead of impairment (Figure 13.4).

When first attempting ADL, the focus should be on accomplishing simple skills, such as holding a spoon with an enlarged handle or getting a cup to the mouth. Initially, self-care tasks should be simplified with adaptive aids as needed, to ensure patient participation and success, which provide the patient with a sense of accomplishment and control. As the patient progresses with ROM, strength, and endurance goals, use of aids should be reduced as more challenging and complex tasks are introduced to the patient's routine. Although considerable time and patience may be involved when using this approach, the patient's general endurance and confidence will be enhanced for later attempts with complex IADL tasks.

Activities as Exercise

The need for immobilization after surgical procedures will periodically limit activity participation and independence. Before surgery, the patient should be informed that a defined period of immobilization will follow the procedure but that under supervision, certain rehabilitation activities will continue. For example, if a patient's hand and forearm burns are surgically excised and grafted, the therapist may still provide shoulder activities at the patient's bedside during the postoperative immobilization period. When a patient's hands are in postoperative dressings, self-feeding may be possible only with adaptive equipment. If adaptations are used to enhance post-operative participation in activities, the patient should understand that they are only temporary.

Loss of strength and endurance and the resulting decrease in daily activity are frequently a consequence of prolonged bed rest. Severe burns also increase metabolism, placing further demands on the body's general physical condition. To limit deconditioning, acute burn patients should be involved in active exercise, structured activities, and ambulation throughout the day. A combination of AAROM, composite and individual joint stretching, and purposeful activities should be used. The therapist should communicate daily with the burn team to help determine when to increase or decrease the patient's activity schedule. If the patient is confined to bed due to lower-extremity grafts, ADL activities, such as self-feeding, simple hygiene tasks, and upper-body grooming, and a modified exercise program should still be performed. Bedside activities that require a variety of fine and gross motor skills can promote upper-extremity flexibility and general strength as well as provide opportunities for socialization. Such activities could include progressing from hitting a balloon back and forth to tossing a beach ball, Velcro® darts, or basketball to promote gross motor coordination and strengthening. Playing cards or board games, crafts, and computer activities help promote fine motor skills. Whenever possible, activities should include current leisure interests or previous pastimes of the patient.

When the patient is medically cleared to ambulate, the intervention program should be adjusted to include out-of-bed exercise and activity. Walking or standing to do exercises, sitting up in a chair for all meals, and standing at a sink for grooming tasks all help promote general conditioning. Patients often complain of fatigue during this phase of increased activity. They will need ongoing support and encouragement to ambulate, perform their exercise program, and complete their self-care tasks independently.

During acute care, a formal schedule may be needed to provide structure, support appropriate patient behaviors, and emphasize treatment objectives. The schedule should include morning and afternoon therapy sessions; dressing changes and nursing procedures; periods for ADL, including ambulation, grooming, eating, and dressing; and *sacred* free time for visitors and rest periods. The schedule should be developed in agreement with the patient, and the entire burn team should adhere to it. Defining daily expectations in advance gives patients a sense of control, reduces anxiety, and fosters active involvement in the rehabilitation process.

Inpatient and Outpatient Rehabilitation Phases: Evaluation

During the inpatient and outpatient rehabilitation phases, the therapist reevaluates ROM, strength, activity tolerance, self-care abilities, work skills, skin and scar condition, and social and emotional adaptation. Goniometric measurements should be made weekly, biweekly, or as needed, depending on the frequency of treatment or need to document changes. Muscle strength, dexterity, and endurance can be evaluated by manual muscle testing and other evaluative tools or by using treatment modalities such as a Baltimore Therapeutic Equipment (BTE) Work Simulator®. When the patient has hand burns, dynamometer recordings of grip strength and measures of pinch strength also should be made at regular intervals. Chronic edema of the hands can be documented using circumferential and volumetric measurements.

Improvement in general endurance and activity tolerance also should be documented. The therapist should quantify the patient's activity tolerance during self-care activities by monitoring and recording the following factors:

- The position in which the task is performed
- The grade or level of physical exertion the task demands
- The amount of assistance needed
- Adaptations or assistive devices required to complete the task
- The duration of participation prior to signs of fatigue
- The frequency and the length of needed rest breaks or percentage of the total treatment session spent resting.

Hypertrophic scars and contractures require close monitoring because they often affect the patient's ability to maintain adequate mobility to perform everyday tasks. When assessing a scar, it is important to notice changes in appearance, texture, and flexibility. The therapist should note the location of any scars that restrict end-range movement in single or combined joint motions. Tight or thick scars near joints restrict mobility and cause discomfort as the patient tries to stretch to the end ranges of the involved joint's motion. Scarring on the face often results in facial distortion, incomplete eye closure, or constriction of nasal and oral passages that impairs breathing and eating abilities.

Early recognition and therapeutic intervention often can stretch developing contractures and help reduce the likelihood of surgical intervention. Some scar bands, however, may be unstable and break down during exercise, which will result in prolonged inflammation with further scarring and progressive loss of mobility. Patients with tight, unstable scar bands should be referred to a surgeon for possible release of the scar band and repair of the defect with more durable, grafted skin.

The occupational therapist must continually reevaluate the burn patient's occupational performance. The patient should be observed during self-care activities and watched for unnecessary exertion or use of abnormal posturing and movements. Therapy intervention should include instruction in energy-conservation techniques and demonstration of methods for performing the task in normal movement patterns. For example, a patient with burns involving the trunk and extremities may become frustrated and fatigued during upper-body dressing activities and feel incapable of correctly completing the task without excessive posturing or unnecessary assistance. The occupational therapist should closely monitor the patient's ability to integrate correct motions for the activity and encourage the patient's creativity in problem solving to accomplish the task.

Awareness of the patient's emotional status is important throughout recovery. Because of pain, fatigue, frustration, and other difficulties encountered with rehabilitation activities, patients may experience extreme anxiety and emotional distress, especially during painful procedures or exercises. The therapist should be aware of a patient's coping abilities and report noticeable declines in affect to the burn team. As appropriate, the patient should be encouraged to discuss problems with the burn team's social worker, psychiatrist, or chaplain.

Inpatient Rehabilitation Phase: Intervention

During the inpatient rehabilitation phase, the patient's role in self-care increases as the need for wound care and nursing procedures decreases. The goal is for the patient to complete self-care activities (i.e., feeding, grooming, and dressing) as independently and with as little adaptation as possible. Continued patient education should stress the importance of resuming preinjury activities and emphasize the daily routines and habits that will give the patient more control over his or her care. Decreased ROM, flexibility, strength, and activity tolerance, however, may interfere with performance of relatively demanding ADL, such as bathing or dressing in regular street clothes. Decreased dexterity or poor sensation may interfere with the completion of fine motor tasks, such as fastening clothing, and may put the patient at increased risk for reinjury. Poor strength and decreased activity tolerance and endurance may prevent the patient from performing repetitive activities or completing ADL tasks within acceptable time limits.

Physical Reconditioning

To promote ROM, strength, and endurance, a variety of treatment modalities and activities should be used (Humphrey, Richard, & Staley, 1994). An exercise program should include stretching and flexibility exercises for the face, neck, trunk, and all extremities as well as strengthening activities. When possible, exercises should be performed in front of a mirror so that patients can self-monitor their posture and progress. Stretching should be performed slowly and should be prolonged at the point where the scar blanches. For scars that extend over more than one joint, the extremity should be involved in a multijoint stretch to elongate the scar fully. AROM should progress to resistive ROM as early as tolerated. Independent exercise programs may start with soft sponges for hand exercises and progress to therapy putty, Theraband® exercises, pulleys, and free weights. When establishing an independent exercise program, special attention should be given to the proximal shoulder and hip muscle groups, which often are particularly weak from disuse or immobilization following surgery.

Scarring, decreased sensitivity, and muscle atrophy can impair fine motor skills and hand coordination. Hand dexterity and sensitivity can be monitored and improved with tasks that require manipulation of small items of various sizes and textures. These activities could include the Minnesota Rate of Manipulation Test©; the Purdue Pegboard©; computer-based tests (which will also provide documentation); and working with items familiar to the patient including pens, pencils, keys, clothespins, paper clips, coins, small tools, cell phones, and other small electronic devices. Fine motor activities of personal interest should be incorporated into the patient's independent exercise program; examples include playing card or board games, completing jigsaw puzzles, doing needlework or other previous hobbies, doing crossword puzzles, and corresponding with family to improve writing dexterity.

Aerobic activities should be incorporated into the patient's comprehensive exercise program to enhance the cardiovascular system and gain endurance. Ideally, the patients should be able to tolerate at least 20 minutes of exercise or rhythmic activity at 60% of maximum heart rate at least 3 times per week by discharge (Breines, 2001). Endurance can be promoted by encouraging the patient to participate in independent strengthening activities such as progressively paced ambulation around the hospital, riding a stationary bike, using an upper-body ergometer, climbing stairs, and standing at the sink for hygiene tasks. Equipment such as a BTE Work Simulator® can imitate functional motions to increase upper-body ROM, strength, and endurance as well as provide written results to monitor patient performance. Other equipment, such as West II and Valpar Work Samples, also is helpful when reproducing functional activities or assessing and simulating work skills (Figure 13.5). A comprehensive circuit-training program that includes stretching, strengthening, endurance, and work-hardening activities in a gym setting promotes patient independence with his or her exercise program in preparation for discharge.

Modalities

Therapists using modalities with patients must have the required training and experience outlined by the American Occupational Therapy Association (AOTA) and state licensing agencies. Modalities can be used as an adjunct to or preparation for occupational performance (AOTA, 1997). Certain modalities may be of benefit in the treatment of burn

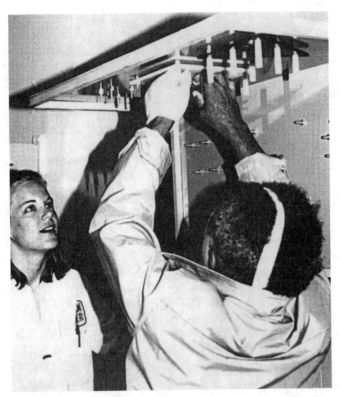

Figure 13.5. Work conditioning equipment can be used to increase active range of motion and general endurance.

scars, but because of altered vascularity and sensitivity in the burn sites, special care must be taken when using modalities with burn patients. Cold modalities, such as ice massage or ice packs, are contraindicated because the accompanying vasoconstriction makes the scars stiffer and less pliable and the cold temperature is usually tolerated poorly by the patient when applied over a burn scar.

Heat modalities may be of benefit but should be used with close supervision. Some hypertrophic scars dissipate heat more slowly and have decreased sensation and therefore may be at increased risk for reinjury. Hot packs should have additional towel layers, and ultrasound settings should be set at a low intensity. Fluidotherapy® can be used with close supervision, but only after all open areas are completely healed. Therapists should exercise caution when using electrical stimulation with newly healed burns, because the injured areas may still have unmyelinated nerve endings and be extremely sensitive to electrical current. Paraffin, if used at a low temperature, works well to heat and relax collagen fibers, and the mineral oil lubricates and softens the scars for stretching. Because gauze can be dipped into the paraffin and layered onto any scar band, this modality is an effective heat treatment with any

area that requires sustained, low-load stretching of contractures. Some patients continue using paraffin as part of their home therapy program after discharge.

Skin Care

Newly healed skin is extremely fragile and prone to breakdown. Problems include hypersensitivity, blisters, and excoriation resulting from friction or even minor trauma. Reduced numbers of oil and sweat glands lead to excessive dryness and possible splitting of the skin when aggressively stretched. Skin-conditioning education and activities should be initiated as soon as wounds are well healed and should include massage, frequent application of appropriate moisturizing products, and safe donning of intermediate and custom-made pressure garments.

Massage

Patients should be taught to massage their healed burns, graft sites, and donor site scars with a moisturizing lotion at least 4 times per day. Massage should be performed only with lotion to prevent shearing friction, and pressure should be just firm enough to cause blanching of the skin. Ideally, scars should be massaged and moisturized prior to and during stretching exercises and whenever the scars feel dry or itchy. Keeping the scars well moisturized helps prevent skin tears, which may occur in dry scars during exercise or activity. The mechanical action of massage helps soften the scars by promoting collagen remodeling while reducing hypersensitivity.

Scar Management

Early compression therapy should be used to provide continuous external vascular support and to reduce the potential for hypertrophic scarring. The presence of edema in the limb and vascular pooling (as evidenced by erythemic skin color) indicate poor venous return in burned extremities. Edema can increase in dependent extremities without external venous support, especially when the patient is inactive. Vascular stockings or elastic wraps should be applied to the feet and legs to aid venous return, whenever the patient's legs are resting in a dependent position, but especially when the patient is out of bed or ambulating. Because the hands and feet are especially prone to edema and contractures, they always should be elevated when at rest, and web-space pads and compression wraps should be applied as soon as initial healing occurs.

A variety of transitional compression techniques and products can be used for early scar-compression therapy. For the torso and extremities, products include elastic bandages, such as Ace® wraps; vascular stockings; and tubular support bandages, such as Tubigrip®. For the hands and digits, compression can be provided using temporary gloves, such as Isotoner® gloves, for lower pressure and prefabricated intermediate gloves, such as Tubigrip™ gloves, for higher pressure; or combinations of digit-sized tubular support bandages, such as Tubiton™ bandages and self-adherent elastic dressings such as Coban and Cowrap (Ward, Reddy, Brockway, Hayes-Lundy, & Mills, 1994). All flexion creases, web spaces, skin cleavages, and other skin surface concavities should be padded under the wraps to ensure adequate pressure.

Special care is needed when applying any elastic or compressive dressing. Dressings should be applied with slight tension, using a figure 8 pattern starting at the distal extremity and wrapping proximately. To apply a self-adherent compression wrap to the hand, inch-wide strips of Coban™ wrap are first placed through the web spaces over padding and attached to a band around the wrist. Silicone gel pads can be used under the Coban wrap to provide added pressure to thicker scars while protecting the skin from irritation. Inch-wide Coban strips are then applied around individual fingers in a distal-to-proximal manner, and the

hand is wrapped. The fingertips should be slightly exposed and appear slightly erythemic or rosy in color. Care should be taken to avoid wrapping too tightly; doing so would impair circulation, as evidenced by blanched, cyanotic, or cold fingertips or by the patient's report of discomfort, numbness, or tingling. The self-adherent elastic wraps should cover the thumb, all fingers, the web spaces, and hand and should extend to at least 2 in. above the wrist. Exercises and ADL should be performed with the Coban wrap intact. If the wrap is applied correctly, hand use will not be restricted. For self-feeding, the Coban wrap can be covered with a rubber glove. Persistent edema that does not respond to Coban wraps also may be treated with intermittent compression-pump therapy.

After most wounds are healed and the patient's weight and areas of edema have stabilized, the patient can be measured for long-term, customized scar-compression garments. The patient's first set of customized compression garments should be fitted to the patient prior to discharge. Most customized scar-compression garments are lightweight, are 60% porous, and provide a more even, higher grade of compression than temporary compression techniques. The pressure provides venous support, which helps the collagen fibers reorganize into a flatter pattern, resulting in a thinner, more flexible, and more cosmetically acceptable scar than if allowed to heal with no compressive therapy. To be effective, compression garments should be worn an average of 23 of every 24 hours until the underlying scars are mature (an average of 18 to 24 months). For this reason, it is recommended that two sets of compression garments be obtained so that one set may be worn while the other is laundered. Ideally, the garments should be removed only for bathing, skin care, and sexual intimacy. Face masks and gloves also may be removed for meals. Patients can perform most ADL tasks and participate in most recreational activities and work environments without interference from the garments (Ward, Hayes-Lundy, Reddy, Brockway, & Mills, 1992); however, patients may experience excessive warmth during outside activities in warmer climates. Patients should be educated early regarding the purpose of the pressure garments and the need to adhere consistently to the wearing schedule if the best results are to be obtained and additional corrective surgeries avoided. When it is time to measure patients for garments, they will recognize scar-compression therapy as a step toward their full recovery (Stewart, Bhagwanjee, Mbakaza, & Binase, 2000).

Customized garments require underlying conformers to equalize pressure over concavities and to increase pressure over areas of heavy scarring. Conformers can be made from a variety of materials, including Velfoam® foam strap padding silicone gel sheets; 1/16-in.-thick Aquaplast®; and custom-molded conformers made from Silastic Elastomer® silicone and prosthetic foam combinations, Oto-form-K® silicone putty, or any number of products on the market. Even with the conformers, however, customized garments are less bulky than pressure wraps or temporary compression techniques and allow the patient to move more freely. Wearing personal clothing over the scar-compression garments should be encouraged to promote a return to "normal" habits and routines and to give the patient practice in donning both compression garments and street clothes (Figure 13.6). Clothing should be casual, loose fitting, comfortable, and made primarily of cotton.

ADL

Independence in performing ADL is the ultimate goal for burn patients, and achieving it may require not only regaining physical skills but also making adaptations in the patient's environment and routines. Some adaptations may be temporary, but permanent loss of physical ability may mean changes in the patient's lifestyle and roles. Uncontrolled scarring or noncompliance with exercise programs often results in contractures, which impair motion and skin flexibility. When this situation occurs, previous performance patterns cannot be completed without compensatory techniques or adaptive equipment. Impaired trunk or hip mobility may prevent a patient from donning pants, underwear, socks, and shoes unless a dressing stick, sock aid, or long-handled shoehorn is provided. Impaired shoulder or elbow mobility will make donning and doffing shirts more difficult, and adaptive techniques or modified clothing styles with special fasteners may be needed. For patients with contractures of the hands and fingers, feeding utensils or drinking cups with easy-to-grip handles may be needed, as well as adapted writing implements, button aids, adapted zippers, and elastic shoelaces. As soon as the patient is able to attempt basic self-care tasks, family members should be asked to bring the patient's own clothes and personal grooming items from home so that the items can be modified if needed.

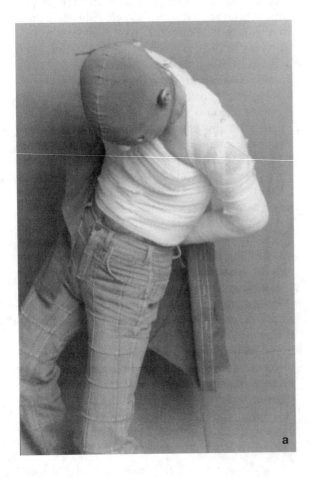

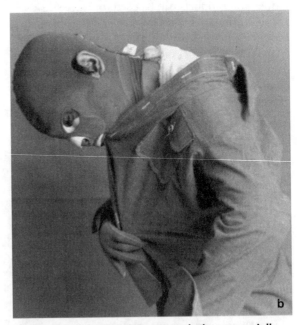

Figure 13.6. (a) Donning street clothes, especially over dressings, can be difficult. (b) Patients should be given the opportunity to problem solve ways to perform tasks independently before adaptive equipment is used.

Despite the extra time and effort it may take, patients should be encouraged to first attempt self-care activities with minimal reliance on compensatory motions or use of adaptive equipment. Recognizing that motivation cannot be maintained without successful task completion, however, the occupational therapist should intervene and modify the task before the patient becomes too frustrated or fatigued. Otherwise, the patient may lose motivation and refuse further attempts. This loss of motivation is especially true for small children (Figure 13.7).

As in the acute phase, the therapist should encourage self-care tasks that promote both independence and self-confidence. Attempting a task using only adaptive techniques before providing adaptive devices allows the patient to have an active part in the problem-solving process. This approach provides the patient with an empowering experience of overcoming difficulties through learning new abilities; in contrast, providing potentially unnecessary devices sends a message of continuing disability. When an adaptive aid is required for task completion, the goal is to improve function to the point that the aid will eventually not be needed. The device should be modified or discontinued as active motion and activity tolerance increase, and the changes should be presented to the patient as signs of progress.

Patients who were injured while bathing or cooking or at work may be reluctant to perform

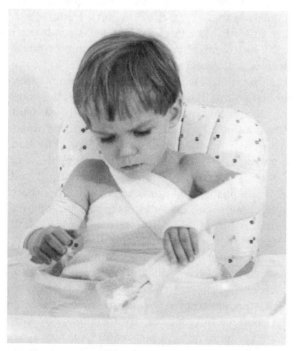

Figure 13.7. Like adults, a small child can be motivated to use his hands if the task is one that holds his interest, such as feeding himself ice cream.

tasks related to those activities. It is crucial that their fears be identified and addressed. Intervention activities should include education in safety precautions and performance of the fear-provoking tasks with therapist supervision. Safety precautions should be discussed before the intervention session so that they can be practiced during the activity.

Prior to discharge, the patient and therapist should address any significant permanent impairment (e.g., amputations from electrical injuries or trauma-related permanent neurological injuries) that will interfere with resumption of previous or modified life roles. The need for wheelchairs, customized prosthetic devices, household modifications, adaptive driving equipment, computerized home-technology assistive devices, or other durable medical equipment should be addressed and ordered so that the items can be available for use during the outpatient rehabilitation phase.

Discharge Planning

The rehabilitation phase of burn recovery is greatly influenced by the patient's previous performance patterns. Extended hospitalization and postdischarge daily outpatient treatment schedules can prevent a patient from resuming familiar roles as family member, student, or provider. It is important in this phase that patients recognize their progress and begin to assume previous roles on at least a part-time basis in preparation for discharge.

Burn patients and their family members must be educated about anticipated home care activities before discharge from the hospital. Throughout hospitalization, education about what can be expected after discharge can aid this process. Home care booklets, classes, and videotapes are some methods burn care facilities use to reinforce this information (Adriaenssens, 1988; Mason & Forshaw, 1986; Yurko & Fratianne, 1988). Discharge education and training should involve the entire burn team and should cover a broad range of topics (Kaplan, 1985).

Before discharge, the patient and caregivers should have opportunities to practice dressing changes, skin care, and application of compression garments and splints. Written instructions for the following home program activities should be provided, reviewed, and practiced:

- Wound and skin care
- Use of medications, moisturizers, and sunblock lotions
- Positioning recommendations
- Home exercise programs (including both therapeutic and recreational activities)
- Use and care of splints and self-help devices

- Scar-compression garments and conformers
- Sun and trauma precautions
- Need for environmental modifications (as appropriate for home, school, work and social settings).

The patient and family members should demonstrate a thorough understanding of the purpose and content of the home program well before discharge. A list of contacts and phone numbers also should be provided in case questions or concerns arise before the first outpatient appointment.

Outpatient Rehabilitation Phase: Intervention

Current views of occupational therapy practice (e.g., Christiansen, 1991; Kielhofner, 1995; Law et al., 1996) recognize the client as constantly changing within a dynamic set of environmental circumstances. Life satisfaction depends on a complex array of conditions, including motivation, experiences, social role expectations, and physical and cognitive capacities. Change in any one of these conditions affects the other areas.

During the outpatient rehabilitation phase of recovery, burn patients may go through countless physical and emotional changes, despite continual and comprehensive patient education. Once home, they truly begin to experience both the functional and social consequences of a serious burn injury. Changes in self-image, loss of previous work roles, and altered social relationships directly affect motivation and compliance with therapy recommendations. Although clients may eat and dress independently at discharge, they may return to the clinic unable to raise a spoon to their mouth. Providing adaptive equipment should not be the first response and may not resolve the problem, because many factors can contribute to such changes in activity performance. Identifying the underlying cause behind a lost ability is the first step toward developing an appropriate intervention response. Although scar contracture is the most common cause, other physical and emotional factors can contribute to performance problems. Some patients may suffer from posttraumatic stress disorders (Perry & Difede, 1992), and others must contend with emotional consequences related to preinjury psychological problems (Malt & Ugland, 1989; Tucker, 1986).

Before discharge from the hospital, a patient's strength and endurance may be adequate for independence in daily living. Once the patient returns home, however, differences between the hospital and home environments may be so great that fatigue sets in before noon. This feeling of fatigue may be caused by a lack of emotional as well as physical energy. The normal reaction is to rest instead of participating in home activities and outpatient therapy. The patient may lose his or her momentum, and as a result, strength may remain poor or decrease; scars may tighten, causing decreased flexibility; and the patient may become increasingly dependent on others. For that reason, outpatient visits should be scheduled to begin shortly after discharge. Follow-up visits should be frequent, so that patients can receive the physical and emotional support they often need to get them through this difficult adjustment period.

Outpatient treatment activities are similar to those used during inpatient rehabilitation, but their intensity and frequency increase. They should include a daily exercise program that emphasizes massage and stretching followed by flexibility and strengthening activities. Although all activities should be done frequently throughout the day, scar massage and stretching can improve a patient's participation in all activities, especially if done prior to the activities.

Scar contracture is the usual cause of most performance problems. When burn scars extend over joint surfaces, a progressive loss of AROM occurs as the skin tightens. If left untreated, secondary muscle shortening and fibrous contracture of the joint capsule can occur (Abston, 1987). The primary goal of a scar-treatment program is to manage scar development so that as scar tissue matures, minimal surface distortions or loss of active ROM result from tight scar bands, hypertrophic scarring, or adhesions to underlying structures.

Scar-compression therapy continues after discharge; the therapist closely monitors the compression garments for proper fit, signs of garment deterioration, the need for underlying conformers or inserts, and effectiveness (as evidenced by flat, smooth scars). Although pressure garments and conformers are used to minimize scar height and maintain pliability, continuous activity is necessary to oppose the contractile forces of the scar. Splints, serial casting, end-range stretching exercises, and activities that accentuate flexibility all are effective treatments for contractures (Daugherty & Carr-Collins, 1994; Rivers, 1987). Sometimes, a scar contracture is so strong that prevention of further loss of motion may seem to be the only goal. A scar band may become unstable and tend to break down repeatedly. Immobilizing such contractures with serial casting in a position of gentle tension often allows the open wound to heal and improves ROM. Contractures that chronically break down, however, eventually will require surgical intervention to restore active mobility and scar durability.

Because scar control and remodeling are easier during the early stages of wound maturation, limitations in self-care ability can be resolved if appropriate treatments are implemented promptly and the patient participates actively. In addition to other outpatient treatment activities, performing basic self-care is an effective, practical, and meaningful way to increase strength, endurance, flexibility, and coordination.

In some cases, burn depth, extent, and involvement of underlying structures are so severe that long-term adaptations are necessary for the patient to perform tasks independently. The adaptations should be simple and designed to use all available AROM. As scars mature and soften, performance skills should gradually improve. Tendon and joint adhesions also should eventually resolve if patients use all their available motion and continue with stretching exercises.

Once scars mature, they no longer require positioning, splinting, or exercise but still require life-long precautions. Burn scars are at higher risk for developing skin cancers years into the future (Ozek et al., 2001), especially if they are chronically inflamed by trauma or excessive sun exposure. In addition, because the skin helps regulate body temperature through perspiration, the loss of sweat and oil glands in large areas of deep burns and grafted areas can increase the risk of heat stroke despite the body's attempt to compensate by increasing perspi-

ration in unburned areas. The client is at risk of dehydration and will need increased fluid intake when in warm environments. Clients must protect all burn, graft, and donor sites from sun exposure using hats, lightweight cotton clothing, and sunblock lotion. Unprotected depigmented scars will sunburn rapidly, and all scars are at risk for uneven hyperpigmentation, which will result in undesirable cosmetic results. Therefore, it is recommended that burn patients use an oil-free, PABA-free, UVA/UVB sunscreen lotion with a SPF rating of 15 or higher. Full-length pants, long-sleeved shirts, and hats also are recommended to protect the scars from both reflected and direct sun exposure.

Depending on their personalities and coping skills, many burn patients with permanent physical limitations develop their own adaptive methods to accomplish specific tasks (Figure 13.8). They may consider extensive adaptations to be an encumbrance or an embarrassment, and if they have to use adaptive equipment, it tends to be small enough to fit in a pocket or purse, such as a button aid (Figure 13.9). This positive change of perspective usually occurs during the outpatient rehabilitation phase and is a sign that the patient is accepting permanent in his or her life context and is developing new performance patterns.

Early in the outpatient rehabilitation phase, patients may have little interest in activities because of the emotional effects of the injury. Depression and anxiety are common during recovery and are often manifested in noncompliance or apathy, both of

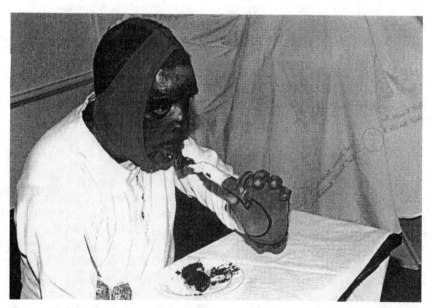

Figure 13.8. Extended handles should be gradually shortened as range of motion improves.

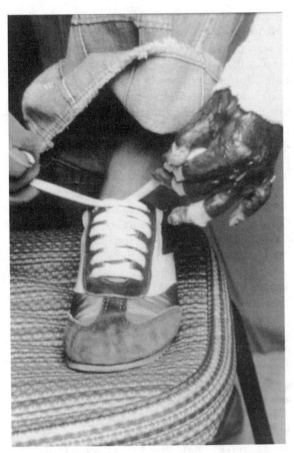

Figure 13.9. Patients should be encouraged to develop strength and dexterity for later task completion.

which slow progress toward functional and emotional independence. During this adjustment period, burn patients may receive comfort and encouragement by talking with other burn patients or by attending a support group. Talking with previously burned patients facilitates understanding by sharing personal perspectives and offering physical evidence that things will get easier and better with time and continued effort.

During the outpatient rehabilitation phase, therapy should include opportunities to engage in activities that incorporate past skills and current interests related to employment, home management, education, and play. Depending on the patient's length of hospital stay, some of these activities already may have been initiated during the inpatient rehabilitation phase. Starting with the first outpatient visit to therapy and continuing until discharge, each therapy session should begin with the patient and therapist reviewing current difficulties and addressing possible adaptations to work or home schedules, physical en-

vironments, and independent home programs. Practicing specific tasks improves the patient's performance of the task itself as well as the underlying performance components. For example, a homemaker may complain of fatigue and inability to complete domestic tasks. She may practice cooking skills during a treatment session to build her standing endurance and activity tolerance. Cooking also provides opportunities to learn and practice safety techniques to help resolve fear of heat, especially if the burns were related to a house fire or cooking. Fine motor skills and activity tolerance are improved by practicing specific tasks related to work roles, not just by using a work simulator or traditional exercise equipment (Figure 13.10). Activities that support current leisure and social interests should be incorporated into intervention sessions so that a balance of work and play are fostered as IADL are resumed.

When possible, the patient's personal home- and work-related equipment, such as cleaning supplies, hand tools, work station materials, cell phones, laptop computers, and motor vehicles, should be brought to therapy sessions so that the therapist can analyze task technique and suggest any needed adaptations. Often, only simple, temporary adaptations are required, such as knob adaptations for a washing machine, computer software modifications, or a padded steering wheel and large gearshift knob for a patient with stiff or fused finger joints. A patient with minimal elbow movement due to heterotopic ossification may need to continue using long-handled devices to perform independent self-feeding, dressing, and personal grooming tasks until surgical intervention is possible (Figure 13.11). Patients with severe functional loss, as with limb amputations or permanent neurological deficits, may need prostheses and costly modifications, such as foot-powered driving controls, bathroom safety equipment, installation of home entry ramps, or computerized home environment control systems. When the need for such equipment is anticipated, the social worker or case manager should be notified of those needs before the patient's discharge from the hospital, especially when funds are limited.

Leisure interests and social roles should not be neglected during the rehabilitation phases. If a previous leisure activity has been discarded due to permanent functional loss, it should be promptly replaced with a new social or recreational activity. Replacement activities may involve learning new skills, such as using public transportation for the first time or strategies for facing the public after a disfiguring burn. Leisure activities should be incor-

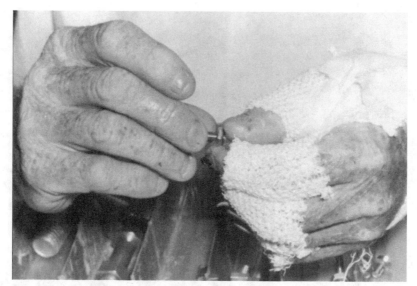

Figure 13.10. This mechanic develops his finger dexterity by working with various sizes of nuts and bolts.

porated into therapy routines as early as possible because of their physical and emotional therapeutic value (Figure 13.12).

If permanent disability precludes resumption of previous work roles, leisure roles take on more importance, and past interests should be encouraged.

An uncomfortable motion is often better tolerated when performed during a leisure activity or play activity (Melchert-McKearnan, Deitz, Engel, & White, 2000). The therapist should be careful not to suppress the patient's interest by turning the leisure task into an "exercise."

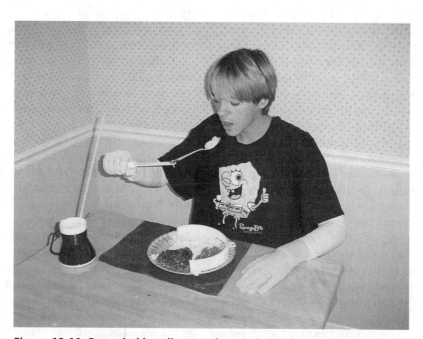

Figure 13.11. Extended handles may be needed long-term when heterotopic ossification or scarring limits elbow motion but should be gradually shortened as range of motion improves or discarded after the elbow is surgically released.

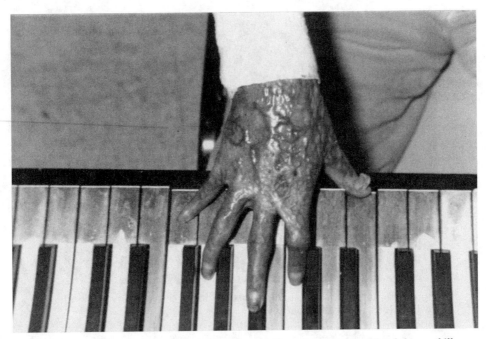

Figure 13.12. A patient stretches tight web spaces and regains a prior leisure skill while practicing on a piano.

During the outpatient rehabilitation phase, the patient's need for ongoing therapy should diminish. When the patient's return to part-time work or attendance at school will promote occupational recovery, outpatient therapy appointments should gradually be reduced in frequency. When the patient achieves the skills needed to live independently at home and can return to school or work full-time, then he or she should be discharged from ongoing outpatient therapy. Because scar maturation may not occur until 18 or more months after injury, however, a patient may continue to wear pressure garments or night splints even after resuming a preinjury routine. Pressure garments and splints need to be checked for excessive wear and possible modification at least every 2 to 3 months, possibly during the patient's return visits to the burn outpatient clinic. On those occasions, the patient should be reevaluated to monitor the status of maturing scars, performance skills, and psychosocial adjustment.

Psychosocial adjustment continues during the outpatient phase of burn recovery; during this process, the patient examines personal interests and values. The patient may grieve for lost roles and abilities before accepting the permanent changes resulting from the burn. Losses often include not only vocational and leisure skills but also past social roles and body image. These issues must be addressed throughout the rehabilitation process.

Facial Scars

In addition to limiting jaw and neck ROM, distortions in facial structures caused by contracting scars and hypertrophy can produce severe disfigurement, including altered nasal contours, everted eyelids (i.e., *ectropion*) that expose the conjunctivae, everted lips and contracted oral commissurae, and missing features such as the nose and ears. Eye contractures can adversely affect sight and cause corneal dryness, which may lead to excessive tearing and nasal drainage. Microstomia cause problems with talking, eating, and excessive salivation and interfere with oral hygiene. Any of these conditions can have a devastating effect on the patient's ability to function in society and may be difficult to correct later. For this reason, early and frequent facial exercises are critical to reduce the potential for tight facial skin (Table 13.2).

Two primary treatment methods are available for compressing facial scarring: a custom-made, elastic face mask with underlying conformers or a rigid, total-contact, transparent facial orthosis (Rivers, 1987). Elastic face masks are combined with thin, flexible conformers to flatten and shape developing facial and head scars and maintain normal feature contours. The garments are custom made and should be checked and, possibly, replaced every 6 to 8 weeks to ensure correct compression. They are usually worn with underlying silicone gel, elastomer, or thermoplastic inserts to distribute the pressure over and around facial contours and an overlying chin strap to maintain neck contours.

Transparent facial orthoses are molded of high-temperature plastic, fit directly to the face, and are held in place with elastic straps. Fabrication of such devices involves taking a negative impression of the patient's face, making a positive plaster cast of the impression, heating and molding the transparent plastic over the cast, finishing the edges, applying adjustable straps, and fitting it to the patient (Rivers, 1984). Because the orthosis is transparent, the therapist can see and check the scars for blanching as it is fitted. Blanching indicates that the scars are being adequately compressed.

Regardless of the method chosen for facial compression, a positive mold of the patient's face should be made early in the healing process, before contractures alter the patient's features. The facial mold can be used to fabricate either a clear orthosis or face mask conformers. It also allows for precise fitting and alteration of the devices. If the plaster mold is cast after scars have developed, the mold can be modified by sculpting and smoothing the plaster to lower the surface where scars are located, before the conformers and mask are formed. This process is used to increase scar compression to specific areas under the mask. An unaltered facial mold also may serve as a three-dimensional model against which any developing facial scarring or distortion can be monitored.

Some therapists and patients prefer a combination of the two techniques, using the clear mask during the day or social activities and the elastic mask with conformers at night or when at home. The elastic mask with conformers has the advantage of multidirectional compression and dynamic fit that is less affected by facial movement or changes in position (i.e., upright versus supine). The clear facial orthosis does not conceal the patient's face, allowing the patient to retain some personal identity.

Early education is critical to preparing the patient for the fabrication and fitting process and for long-term compliance with the facial compression and exercise program. Education also should include training in skin lubrication and massage techniques, to ensure that correct pressure is applied during massage to desensitize scars and to help stretch tight skin. An exercise program to stretch tight facial skin should be initiated during inpatient treatment and continued as an outpatient. To be effective, all compression devices, including face masks, should be worn almost continuously until

the scars mature. Face masks should be removed only for brief periods for meals, hygiene, skin care, exercises, scar massage, and sexual activity.

To avoid misunderstandings with people who are unfamiliar with their condition, adult patients should be advised to remove all facial coverings before entering any store, bank, government building, airport, or any business where they are not well known. They should be aware of any local laws or ordinances prohibiting face coverings in public and carry an identification card or letter that verifies the medical necessity for the mask.

People wearing either type of mask often report feelings of self-consciousness, isolation, poor self-esteem, and loss of personal identity (Figure 13.13). These perceptions need to be acknowledged and addressed by the people close to the patient. Many patients benefit from counseling and from speaking with someone else who is wearing or has worn a facial mask or orthosis.

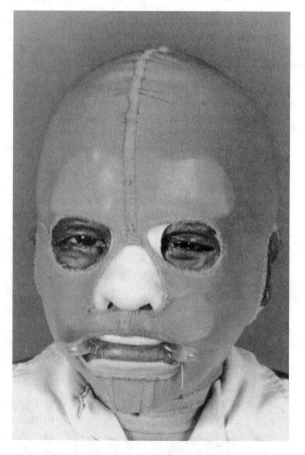

Figure 13.13. Patients with severe facial burns experience a loss of personal identity and must reconcile themselves to a new body image, first with a mask and then without it.

Various reconstructive procedures may improve facial mobility and appearance. When facial distortion caused by scarring is extensive, scar excision and autografting usually can improve appearance once scar maturation is complete. Preburn skin appearance can never be achieved after a severe burn, but the illusion of normal skin may be possible with creative use of special scar-concealing cosmetics (Salisbury, Petro, & Winski, 1987). When the wounds are mature, the patient should be referred to a cosmetologist who has training in corrective makeup blending for the face or other body areas. Although the appearance of facial scars may be improved with surgical reconstruction and the use of special camouflaging makeup, patients eventually must come to the realization that they will never look the same as before the injury. With the support of others, they can learn to accept their new body image.

Neuromuscular and Heterotopic Ossification Complications

Heterotopic ossification is an abnormal calcification process occurring at damaged joints that can severely limit joint movement and interfere with the ability to perform everyday tasks. The best intervention is to preserve as much range of motion as possible through nonaggressive AAROM, frequent AROM, and splinting. Adaptive devices also may be indicated for performing everyday activities.

Peripheral neuropathy is a common complication of severe burn injury in patients who are older, are critically ill, have an electrical injury, or have a history of alcohol abuse (Kowalske, Holavanahalli, & Helm, 2001). Polyneuropathy is most common among patients who have burns greater than 15% full thickness, are older than 40 years of age, and stay in the intensive care unit for more than 20 days. Patients with electrical burns may have a direct electrical injury to the nerve or may develop neuropathy from postinjury edema. Patients with a history of alcohol abuse may have a mild underlying abnormality of nerve function that would predispose them to postburn neuropathies. Peripheral nerve damage can be caused by infections, neurotoxicities, and metabolic abnormalities and are evident as a symmetrical distal weakness that slowly improves over time. Localized stretch or compression nerve injuries can occur because of improper or prolonged positioning in bed or during surgery. Prolonged tourniquet use or extreme edema, combined with tight dressings, also can contribute to neuropathy and should be avoided. The most common

injury sites are the brachial plexus and the ulnar and peroneal nerves (Helm, 1984). Diligent proper positioning can prevent most of these injuries. Positioning should avoid prolonged elbow flexion, maintain the lower extremities in neutral rotation and knee extension (to prevent the frog leg position), and avoid prone positioning with arms overhead.

When neuropathies persist and do not spontaneously resolve, it is important that strength and sensory recovery be reevaluated periodically throughout rehabilitation. To promote sensory recovery, the patient should be taught sensory-reeducation techniques. ADL-related safety precautions also should be practiced to avoid further injury that could result from residual weakness or decreased protective sensation.

Age-Related Considerations

Small children tend to heal and scar differently from older children and adults. Children younger than 5 years of age have higher potential for hypertrophic scarring of burn and donor sites because of prolonged scar maturation. Small muscles, hypermobile joints, and inability to cooperate place young children at higher risk for contractures than adults. Contractures and the binding properties of tight scars also may inhibit normal growth in small children, especially in the hands and feet. The surgical team therefore may intervene earlier with surgical releases and reconstruction for children than they would for adults with similar scars.

Children are more likely to experience emotional regression, especially during the acute phase of recovery. The physical and social restrictions resulting from contractures and disfigurement can interfere with meeting developmental milestones. For this reason, it is helpful to obtain information from parents and family members regarding developmental milestones met by children before the burn, so that if regression occurs, appropriate interventions can be initiated while the patient is still in the hospital.

For school-age children, a school reentry program should be initiated before discharge. With such programming, the teacher, classmates, and, in some cases, the school-based therapist can become well acquainted with the appearance and special needs of the injured child before he or she returns to school (Meyer, Barnett, & Gross, 1987; Rosenstein, 1987). Videotaped messages from the burned child to his or her classmates explaining child-to-child what happened can be effective. The tape, which should be delivered by a family member or health care professional, allows the classmates to see the child's appearance (when appropriate, with and without the compression garments) and ask questions freely. Such foreknowledge helps ease the resumption of the student role for the child and can help improve acceptance by other children who may not otherwise understand the cause of the disfigurement and the need for splints, adaptive equipment, and scar-compression garments. Summer camps for burned children, often sponsored by local firefighter organizations, also help children adjust by placing them in settings where they can socialize with peers who also have been burned.

Elderly patients may not form hypertrophic scars as readily as younger patients, but their scars may stay fragile longer and may heal more slowly. Degenerative joint disease, osteoporosis, cardiopulmonary complications, diabetes, deconditioning, and other preexisting conditions in the elderly person may further complicate the rehabilitative process. Care must be taken during AAROM or PROM exercises not to overstretch joints that may have been restricted by age-related joint disease even before the burn injury.

Sexuality

Sexual activity is an occupational performance area that should be addressed during the inpatient rehabilitation phase of recovery well before discharge. Following a serious burn, multiple factors can interfere with sexual activity, including decreased mobility due to scar contractures or limited joint ROM, decreased physical strength and poor endurance, loss of sensation, hypersensitivity or pain, fragile skin and skin inflexibility, and penile erectile dysfunction due to scarring. Pain, poor body image, depression, performance anxiety, and lack of information also are serious deterrents to resumption of sexual activity. The therapist should obtain a history from the patient regarding his or her basic understanding of sexual practices and related issues (including birth control, safe sex practices, hygiene, and social and cultural influences) and personal preferences regarding sex-related issues. The occupational therapist should conduct an activity analysis to assess the patient's positioning and educational needs. Information regarding sexual performance should be provided on several occasions along with copies of or recommendations for printed information and books relating to sexual performance. The therapist can offer solutions for specific anticipated problems related to physical disability, such as the need for positional adaptations,

lubrication and skin care, hygiene, or use of adaptive aids. Only a sexual counselor or professional with advanced training in sexual counseling, however, should provide in-depth sexual therapy (Burton, 2001).

Community Mobility

If a burn patient has a permanent functional impairment that prevents driving a standard vehicle, he or she will need to consider options for personal transportation in the community. The local public transportation department may offer ample services for people with physical impairments. Use of these services should be investigated as an economic alternative before ordering costly personal transportation adaptations.

Should personal vehicle adaptation be preferred, the occupational therapist must consider the patient's physical and cognitive capabilities for driving and transferring in and out of the vehicle, the types of adaptations that will be needed, and the extent of driver education needed for safe driving. This assessment should be performed by a professional with special training and experience in determining what kind of vehicle or equipment is appropriate. Efforts should be made to prescribe the least amount of modification possible so that the patient can safely make maximum use of his or her capabilities. The occupational therapist or evaluator then issues a prescription for use by the equipment or vehicle supplier. The prescription also may be necessary for insurance or state agencies that may be contributing funding toward the purchase or modification of equipment. The cost of vehicle modifications varies widely, depending on the type of adaptive equipment needed. The patient should take advantage of services and organizations that provide funding for adaptive vehicles and equipment, such as insurance companies, state rehabilitation service agencies, and local service organizations. The U.S. Department of Veterans Affairs provides grants and reimbursement for adaptive equipment prescribed for people with service-related disabilities and may also provide financial aid for non-service-related disabilities. Most car manufacturers offer some type of reimbursement program or financial assistance for reducing the cost of a new or used adapted vehicle.

Summary

To obtain optimal outcomes after severe burns, it is necessary to consider not only the client's phase of recovery, physical limitations, compliance with treatment, and psychological adjustment but also his or her personal goals and priorities. It is the therapist's responsibility to anticipate and prevent physical limitations, emotional dependence, and social isolation through prompt therapeutic intervention, psychosocial support, and referral to appropriate ancillary services and community resources. The ultimate objective of occupational therapy is to enable the burn patient to achieve functional independence in his or her chosen roles, life context, and environment.

Study Questions

1. What are the major potential problems for superficial and deep partial burns?
2. Why is patient–caregiver education important, and when should it be initiated?
3. What is the general rule for positioning and splinting a contracting scar?
4. What is the ADL task that typically carries the most significance for the patient, regardless of age?
5. What are the wearing and removal requirements for scar compression face masks and garments to achieve the most successful outcome?
6. How does age affect the development of hypertrophic scars?
7. When should ongoing outpatient burn therapy be discontinued?

References

Abston, S. (1987). Scar reaction after thermal injury and prevention of scars and contractures. In J. Boswick (Ed.), *The art and science of burn care* (pp. 359–371). Gaithersburg, MD: Aspen.

Adriaenssens, P. (1988). The video invasion of rehabilitation. *Burns Including Thermal Injuries, 14,* 417–419.

Alvarado, M. I. (1995). Burns. In C. Trombly (Ed.), *Occupational therapy for physical dysfunction* (4th ed., pp. 832–848). Baltimore: Williams & Wilkins.

American Occupational Therapy Association. (1997). Physical agent modalities: A position paper. *American Journal of Occupational Therapy, 51,* 870–871.

Breines, E. B. (2001). Therapeutic occupations and modalities. In L. W. Pedretti & M. B. Early (Eds.), *Occupational therapy: Practice skills for physical dysfunction* (5th ed., pp. 503–525). St. Louis: Mosby.

Burton, G. U. (2001). Sexuality and physical dysfunction. In L. W. Pedretti & M. B. Early (Eds.), *Occupational therapy: Practice skills for physical dysfunction* (5th ed., pp. 212–225). St. Louis: Mosby.

Carvajal, H. F. (1988). Resuscitation of the burned child. In H. F. Carvajal & D. H. Parks (Eds.), *Burns in children: Pediatric burn management* (pp. 78–98). Chicago: Year Book.

Cheng, S., & Rogers, J. C. (1989). Changes in occupational role performance after a severe burn: A retrospective study. *American Journal of Occupational Therapy, 43,* 17–24.

Christiansen, C. (1991). Intervention for life performance. In C. Christiansen & C. Baum (Eds.), *Occupational therapy: Overcoming human performance deficits* (pp. 1–43). Thorofare, NJ: Slack.

Christiansen, C. H., & Baum, C. M. (1997). Person-environment occupational performance: A conceptual model for practice. In C. Christiansen & C. Baum (Eds.), *Occupational therapy: Enabling function and well-being* (pp. 47–70). Thorofare, NJ: Slack.

Daugherty, M. B., & Carr-Collins, J. A. (1994). Splinting techniques for the burn patient. In R. Richard & M. Staley (Eds.), *Burn care and rehabilitation: Principles and practice* (pp. 242–323). Philadelphia: F. A. Davis.

Fleet, J. (1992). The psychological effects of burn injuries: A literature review. *British Journal of Occupational Therapy, 55,* 198–220.

Hartford, C. (1984). Surgical management. In S. Fisher & P. Helm (Eds.), *Comprehensive rehabilitation of burns* (pp. 28–63). Baltimore: Williams & Wilkins.

Helm, P. A. (1984). Neuromuscular considerations. In S. Fisher & P. Helm (Eds.), *Comprehensive rehabilitation of burns* (pp. 235–241). Baltimore: Williams & Wilkins.

Helm, P. A., & Fisher, S. (1988). Rehabilitation of the patient with burns. In J. DeLisa, D. Currie, & B. Gans (Eds.), *Rehabilitation medicine: Principles and practice* (pp. 821–839). Philadelphia: Lippincott.

Helm, P. A., Walker, S. C., & Peyton, S. A. (1986). Return to work following hand burns. *Archives of Physical Medicine and Rehabilitation, 67,* 297–298.

Humphrey, C., Richard, R. L., & Staley, M. J. (1994). Soft tissue management and exercise. In R. Richard & M. Staley (Eds.), *Burn care and rehabilitation: Principles and practice* (pp. 324–360). Philadelphia: F. A. Davis.

Kaplan, S. H. (1985). Patient education techniques used at burn centers. *American Journal of Occupational Therapy, 39,* 655–658.

Kielhofner, G. (1995). *A model of human occupation: Theory and application* (2nd ed.). Baltimore: Williams & Wilkins.

Kowalske, K., Holavanahalli, R., & Helm, P. (2001). Neuropathy after burn injury. *Journal of Burn Care and Rehabilitation, 22,* 353–357.

Law, M., Cooper, B., Strong, S., Stewart, D., Rigby, P., & Letts, L. (1996). The person-environment-occupation model: A transactive approach to occupational performance. *Canadian Journal of Occupational Therapy, 63,* 9–23.

Lund, C., & Browder, N. (1944). The estimation of area of burns. *Surgical Gynecology and Obstetrics, 79,* 352–355.

Malt, U. F., & Ugland, O. M. (1989). A long term psychosocial follow-up study of burned adults. *Acta Psychiatrica Scandinavia, 80*(Suppl. 355), 94–102.

Mason, S., & Forshaw, A. (1986). Burns after care: A booklet for parents: Your child at home after injury. *Burns Including Thermal Injuries, 12,* 343–350.

Melchert-McKearnan, K., Deitz, J., Engel, J. M., & White, O. (2000). Children with burn injuries: Purposeful activity versus rote exercise. *American Journal of Occupational Therapy, 54,* 381–390.

Meyer, D. O., Barnett, P. H., & Gross, D. J. (1987). A school reentry program for burned children. Part II: Physical therapy contribution to an existing school reentry program. *Journal of Burn Care and Rehabilitation, 8,* 322–324.

Ozek, C., Cankayali, R., Bilkay, U., Guner, U., Gundogan, H., Songur, E., et al. (2001). Marjolin's ulcers arising in burn scars. *Journal of Burn Care and Rehabilitation, 22,* 384–389.

Perry, S., & Difede, J. (1992). Predictors of posttraumatic stress disorder after burn injury. *American Journal of Psychiatry, 149,* 931–935.

Petro, J., & Salisbury, R. (1986). Rehabilitation of the burn patient. *Clinics in Plastic Surgery, 3*(1), 145–149.

Pullium, G. F. (1984). Splinting and positioning. In S. Fisher & P. Helm (Eds.), *Comprehensive rehabilitation of burns* (pp. 64–95). Baltimore: Williams & Wilkins.

Reeves, S. U. (2001). Burns and burn rehabilitation. In L. W. Pedretti & M. B. Early (Eds.), *Occupational therapy: Practice skills for physical dysfunction* (5th ed., pp. 898–923). St. Louis: Mosby.

Reilly, M. (1962). Occupational therapy can be one of the great ideas of the 20th century. *American Journal of Occupational Therapy, 16,* 1–9.

Rivers, E. (1984). Management of hypertrophic scars. In S. Fisher & P. Helm (Eds.), *Comprehensive rehabilitation of burns* (pp. 177–217). Baltimore: Williams & Wilkins.

Rivers, E. (1987). Rehabilitation management of the burn patient. *Advances in Clinical Rehabilitation, 1,* 177–213.

Rosenstein, D. W. L. (1987). A school reentry program for burned children. Part I: Development and implementation of a school reentry program. *Journal of Burn Care and Rehabilitation, 8,* 319–322.

Salisbury, R., Petro, J., & Winski, F. (1987). Reconstruction of the burn patient. In J. Boswick (Ed.), *The art and science of burn care* (pp. 353–357). Gaithersburg, MD: Aspen.

Solem, L. (1984). Classification. In S. Fisher & P. Helm (Eds.), *Comprehensive rehabilitation of burns* (pp. 9–15). Baltimore: Williams & Wilkins.

Stewart, R., Bhagwanjee, A., Mbakaza, Y., & Binase, T. (2000). Pressure garment adherence in adult patients with burn injuries: An analysis of patient and clinician perceptions. *American Journal of Occupational Therapy, 54,* 598–606.

Trombly, C. A. (1995). Theoretical foundation for practice. In C. A. Trombly (Ed.), *Occupational therapy for physical dysfunction* (4th ed., pp. 15–28). Baltimore: Williams & Wilkins.

Tucker, P. (1986). The burn victim: A review of psychosocial issues. *Australian and New Zealand Journal of Psychiatry, 20,* 413–420.

Wachtel, T. (1985). Epidemiology, classification, initial care, and administrative considerations for critically burned patients. In T. Wachtel (Ed.), *Critical care clinics* (pp. 3–26). Philadelphia: Saunders.

Ward, R. S., Hayes-Lundy, C., Reddy, R., Brockway, C., & Mills, P. (1992). Influence of pressure supports on joint range of motion. *Burns, 18,* 60–62.

Ward, R. S., Reddy, R., Brockway, C., Hayes-Lundy, C., & Mills, P. (1994). Uses of Coban self-adhesive wrap in management of postburn hand grafts: Case reports. *Journal of Burn Care and Rehabilitation, 15,* 364–369.

Yurko, L., & Fratianne, R. (1988). Evaluation of burn discharge teaching. *Journal of Burn Care and Rehabilitation, 9,* 643–644.

Chapter 14

Everyday Living for People With Cognitive Deficits After Alzheimer's Dementia and Traumatic Brain Injury

BEATRIZ C. ABREU, PHD, OTR, FAOTA

KEY TERMS

Alzheimer's dementia (AD)

Alzheimer's dementia stages

brain cortex lobes

cognitive rehabilitation

Glasgow Coma Scale (GSC)

Mini-Mental Test

Post-traumatic Amnesia Scale (PTA)

traumatic brain injury (TBI)

traumatic brain injury stages

OBJECTIVES

Upon completion of this chapter, the reader will be able to

- Define Alzheimer's dementia (AD) and traumatic brain injury (TBI);

- Describe the physiological basis for cognitive disabilities in AD and TBI;

- Describe the stages of cognitive decline in AD and stages of recovery in TBI;

- Outline evaluation strategies for people with AD and TBI;

- Describe the challenges to occupational performance (i.e., everyday living) experienced by people with AD and TBI; and

- Describe adaptive strategies equipment or environmental modifications useful for optimal performance of everyday activities.

This chapter describes the challenges to occupational performance (i.e., activities of daily living [ADL]) experienced by people with cognitive disabilities as a result of Alzheimer's dementia (AD) and traumatic brain injury (TBI); illustrates evaluation strategies; and describes adaptive strategies, equipment, and environmental modifications useful for optimal performance of ADL for people with AD or TBI.

Alzheimer's Dementia and Traumatic Brain Injury

Most countries have a large and increasing population of people who are affected by cognitive deficits after AD and TBI (Glueckauf & Loomis, 2003; Thurman, Alverson, Dunn, Guerrero, & Sniezek, 1999). In the United States, about 4 million people have AD (BIOTA, 1998), and more than 2 million head injuries occur each year (Thurman et al., 1999). Cognitive deficits caused by AD and TBI influence the ability to perform ADL and increase the need for occupational therapy services in both institutional and home settings. In addition, occupational therapists and occupational therapy assistants work with people with other diagnoses, such as schizophrenia, stroke, brain tumors, and cerebral palsy, which also involve cognitive deficits and everyday living management issues. With this increased demand for services, occupational therapists and occupational therapy assistants need to understand more fully the effects of such cognitive impairments on ADL to provide effective evaluation and intervention strategies.

The relationship between cognition and everyday living for clients with cognitive deficits is complex, dynamic, and difficult to comprehend. Although no simple answers exist for dealing with AD and TBI, this chapter presents a practical approach for evaluation and intervention. One general (and, perhaps, obvious) principle that may be applied to the relationship between cognition and ADL skills is that the more severe the cognitive deficit, the more dependent the person will be. Extensive information is available about cognition and cognitive impairments in both the cognitive psychology and neuropsychology literature, but a review of this knowledge is beyond the scope of this chapter.

Evidence-Based Practice for People With AD and TBI

Since the late 1990s, the occupational therapy literature has identified the use of evidence-based practice (EBP) as a critical factor for evaluation and intervention (Law, 2002; Taylor, 1997). EBP is the umbrella term that describes a critical process for searching, evaluating, rejecting or accepting, and integrating research findings into clinical decision making. EBP enables practitioners to upgrade their knowledge, improve their understanding of research methods, become more critical when using research information, and improve their confidence in practice. Research findings in EBP are not the only answer for clinical problem solving and decision making, but they can help. At times, clinical decisions are based on habits, traditions, opinions, protocols, and professional or institutional authority (Abreu, 2003).

In addition to using EBP, occupational therapists need to be aware of the role of diverse research methodologies that provide different types of research findings (Morse, Swanson, & Kuzel, 2001). Qualitative research investigates research participants' meaningful information, and quantitative research investigates research participants' measurements and numerical information. Occupational therapists need to combine both qualitative and quantitative findings into their practice while remembering that most evidence in health care is provisional, lacking, emergent, and incomplete.

Using an evidence-based approach will not inevitably lead to support for a given technique or treatment. Indeed, EBP may show that the treatment does not improve human impairment, activity, or social participation, or it may support a different approach to practice. At this stage, limited evidence validates the use of occupational therapy interventions for either AD or TBI. Although much research on occupational therapy intervention for clients with these conditions has been published, many of the studies used weak methodological designs, small sample sizes, and no control group, flaws that limit their generalization to practice.

Research information as well as neuroanatomical information guide occupational therapy practice. The following section briefly describes the neuroanatomical impact of AD and TBI on clients as well as their caregivers.

Challenges to Everyday Living for People With AD and TBI

When cognitive changes first appear as a result of AD and TBI, individuals and families may not fully realize the devastating effect that these conditions will have on their entire social support system and their community integration (Minnes et al., 2003). The behavioral changes caused by such deficits extend far beyond the person who has incurred the disability. Family groups, including immediate family members, friends, and others, spend a tremendous amount of time assisting cognitively impaired people with managing their ADL. The group members must become caregivers, and they frequently become overworked and stressed when faced with their new role responsibilities (McGrath, Mueller, Brown, Teitelman, & Watts, 2000). As a result, the emotional state of the group members is adversely affected, and they themselves become candidates for counseling and guidance. Occupational therapists and occupational therapy assistants, as part of a multidisciplinary health care team, may be able to use purposeful activity and ordinary occupation to promote health and achieve functional outcomes for both clients and family groups by using retraining and compensatory strategies.

Two of the most common mental dysfunctions associated with AD and TBI are in the areas of cognitive integration and cognitive components: impairment of memory and the lack of awareness of disability (Abreu et al., 2001; Dirette, 2002; Katz, Fleming, Keren, Lightbody, & Hartman-Maeir, 2002; Roche, Fleming, & Shum, 2002; Toglia & Kirk, 2000). These deficits often lead to unsafe personal behaviors that create additional stressors for family groups. Practitioners and other members of the health care team may become burned out with the chronicity, decline, and maladaptive behaviors that are prevalent with such diagnoses. At times, people with TBI and AD may require intense cueing and repetition to perform ADL. In addition, they may be socially and sexually disinhibited, thus requiring caretakers to expend extra energy to avoid negative repercussions. Cognitive deficits, whether minimal, moderate, or severe, have far-reaching consequences on the total social support network.

AD and TBI are acquired, persistent conditions that affect multiple areas of cognitive function. AD and TBI follow quite different trajectories, however. In AD, clients show deterioration in thinking, behavior, and occupational performance over time. In TBI, clients show recovery, followed by a plateau in thinking, behavior, and functional ability over time. Rehabilitation for both AD and TBI includes occupational therapy intervention approaches of (1) establishing, restoring, and remediation and (2) adaptive techniques, equipment, or environmental modifications. The primary focus for AD is on adaptive strategies and environmental modification. For example, strategies for memory deficits may involve external cues in the environment to trigger a client's recall. Specific changes in the behavior of clients who have AD are addressed by retraining and compensatory strategies.

For TBI, the treatment emphasis includes restoring lost skills and adapting the task or the environment. For example, the restoration approach may use paper-and-pencil tasks to retrain people who experience math and money management skill impairments following TBI.

Behavior Changes Associated With Brain Damage

All functional behavior is controlled by the nervous system and, in particular, the brain. The nervous system is an organized group of nerve and other nonneural cells that function to receive, integrate, and transmit information. The brain is the part of the nervous system that is most significantly damaged by AD and TBI. The four major structures of the brain that are commonly affected by AD and TBI are the frontal, parietal, temporal, and occipital lobes (Figure 14.1). The following sections summarize the performance-component impairments related to each brain lobe.

Frontal Lobes

The frontal lobes are located in the most forward section of the brain, one on each side of the midline. Damage to the frontal lobes causes both cognitive and motor dysfunction. Cognitive impairment demonstrated by symptoms such as lack of alertness and motivation, poor judgment, flat affect, and memory problems. Broca's aphasia may occur with damage to the lower portion of the lobe, resulting in the inability to speak or understand spoken or written language. Decline in the function of the frontal lobes may result in occupational performance challenges of deceased concern for personal hygiene, poor insight, difficulty in problem solving, emotional dullness, and social withdrawal. In addition, certain pathological motor responses, such as grasp reflex and groping responses with the hands, may occur, which present a challenge for functional hand use for ADL. People with injury to the frontal lobes may experience deficits in how to position the hand for grasping familiar or unfamiliar objects, or they may overshoot or undershoot when reaching for objects.

Parietal Lobes

The parietal lobes are located between the frontal and the occipital lobes. Damage to the parietal lobes may result in a decreased ability to engage and disengage in tasks such as dressing or grooming. In addition, clients may experience reduced ability to

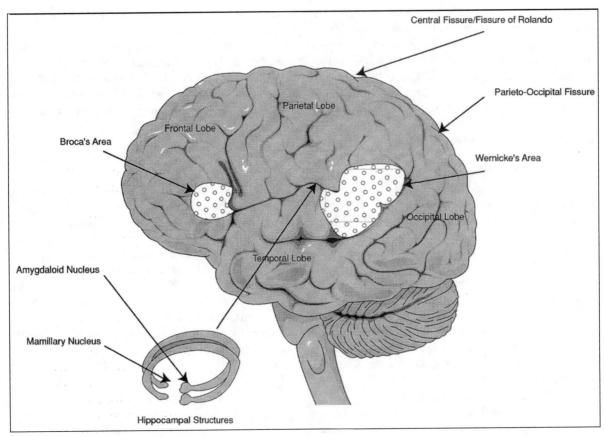

Figure 14.1. The lateral view of the brain, showing the locations of the structures affected by AD and TBI.

detect spatial orientation. Common occupational performance challenges associated with this condition are getting lost, bumping one's wheelchair into walls, and inadvertently hitting affected extremities against walls and furniture. Clients with this sort of brain damage may be unsafe and require supervision from family and caretakers.

Temporal Lobes

The temporal lobes are located below the frontal and parietal lobes. Damage to the temporal lobes can result in decreased visual and auditory memory and impairment of emotional memories, particularly with damage to the hippocampus or the amygdala, both of which are located within the temporal lobes. A second area in the posterior portion of the left frontal lobe, Wernicke's area, affects speech and language. Damage to this area can result in Wernicke's aphasia, which is the loss of comprehension of the spoken and, often, the written word. The effect on occupational performance is the disorganization of everyday living; inability to understand instructions; and forgetfulness during ADL, instru-

mental ADL (IADL), work, play, and leisure. Although clients can speak, their statements are disorganized, illogical, and without context.

Occipital Lobes

The occipital lobes are located behind the parietal and temporal lobes. Damage to the occipital lobes may cause visual field cuts, spatial memory problems, and problems with object identification. Clients may be able to see, but their level of pattern recognition and visual memory may be impaired. The occupational performance challenges associated with this area of impairment include decreased safety in ADL, IADL, work, play, and leisure activities (e.g., reading, driving, and writing).

Specific Changes in Cognition and ADL After AD

AD is a progressive, degenerative disease of uncertain causes that manifests itself in damage to the brain. Rombouts et al. (2003) and Silverman et al. (2003) are among the researchers who have proposed a multitude of causes for AD, including injury from neurochemicals, other toxins, and abnormal proteins, and immunological, viral, and genetic causes. AD is named after Alois Alzheimer, who first described the disease in 1907. The brains of people with AD typically show pathology of the cytoskeleton of neurons in the cerebral cortex, a structure that is crucial to cognitive function. Postmortem microscopic analysis of the brain in people with AD shows dead neurons. AD causes changes in the neuron nucleus and cytoplasm; the damaged neurons eventually disappear with the advancement of the disease. A chemical transformation in neurons leads to abnormal secretion of brain proteins (i.e., the tau and amyloid proteins), which results in formation of a tangle bundle of fibrils that emerge in place of the damaged neurons. The fibril tangles are called "tombstones" of neurons (Bear, Connors, & Paradiso, 2001). AD is the fourth leading cause of death in people older than 65 years of age; incidence of the disease increases in people older than 85 years of age.

AD is marked by a loss of cognitive abilities that is not considered part of the normal aging process. Dementia has been classified according to the area of damage. The classifications include (1) cortical damage, including damage from AD and Picks disease; (2) subcortical damage secondary to Huntington's and Parkinson's disease; and (3) mixed type, such as multiinfarct dementia. Readers should refer to the *Diagnostic and Statistical Manual of Mental Disorders,* 4th Edition, Text Revision, for a further classification of dementia (American Psychiatric Association, 2000).

Specific behavior changes in people with AD go beyond basic ADL skills. People with AD may express themselves in intimate and sexual ways while living in care facilities, creating dilemmas for staff members and families (Kuhn, 2002). The earliest and most frequently affected ADL in early AD involve a reduction in social and leisure activities (Derouesne et al., 2002). Other areas exhibiting early declines in people with AD involve handling finances and shopping (Derouesne et al., 2002). For example, someone with early AD may experience difficulties with organization of their shopping task or counting their change at the cash register.

Stages of Cognitive Changes in AD

Cognition and daily living management issues associated with AD have been divided into three stages: mild, moderate, and severe (Reisberg, 1984; Reisberg, Ferris, De Leon, & Crook, 1982). The three stages describe and predict the behaviors that are expected to emerge during the course of the disease; they are not rigidly defined, but they can guide occupational therapy interventions. Unfortunately, they portray a grim picture of dementia. Practitioners may develop a clearer understanding of the complexities involved in treating AD when they better understand the social factors associated with the disease, which include the following issues:

- Social stigma is attached to dementia.
- The diagnostic process frequently is based on subjective factors.
- Clients with AD are sometimes treated in a dehumanizing manner once a diagnosis is made.
- Some disruptive behaviors observed in clients may be viewed as normal reactions to increased anxiety (Herskovits, 1995; Ronch, 1996).

Because of the social phenomena associated with AD, occupational therapists and occupational therapy assistants should seek to understand the factors that contribute to caregiving and strive to promote the preservation of personal identity and compassion.

First Stage of AD: Mild

The first stage begins with the appearance of symptoms that include forgetfulness, repetition of questions, and difficulty in using words. Forgetfulness includes the inability to recall information after brief or extended periods of time (which correspond to short- and long-term memory loss). An example of forgetfulness would be the inability to remember names or recall recent events, conversations, or object placements. Note that age or stress-related forgetfulness does not indicate the presence of AD and does not, like AD, interfere with daily living.

During the first stage of AD, most clients encounter difficulties with the initiation, speed, amount, and quality of performance of ADL and begin to require assistance and supervision. They become forgetful, which begins to affect their job performance. They may get confused about travel directions and begin to miss appointments. Clients experience impaired judgment and problem-solving skills, and may exhibit money management problems. As the clients become more passive and forgetful, family members notice personality and behavioral changes such as episodes of irritability and sleep disturbances. This stage may last from 2 to 4 years, during which time clients usually reside at home.

Second Stage of AD: Moderate

During the second stage, the symptoms worsen, and the need for caregiver supervision and assistance increases. Symptoms include difficulty with short- and long-term memory, leading to *confabulation* (i.e., clients invent stories to fill in the blanks of memory loss). In addition, clients encounter difficulty recognizing family and friends as well as remembering their visits. Clients' difficulty in finding their words increases, and they may be unable to dress and bathe independently. Supervision for mobility and travel is required. Clients exhibit decreased ability to read, write, and perform mathematical calculations. Changes in body weight occur, the client becomes restless and suspicious, and he or she tends to sleep often. At this stage, many people are unable to maintain jobs. The caregivers must offer moderate but constant supervision for the person to perform ADL in a safe fashion. This stage may last from 2 to 10 years and usually leads to the final stage of AD.

Third Stage of AD: Severe

In the final stage of AD, a global decline of all daily functions and a complete loss of judgment occur. In this stage, clients are unable to judge right from wrong and are dependent on 24-hour supervision and maximal assistance. The severe stage may last from 1 to 3 years. Clients have little capacity for self-care; become incontinent; and require help eating, dressing, bathing, and toileting. They sleep more frequently and for longer periods of time. They may groan and scream and become disoriented. Clients are unable to recognize family, friends, and even themselves. Some suffer a marked weight loss. Many family groups are forced to place their loved ones in nursing homes or long-term care institutions, where they can receive the most effective care and intervention.

Clients with dementia who have lost their self-identity and self-care management skills still maintain the capacity for love, affection, satisfaction, joy, pain, fear, and anxiety. Therefore, practitioners need to devise management and coping strategies that will enable the clients and their family groups to gain some relief.

Specific Changes in Cognition and Daily Living After TBI

TBI is nonprogressive, persistent damage to the brain. It is usually caused by a blow to the head from an external object or by internal forces caused by high-speed acceleration or deceleration. In the United States, more than 44% of TBIs are caused by motor vehicle accidents, many of which are alcohol related. The remaining 56% are accounted for by falls, assaults, and sports injuries (Brain Injury Association, 2001). More than two thirds of TBI cases are diagnosed in people younger than 30 years of age. Young men between the ages of 14 and 24 have the highest rate of injury.

Brain injury following head trauma is classified as either a *closed* or a *penetrating* head injury. A closed head injury is one that involves no penetration of the brain by a foreign object. A penetrating head injury involves just such a violation. TBI may include brain contusions, vascular damage, and intracranial pressure changes (Scott & Dow, 1995). Injuries can be *localized* or *diffuse*. Localized injuries are specific to certain areas of the brain (e.g., the frontal lobe). Diffuse injuries involve more generalized effects and many brain structures.

Although personal management skills frequently are affected following brain injury, people with TBI judge their abilities higher than clinician ratings of actual performance in basic and IADL, such as dressing, meal planning, and money management (Abreu et al., 2001). Shopping can be negatively affected in people with TBI who exhibit memory dysfunction and initiation problems (Alderman, Burgess, Knight, & Henman, 2003). Deficits in attention, language, and executive functioning associated with brain injury may impair a person's money management skills (Gaudette & Anderson, 2002).

Mobility disability for people with TBI is the result of an interaction of individual and environmental factors (Shumway-Cook et al., 2003). People with physical impairments may be limited in their ability to get around in the community if modifications such as wheelchair ramps and elevators are not available. People with cognitive impairments may be limited in their participation in community mobility if memory deficits impair their orientation. Mazaux et al. (1997) found that the most impaired social abilities in people with TBI included performing administrative tasks and financial management, writing letters and calculating, driving, planning the week, and using public transportation. The Community Mobility Assessment was developed for adolescents with acquired brain injury to determine their ability to safely go out alone in the community (Brewer, Geisler, Moody, & Wright, 1998).

TBI also can affect satisfaction in other areas of life, such as leisure or sexual enjoyment. In a study assessing life satisfaction of patients with severe TBI, Quintard and colleagues (2002) found that 36% were dissatisfied with their leisure activities and

32% were dissatisfied with their sexual life. Compared with people without disability, people with TBI reported more frequent physiological difficulties influencing their energy for sex, sex drive, and ability to initiate sexual activities as well as physical difficulties influencing body positioning, body movement, and sensation (Hibbard, Gordon, Flanagan, Haddad, & Labinski, 2000). Psychosocial disability in people with TBI may result in a lack of involvement in leisure activities (Hall et al., 1994).

Stages of Recovery After TBI

TBI is a complex diagnosis; this chapter uses three stages of cognitive function to describe the recovery of abilities as well as the progression and leveling off of thinking and behavior. In TBI, the trajectory of recovery generally is upward, as opposed to the regression shown in AD. TBI clients may advance from the severe to the moderate to the mild stage. Some of the symptoms may diminish over time, but others may persist.

Two of the most common scales used to characterize particular aspects of recovery after TBI are the Glasgow Coma Scale (GCS; Teasdale & Jennett, 1974) and the Post-Traumatic Amnesia (PTA; Giacino, Kezmarsky, DeLuca, & Cicerone, 1991) measures. The GCS is based on the duration of prolonged unconsciousness or deep sleep, whereas the PTA is based on the duration of memory loss of the period preceding the injury (i.e., *retrograde amnesia*). These scales can be used to categorize and predict the functional outcome for clients.

The GCS consists of a 15-point scale used to rate eye opening and motor and verbal responses. The PTA is a measurement obtained by estimating the duration of the memory loss from the moment of trauma to the time of evaluation (i.e., the point at which clients are able to demonstrate the ability to communicate about memory).

The GCS and PTA are used to classify TBI clients into five categories. In general, lower scores on the GCS and a greater PTA duration indicate a more severe injury. The five classifications of TBI are mild, moderate, severe, very severe, and extremely severe. The mild category includes clients who may not have been rendered unconscious, achieved GCS scores ranging from 13 to 15, and had a memory loss after trauma lasting from 5 minutes to 1 hour, as measured by the PTA. The moderate category refers to clients who endured a period of unconsciousness, achieved a GCS score of 9 to 12, and had a PTA duration of less than 24 hours. The severe classification includes clients who have sustained coma with GCS scores below 8 and a PTA duration

of more than 24 hours. The very severe classification includes clients who sustained coma, had a GCS score of 5 points, and a PTA duration of 4 weeks. Finally, the extremely severe category includes those with sustained coma, a GCS below 5 points, and a PTA of more than 4 weeks.

The five TBI classifications also are used to predict functional outcomes. Although the outcomes for very severe and extremely severe TBI are projected to be poor, many such clients have regained functional self-care and some productive employment. The reader is cautioned not to confuse the classifications of TBI outcomes using GCS and PTA with the stages of recovery described in the following section.

First Recovery Stage: Severe

Damage from TBI varies with the nature of the blow or forces applied to the head and brain. Many TBI clients incur severe damage and begin their recovery in this first stage. Some clients may have survived only due to advances in medical technology (Thurman et al., 1999). As a result, their family group must confront the ethical challenge of prolonged life in a coma or vegetative state. Although many people hope for functional improvement, some clients will remain totally dependent. The first stage of recovery has three levels: coma, persistent vegetative state, and reactive level. During coma, patients are bedridden and lack meaningful interaction with people and the environment. They have a sleep-and-wake rhythm pattern and may be able to move reflexively, showing grasping, chewing, sucking, and postural reflexes. During this period, clients are totally dependent in self-care. From coma, patients may move to a persistent vegetative level, in which they are able to control respiration, blood pressure, and digestive and excretory functions but are still totally dependent on others for self-care. After the vegetative state, patients may progress to the final level of the first stage, in which they become responsive and begin to interact with the environment. The range of physical and cognitive skills for individual clients in the reactive-level stage may vary greatly. The rate of recovery of physical skills does not necessarily correlate to the rate of recovery of cognitive skills. Clients may exhibit the physical capability to perform self-care but may be unable to do so because of low arousal, severe impairment in awareness of disability, poor judgment, and limited problem-solving skills. Regardless of their apparent physical recovery, clients may be confused and agitated and unable to take care of themselves in a safe fashion. They may need help bathing, dressing, eating, and going to the toilet and require assistance with mobility. Clients may be able to talk, yet have communication problems because they are disoriented in time, person, and place. Many symptoms are reversible, and many clients advance to the second stage of recovery.

Second Recovery Stage: Moderate

In the second stage of recovery, clients may increase their cognitive and physical capabilities and require less assistance and supervision than they previously did. As in the first stage, recovery of the cognitive does not go hand in hand with recovery of physical capabilities. Some clients may show moderate cognitive improvement but minimal physical or motor recovery of the upper or lower extremities. In the second stage, clients are more purposeful and interact more appropriately with the environment, and they may be able to follow instructions; however, they may demonstrate difficulty with detecting, processing, and responding to stimuli. Their behaviors are characterized as distractible, impulsive or slow, hyperactive or hypoactive, and repetitive (i.e., perseverative). They may have difficulty with short- and long-term memory, including recall and recognition of names, faces, objects, and locations. Clients also may be unable to remember family and friends, when they ate, when or whether they took a shower, and whether they had traveled. They may have problems reading, writing, and doing simple math. Many may be able to perform cash transactions independently but require supervision in budgeting and banking.

Clients in this stage often exhibit emotional changes that affect their relationships with others. They may become irritable, short-tempered, and disinhibited, leading to cursing and sexually inappropriate behavior. TBI clients are likely to express emotional distress after injury and have sleep disturbances. They may have verbal as well as nonverbal speech and language problems. Their language problems can take the form of responses that are inappropriate to the situation, are irrelevant, are incoherent, or demonstrate misunderstanding of the intentions of others. Some clients also experience difficulty with intonation and gesture. Their speech may not have the inflection necessary to communicate meaning, and they may sound robotic.

During this stage, caregivers must provide constant supervision in order to provide a safe environment for self-care. Clients may not regain their former employment status, but they may be able to perform other productive activities. Some people progress to the third stage of recovery, but many clients remain fixed at this level for the rest of their lives.

Third Recovery Stage: Mild

The third stage of recovery includes clients who have successfully completed the second stage and those who have experienced a mild closed-head injury. Clients who sustain mild TBI may not experience coma; if they have posttraumatic memory loss, it is of brief duration. Clients who reach this stage may persist in having mild chronic symptoms, reverse some of the symptoms, or achieve total recovery. In this final stage, global improvement of cognition and performance of ADL occurs. Clients may be distractible and mildly forgetful, and they may need self-monitoring, organization, and structure. They also may complain about headaches, sensitivity to light and sound, lack of sleep, and sexual disturbances. Some clients appear fatigued, apathetic, passive, and indifferent. Others may experience loss of role identity; have reduced leisure interest; and become socially isolated, withdrawn, and depressed. Many clients are able to walk, talk, and perform basic self-care management independently. Others may have discrepancies between cognitive and motor skills and thus require a wheelchair user for motor performance, despite a high level of cognition. In addition, with the use of compensatory strategies, many clients are able to shop, clean, cook, and go to school. Most are able to regain productive employment and reshape and simplify their responsibilities. Some people are able to reconstruct and find more meaning in their lives. Often, clients turn to religion, become active in the community, and advocate for brain injury awareness.

The three stages described are intended to provide general guidelines that may help practitioners describe and predict the behaviors that emerge during recovery. The stages are not homogeneous across or within cognitive or functional areas. For example, the recovery of short- and long-term memory may not be the same for any given client. In addition, clients may not achieve the same level of proficiency in feeding and bathing. The stages present a hopeful picture for TBI clients. As practitioners consider the persistent nature of symptoms and their impact on clients' self-image and support system, understanding the stages should help them appreciate the psychological and social consequences of TBI on clients and their families.

Evaluation of Cognition Performance Components and Occupational Performance

One objective of occupational therapy evaluations is to gather information that can guide intervention, whether it is remedial or adaptive. In evaluating cognition and self-care function, practitioners should administer the measurement instruments frequently in order to discover how clients respond to cues and repetition. When interpreting results, a client's improvement in responding to cues and repetition will have more clinical significance than a change in the client's standardized norm scores will. Observed changes in cognition and self-care may be used in the development of intervention strategies.

General Evaluation Strategies

The use of standardized and nonstandardized measurement instruments for evaluating cognition and ADL skills is common in the rehabilitation process. Measurement strategies are used to describe, classify, and assign numbers to behaviors to establish a baseline for intervention, monitor changes, and provide information useful for discharge planning. Two approaches—bottom up and top down—may be used (Abreu, 1998). The bottom-up perspective is used to measure specific impairment within performance components, such as cognition. The top-down perspective is used to measure and describe performance in everyday activities. Successful rehabilitation results from a confluent, free-flowing application of both perspectives. In therapeutic practice, *confluence* denotes a fluid, back-and-forth movement between perspectives (Peloquin, 1996), which results in simultaneous attention being given to both performance components and everyday living occupations and habits. This evaluation model balances an understanding of the specific nature of impairments with an understanding of people as occupational beings. It rejects the common assumption that practitioners must choose between holism and reductionism and instead promotes the use of both related perspectives (Abreu, 1998). No causality or directional relationship is implied or necessary for this model to be effective (Wood, Abreu, Duval, & Gerber, 1994).

During evaluation, practitioners must analyze the processing strategies clients use during task performance. In addition, they must examine the conditions that can affect the performance positively or negatively, including the use of cues and test repetition (Abreu & Toglia, 1987; Toglia, 1991). This analysis can be accomplished by using a process-oriented approach to probe clients and assess their ability to change with practice and with benefit from instructions and cues.

Identifying Cognitive Performance Necessary for Everyday Living

Therapists can use standardized and nonstandardized measures to identify clients' remaining cognitive skills and determine the degree of change in performance. Examples of evaluation strategies in this area are test repetition; external cueing; and environment modifications, such as strategically placed reminder signs. Therapists using these strategies can measure the client's cognitive deficits and determine the conditions that improve or cause deterioration in performance (Abreu & Toglia, 1987). Standardized measures use scores to indicate how well the client performs relative to norms. In contrast, nonstandardized measures do not incorporate norms. Tables 14.1, 14.2, and 14.3 show examples of measures used for both AD and TBI.

Therapists should select various standardized and nonstandardized measurement tools to survey at least four different performance components:

1. *Cognitive function,* or the manner in which clients gather information from the environment. This component includes attention, memory, and problem solving. Therapists may use a cancellation test, which assesses both speed and accuracy, to evaluate attention. Memory can be tested with a simple recall schema for auditory and visual memory. Simple mathematics problems may be used for problem solving.
2. *Awareness of disability,* which may be tested using an interview process. Therapists may ask clients if they are aware of any problems, determine whether they recognize errors, and see whether they predict that they are going to have any problems in the future.
3. *Movement and postural control.* These components may be tested when practitioners observe people performing arts, crafts, or other activities.
4. *Body alignment,* examined through observation while the body is in action or at rest.

The evaluation of both cognitive and motor components is essential because motor performance is a reflection of cognitive processes.

Evaluating Everyday Living Skills

The evaluation of ADL skills is designed to identify and describe a client's level of abilities and subjective sense of satisfaction with performance after TBI. Evaluation from this perspective assumes a humanistic orientation, wherein therapists become active observers, recorders, and collaborators. Therapists use narrative and performance analysis to explain and predict behavior based on four client characteristics: lifestyle status, life stage, health status, and level of disadvantage. Therapists interview clients

Table 14.1. Global Deterioration Scale (GDS)

GDS Scale	Cognitive Function	Clinical Phase and Characteristics
1	No cognitive decline	Normal phase. No subjective memory complaints.
2	Very mild decline	Forgetfulness phase. Subjective memory complaints such as forgetting where common objects have been placed or forgetting names of personal acquaintances.
3	Mild decline	Early confusional phase. First explicit evidence of cognitive disturbance. Decreased retention and concentration, misplaces objects, and exhibits anomia. Performance decreases when placed in stressful employment or social settings. Denial and mild-to-moderate anxiety is observed.
4	Moderate decline	Late confusional phase. Topographical apraxia, decreased knowledge about current and recent events, possibly decreased memory in relation to personal history, and is unable to perform complex tasks. Orientation to person and place or recognizing familiar faces or persons may not be disturbed. Displays a flattened affect and tends to withdraw from stressful or challenging situations.
5	Moderately severe decline	Early dementia phase. Dependent on others to survive. Disoriented. Independent in toileting and eating but has difficulty dressing self. Able to retain major personal and family facts.
6	Severe decline	Middle dementia phase. Requires moderate-to-maximal assistance with ADL tasks, disoriented, may become incontinent, and begins to display behavioral and psychological deficits such as paranoia, obsessive-compulsive behaviors, anxiety, agitation, or cognitive abulia.
7	Very severe decline	Late dementia phase. Unable to verbally communicate, ADL dependent, loss of psychomotor skills, and may display generalized cortical or focal neurologic signs symtomatology.

Note: ADL = activities of daily living.
From "The Global Deterioration Scale for Assessment of Primary Degenerative Dementia," by B. Reisberg, S. H. Ferris, M. J. DeLeon, & T. Crook, 1982, *American Journal of Psychiatry, 139,* 1136–1139. Adapted with permission.

and family groups about each characteristic. Questions about lifestyle focus on communication, work, and day-to-day activities, including personal characteristics and the use of economic resources. A sample question is, "How would you describe your lifestyle before your accident?" Life stage status is examined by a description of the physical, emotional, and spiritual characteristics of one's life. Relevant factors include age, marital status, accomplishments, and losses (e.g., "What was your latest accomplishment?"). Occupational therapists survey the client's health status, including premorbid conditions and changes in behavior or condition fol-

lowing the accident or illness (e.g., "How was your health before the illness?").

To determine the level of disadvantage experienced by the client, therapists investigate the client's personal and social restrictions (e.g., a client's inability to attend movies, shop, cook, or provide in any way for family members or others) by asking questions such as, "What support system does your community offer to people with brain injury?" Therapists evaluate the client's motivation, goals, actions, and capacity by analyzing his or her performance of ordinary occupations and activities. Therapists use both standardized and nonstandard-

Table 14.2. Assessments for Alzheimer's Disease

Test	Purpose	Reference
Alzheimer Home Assessment	To evaluate the home environment to ensure safety	Painter, J. (1996). Home environment considerations for people with Alzheimer's disease. *Occupational Therapy in Healthcare, 10,* 45–63.
Cleveland Scale of Daily Living (CSADL)	To measure physical disability, instrumental activities of daily living, communication skills, and social behaviors	Patterson, M. B., Mack, J. L., Neundorfer, M. M., Martin, R. J., Smyth, K. A., & Whitehouse, P. J. (1992). Assessment of functional ability in Alzheimer's disease: A review and a preliminary report on the Cleveland Scale of Activities of Daily Living. *Alzheimer's Disease and Associated Disorders, 6,* 145–163.
Clifton Assessment Procedures for the Elderly (CAPE)	To measure physical disability, apathy, communication, and disturbances	Pattie, A. H., & Gilleard, C. J. (1979). *Clifton Assessment Procedures for the Elderly (CAPE).* Sevenoaks, Kent: Hodder & Stoughton.
Clinical Dementia Rating (CDR)	To measure and follow the natural history (i.e., regardless of intervention) of senile dementia of the Alzheimer's type	Morris, J. C. (1993). The Clinical Dementia Rating (CDR): Current version and scoring rules. *Neurology, 43,* 2412–2414.
Echelle Comportment et Adaption (ECA)	To measure physical independence, social integration, occupation, orientation, mobility, and language	Ritchie, K., & Ledesert, B. (1991). The measurement of incapacity in the severely demented elderly: The validation of a behavioral assessment scale. *International Journal of Geriatric Psychiatry, 6,* 217–226.
Global Deterioration Scale (GDS)	To assess the clinically identifiable ratable stages of primary degenerative dementia and age-associated memory impairment	Reisberg, B., Ferris, S. H., De Leon, M. J., & Crook, T. (1982). The Global Deterioration Scale for assessment of primary degenerative dementia. *American Journal of Psychiatry, 139,* 1136–1139.
Kitchen Task Assessment (KTA)	A functional measure that records the level of cognitive support required by a person with Alzheimer's disease	Baum, C., & Edwards, D. F. (1993). Cognitive performance in senile dementia of Alzheimer's type: The Kitchen Task Assessment. *American Journal of Occupational Therapy, 47,* 431–436.
London Psychogeriatic Rating Scale (LPRS)	To measure mental disorganization, confusion, physical disability, socially irritating behavior, and disengagement	Hersch, E. L., Kral, V. A., & Palmer, R. B. (1978). Clinical value of the London Psychogeriatric Rating Scale. *Journal of American Geriatrics Society, 26,* 348–354.
Structured Assessment of Independent Living Skills (SAILS)	To measure language, orientation, money-related skills, instrumental activities, and social interaction	Mahurin, R. K., De Bettignes, B. H., & Pirozzolo, F. J. (1991). Structured Assessment of Independent Living Skills: Preliminary report of a performance measure of functional abilities in dementia. *Journal of Gerontology: Psychological Sciences, 46,* 48–66.

ized measures to assess clients' ability in daily living activities. Such measures are based on a performance level of 100%. Clients are classified as independent or as requiring mild, moderate, or maximum assistance.

People with AD and TBI appear to retain procedural memory (i.e., "knowing how" to do particular activities) better than declarative memory (i.e., "knowing what"; Cooke, Fisher, Mayberry, & Oakley, 2000). These differences are used for evaluation

Table 14.3. Assessments for Traumatic Brain Injury

Test	Purpose	Reference
Coma/Near Coma Scale (CNC)	Monitors responsivity to stimulation, indicating the severity of sensory, perceptual, and primitive response deficits at the coma level	Rappaport M., Doughtery, A. M., & Kelting D. L. (1992). Evaluation of coma and vegetative states. *Archives of Physical Medicine and Rehabilitation, 73,* 628–634.
Coma Recovery Scale (CRS)	Monitors responsivity to stimulation, indicating the severity of sensory, perceptual, and primitive response deficits at the coma level	Giacino, J. T., Kezmarsky, M. A., DeLuca, J., & Cicerone, K. D. (1991). Monitoring rate of recovery to predict outcome in minimally responsive patients. *Archives of Physical Medicine and Rehabilitation, 72,* 897–900.
Sensory Stimulation Assessment Measure (SSAM)	Monitors responsivity to stimulation, indicating the severity of sensory, perceptual, and primitive response deficits at the coma level	Rader, M. A., Alston, J. B., & Ellis, D. W. (1989). Sensory stimulation of severely brain-injured patients. *Brain Injury, 3,* 141–147.
Western Sensory Stimulation Profile (WNSSP)	Monitors responsivity to stimulation, indicating the severity of sensory, sensory stimulation perceptual, and primitive response deficits at the coma level	Ansell, B. J., & Keenan, J. E. (1989). The western neuro profile: A tool for assessing slow-to-recover head injury patients. *Archives of Physical Medicine and Rehabilitation, 70,* 104–108.
Awareness Questionnaire	Measures cognitive, behavioral/affective, and motor/sensory factors	Sherer, M., Bergloff, P., Boake, C., High, W., Jr., & Levin, E. (1998). The Awareness Questionnaire: Factor structure and internal consistency. *Brain Injury, 12,* 63–68.
Self-Awareness Deficits Interview	Qualitative methods to evaluate self-awareness	Fleming, J. M., Strong, J., & Ashton, R. (1996). Self-awareness of deficits in adults with traumatic brain injury: How best to measure? *Brain Injury, 10,* 1–15.
Community Integration Questionnaire (CQI)	Measures handicap in homelike settings, social networks, and integration into productive activities	Willer, B., Ottenbacher, K. J., & Coad, M. L. (1994). The Community Integration Questionnaire: A comparative examination. *Archives of Physical Medicine and Rehabilitation, 73,* 103–111.
Functional Independence Measure (FIM)	Measures disability, using average daily minutes of assistance needed from another person	Corrigan, J., Smith-Knapp, K., & Granger, C. V. (1997). Validity of the Functional Independence Measure for persons with traumatic brain injury. *Archives of Physical Medicine and Rehabilitation, 78,* 828–834.
Head Injury Symptom Checklist	Measures impairment in mild traumatic brain injury	McLean, A., Dikmen, S., Temkin, N., Wyler, A. R., & Gale, J. I. (1984). Psychosocial functioning at one month after injury. *Neurosurgery 14,* 393–399.
Medical Outcome Study, SF-36	Measures physical health and role limitations	Ware, J. E. (1993). *SF-36 health survey manual and interpretation guide.* Boston: Health Institute, England Medical Center.
Assessment of Motor and Process Skills	Evaluates household task performances	Darragh, A. R., Sample, P. L., & Fisher, A. G. (1998). Environment effect of functional task performance in adults with acquired brain injuries: Use of the Assessment of Motor and Process Skills. *Archives of Physical Medicine and Rehabilitation, 79,* 418–423.

and intervention directed toward increasing functional independence. It is unclear, however, how cognitive performance components relate and affect ADL and IADL (Nygard, Amberla, Bernspang, Almkvist, & Winblad, 1998). Therefore, it is important to continue to evaluate and study their relationship.

Approaches to Intervention

Intervention alternatives for people with cognitive deficits are varied and complex. The goals are to (1) maintain, restore, and improve everyday living; (2) promote health; (3) modify through compensation and adaptation (Moyers, 1999); and (4) prevent further deterioration. The use of cueing and the repetition of tasks continue as a basic theme in the intervention strategies, whether the intervention is for remediation or compensation. Cues and repetitions are used to determine the most efficient methods of instruction and training.

General Intervention Strategies

The following sections describe four dynamically interrelated intervention strategies that are used for both AD and TBI (Figure 14.2): drugs and medications, cognitive rehabilitation, human connection, and caregiver education.

Drugs and Medications

Drugs and medications may be used to calm clients, increase attention, and foster the success of cognitive rehabilitation. They can reduce symptoms and enhance function for AD and TBI clients (Parenté & Herrmann, 1996; Wolf-Klein, 1993). Hidergine, Vasopressin, and Cognex can increase cognitive function; Prozac and Zoloft can calm agitated and depressed clients; Xanax can relieve anxiety and agitation; and Haldol can reduce paranoia and hallucinations. In addition, some investi-

gators advocate the use of herbs including ginseng and ginko biloba for treatment. These drug interventions may assist in the improvement or retainment of self-care skills.

Cognitive Rehabilitation

Cognitive rehabilitation approaches are designed to remediate or compensate for cognitive deficits; therapists use these approaches to design programs for people with AD and TBI (Katz, 1998). Cognitive learning strategies, which are based on cognitive psychology, are used to treat deficits, including memory and problem-solving problems, that cannot be directly observed. Using these strategies, therapists teach clients to process, structure, and modify information from the environment to improve performance in everyday living skills. Therapists prescribe specific tasks, situations, and rules of behavior for clients and teach them to use imagery, conscious awareness, and self-monitoring techniques (e.g., using checklists, slowing down before rechecking answers, and self-talk). The assumption when using cognitive strategies is that clients' motivation to successfully perform ADL is rooted in their desire to master competency and enjoy inde-

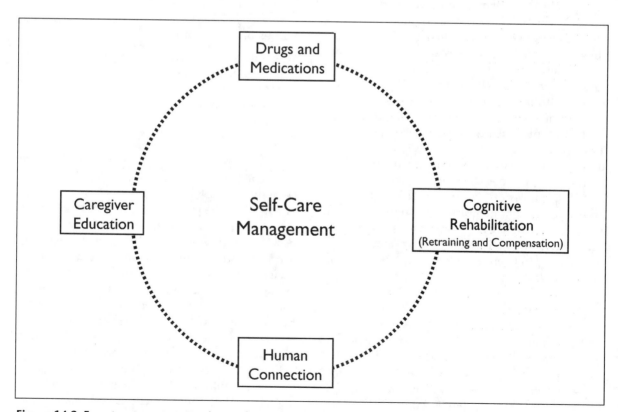

Figure 14.2. Four treatment strategies as they relate to self-care management.

pendence. Cognitive learning strategies are limited by the client's ability to use conscious awareness and self-monitoring techniques.

Behavioral learning strategies are based on behavior modification principles (Giles & Clark-Wilson, 1993; Jacobs, 1993). Therapists use behavioral learning strategies to treat deficits that can be directly observed, such as problems with ADL tasks (e.g., when a client voids in an inappropriate container instead of the toilet). Therapists identify possible functional relationships of cause and effect to shape specified behaviors. The assumption is that positive or negative environmental reinforcements can motivate clients to perform self-care. Behavioral learning strategies are limited by the fact that they require a rigorous program involving the entire health care team. Most practitioners use a combination of cognitive and behavioral learning strategies. Table 14.4 lists samples of cognitive and behavioral learning strategies.

Human Connection

Human connection strategies are based on universal principles of wellness, social science, and occupational science. They are used to regain or preserve clients' meaningful and emotional experiences (Wilcock, 1998; Zemke & Clark, 1996). Therapists need to use human connection strategies for everyday living skill management because these emotional experiences are essential to the achievement of a holistic intervention. Therapists must recognize that clients are meaningfully connected within society and that there is hope for them to maintain a sense of well-being regardless of their cognitive deficits (Abreu, 1998; Hasselkus, 1998; Herskovits, 1995). Therapists must try to understand the experience of disability, the trajectory of illness, the loss of well-being, and the disruption of self. Examples of human connection strategies are empathic communication; caring touch; and the reconstruction of rituals and habits, such as the morning routine, television viewing, and outings (Clark, 1993; Crepeau, 1995; Peloquin, 1995; Zemke, 1995).

Caregiver Education

Caregiver education strategies include identifying and describing the needs and characteristics of clients for the family group. These strategies are used to prepare caregivers for their new role in society. Although numerous reports on family-focused intervention have been published, limited guidelines exist for these strategies. Therapists must use sociological principles to develop an approach to caregiving and consider cultural differences. Haley et al. (1996) have shown that African-American caregivers often report less depression than White family groups when assisting clients with AD. Other studies suggest that Hispanic caregivers are strongly governed by familial relationships, values, and norms (Cox & Monk, 1993).

For clients with AD, therapists must educate family groups about how to deal with fear of genetic linkages, puzzlement, and the responsibilities of caregiving for a person with substantial cognitive deficits. In addition, therapists must inform caregivers about the need for respite services and support groups. In the later stages of dementia, caregivers must be prepared to deal with nursing care decisions, guardianship, and informed consent.

For clients with TBI, therapists must educate family groups about confusion, awareness of disability, and other effects of cognitive impairment. Therapists should inform clients and family groups about community resources and support groups. In cases involving chronic and severe impairment, placement, guardianship, and informed consent should be addressed. Many caregivers become advocates for their significant others diagnosed with AD or TBI.

Stages of Intervention

Most intervention involves three phases: preparation, performance, and review. To be effective, each phase requires collaboration among practitioners, clients, and family groups.

Preparation Phase

In the first phase, the therapist works with the client and family group to establish emotional and social connections and to enable the client to express his or her goals. The preparation phase has three parts. First, the therapist, client, and family group establishes a trusting and relaxed rapport through conversation, stress reduction, and meditation techniques. Next, the therapist helps the client become aware of and focus on the goals and projected outcomes of intervention. Therapists may use instruction and cueing with multiple senses to increase the awareness of intervention (e.g., visual and auditory instructions). Finally, the therapist and client develop strategies to maximize the ability to organize and process information in preparation for self-care and other ADL. The instructional information may have to be divided into small steps to make it more understandable.

Table 14.4. Treatment Strategies for Self-Care Management

Action	Retraining for Mild Cognitive Impairment	Compensation for Moderate Cognitive Impairment	Total Caregiving for Severe Cognitive Impairment
Personal hygiene Unable to brush hair	Clients are taught to simplify and organize task in parts: right side, left side, and front. Therapists' cues match clients' most beneficial sensory modality (auditory, visual, tactile, or kinesthetic). Clients are taught to say steps aloud before and during task.	Clients are given checklist with steps and sequences. Clients are taught one-handed techniques. Therapists appropriately modify brushes: larger or smaller, heavier or lighter, bright colors. Therapists appropriately modify location of brush: constant, nonrotated location to match any perceptual or cognitive loss. Therapists appropriately modify mirror location and size.	Use caregiver assistance for part or whole task.
Unable to perform oral hygiene	Clients are taught to use toothbrush and floss in parts: front teeth first, followed by left, right, and back teeth.	Battery-operated toothbrushes, one-handed flossing.	Use caregiver assistance for part or whole task.
Unable to bathe and shower	Clients are taught to simplify and organize task in steps: Temperature control (cold water before hot) regulation, remember to clean critical body areas.	Clients are given checklist with steps and sequences. Clients are given bathtub and shower seats, adapter shower handles, soap on a rope, rubber mats, and handrails.	Use caregiver assistance for part or whole task.
Dressing Unable to perform upper-extremity dressing	Clients are taught to arrange garments in a specific order and dress in a specific sequence. Clients are taught to say steps aloud before and during task.	Clients are given checklist with correct steps and sequences. Clients are given pictures or photos of correct steps as cues. Clients are taught one-handed techniques. Therapists appropriately modify clothing: larger sizes, Velcro® snaps, button aids, zipper aids.	Use caregiver assistance for part or whole task.
Unable to perform lower-extremity dressing (e.g., unable to put shoes on feet; unable to put on prosthetic devices)	Clients are taught to arrange garments in a specific order and dress in a specific sequence; in addition to postural control training in bed, sitting on a chair, or standing. Clients are taught to say steps aloud before and during task.	Clients are given checklist with correct steps and sequences. Clients are given pictures or photos of correct steps as cues. Clients are taught one-handed techniques. Therapists appropriately modify clothing: elastic pants, Velcro® snaps, button aids, zipper aids, long-handled shoehorns, shoe aids, stocking aids.	Use caregiver assistance for part or whole task.

Continued

331

Table 14.4. *Continued*

Action	Retraining for Mild Cognitive Impairment	Compensation for Moderate Cognitive Impairment	Total Caregiving for Severe Cognitive Impairment
Eating Unable to indicate food needs	Clients are taught to remember the specific time schedule.	Clients are taught to set alarm clocks to remember schedules. Clients are taught to use a memory notebook or visual aids to point out needs to others.	Use caregiver assistance for part or whole task.
Unable to get or set up food	Clients are taught mobility techniques to get food within reach. Clients are taught to organize and arrange utensils within their visual field and easy reach (low placement).	Clients are taught appropriate techniques: use a one-handed technique, switch handedness, or use two hands in a specific way. Therapists set up food location to help client.	Use caregiver assistance for part or whole task.
Unable to select or use utensils	Clients are taught to organize and arrange utensils within their visual field and easy reach before starting to eat. Clients are taught to look over the entire place setting to locate utensils before starting to eat.	Therapists set up utensil location to help clients. Therapists arrange kitchen drawers with utensil facing open end of drawer and handles pointing toward rear. Therapists appropriately modify utensils: large or small handles, heavier or lighter, colorful. Clients are provided one-handed knives.	Use caregiver assistance for part or whole task.
Unable to eat or drink	Clients are taught oral–motor retraining. Clients are taught swallowing retraining. Clients are taught to take small bites and to drink fluids to encourage swallowing (refer to neurodevelopmental motor techniques).	Therapists appropriately modify consistencies: make liquid thicker consistencies, use straws. Therapists appropriately modify drinking cups: larger, smaller, heavier, lighter, colorful, personalized with picture or name. Therapists appropriately modify use of napkins as bibs. Modify for motor incoordination: scoop dish, plate guard, nonskid mat.	Use caregiver assistance for part or whole task.
Unable to finish eating in a timely manner	Clients are taught self-monitoring: estimating time and speed of eating routine to slow down or speed up the process. Clients are taught to self-question: "Am I eating slow enough?" "Am I eating fast enough?"	Clients are taught to set alarm clocks to remember timing. Clients are taught to keep a log of when they started eating and at what time they finished eating.	Use caregiver assistance for part or whole task.

Performance Phase

In the performance phase, the goal is to improve or compensate for the client's memory and learning ability and increase his or her satisfaction. This phase involves the use of practice, feedback, and environmental modification, the nature of which is determined according to the occupational therapist's evaluation of the client and the client's goals. The therapist, client, tasks, exercises, and occupations all contribute to the environmental change or contextual modification during intervention (Figure 14.3). Practice consists of planned repetition of clients' actions and behaviors at a predetermined frequency for a predetermined duration. An example would be for clients to repeat the action of putting on a sweater 3 times in a half-hour 3 times per week. Therapists and caregivers use feedback to provide helpful responses to clients during practice. The frequency varies depending on the clients' cognitive and physical recovery level, as determined through the use of performance tests. Clients may be independent or require mild, moderate or maximum assistance. If the baseline performance is established at less than 50% of optimum performance, therapists will use constant feedback. If the baseline is established above the 50% level, the frequency of feedback will be less and will decline as the clients improve. Environmental modifications include adaptation by clients, therapists, and family groups to their surroundings and the changing of the objects within that environment.

Environments are one of two types. A *congruent* environment is one that is simple and familiar and requires minimal cognitive-processing demands (e.g., making soup from a can in the client's home kitchen under no time constraints). A *contextual interference* environment is a complex one that requires maximum processing demands (e.g., making full-course meals in an unfamiliar kitchen with a time limit). Contextual interference makes the immediate intervention goal more difficult to achieve; if used properly, however, such environments can strengthen the learning pattern. Such an environment is used for those clients whose performance requires mild assistance. A congruent environment is used for clients who require moderate and maximum assistance.

Review Phase

At the end of each intervention session, therapists bring closure by documenting client progress and comparing current with prior performance. On the basis of this constant reevaluation, therapists, clients, and family groups readjust their goals and timetables. Chronic clients who are maximally dependent in daily activities such as self-care may not achieve significant functional progress. With such clients, the focus must be on humanistic connection and well-being.

Examples of strategies used in each phase are provided in Table 14.5. Tables 14.6 and 14.7 list examples of intervention strategies for AD and TBI.

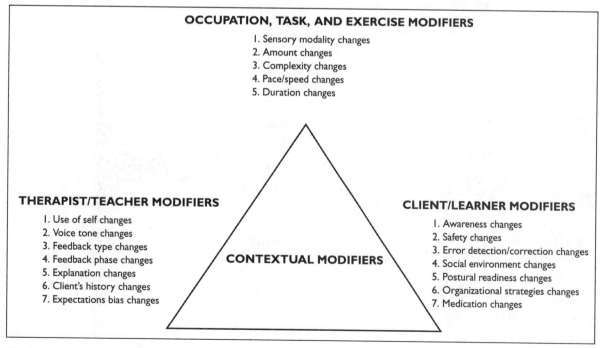

OCCUPATION, TASK, AND EXERCISE MODIFIERS
1. Sensory modality changes
2. Amount changes
3. Complexity changes
4. Pace/speed changes
5. Duration changes

THERAPIST/TEACHER MODIFIERS
1. Use of self changes
2. Voice tone changes
3. Feedback type changes
4. Feedback phase changes
5. Explanation changes
6. Client's history changes
7. Expectations bias changes

CONTEXTUAL MODIFIERS

CLIENT/LEARNER MODIFIERS
1. Awareness changes
2. Safety changes
3. Error detection/correction changes
4. Social environment changes
5. Postural readiness changes
6. Organizational strategies changes
7. Medication changes

Figure 14.3. Sources of environmental change.

Table 14.5. Treatment Phases

Preparation Phase	Performance Phase	Review Phase
Identify language regulators • Verbal instructions: language used, level, volume, speed, inflections, concreteness, complexity, general cues, specific cues, give-away cues, hierarchy • Written instructions: language used, level, speed of presentation, size, concreteness, complexity, general cues, specific cues, give-away cues • Gestural instructions: language used, speed, concreteness, general cues, specific cues, give-away cues • Pictorial instructions: line drawings, black and white pictures, color pictures, two-dimensional, three-dimensional • Tactile or kinesthetic instructions: amount of hand guidance, tactile proprioceptive pressure used, speed of movement, general cues, specific cues, give-away cues Identify sociocultural regulators: client's value judgment on the meaningfulness of the skill Identify physical regulators: physical attributes that control actions of that skill, such as temporal and spatial attributes (location and target speed) Identify physical appearances: physical affordances and attributes that may or may not control action; they can conceal or make the goal of the skill more salient, such as color, texture, size Schedule practice location: the practice setting; real-life or simulated environments (client's room, gym, unit kitchen, bathroom, gift shops) Schedule practice frequency and intensity: amount of repetition of specific skill and time of analysis dedicated to the practice of each skill in one training session Identify the nature of feedback: verbal, nonverbal, general, specific, give-away, or face-saving hierarchy Schedule feedback frequency and intensity: constant, immediate, delayed, infrequent (e.g., 100% feedback = every trial, 50% = 5 times out of every trial)	List goals by common denominator Analyze underlying skills for each goal Analyze pretreatment, concurrent, and post-treatment practice strategies Bottom-up (micro) goals • Able to orient eyes, head, and neck 100% of the time during a variety of postures in 1 week • Able to realign and adjust to self-initiated postural control during dressing tasks 75% of the time in 2 weeks • Able to realign and adjust to externally initiated postural control during dressing tasks 75% of the time in 3 weeks • Able to increase body response during self-care from 12 seconds to 7 seconds in 1 week Top-down (macro) goals • Client is able to perform favorite occupation safely in 3 weeks, while standing. • Client is able to perform more than one activity, task, or role safely in 2 weeks. • Client is able to engage in favorite social recreation (e.g., dancing) in 2 weeks. Example • Orienting activities and tasks that elicit eye, head, and neck movement in a variety of positions and locations General Rules • Instruct learners on the importance of practice as it relates to posture (i.e., home, institution, and community safety). • Involve family during practice; they can help you validate responses. • During the initial trial, allow client to respond without modification; then adapt the modification strategies during the next trials. • Notice and recognize improvement from gross to subtle changes in visual, auditory, vestibular, and proprioceptive stimuli.	Performance tested after interval long enough to have practice effects dissipated Question client or family about their satisfaction with the results of the treatment session Question client or family about their dissatisfaction with the results of the treatment session Adjust, expand goals in an interdisciplinary context Determine the performance effect of random, variable, and blocked practice

Table 14.6. Treatment Strategies for Alzheimer's Disease

Strategy	Purpose	Resource
Cognitive and behavioral strategies	Establish cognitive disability perspective	Levy, L. L. (1986). A practical guide to the care of the Alzheimer's disease victim: The cognitive disability perspective. *Topics in Geriatric Rehabilitation, 1,* 16–26.
Behavioral strategies	Regain and retain meaningful life skills Assess motor and process skills	Josephsson, S., Bäckman, L., Borell, L., Nygård, L., & Berspång, B. (1995). Effectiveness of an intervention to improve occupational to improve occupational performance in dementia. *Occupational Therapy Journal of Research, 15,* 36–49.
	Use morning bright light for disturbed sleep and behavior disorders	Van Someren, E. J., Kessler, A., Mirmiran, M., & Swaab, D. F. (1997). Indirect bright light improves circadian rest–activity rhythm disturbances in demented patients. *Biological Psychiatry, 41,* 955–963.
		Mishima, K., Okawa, M., Hishikawa, Y., Hozumi, S., Hori, H., & Takahashi, K. (1994). Morning bright light therapy for sleep and behavior disorders in elderly patients with dementia. *Acta Psychiatrica Scandinavica, 89,* 1–7.
	Address cognitive deficits	Bellus, S. B., Kost, P. P., Vergo, J. G., & Dinezza, G. J. (1998). Improvements in cognitive functioning following intensive behavioral rehabilitation. *Brain Injury, 12,* 139–145.
	Strengthen physical and social cues in the environment Preserve stability in physical and social environment	Roberts, B. L., & Algase, D. L. (1988). Victims of Alzheimer's disease and the environment. *Nursing Clinics of North America, 23,* 83–93.
Cognitive strategies	Use memory wallets to prompt factual information during prompted conversations	Zanetti, O., Binetti, G., Magni, E., Rozzini, L. Bianchetti, A., & Trabucchi, M. (1997). Procedural memory stimulation in Alzheimer's disease: Impact of a training programme. *Acta Neurologica Scandinavica, 95,* 152–157.
		Bourgeois, M. S. (1992). Evaluating memory wallets in conversations with persons with dementia. *Journal of Speech and Hearing Research, 35,* 1344–1357.
	During group therapy for orientation, employ strategies for reminiscence through recollection; strategies for reality orientation through time, place, and person; and strategies for remotivation through discussion, thought, and deduction	Zanetti, O., Frisoni, G. B., De Leo, D., Dello Buono, M., Bianchetti, A., & Trabucchi, M. (1995). Reality orientation therapy in Alzheimer disease: Useful or not? A controlled study. *Alzheimer Disease and Associated Disorders, 9,* 132–138. Koh, K., Ray, R., Lee, J., Nair, A., Ho, T., & Ang, P.C. (1994). Dementia in elderly patients: Can the 3R mental stimulation programme improve mental status? *Age and Ageing, 23,* 195–196.
Human connection strategies	Promote calmness by playing classical music an the favorite music of the patient	Casby, J. A., & Holm, M. B. (1994). The effect of music on repetitive disruptive vocalizations of persons with dementia. *American Journal of Occupational Therapy, 48,* 883–889.
	Understand the style and preference of the caregiver through qualitative analysis	Corcoran, M. A. (1994). Management decisions made by caregiver spouses of persons with Alzheimer's disease. *American Journal of Occupational Therapy, 48,* 38–45.

Table 14.7. Treatment Strategies for Traumatic Brain Injury

Strategy	Purpose	Resource
Cognitive retraining	Attentional retraining using microcomputers to assist TBI clients in a hospital	Gray, J. M., Robertson, I., Pentland, B., & Anderson, S. (1992). Microcomputer-based attentional retraining after brain damage: A randomized group controlled trial. *Neuropsychological Rehabilitation, 2*, 97–115.
	Changing physical traits and using clients' communication skills and self-awareness of brain injury clients	Toglia, J. P. (1991). Generalization of treatment: A multi-context approach to cognitive perceptual impairment in adults with brain injury. *American Journal of Occupational Therapy, 45*, 505–516.
	Metacognitive training	Abreu, B. C., & Toglia, J. P. (1987). Cognitive rehabilitation: A model for occupational therapy. *American Journal of Occupational Therapy, 41*, 439–448.
	Compensatory strategies checklist and phone calls to assist clients with TBI in home settings	Schwartz, S. M. (1994). Adults with traumatic brain injury: Three case studies of cognitive rehabilitation in home setting. *American Journal of Occupational Therapy, 49*, 655–667.
	Verbal information retraining using mnemonic strategy	Gasquoine, P. G. (1991). Learning in post-traumatic amnesia following extremely severe closed head injury. *Brain Injury 5*, 156–175.
		Neistadt, M. E. (1994). Perceptual retraining for adults with diffuse brain injury. *American Journal of Occupational Therapy, 48*, 225–233.
	Reaction time training after TBI using feedback	Deacon, D., & Campbell, K. B. (1991). Decision making following closed-head injury: Can response speed be re-trained? *Journal of Clinical and Experimental Neuropsychology, 13*, 639–651.
	Scaffolding: previous skills used serve as a platform for the acquisition of new skills (e.g., scanning training leads to wheelchair use) Metacognition: personal control use, introspection, talking aloud to self-monitor; awareness training	Ben-Yishay, Y., & Diller, L. (1993). Cognitive remediation in traumatic brain injury: Update and issues. *Archives of Physical Medicine and Rehabilitation, 74*, 204–213.
	Self-monitoring instructions to increase interpersonal skills	Schloss, P. J., Thompson, C. K., Gajar, A. H., & Schloss, C. (1985). Influence of self-monitoring on heterosexual conversational behaviors of head trauma youth. *Applied Research in Mental Retardation, 6*, 269–282.
	Postural control training for vestibular pathologies after TBI	Shumway-Cook, A. (1994). Vestibular rehabilitation in traumatic brain injury. In S. J. Herdman (Ed.), *Vestibular rehabilitation* (pp. 347–359). Philadelphia: F. A. Davis.
Cognitive retraining and human connection	Information processing, teaching learning, neurodevelopmental, biomechanical strategies for cognitive and postural control training Narrative, storytelling for personalized and meaningful training	Abreu, B. C. (1998). The quadraphonic approach: Holistic rehabilitation for brain injury. In N. Katz (Ed.), *Cognition and occupation in rehabilitation: Cognitive models for intervention in occupational therapy* (pp. 51–97). Bethesda, MD: American Occupational Therapy Association. Abreu, B. C. (in press). The reasoning behind assessment and treatment of memory and learning. In C. Unsworth (Ed.), *Cognitive and perceptual dysfunction: A clinical reasoning approach to assessment and treatment.* Philadelphia: F. A. Davis.

Continued

Table 14.7. *Continued*

Strategy	Purpose	Resource
Human connection	Structuring of the volunteer role, structured failure experiences videotaped and replayed for reinforcement Family and client education to develop a new identity rather than reproducing the old identity	Krefting, L. (1989). Reintegration into the community after head injury: The results of an ethnographic study. *Occupational Therapy Journal of Research, 9, 67–83.*
	Peer group experiences to assist clients with TBI, provide support, self-advocacy, and fellowship network with other clients with TBI	Schwartzberg, S. L. (1994). Helping factors in a peer-developed support group for persons with head injury. Part 1: Participant observer perspective. *American Journal of Occupational Therapy, 48, 297–304.*
		Schollz, C. H. (1994). Helping factors in a peer-developed support group for persons with head injury. Part 2: Survivor interview perspective. *American Journal of Occupational Therapy, 48, 305–309.*
Behavioral	Washing and dressing retraining	Giles, G. M., Ridley, J. E., Dill, A., & Frye, S. (1997). A consecutive series of adults with brain injury treated with a washing and dressing retraining program. *American Journal of Occupational Therapy, 51, 256–266.*
	Repetition, multisensory input, and human connection	Zencius, A. H., Wesolowski, M. D., & Rodriguez, I. M. (1998). Improving orientation in head injured adults by repeated practice, multi-sensory input, and peer participation. *Brain Injury, 12, 53–61.*
Sensory stimulation	Uncertain evidence for effectiveness of sensory stimulation to promote recovery from coma	Giacino, J. T. (1996). Sensory stimulation: Theoretical perspectives and the evidence for effectiveness. *Neurorehabilitation, 6, 69–78.*

Measuring Intervention Outcomes

Outcome measurement is an attempt to quantify the quality of therapeutic services in terms of effectiveness (i.e., achievement of goals), efficiency (i.e., optimal rate of progress), and value (i.e., cost containment; Foto, 1996). Both standardized and nonstandardized measures may be used to quantify results. AD and TBI clients in the severe phase may not achieve functional improvement; therefore, functional outcomes are not always appropriate. A critical outcome for these clients is physical, mental, and spiritual wellness. Other tools at the community and participation level may be appropriate.

Summary

Management of AD and TBI is a collaborative effort that requires the coordinated efforts of the entire rehabilitation team, the client, and the family group. This collaboration allows constant monitoring of ADL skills and enrichment through cultural diversity. Health is more than the absence of illness: It includes social and cultural factors such as awareness of community awareness integration. Such integration provides an opportunity to develop healthy lifestyles for clients and family groups (Wilcock, 1998). The interventions can enable clients to increase their sense of connection with others, sense of power, self-control, self-reconstruction, and meaningful occupations. Daily living management for people with cognitive deficits stemming from AD and TBI remains both an art and a science.

Acknowledgments

I would like to express my gratitude to Joanne Jones and Renee Pearcy of the research/editorial team for their help with the preparation of this chapter. National Institutes of Health Grant 3R01AG17638-01A1S1 and Moody Foundation Grant 78 sponsored the work in this project.

Study Questions

1. Identify common impairments affecting everyday living in people with TBI and AD.

2. Describe the degree of evidence currently available for occupational therapy treatment of both populations.

3. Compare and contrast the stages of recovery in TBI and AD.

4. Describe the factors that interact to affect community mobility in people with TBI.

5. Identify the IADL that typically demonstrate the earliest decline in people with AD.

References

Abreu, B. C. (1998). The quadraphonic approach: Holistic rehabilitation for brain injury. In N. Katz (Ed.), *Cognition and occupation in rehabilitation: Cognitive models for intervention in occupational therapy* (pp. 51–97). Bethesda, MD: American Occupational Therapy Association.

Abreu, B. C. (2003). Evidence-based practice. In G. McCormick (Ed.), *The Occupational Therapy Manager* (4th ed., pp. 351–373). Bethesda, MD: American Occupational Therapy Association.

Abreu, B. C., Seale, G., Scheibel, R. S., Huddleston, N., Zhang, L., & Ottenbacher, K. J. (2001). Levels of self-awareness after acute brain injury: How patients' and rehabilitation specialists' perceptions compare. *Archives of Physical Medicine and Rehabilitation, 82,* 49–56.

Abreu, B. C., & Toglia, J. P. (1987). Cognitive rehabilitation: A model for occupational therapy. *American Journal of Occupational Therapy, 41,* 439–448.

Alderman, N., Burgess, P. W., Knight, C., & Henman, C. (2003). Ecological validity of a simplified version of the multiple errands shopping test. *Journal of the International Neuropsychological Society, 9*(10), 31–44.

American Psychiatric Association. (2000). *Diagnostic and statistical manual of mental disorders* (4th ed., text rev.). Washington, DC: Author.

Bear, M. G., Connors, B., & Paradiso, M. (2001). *Neuroscience: Exploring the brain.* Baltimore: Lippincott Williams & Wilkins.

BIOTA Holdings. (1998). *Fact sheet 001: Alzheimer's disease.* Retrieved from http://www.biota.com.au/announcements/factsheets/sheet001.html.

Brain Injury Association, Inc. (2001). *Brain injury fact sheet: Brain injury.* Retrieved from httpwww.biausa.org/Pages/facts_and_stats.html.

Brewer, K., Geisler, T., Moody, K., & Wright, V. (1998). A community mobility assessment for adolescents with an acquired brain injury. *Physiotherapy Canada, 50*(2), 118–122.

Clark, F. (1993). Occupation embedded in real life: Interweaving occupational science and occupational therapy [1993 Eleanor Clark Slagle Lecture]. *American Journal of Occupational Therapy, 47,* 1067–1068.

Cooke, K. Z., Fisher, A. G., Mayberry, W., & Oakley, F. (2000). Differences in activities of daily living process skills of persons with and without Alzheimer's disease. *Occupational Therapy Journal of Research, 20,* 87–105.

Cox, C., & Monk, A. (1993). Hispanic culture and family care of Alzheimer's patients. *Health and Social Work, 18*(2), 92–100.

Crepeau, E. B. (1995). Lesson 6: Rituals. In C. B. Royeen (Ed.), *AOTA self-study series: The practice of the future: Putting occupation back into therapy.* Rockville, MD: American Occupational Therapy Association.

Derouesne, C., Thibault, S., Lozeron, P., Baudouin-Madec, V., Piquard, A., & Lacomblez., L. (2002). Perturbations des activities quotidiennes au cours de la maladie d'Alzheimer. Etude chez 172 patients a l'aide d'un questionnaire rempli par le conjoint. [Perturbations of activities of daily living in Alzheimer's disease. A study of 172 patients using a questionnaire completed by caregivers]. *Revue Neurologique, 158*(6–7), 684–700.

Dirette, D. (2002). The development of awareness and the use of compensatory strategies for cognitive deficits. *Brain Injury, 16,* 861–871.

Foto, M. (1996). Nationally speaking: Outcome studies: The what, why, how, and when. *American Journal of Occupational Therapy, 50,* 87–88.

Gaudette, M., & Anderson, A. (2002). Evaluating money management skills following brain injury using the assessment of functional monetary skills. *Brain Injury 16,* 133–148.

Giacino, J. T., Kezmarsky, M. A., DeLuca, J., & Cicerone, K. D. (1991). Monitoring rate of recovery to predict outcome in minimally responsive patients. *Archives of Physical Medicine and Rehabilitation, 72,* 897–900.

Giles, G. M., & Clark-Wilson, J. (1993). *Brain injury rehabilitation: A neurofunctional approach.* San Diego, CA: Singular Publishing Group.

Glueckauf, R. L., & Loomis, J. S. (2003). Alzheimer's caregiver support online: Lessons learned, initial findings and future directions. *NeuroRehabilitation, 18,* 135–146.

Haley, W. E., Roth, D. L., Coleton, M. I., Ford, G. R., West, C. A. C., Collins, R. P., et al. (1996). Appraisal, coping, and social support as mediators of well-being in black and white family caregivers of patients with Alzheimer's disease. *Journal of Consulting and Clinical Psychology, 64,* 121–129.

Hall, K. M., Karzmark, P., Stevens, M., Englander, J., O'Hare, P., & Wright, J. (1994). Family stressors in traumatic brain injury: A two-year follow-up. *Archives of Physical Medicine and Rehabilitation, 75,* 876–884.

Hasselkus, B. R. (1998). Occupation and well-being in dementia: The experience of day-care staff. *American Journal of Occupational Therapy, 52,* 423–434.

Herskovits, E. (1995). Struggling over subjectivity: Debates about "self" and Alzheimer's disease. *Medical Anthropology Quarterly, 9,* 146–164.

Hibbard, M. R., Gordon, W. A., Flanagan, S., Haddad, L., & Labinski, E. (2000). Sexual dysfunction after traumatic brain injury. *NeuroRehabilitation, 15,* 107–120.

Jacobs, H. E. (1993). *Behavior analysis guidelines and brain injury rehabilitation: Peoples, principles, and programs.* Gaithersburg, MD: Aspen.

Katz, N. (Ed.). (1998). *Cognition and occupation in rehabilitation: Cognitive models for intervention in occupational therapy.* Bethesda, MD: American Occupational Therapy Association.

Katz, N., Fleming, J., Keren, N., Lightbody, S., & Hartman-Maeir, A. (2002). Unawareness and/or denial of disability: Implications for occupational therapy intervention. *Canadian Journal of Occupational Therapy, 69,* 281–292.

Kuhn, D. (2002). Intimacy, sexuality, and residents with dementia. *Alzheimer's Care Quarterly, 3*, 165–173.

Law, M. (Ed.). (2002). *Evidence-based rehabilitation*. Thorofare, NJ: Slack.

Mazaux, J.-M., Masson, F., Levin, H. S., Alaoui, P., Maurette, P., & Michel, B. (1997). Long-term neuropsychological outcome and loss of social autonomy after traumatic brain injury. *Archives of Physical Medicine and Rehabilitation, 78*, 1316–1320.

McGrath, W. L., Mueller, M. M., Brown, C., Teitelman, J., & Watts, J. (2000). Caregivers of persons with Alzheimer's disease: An exploratory study of occupational performance and respite. *Physical and Occupational Therapy in Geriatrics, 18*, 51–69.

Minnes, P., Carlson, P., McColl, M. A., Nolte, M. L., Johnston, J., & Buell, K. (2003). Community integration: A useful construct, but what does it really mean? *Brain Injury, 17*, 149–159.

Morse, J. M., Swanson, J. M., & Kuzel, A. J. (2001). *The nature of qualitative evidence*. Thousand Oaks, CA: Sage.

Moyers, P. A. (1999). The guide to occupational therapy practice. *American Journal of Occupational Therapy, 53*, 247–322.

Nygard, L., Amberla, K., Bernspang, B., Almkvist, O., & Winblad, B. (1998). The relationship between cognition and daily activities in cases of mild Alzheimer's disease. *Scandinavian Journal of Occupational Therapy, 5*, 160–166.

Parenté, R., & Herrmann, D. (1996). *Retraining cognition: Techniques and applications*. Gaithersburg, MD: Aspen.

Peloquin, S. M. (1995). The fullness of empathy: Reflections and illustrations. *American Journal of Occupational Therapy, 49*, 24–31.

Peloquin, S. M. (1996). Using the arts to enhance confluent learning. *American Journal of Occupational Therapy, 50*, 148–151.

Quintard, B., Croze, P., Mazaux, J.M., Rouxel, L., Joseph, P.A,. Richer, E., et al. (2002). Satisfaction de vie et devenir psychosocial des traumatisés crâniens graves en Aquitaine. [Life satisfaction and psychosocial outcome in severe traumatic brain injuries in Aquitaine]. *Annales de Readaptation et de Medecine Physique, 45*, 456–465.

Reisberg, B. (1984). Alzheimer's disease: Stages of cognitive decline. *American Journal of Nursing, 84*, 225–228.

Reisberg, B., Ferris, S. H., De Leon, M. J., & Crook, T. (1982). The Global Deterioration Scale for assessment of primary degenerative dementia. *American Journal of Psychiatry, 139*, 1136–1139.

Roche, N. L., Fleming, J. M., & Shum, D. H. K. (2002). Self-awareness of prospective memory failure in adults with traumatic brain injury. *Brain Injury, 16*, 931–945.

Rombouts, S. A. R. B., van Swieten, J. C., Pijnenburg, Y. A. L., Goekoop, R., Barkhof, F., & Scheltens, P. (2003). Loss of frontal fMRI activation in early frontotemporal dementia compared to early AD. *Neurology, 60*, 1904–1908.

Ronch, J. L. (1996). Assessment of quality of life: Preservation of the self. *International Psychogeriatrics, 8*, 267–275.

Scott, A. D., & Dow, P. W. (1995). Traumatic brain injury. In C. A. Trombly (Ed.), *Occupational therapy for physical dysfunction* (4th ed., pp. 705–731). Baltimore: Williams & Wilkins.

Shumway-Cook, A., Patla, A., Stewart, A., Ferrucci, L., Ciol, M. A., & Guralnik, J. M. (2003). Environmental components of mobility disability in community-living older persons. *Journal of the American Geriatric Society, 51*, 393–398.

Silverman, J. M., Smith, C. J., Marin, D. B., Mohs, R. C., & Propper, C. B. (2003). Familial patterns of risk in very late-onset Alzheimer disease. *Archives of General Psychiatry, 60*, 190–197.

Taylor, M. L. (1997). What is evidence-based practice? *British Journal of Occupational Therapy, 60*, 470–473.

Teasdale, G., & Jennett, B. (1974). Assessment of coma and impaired consciousness: A practical scale. *Lancet, 2*, 81–84.

Thurman, D. J., Alverson, C., Dunn, K. A., Guerrero, J., & Sniezek, J. E. (1999). Traumatic brain injury in the United States: A public health perspective. *Journal of Head Trauma Rehabilitation, 14*, 602–615.

Toglia, J. P. (1991). Generalization of treatment: A multicontext approach to cognitive perceptual impairment in adults with brain injury. *American Journal of Occupational Therapy, 45*, 505–516.

Toglia, J., & Kirk, U. (2000). Understanding awareness deficits following brain injury. *NeuroRehabilitation, 15*, 57–70.

Wilcock, A. A. (1998). *An occupational perspective of health*. Thorofare, NJ: Slack.

Wolf-Klein, G. P. (1993). New Alzheimer's drug expands your options in symptom management. *Geriatrics, 48*(8), 26–36.

Wood, W., Abreu, B., Duval, M., & Gerber, D. (1994). Lesson 9: Occupational performance and the functional approach. In C. B. Royeen (Ed.), *AOTA self-study series: Cognitive rehabilitation*. Rockville, MD: American Occupational Therapy Association.

Zemke, R. (1995). Lesson 9: Habits: In C. B. Royeen (Ed.), *AOTA self-study series: The practice of the future: Putting occupation back into therapy*. Rockville, MD: American Occupational Therapy Association.

Zemke, R., & Clark, F. (Eds.). (1996). *Occupational science: The evolving discipline*. Philadelphia: F. A. Davis.

Chapter 15

Adaptive Living Strategies for People With Psychiatric Disabilities

CAROL A. HAERTLEIN, PHD, MS, BS

VIRGINIA C. STOFFEL, MS, BS

KEY TERMS

assertive community treatment

case management

clubhouse models

community support program (CSP)

dual diagnoses

empowerment models

procovery

psychoeducational approaches

serious mental illness/psychiatric disability

OBJECTIVES

Upon completion of this chapter, the reader will be able to

- Describe the impact of the major psychiatric disabilities on occupational performance;

- Identify the role of occupational therapy in achieving desirable outcomes for people with psychiatric disabilities;

- Identify useful assessments for people with psychiatric disabilities;

- Identify strategies that enable enhancement of occupational performance, including the psychoeducational approach, case management, assertive community treatment, empowerment models, psychiatric rehabilitation, and building community supports; and

- Discuss research on outcomes of intervention for people with psychiatric disabilities.

The quotation at the right reflects the hopes and dreams of dozens of people whom we serve every day. We (the authors of this chapter) are currently university professors, and the people with whom we work are university students. Their aspirations are not much different from those of the hundreds of people with psychiatric disorders with whom we have worked over the past two decades. Just as we strive to help our students reach their goals, how can we, as occupational therapists and occupational therapy assistants, support the millions of people with psychiatric disorders in their efforts to reach those same goals?

The *Occupational Therapy Practice Framework* (American Occupational Therapy Association [AOTA], 2002) provides a clear statement of the domain of concern for the profession as "engagement in occupation to support participation in context or contexts" (p. 610). This definition reflects a focus on helping people to become full participants in community life through active engagement in their meaningful occupations in the contexts of their choice. One apparent participation restriction for people with mental illness is that of stigma; that is, public perception plays a role in opening and closing doors of opportunity to people who seem to "belong" or "not belong." For occupational therapists and occupational therapy assistants to have an impact on promoting full participation in community life, they must be prepared to make changes in the environment through advocacy and public policy, through participation in antistigma campaigns, and through public information and awareness. Kathleen Crowley (2000), in her book *The Power of Procovery in Healing Mental Illness: Just Start Anywhere,* suggested that hope and the taking of practical, everyday steps toward living a productive and fulfilling life by starting *anywhere* are key elements of the "procovery" process. Creating supportive environments and addressing participation restrictions goes hand in hand with helping the client create a life beyond mental illness and rebuilding his or her dreams. This expanded focus of recovery from mental illness guides this chapter on adaptive strategies for people with psychiatric disabilities in all areas of occupation.

Occupational Therapy Role

Occupational therapists and occupational therapy assistants can provide a wide range of services for people with psychiatric disabilities (also referred to as *consumers*). Occupational therapy services are designed to address areas of occupation (activities of

> *Speaking of fantasies, I once had one: That I was one of millions of mental health clients who all lived in the communities of our choice, in our own places, with our own kitchens, our own furniture, our own bathrooms, our own food and clothing.... We shared our communities with all kinds of people...we did things together, helped each other, and laughed and cried with each other...we all had decently paying, fulfilling jobs.*
>
> Howie the Harp, 1995, p. xiii

daily living [ADL], instrumental activities of daily living [IADL], education, work, play, leisure and social participation), performance skills, performance patterns, contexts, activity demands, and client factors. Services for people with psychiatric disabilities may focus on one or more of these areas. The emphasis may be on evaluating and restoring performance patterns, modifying activity demands, or establishing the performance skills necessary to support occupational performance. The context in which the consumer participates is often overlooked, but it may be the most critical influence on successful adaptation to the demands of daily life.

Case study 15.1 illustrates how areas of occupation, performance skills and patterns, context, and activity demands all interact to affect the quality of occupational therapy services for one consumer.

This chapter focuses on adaptive strategies for people with a psychiatric disability. It emphasizes the occupational needs of people with serious mental illnesses, particularly schizophrenia, but it also reviews other conditions, such as mood disorders, personality disorders, and substance abuse. It is the authors' belief that occupational therapy intervention for people with psychiatric disabilities should be targeted to the level of occupational performance and should occur within the communities in which the consumers live.

Psychiatric Disorders

Among adults seen by occupational therapists and occupational therapy assistants for treatment related to a psychiatric disorder, the most common such disorders are schizophrenia, mood disorders, personality disorders, and substance-use disorders (Table 15.1).

Schizophrenia is a pervasive and usually chronic disorder that is diagnosed when a person shows deterioration from a previous level of function in per-

Case Study 15.1. B. T.

B. T. is a 40-year-old man with a 22-year history of mental illness, specifically chronic schizophrenia and dependent personality disorder. He had his first psychotic incident during exam week of his first semester in college. Following a hospitalization of several months, he returned to the university to continue his education. For about 3 years, he was able to live on his own and attend classes with the help of two roommates and his mother.

As the time approached to make an employment decision, and when his roommates graduated and moved away, B. T. experienced another psychotic episode and severe depression. That hospitalization was for a longer period, which was extended by his setbacks any time a trial discharge or extended home pass occurred.

The intervening years—until age 37—consisted of several hospitalizations, group home placements, and brief periods of living with his mother. Each setting seemed only to increase his dependency and his belief that he was unable to meet his most basic self-care needs.

At age 37, B. T. was admitted to a community support program (CSP), where he initially attended groups in a day treatment setting. The groups focused on learning the skills that would lead to more

independence in his daily life (e.g., personal hygiene, meal preparation, grocery shopping, financial management, and home management). Once he found an apartment, with the help of his occupational therapist, who was also his case manager, he began to do those activities independently.

An occupational therapy assistant now meets with B. T. every other week to help him with his grocery shopping. He prepares his own meal plan and shopping list prior to the trip. The therapist reports that B. T. is independent in most tasks but needs some encouragement and support to deal with difficult situations, such as the crowds at the grocery store or confronting the landlord about repairs.

B. T. credits the one-on-one feedback and the constant encouragement from his occupational therapist/case manager and other CSP staff with his ability to live on his own for the past 3 years. He says "I thought I took care of myself before, but I really didn't know how. I only knew how to get others to take care of me. With the help of my occupational therapist I now know that I can take care of myself and my apartment. I'm even budgeting my money so I can take a trip soon!"

As B. T. acquired the knowledge and skills necessary for living on his own, his self-esteem and motivation increased to the point where he was willing to engage in the necessary occupational behaviors.

sonal care, social relationships, or work and education. A wide range of characteristics may occur in schizophrenia, not all of which are found in everyone diagnosed with the condition.

Mood disorders include a wide range of conditions, from depressed mood secondary to bereavement to severe depressive and bipolar disorders. Impairment in areas of occupation vary considerably between conditions of depression and mania.

People with *personality disorders* have exaggerations of traits found in people without psychiatric disturbances, such as detached and limited emotional responses (schizoid disorder), distrust and suspiciousness (paranoid disorder), grandiosity and self-absorption (narcissistic disorder), and orderliness and perfectionism (obsessive–compulsive disorder). People with personality disorders typically have long-term behavioral patterns that are dysfunctional throughout life; the affected person learns little or nothing from life experiences. Only when the personality decompensates in the face of a crisis or the person seeks help for another psychiatric condition is the disorder typically diagnosed.

People who have histories of *substance-use disorders* often have other psychiatric diagnosis (e.g., the person with depression who drinks to avoid feelings of hopelessness) or have a situational response to a physical condition (e.g., the person who abuses prescription drugs to cope with pain and develops a physical and psychological dependence on them). Abuse is defined as recurrent use that interferes with some aspect of functioning, such as fulfilling role obligations, or use that is physically hazardous, such as driving while impaired (O'Farrell, 2001). Dependence is more severe than abuse; it interferes with most aspects of function and includes increased tolerance for the substance, unsuccessful efforts to decrease use, and possible elicitation of withdrawal symptoms upon cessation of use (O'Farrell, 2001).

Dysfunction in Occupational Performance

Occupational performance is a highly complex process that may include aspects such as the person's performance skills and patterns, physical and social

Table 15.1. Primary Psychiatric Disorders Seen by Occupational Therapists and Occupational Therapy Assistants

Disorder or Condition	Symptoms	Onset and Duration	Prognosis and Treatment
Schizophrenia	Two or more of the following for 1 month: Delusions, hallucinations, disorganized speech, disorganized or catatonic behavior, negative symptoms, social or occupational dysfunction below level achieved prior to onset.	Late adolescence or early adulthood onset with an acute episode; fluctuating remissions and exacerbations throughout life span.	Majority have chronic disability and marginal functioning; prognosis improves with late onset. Treatment includes medications, social skills training, psychoeducational approaches, family support, and community support programs.
Mood disorder: Depressive disorder	Five or more of the following for 2 weeks: Depressed mood; diminished interest in activities; weight loss or gain; insomnia or hypersomnia; psychomotor agitation or retardation; loss of energy; restlessness; irritability; feelings of worthlessness, guilt, or helplessness; poor concentration; and recurrent thoughts of death.	Onset at any age between childhood to older adult, with highest incidence for ages 25–34; one or more factors—genetic, psychological, and environmental—linked to cause; duration is dependent on the severity, with most people experiencing long periods of depression that are recurrent throughout their life span.	Recurrent episodes likely to occur throughout life span. Treatment includes psychotherapy and medications, specifically selective serotonin reuptake inhibitors (SSRIs) and monoamine oxidase inhibitors (MAOIs).
Mood disorder: Bipolar disorder	Depressive episode alternating with a distinct period of expansive, elevated, or irritable mood of 1 week duration with three or more of the following: Grandiosity, decreased need for sleep, pressured speech, flight of ideas, distractibility, increase in goal-directed activity or psychomotor agitation, excessiveness in activities with potential negative results.	Onset can occur from childhood to adulthood, with episodes of mania and depression recurring throughout one's life; most who suffer from bipolar disorder are free of symptoms between episodes (average interval of 2.5 yrs); a small percentage experience chronic constant symptoms.	Severity of symptoms determines seriousness of impact. Treatment includes medications (mood stabilizers [e.g., lithium] and anti-depressants) and psychotherapy, including cognitive/behavioral and psychoeducational approaches and family therapy.
Personality disorders	Characterized by an enduring pattern of inner experience and behavior that deviates from expectations of culture in two of the following areas: Cognition, affect, interpersonal functioning, and impulse control. The pattern is inflexible and pervasive, leading to significant impairment in social or occupational functioning.	Adolescence or early adulthood onset; patterns of behavior are stable and of long duration.	The course of the disorder is lifelong, and prognosis is unpromising due to resistance to treatment. Treatment approaches include pyschodynamic therapy, cognitive therapy, dialectical behavioral therapy, social skills training, assertiveness training, and psychoeducational approaches.
Substance-use disorders	Dependence characterized by maladaptive patterns causing significant impairment with three of the following over 12 months: Increased tolerance; withdrawal symptoms; unintended excessiveness; unsuccessful efforts to control use; excessive focus on use; changes in social, occupational, or recreational function; continued use despite knowledge of problems. Abuse characterized by one of the following over 12 months: Failure to fulfill major role obligations, recurrent use in dangerous situations, legal problems, and continued use despite knowledge of problems.	Adolescence to adulthood onset. Higher risk noted for males with less education, unmarried, separated or divorced more than once, and younger age. Duration can be lifelong, with frequent remissions and can include abuse of substances. Course and family/genetic patterns vary considerably among substances used.	Prognosis varies among substances used; prevalence drops with age; up to 35% do not improve or progressively deteriorate until death; up to 25% have stable remission via long-term abstinence or nonproblem drinking; up to 40% alternate between short-term abstinence and problem drinking. Treatment includes 12-step programs, medications, group and individual psychotherapy, and community interventions.

Note. Data from (1) *Desk Reference to the Diagnostic Criteria From DSM-IV-TR,* by American Psychiatric Association, 2000, Washington, DC: American Psychiatric Association, and (2) *Advanced Abnormal Psychology* (2nd ed.), by M. Hersen and V. B. Van Hasselt, 2001, New York: Kluwer Academic/Plenum.

context, societal norms, and other people. Doing an ADL such as bathing is associated with knowledge of hygiene, healthy behavior, and use of the supplies and equipment necessary for safe bathing; the motivation to respond to sociocultural norms of acceptable cleanliness; routines and habits that support daily hygiene; and the ability to recognize and respond to feedback from others regarding the practice of adequate bathing routines. It also requires sufficient motor coordination to manipulate faucets and shampoo bottles; strength, mobility, and balance to enter and exit the tub; sensitivity to temperature so as to regulate warmth of water; kinesthetic awareness to wash all body parts; and judgment and sequencing ability to organize bathing tasks.

A person with a psychiatric disorder is unlikely to bathe if he or she is indifferent to social and cultural expectations and feedback from others, lacks sufficient self-esteem to maintain his or her own health, lacks the sensory or neuromusculoskeletal abilities and skills to use equipment and supplies in a particular environment, or is unable to cognitively process the demands of bathing. Difficulty in carrying out ADL may increase when one has impairments in habits, routines, and interpersonal skills (e.g., seeking help) or lacks meaningful life roles.

The same parameters that influence the ability to bathe can be applied to activities across the spectrum of the areas of occupation, work, education, play, leisure, and social participation. For example, employment seeking and acquisition require knowledge of resources for job opportunities, cognitive and process functions to understand and complete job applications, information exchange and relational skills to participate in an interview, and sufficient self-knowledge to match a job opportunity with one's best interests. Participation in family life requires clear understanding of one's roles within the family; communication and interpersonal skills to convey needs, wants, and expectations; and sensitivity to and knowledge of the social context of the family.

Impairment in areas of occupation may appear as total lack of performance, partial or incomplete performance, performance that does not meet socially accepted standards, or performance that is insufficient to meet the person's needs. The impact of impaired performance in ADL and IADL may be particularly distressing for people with psychiatric disabilities because they include the very essence of survival on a daily basis and the foundation skills (acceptable personal hygiene, adequate nourishment, health management, and awareness of safety and emergency responses) needed to be successful in the occupations of work, education, leisure, and social participation.

The impairments seen in ADL and IADL of people with psychiatric disabilities are the focus of this chapter. The manifestation of impairments differs with the type of psychiatric disability.

ADL Impairments

Changes in personal care and hygiene may be among the most noticeable early symptoms for people with schizophrenia and mood disorders. They typically appear as a person moves from substance abuse to a substance dependence disorder. Dysfunction in ADL is not characteristic of people with personality disorders. When it is present, dysfunction represents not a deficit in performance skills but a symptom of the disorder (e.g., the exaggerated trait that characterizes the particular disorder, such as unkempt appearance in a person with socially isolated schizoid personality).

Early in the disease process of schizophrenia, the person may cease or change personal hygiene and grooming habits. Women may adopt inappropriate and attention-seeking uses of makeup (e.g., excessive eye shadow and liner or unusual lipstick color and application). Changes in dress are common, and the person often becomes unkempt, slovenly, or dirty. Inappropriate attire is often seen, such as clothes that are too casual or dressy for the occasion or are inappropriate for the weather—especially for people with a long history of the disease. Changes in dress sometimes occur in response to hallucinations or delusional thinking as described in case study 15.2.

A typical secondary effect of deterioration in personal hygiene and grooming is adverse responses from other people. Family and friends may react with concern or denial, but strangers almost always will respond with avoidance, contributing to the person's delusional thought processes, social withdrawal, or other symptomatic behavior. The

---

Case Study 15.2. R. F.

R. F. is a 40-year-old man diagnosed with continuous paranoid schizophrenia who always wears a long-sleeved shirt, and often a sweater or jacket too, even in hot weather. He feels he must do this to keep the panther tattooed on his forearm from biting him or from coming alive and attacking someone else.

interaction of declining hygiene and grooming and interpersonal rejection becomes a self-perpetuating, downward cycle for people with schizophrenia.

Eating habits of people with schizophrenia may deteriorate, and they may have a total disregard for good nutrition. They may start overeating at meals, eat junk food in excess, or avoid certain foods or meals secondary to delusions or hallucinations. People with early signs of the illness (occurring in late adolescence through early adulthood) may never have developed the process skills that facilitate good self-care (e.g., temporal organization and adjustment to social norms). More often, those who have had frequent or long-term hospitalizations lose performance skills (Bonder, 1995) along with motivation and interest in maintaining performance patterns of care routines, and they stop responding to external cues in the environment (e.g., time, events, and temperature).

The range of ADL dysfunction in people with mood disorders is wide, from no apparent changes to the inability to get out of bed and engage in any occupational behaviors. The deficits seen in personal hygiene and grooming care are not from loss of performance skills and patterns or actual changes in mental or physical functions; rather, they are secondary symptoms of the altered mood, and subsequent behavioral and thought disturbances. Because of the habitual nature of the performance of most ADL, however, direct intervention at the level of occupational performance not only can reestablish performance patterns but also can improve self-perceptions and encourage the actual use of performance skills as the client engages in occupations.

Altered appetite is a fairly common change in ADL for people with depression. This change may appear as decreased eating, which results in weight loss and potentially inadequate nutrition, or increased appetite secondary to agitation, resulting in weight gain. Personal hygiene, grooming, and dressing may be neglected as a result of depressed mood, loss of interest, impaired concentration, and lethargy.

In contrast, people in the manic episode of a bipolar disorder may change their dress or appearance as they act on increased goal-directed activities in the areas of work or social or sexual activities (e.g., a woman who starts engaging in sexual indiscretions wears provocative clothing, or a man who makes a sudden job switch or changes his social circle grows a beard and long hair). Changes in patterns of sleep and rest also are characteristic of a manic episode.

The ADL dysfunctions seen among people who have personality disorders involve enduring deviations from their cultural expectations and are consistent with the particular type of disorder. For example, a woman with narcissistic personality disorder may use excessive makeup and dress seductively as part of attention-seeking behavior (Bonder, 1995). The impulsivity of a person with borderline personality disorder may lead to abandonment of hygiene and eating routines as value systems fluctuate and relationships waiver.

People with substance-use disorders may exhibit ADL impairment as loss of interest in eating or lack of attention to personal hygiene, grooming, and other daily self-care as the need for the substance supersedes all other occupations. Central nervous system changes are most apparent during intoxication but may persist; if abuse continues, the changes may cause impairment in performance skills, which in turn will lead to deficits in all areas of occupation.

IADL Impairments

Because IADL are "oriented toward interacting with the environment and . . . are often complex" (AOTA, 2002, p. 620), they put considerably more demands on underlying performance skills, particularly process skills, communication and interaction skills, and performance patterns necessary for satisfactory function. Again, the manifestations of dysfunction will vary depending on the psychiatric disorder that is present.

For people with schizophrenia, especially that of a more severe and enduring nature, IADL that are particularly problematic include financial management, health management and maintenance, home management, meal preparation and cleanup, and safety procedures and emergency responses. Daily medication management is often difficult and usually has to be supervised by someone else. Reminders of appointments for medication checkups or physical health assessments also may be needed. Because of impairments in communication and interaction skills, shopping and community mobility may suffer. The tendency toward social isolation also interferes with functional communication and, consequently, getting need fulfillment at several levels. For example, even though he or she experiences hunger, someone with schizophrenia living in a group home environment may not seek information from others regarding the time of the next meal. This lack of initiative may cause him or her to miss the call or reminder for that meal. Instead of eating a meal, the person typically will find their way to the vending machine and fill up on junk food. Consequently, adequate nutritional needs go unmet.

When a person experiences a depressive disorder, IADL impairments will be most obvious for activities requiring processing and communication and interaction skills. Managing daily medications may be impaired because of lowered concentration. Appearance of clothes may suffer due to disinterest and disorganization. Care of others, financial management, meal planning and preparation, home management, and shopping—all of which require considerable energy, initiation, and organization—will become difficult, if not impossible for the person with depression to accomplish. Functional communication may be impaired as the depressed mood, loss of interest, and behavioral manifestations elicit negative reactions and avoidance responses from others. The impulsivity and excessiveness seen in a manic episode will interfere with the person's ability to attend to the complexities inherent in completing many IADL. Inability to carry out tasks related to care of others, managing one's finances or home, or abiding by safety procedures may ultimately result in the complete upheaval of daily life for someone with bipolar disorder who is experiencing either mania or depression.

For many people with personality disorders, the potential for dysfunction exists in carrying out complex IADL, particularly in money management, care of the home, and care of other people. A common feature among people with personality disorders is impaired interpersonal relationships. The IADL that require interactions with others will likely be impaired in people with personality disorders.

As people with substance-use disorders focus on obtaining substances, they may experience a loss of motivation and eventual loss of the performance patterns and skills necessary for IADL such as care of others, financial management, meal planning and preparation, home management, and shopping. The disruption they eventually experience in home life will likely alter the entire spectrum of their daily life activities and carry over into other areas of occupational performance.

Education

Participation in all "activities needed for being a student and participating in a learning environment" (AOTA, 2002, p. 620), the occupational area of education, presents unique challenges for people with psychiatric disabilities. The onset of several of the adult psychiatric disabilities occurs in late ado-

lescence and early adulthood, often disrupting educational plans and endeavors. The current literature does not report any studies on the impact of psychiatric disability specifically on educational activities, but some of the impairments in performance skills and patterns associated with the various disorders are likely to preclude the kind of planning and goal-directed activity necessary for success in educational occupations. For example, the disorganized thought processes and delusional ideation associated with schizophrenia may prevent use of the communication and interaction skills necessary to plan an academic course of study or participate in a classroom environment.

Mood disorders are characterized by disruptions in performance patterns, particularly maintenance of routines, which makes it difficult to comply with the schedule and routine of being a student. Among people with the psychiatric disabilities reviewed in this chapter, however, educational achievements are typically highest among those with mood disorders (Tse, 2002).

The impairments in process skills (e.g., use of knowledge and ability to adapt) and in relational skills (e.g., focus on self) that are characteristic of many personality disorders will likely interfere with making realistic educational plans and following through on them. Such impairments also prevent people with personality disorders from accurately judging the social norms and role expectations associated with being a student and functioning in an educational setting.

Alcohol abuse among college students often interrupts the educational plans of young adults; for a subset of that population who are especially at risk, alcohol abuse may lead to lifelong problems with substances (Larimer & Cronce, 2002). Once the habit of substance abuse is established, it dominates daily life and overrides the performance skills and patterns needed for engagement in education occupations (Moyers & Stoffel, 2001).

The presence of a psychiatric disability does not preclude a person from high levels of educational achievement, as evidenced by such accomplished people as Abraham Lincoln (lawyer and president), Virginia Woolf and Ernest Hemingway (writers), Beethoven and Schumann (composers), and John Nash (mathematician and Nobel Prize winner; NAMI, n.d.).

Work

Entering or reentering the workforce is a highly desired yet often unattainable goal for people with psychiatric disabilities (Nagle, Cook & Polatajko, 2002).

It has been reported that people with a major psychiatric disability generally do not work and thus experience a sense of uselessness and diminished meaning in life (Lloyd & Samra, 2000). A growing body of literature addresses work and employment issues for people with all types of disabilities, including the psychiatric disabilities reviewed here.

The onset of schizophrenia in late adolescence or young adulthood may disrupt early work opportunities and vocational development. If one of the most consistent predictors of vocational function for people with mental illnesses is their employment history (Lloyd & Samra, 2000; Tsang, Ng, & Chiu, 2002; Gioia & Brekke, 2003), the person with schizophrenia may be particularly disadvantaged in never having the opportunity to develop the employment-seeking and -acquisition skills or vocational performance patterns that are critical to success. A study of 20 young men and women with schizophrenia in the United States (Gioia & Brekke, 2003) found that they had greater vocational success when requesting "job accommodations" (through the Americans With Disabilities Act), such as status quo job assignments and flexibility of job hours to respond to unexpected symptoms, rather than climbing the employment ladder. The difficulty in communication and interaction skills seen in people with schizophrenia, however, may make requesting those accommodations difficult. The involvement of a suitable support system—a family member, case manager, or supported employment counselor—may be necessary for even that first step toward returning to employment. Possibly one of the most socially debilitating effects of schizophrenia—the side effects of foot tapping or pin-rolling finger motions that appear when symptoms are managed with medications (Bonder, 1995)—may bring embarrassing attention from others and entirely preclude entering and sustaining employment in the competitive job market.

People with mood disorders may have higher educational levels than what is seen in other psychiatric disabilities; consequently, they are more likely to have vocational histories and job-performance skills. Practice guidelines from New Zealand for people with bipolar disorder emphasize quick job placement (Tse, 2002) and the "place-then-train" supported employment model over the "train-then-place" approach that emphasizes protected employment options and typically low-skill level jobs. Because job histories may not match educational achievement in people with bipolar disorder, the emphasis in occupational therapy should be on maintaining a sense of hope; increased self-aware-

ness; and good fit among the client, the job, the support system, and the wider context (Tse & Walsh, 2001; Tse & Yeats, 2002).

Personality and substance-use disorders present patterns of behaviors that are not conducive to success in employment, although the patterns may be disruptive at different points in the person's life. Because personality disorders endure over a lifetime, they will affect early employment experiences and may lead to similar situations of unemployment or underemployment as with other psychiatric disabilities. Substance-use disorders in the stage of abuse may not initially cause problems in the occupational area of work. As dependence develops, job-performance skills will be compromised and role fulfillment in employment situations will become impaired.

Little attention has been paid to the context of employment for people with psychiatric disabilities. Swedish authors have described a strategy to address the problem of workforce reentry for people with psychiatric disabilities (Gahnstrom-Strandqvist, Liukko, & Tham, 2003). The "social working cooperative" provides a setting for psychiatric rehabilitation that incorporates real work activities and opportunities for social connection. Such cooperatives are based on principles of democracy, responsibility, permissiveness, and communality: "living-learning situations."

Finally, concepts such as "return to work," work hardening, work outcomes, and work disability have not been developed for people with psychiatric disabilities as much as for those with physical impairments. It has been suggested that work capacity evaluation and subsequent work-preparation and work-hardening programs be made available to people with psychiatric disabilities, given the employment issues seen with this population (Tsang et al., 2002).

Play and Leisure

Although games and leisure activities typically are used as treatment modalities for people with psychiatric disorders, the literature gives little attention to the play and leisure occupations of people with psychiatric disorders. Yet, "leisure is considered to be an important part of life for every individual. This is even more so for people with limited employment prospects and life options" (Lloyd, King, Lampe, & McDougall 2001, p. 107).

Many types of play and leisure participation require motor, process, and communication and interaction skills that become impaired with many psychiatric disabilities. For example, as a result of the side effects of medications mentioned earlier, a person with schizophrenia may be unable to engage in games requiring mobility and coordination skills. Someone in the manic phase of a bipolar disorder may have unrealistic expectations of his or her ability to succeed in competitive games. People with personality disorders may pursue play and leisure activities that minimize interaction with others, such as computer games, collecting items that can be done individually, and noncompetitive sports activities. Substance use typically is the focus of leisure participation in the stage of abuse, and it replaces other leisure and play participation as abuse becomes dependence. Unemployment or underemployment also affects play and leisure participation because it results in reduced financial resources.

The timing of the onset of several psychiatric disabilities may prevent the development of many of the play and leisure interests that adults pursue. Yet, people in a mental health rehabilitation program reported that their leisure participation was a source of intellectual stimulation, enjoyable relationships with others, and relaxation at a higher level than that reported by a population without diagnosed mental illness (Lloyd et al., 2001). For people with a dual diagnoses of a mental illness and substance-use disorder, leisure participation is complicated by the need to replace old activities associated with "using" and to change social contacts (Hodgson, Lloyd, & Schmid, 2001). Leisure participation is important for the recovery process and to prevent relapse (Hodgson & Lloyd, 2002).

Occupational Therapy Evaluation

The first consideration in evaluating a person with a psychiatric disability is deciding just what to assess: occupational performance, performance skills and patterns, the context or contexts in which occupational performance will occur, activity demands, or client factors. The *Occupational Therapy Practice Framework: Domain and Process* (AOTA, 2002) suggests that an occupational profile be conducted to ascertain the person's occupational history and experiences; gain an awareness of their typical patterns of daily living; and determine their interests, values, and needs with regard to current and future occupational goals. Once the client-identified priorities are established, specific evaluations can be selected to provide a clear picture of the client's occupational performance in selected contexts. Naturalistic observation of actual performance in the areas of occupations in which the person is currently engaged, combined with a structured interview, such as the Canadian Occupational Performance

Measure (COPM; Law, Baptiste, Carswell, McColl, Polatajko, & Pollock 1998), can help identify areas of performance or environments needing further evaluation and highlight client factors and performance skills. Use of the COPM has been recommended for use in mental health practice (Warren, 2002) to measure outcomes associated with changes in occupational competence of clients with mental health problems (Chesworth, Duffy, Hodnett, & Knight, 2002).

Evaluation of the client and his or her chosen environments is consistent with the psychiatric rehabilitation assessment process as described by Mac-Donald-Wilson, Nemec, Anthony, and Cohen (2001), who suggested that the skills and resources present and needed by the person to achieve his or her rehabilitation goal should be the focus of such an evaluation. Useful assessment instruments should be "clear, brief, environmentally specific, and skills- and/or resources-oriented" (p. 430).

The underlying client factors and performance skills affecting occupational performance may include impaired attention, memory, or thought; altered body awareness and self-concept; and lack of knowledge and judgment. These factors often can be analyzed simultaneously with occupational performance. Evaluation should begin at the level of performance; client factors, contexts, and performance skills and patterns can be considered as necessary. This perspective allows the therapist to assist someone with psychiatric disabilities to focus on what is "necessary and fulfilling" (Bonder, 1993, p. 214) to be able to engage in meaningful occupations, not on whether he or she is depressed or isolated. It may be helpful at some level of evaluation and intervention to identify the relationship between the person's social isolation and depression, but it is probably more meaningful to assist in developing financial management and communication skills so that the person can afford to eat one meal a day at the local coffee shop, and in doing so be part of an important social context and experience social participation.

Chapter 3 outlines several instruments that assess occupational performance; many of them can be used with clients with psychiatric disorders. A multitude of assessments that have been developed in the past two decades, such as observational tools, self-report checklists and questionnaires, interviews, and mixed-method assessments, are reported in the occupational therapy literature (Kielhofner, 2002). A number of assessments have been developed to measure ADL and IADL, such as the Milwaukee Evaluation of Daily Living Skills (Leonardelli, 1988) and the Kohlman Evaluation of Living Skills (Kohlman-Thomsen, 1992). Other instruments, such as the Comprehensive Occupational Therapy Evaluation (Brayman & Kirby, 1982), offer a scale upon which to record observation of occupational performance. Other tools have been developed to measure underlying cognitive deficits, such as Allen's Cognitive Level Test (Allen, 1985) and the Routine Task Inventory (Allen, 1992). Practitioners should evaluate the validity, reliability, assessment protocols, clinical applications, and other supporting information for any instrument before using it in an intervention setting.

Other dimensions of participation that might influence engagement in meaningful occupations for people with psychiatric disabilities include life roles, use of time, and perceived quality of life. Instruments useful for assessing function in these areas include the Role Checklist (Oakley, Kielhofner, Barris, & Reichler, 1986), the Occupational Questionnaire (Smith, 1993), and the Wisconsin Quality of Life Index (Becker, Diamond, & Sainfort, 1993). The Wisconsin Quality of Life Index includes items related to housing, neighborhood, access to transportation, physical health status, money, and personal safety. These dimensions of daily life may affect the ability to satisfy self-care needs and should be considered when working with consumers with psychiatric disorders.

Adaptive Strategies for Occupational Performance

Helping clients with psychiatric disabilities develop strategies to manage ADL, IADL, work, education, and the other areas of occupation can take many forms, including psychoeducational approaches, case management, assertive community treatment (ACT), psychiatric rehabilitation, empowerment models, and community supports. Most of the programs found in the occupational therapy literature use an academic or educational model to address ADL and IADL for people with psychiatric disabilities (Eaton, 2002; Fike, 1990; Friedlob, Janis, & Deets-Aron, 1986; Neistadt & Cohn, 1990; Remien & Christopher, 1996; Ziv, 2000). Psychoeducational (PE) models are found outside the occupational therapy literature and often are described in connection with the strategies mentioned earlier.

PE Models

The notion that one can use educational approaches to change occupational performance in ADL and IADL and to change the habits and routines of

clients is grounded in the belief that therapy is learning. This concept is not new; references to teaching and learning in therapy have appeared in the occupational therapy literature since the 1960s (Box 15.1).

Behavioral Approaches

Behavioral approaches consist of cause–effect associations, shaping, reinforcement, behavior modification, habituation, and sensitization and are most effective for people with psychiatric disabilities who also have the following characteristics:

- Their cognitive abilities are impaired by psychoses (e.g., acute schizophrenia, severe depression).
- They have normal attention span and memory abilities (e.g., personality disorders).
- They are in situations in which the environment is unchanging and responses require little or no judgment in determining what to do (e.g., people living in group homes).

Cognitive Approaches

Cognitive approaches focus on teaching how learning occurs, transferring learning, role playing, re-

---

Box 15.1. Strategies and Characteristics of PE Approach

Specific strategies common to PE programs:

- Verbal, written, visual, and experiential learning in various areas of daily living, including technology-based learning
- Community outings to relate learning to real-life experiences and apply the new skills to the real environment
- Role-playing, rehearsal, and education games.

Characteristics suggested for a consumer's successful involvement in a PE program:

- The consumer is able to learn.
- Enrollment in the program is voluntary.
- Participants in the program are seen as students and instructors, not clients and staff.
- Students set their own goals for learning.
- Involvement in the program is time limited so as to impart a sense of urgency for acquiring skills or knowledge.
- Students bear some financial cost (Bakker & Armstrong, 1976; Lillie & Armstrong, 1982).

hearsal, imagery, and memory enhancement techniques and are best used in the following circumstances:

- The client must learn to do situational problem solving (e.g., select appropriate clothing for weather conditions).
- The client has deficits in attention span, memory, or other cognitive abilities (e.g., a person with central nervous system damage such as someone with a long history of substance use).
- The skills being learned need to be generalized or transferred to other situations (e.g., using acceptable eating behaviors in a restaurant).

Case study 15.3 demonstrates how behavioral and cognitive approaches may be combined when helping a client develop socially acceptable standards of personal hygiene.

When implementing the PE approach, it is important to take the "mystique" out of learning; that is, it is important to tell learners that behavior patterns are learned, that everyone goes through essentially the same learning process, and that behavior can be acquired or changed. As Lamb (1976) stated when describing a psychoeducational model for people with long-term psychiatric disorders, it is crucial to help consumers "realize that the basic skills of everyday living are learned skills" (p. 877). The key principle to success is consumer involvement: in establishing the goals for learning, in establishing curriculum, and in taking some responsibility for its implementation. Another key factor is conducting the program away from the site of mental health treatment, if possible. By doing so, the consumer can acquire "a new identity, that of student, and feels he can participate in activities outside of mental health centers just like other people in the community. That, plus the information imparted to him in the course, helps the student move beyond the mental health system" (Lamb, p. 877).

The adoption of PE strategies into occupational therapy services for people with psychiatric disabilities is also described by Crist (1986); Jacobs, Selby, and Madsen (1996); Kielhofner and Brinson (1989); Neistadt and Marques (1984); and Weissenberg and Giladi (1989). For the most part, these programs emphasize complex IADL, work, and education tasks needed in acute and community settings with adults, families, and older adults.

Case Management

Case management has been described as a "service which assists clients in negotiating for services that they both need and want" (Cohen & Nemec, 1988,

---

Case Study 15.3. T. R.

The format of an ADL skills group at a community day treatment setting is open ended and addresses the needs of clients as determined by group members on a day-to-day basis. All consumers in the treatment program attend the ADL group. Consequently, the group's focus varies depending on whose issues are being dealt with on a given day. Group members assume a supportive peer role and give feedback to each other about how to accomplish their goals. For some consumers, the goal is to learn how to plan and cook a nutritious meal. For others it may be to learn how to shop in a grocery store and make appropriate, cost-effective purchase decisions. Still others need feedback on a more basic level.

T. R. joined the program and initially remained a quiet, background participant in most of the activities. Some of the staff and consumers had difficulty approaching T. R. because of his obvious body odor and disheveled appearance. In the context of the ADL group, his peers were able to share with T. R. the effect he had on others and how that was keeping people from approaching and getting to know him. The group used role-playing and rehearsal (i.e., cognitive techniques) to help T. R. improve his personal hygiene and learn how to use the machines at the laundromat. A group shopping trip helped him begin to overcome his anxiety about being in crowds and having a store clerk approach him. After a few weeks he was attending the group in clean clothes and had a more pleasing odor, because he had begun to use the aftershave a fellow group member had given to him as a present (i.e., reinforcement, a behavioral technique).

---

p. 27). Descriptions of case management also may emphasize coordination and allocation of services with limited resources, as is more common with European-based models (Ziguras, Stuart, & Jackson, 2002). An extensive body of literature describes case management approaches and strategies to assist people with psychiatric disabilities. Recent literature describes variations of earlier case management concepts to include strengths-based case management (Brun & Rapp, 2001), intensive case management (Kuno, Rothbard, & Sands, 1999), and the continuous treatment team model (Johnsen, Samberg, Caslyn, Blasinsky, Landow, & Goldman, 1999). One study reported that consumers involved in intensive case management over a 2-year period had fewer emergency visits and increased social networks and that families had experienced a reduced burden of care (Aberg-Wistedt, Cressell, Lidberg, Liljenberg, & Osby, 1995).

Although variations in case management exist, all the models for the most part, have the following characteristics in common: Establishing a close relationship with the consumer; working with the consumer in his or her own environment; assessing skills and training in areas such as self-care, symptom management, money management and so forth; linking consumers to preferred service providers; and advocating for service improvement (Cohen, Nemec, Farkas, & Forbess, 1988). Services may be provided by teams or individuals.

Hodges and Gesler (1997) have developed case management practice guidelines and identified three levels of intensity for case managers, which are based on the needs of the client. Levels I and II case management involve having the case manager teach independent living skills in the client's natural environment; Level III services are primarily directed toward finding the community resources matched to the client's needs.

Occupational therapists and occupational therapy assistants are well suited to the case management of people with psychiatric disabilities. The occupations of ADL, IADL, education, work, and play or leisure are the centerpiece of the occupational therapist's knowledge base. In addition, the occupational therapist's knowledge of activity analysis, therapeutic use of self, the importance of meaningful occupation, and interdisciplinary team approaches provide a solid foundation for the case manager role.

Assertive Community Treatment (ACT)

The Assertive Community Treatment program was developed by Leonard Stein, Mary Ann Test, and Arnold Marx in the early 1970s at Mendota Mental Health Institute in Madison, Wisconsin (Stein & Santos, 1998). This comprehensive, multidisciplinary program offers full-support case management services in the community with a team of staff whose expertise informs group decision making. By working with the community and families as a collaborative process, the model ACT program has had powerful outcomes that demonstrate success in community living and working (summarized in Stein and Santos, 1998). ACT programs have been reviewed and studied extensively in the United States (Becker, Meisler, Stormer, & Brondino, 1999; McGrew, Pescosolido, & Wright, 2003; McGrew, Wilson & Bond, 2002), Canada (Dewa et al., 2003;

Krupa, McLean, Estabrook, Bonham, & Baksh, 2003; Neale & Rosenheck, 2000; Prince & Prince, 2002; Schaedle, McGrew, Bond, & Epstein, 2002), and Europe (Falk & Allebeck, 2002; Ford et al., 2001; Gournay, 1999). The approach is generally accepted as having "shaped the delivery of mental health care over the past 25 years" (Dixon, 2000, p. 759).

Occupational therapy can offer the ACT team concrete expertise in ADL and IADL assessment and training. The typical ACT assessment includes an ADL and IADL assessment that covers food and nutrition skills, maintenance and housekeeping skills, personal hygiene and grooming skills, mobility skills, recreation and leisure skills, social skills, communication skills, interpersonal relationships, money management and banking skills, time management, problem-solving and decision-making skills, and safety skills (Stein & Santos, 1998). Occupational therapists are skilled in assessing the client's capacity for independent living as well as the context needed to support the client's optimal function. Pitts (2001); Auerbach (2002); and Krupa, Radloff-Gabriel, Whippey, and Kirsh (2002) all wrote about the contributions of occupational therapy to ACT programs and agree that the focus on occupations and enhancing community adjustment and quality of life are consistent with desired occupational therapy intervention outcomes for people with psychiatric disabilities.

Personal Assistance in Community Existence

Empowerment models for people with psychiatric disabilities, sometimes referred to as *consumer/ survivor models,* give consumers considerable control over services; in fact, consumers may actually provide services (Ahern & Fisher, 1999; Chinman, Rosenheck, Lam, & Davidson, 2000; Liberman & Kopelowicz, 2002; Spaniol & Koehler, 1994). The Personal Assistance in Community Existence (PACE) philosophy is based on five elements of recovery: relationships, beliefs, self/identify, community, and skills (Ahern & Fisher, 2001). Laurie Ahern, a successful journalist, and Daniel Fisher, a biochemist and psychiatrist, are survivors of mental illness and nationally known writers and speakers on recovery for people who have been labeled with a mental illness. The PACE philosophy that they promote incorporates the fact that people do fully recover from even the most serious mental illnesses and must do so at their own pace. In addition consumers must

- Believe they will recover,
- Have someone who believes in them and also believes they will recover,

- Have economic support and a social identity,
- Have a positive sense of self,
- Be a part of a "collective voice" for security and identity, and
- Acquire self-management and self-help skills.

Other premises of consumer-driven models include the belief that mental illness is caused by severe emotional distress and loss of social roles, rather than a permanent brain disorder, and that the most important relationships are with peers and those who provide encouragement and support, not with mental health professionals. These approaches and beliefs are consistent with interventions and beliefs about serious mental illness in nonindustrial societies, the Vermont Longitudinal Study, and the Soteria Project, as discussed earlier.

Psychiatric Rehabilitation

The literature on psychiatric rehabilitation has become rich with principles and outcomes supporting people with psychiatric disabilities living full lives in their community of choice. The emphasis on rehabilitation over treatment focuses on improved functioning and life satisfaction; present and needed skills and supports; teaching skills; and coordinating and modifying resources instead of focusing on "cure," symptomology, and medications (Anthony, Cohen, Farkas, & Gagne, 2002).

Occupational therapy practitioners are one of several types of professionals who contribute to the rehabilitation process. Tse and Walsh (2001) reflected on the importance of hope in vocational recovery for people with bipolar affective disorder. Brown (2001) suggested that sensory processing self-awareness may help people with mental illness find environments that facilitate optimum occupational functioning.

The basic principles of psychiatric rehabilitation include a focus on improving capabilities and competencies; enhancing the consumer's environmental supports; eclectically using techniques; improving vocational, residential, and educational outcomes; instilling hope; and actively involving the client in the rehabilitation process (Anthony et al., 2002). The State of Wisconsin's Blue Ribbon Commission on Mental Health (1997) applied these principles to its reorganization of the state mental health program and has advocated shifting the paradigm of care from treatment to rehabilitation to recovery. In this vision of recovery, the client attains a productive and fulfilling life regardless of mental illness. Occupational therapists and occupational therapy assistants can help the client build mean-ingful life roles leading to full, active participation in his or her community of choice.

Clubhouse Models

Consistent with a psychiatric rehabilitation model is the clubhouse model of psychosocial rehabilitation, often referred to as the Fountain House Model. The model is based on the New York City institution of the same name established in 1948, where people with serious mental illness joined together to support one another as they adjusted to community living and helped one another find jobs (Fountain House, n.d.). The International Center for Clubhouse Development (ICCD) lists in its 2002 International Directory (available at http://www.iccd.org/NewDirectory.asp) clubhouse programs in 24 countries and more than 170 sites in the United States. The ICCD has established standards and sponsors training and accreditation programs. Clubhouse staff and members work side by side and operate as generalists to meet the needs and interests of the members (Dougherty, 1994). Occupational therapy practitioners are well suited to contribute to clubhouse programs, given the good fit between the domain of the occupational therapy profession (i.e., "engagement in occupation to support participation in context or contexts" [AOTA, 2002, p. 610]) and the following description of what a clubhouse is from the International Center for Clubhouse Development Web site:

> A Clubhouse is a place where people who have had mental illness come to rebuild their lives. The participants are called members, not patients and the focus is on their strengths not their illness. Work in the clubhouse, whether it is clerical, data input, meal preparation or reaching out to their fellow members, provides the core healing process. Every opportunity provided is the result of the efforts of the members and small staff, who work side by side, in a unique partnership. One of the most important steps members take toward greater independence is transitional employment, where they work in the community at real jobs. Members also receive help in securing housing, advancing their education, obtaining good psychiatric and medical care and maintaining government benefits. Membership is for life so members have all the time they need to secure their new life in the community. (see http://www.iccd.org/article.asp?articleID53)

Occupational therapists and occupational therapy assistants are employed at a number of clubhouses throughout the United States.

Community Supports

The integration of people with psychiatric disabilities into the community is a challenge to all people with an interest in community mental health. This group should include consumers, family members, mental health professionals, policymakers, housing professionals, and employers. Paul Carling (1995) and his colleagues at the Center for Community Change have identified several principles that underlie successful integration. Almost 30 years ago, they called for a radical shift in thinking about needs of people with psychiatric disabilities and how they are served. Note that these principles are particularly consistent with those of a client-centered approach in occupational therapy as described by Law (1998). The principles proposed by Carling (1995) and supported by Bonder (1995) may be summarized as follows:

- All people, regardless of any differences, belong in a community.
- People with differences can be integrated into typical neighborhoods, work situations, and community social situations.
- Support is necessary for *all* people and their families (not just those who are "different") and should be offered in regular places in the community.
- Relationships between people with and without labels are crucial; each group has much to teach the other.
- Service users and their families should be involved in the design, operation, and monitoring of all services and should have the power to hold services accountable.
- Success in housing, work, and social relationships is primarily a function of whether a person has the skills and supports that are relevant to that environment or relationship.
- People's needs and relationships change over time; services and supports should be available at various levels of support for as long as a person needs them. (Bonder, 1995)

Issues that must be addressed in communities for full participation of people with psychiatric disabilities include access to and support in housing, employment, education, health and dental care, and resocialization. Occupational therapists and occupational therapy assistants are well suited to address those needs as stated above for mental health con-

sumers. They must position themselves in community agencies, work to establish informal networks for clients, and empower consumers to help themselves.

Intervention Outcomes for People With Psychiatric Disabilities

Occupational therapy outcomes for people with psychiatric disabilities should focus on enhanced occupational performance and role competence, improved adaptation in response to occupational challenge, health and wellness, and satisfactory quality of life (AOTA, 2002).

It has long been known that treatment outcomes for people with serious mental illnesses, particularly schizophrenia, in nonindustrial nations (e.g., Sri Lanka, Nigeria, and India) are superior to those in industrial nations (e.g., Denmark, United Kingdom, United States; Waxler, 1979). The Vermont Longitudinal Study and the Soteria Project (Mosher, 1999) found similar results in the United States as those in nonindustrial nations for people with schizophrenia (Harding, Brooks, Ashikaga, Strauss, & Breier, 1987; DeSisto, Harding, Mc-Cormick, Ashikaga, & Brooks, 1995). The common features of successful intervention approaches are a deemphasis of psychotropic medications; limited inpatient hospitalization (if any); and quick return to the community, which may be the family, the village, or town or, in the case of Soteria House, a supportive, protective residential environment. The approach allows the ill person to resume his or her usual work, IADL, and social occupations and routines as soon as possible. The research makes a compelling case for the resumption of meaningful occupations and occupational roles as soon as possible for anyone diagnosed with a serious mental illness or experiencing a relapse of symptoms.

Several authors have described positive relationships between engagement in occupation, recovery from mental illness, and the desired outcomes of occupational therapy interventions as noted earlier. A study in Montreal confirmed that "perceived competence in daily tasks and rest, and pleasure in work and rest activities are positively correlated with subjective quality of life" (Aubin, Hachey, & Mercier, 1999, p. 53). Another Canadian study found that activities that bring enjoyment to people with serious mental illness also were associated with excitement, a sense of accomplishment, relaxation, social connectedness, and interest, demonstrating a relationship between health and wellness and engagement in occupations (Emerson, Cook, Polatajko, & Segal, 1998).

Likewise, in Sweden it was found that characteristics of meaningful occupations were closely related to support for "living a life approaching normality, and . . . creating a natural arena of social interaction . . . and a sense of well-being" (Hvalsoe & Josephsson, 2003, p. 61). Kelly, McKenna, Parahoo, and Dusoir (2001) studied people with serious mental illness in Northern Ireland and also found a positive correlation between involvement in activities and self-reported quality of life. People with serious mental illness in England reported that the opportunity to engage in occupation at a workshop and a drop-in center was empowering and gave them a sense of purpose and a reason to stay healthy (Mee & Sumison, 2001).

The study of the influence of occupation and its meaning on desired occupational therapy outcomes for people with severe psychiatric disabilities is in its infancy and is currently most active outside the United States. The research to date offers encouraging and compelling evidence that engagement in occupations greatly benefits people whose lives have been disrupted by mental illness.

Study Questions

1. What are the symptoms, onset, duration, prognosis, and treatment of the major psychiatric disabilities?
2. Compare and contrast impairment in occupational performance among people with different types of psychiatric disabilities.
3. What are the desired outcomes of occupational therapy for people with psychiatric disabilities, and what is the role of occupation in achieving them?
4. What are the differences between the PACT and PACE approaches to recovery for people with psychiatric disabilities?
5. Identify how an occupational therapist's professional preparation matches the kinds of programs and focus that a clubhouse program offers.
6. Describe the principles for integrating people with psychiatric disabilities within the community.

References

Aberg-Wistedt, A., Cressell, T., Lidberg, Y., Liljenberg, B., & Osby, U. (1995). Two-year outcome of team-based intensive case management for patients with schizophrenia. *Psychiatric Services, 46,* 1263–1266.

Ahern, L., & Fisher, D. (1999). *Personal assistance in community existence: Recovery at your own PACE.* Lawrence, MA: National Empowerment Center, Inc. Available from www.power2u.org.

Ahern, L., & Fisher, D. (2001, December). An alternative to PACT: Recovery at your own PACE. *Mental Health Special Interest Section Quarterly, 24,* 3–4.

Allen, C. K. (1985). *Occupational therapy for psychiatric diseases: Measurement and management of cognitive disabilities.* Boston: Little, Brown.

Allen, C. K. (1992). Routine Task Inventory (RTI-2). In C. K. Allen, C. A. Earhart, & T. Blue (Eds.), *Occupational therapy treatment goals for the physically and cognitively disabled* (pp. 54–68). Rockville, MD: American Occupational Therapy Association.

American Occupational Therapy Association. (2002). Occupational therapy practice framework: Domain and process. *American Journal of Occupational Therapy, 56,* 609–639.

Aubin, G., Hachey, R., & Mercier, C. (1999). Meaning of daily activities and subjective quality of life in people with severe mental illness. *Scandinavian Journal of Occupational Therapy, 6,* 53–62.

Auerbach, E. (2002). An occupational therapist in an assertive community treatment program. *Mental Health Special Interest Section Quarterly, 25*(1), 1–2.

Bakker, C. B., & Armstrong, H. E. (1976). The adult development program: An educational approach to the delivery of mental health services. *Hospital & Community Psychiatry, 27,* 330–334.

Becker, M., Diamond, R., & Sainfort, F. (1993). A new patient focused index for measuring quality of life in persons with severe and persistent mental illness. *Quality of Life Research, 2,* 239–251.

Becker, R. E., Meisler, N., Stormer, G., & Brondino, M. J. (1999). Employment outcomes for clients with severe mental illness in a PACT model replication. *Psychiatric Services, 50,* 104–106.

Bonder, B. (1993). Issues in assessment of psychosocial components of function. *American Journal of Occupational Therapy, 47,* 211–216.

Bonder, B. (1995). *Psychopathology and function* (2nd ed.). Thorofare, NJ: Slack.

Brayman, S., & Kirby, T. (1982). The comprehensive occupational therapy evaluation. In B. J. Hemphill (Ed.), *The evaluation process in psychiatric occupational therapy* (pp. 221–226). Thorofare, NJ: Slack.

Brown, C. (2001). What is the best environment for me? A sensory processing perspective. *Occupational Therapy in Mental Health, 17*(3/4), 115–126.

Brun, C. & Rapp, R. C. (2001). Strengths-based case management: Individuals' perspectives on strengths and the case manager relationship. *Social Work, 46,* 278–288.

Carling, P. J. (1995). *Return to community: Building support systems for people with psychiatric disabilities.* New York: Guilford.

Chesworth, C., Duffy, R., Hodnett, J., & Knight, A. (2002). Measuring clinical effectiveness in mental health: Is the Canadian Occupational Performance an appropriate measure? *British Journal of Occupational Therapy, 65,* 30–34.

Chinman, M. J., Rosenheck, R., Lam, J. A., & Davidson, L. (2000). Comparing consumer and nonconsumer case management services for homeless persons with serious mental illness. *Journal of Nervous and Mental Disease, 188,* 446–453.

Cohen, M., & Nemec, P. (1988). Trainer orientation. In M. Cohen, P. Nemec, & M. Farkas (Eds.), *Case management training technology.* Boston: Boston University; Center for Psychiatric Rehabilitation.

Cohen, M., Nemec, P., Farkas, M. & Forbess, R. (1988). Training module: Introduction. In M. Cohen, P. Nemec, & M. Farkas (Eds.), *Case management training technology.* Boston: Boston University, Center for Psychiatric Rehabilitation.

Crist, P. H. (1986). Community living skills: A psychoeducational community-based program. *Occupational Therapy in Mental Health, 6*(2), 51–64.

Crowley, K. (2000). *The power of procovery in healing mental illness: Just start anywhere.* Los Angeles: Kennedy Carlisle.

DeSisto, M. J., Harding, C. M., McCormick, R. V., Ashikaga, T., & Brooks, G. W. (1995). The Maine and Vermont three-decade studies of serious mental illness, I: Matched comparison of cross-sectional outcomes. *British Journal of Psychiatry, 167*, 331–342.

Dewa, C. S., Horgan, S., McIntyre, D., Robinson, G., Krupa, T., & Estabrook, S. (2003). Direct and indirect time inputs and assertive community treatment. *Community Mental Health Journal, 39*, 17–32.

Dixon, L. (2000). Assertive community treatment: Twenty-five years of gold. *Psychiatric Services, 51*, 759–765.

Eaton, P. (2002). Psychoeducation in acute mental health settings: Is there a role for occupational therapists? *British Journal of Occupational Therapy, 65*, 321–326.

Emerson, H. A., Cook, J., Polatajko, H., & Segal, R. (1998). Enjoyment experiences as described by persons with schizophrenia: A qualitative study. *Canadian Journal of Occupational Therapy, 65*, 183–192.

Falk, K., & Allebeck, P. (2002). Implementing assertive community care for patients with schizophrenia. *Scandinavian Journal of Caring Sciences, 16*, 280–286.

Fike, M. L. (1990). Considerations and techniques in the treatment of multiple personality disorder. *American Journal of Occupational Therapy, 44*, 984–990.

Ford, R., Barnes, A., Davies, R., Chalmers, C., Hardy, P., & Muijen, M. (2001). Maintaining contact with people with severe mental illness: 5-year follow-up of assertive outreach. *Social Psychiatry and Psychiatric Epidemiology, 36*, 444–447.

Friedlob, S. A., Janis, G. A., & Deets-Aron, C. (1986). A hospital-connected halfway house program for individuals with long-term neuropsychiatric disabilities. *American Journal of Occupational Therapy, 40*, 271–277.

Gahnstrom-Strandqvist, K., Liukko, A., & Tham, K. (2003). The meaning of the working cooperative for persons with long-term mental illness: A phenomenological study. *American Journal of Occupational Therapy, 57*, 262–271.

Gioia, D., & Brekke, J. S. (2003). Use of the Americans With Disabilities Act by young adults with schizophrenia. *Psychiatric Services, 54*, 302–304.

Gournay, K. (1999). Assertive community treatment—Why isn't it working? *Journal of Mental Health, 8*, 427–429.

Harding, C. M., Brooks, G. W., Ashikaga, T., Strauss, J. S., & Breier, A. (1987). The Vermont Longitudinal Study of persons with severe mental illness, I: Methodology, study sample, and overall status 32 years later. *American Journal of Psychiatry, 144*, 718–726.

Hodge, L., & Giesler, L. (1997). *Case management practice guidelines for adults with severe and persistent mental illness.* Ocean Ridge, FL: National Association of Case Management.

Hodgson, S., & Lloyd, C. (2002). Leisure as a relapse prevention strategy. *British Journal of Therapy and Rehabilitation, 9*, 86–91.

Hodgson, S., Lloyd, C., & Schmid, T. (2001). The leisure participation of clients with a dual diagnosis. *British Journal of Occupational Therapy, 64*, 487–492.

Howie the Harp. (1995). Preface. In P. J. Carling, *Return to community: Building support systems for people with psychiatric disabilities* (pp. xiii–xvii). New York: Guilford.

Hvalsoe, B., & Josephsson, S. (2003). Characteristics of meaningful occupations from the perspectives of mentally ill people. *Scandinavian Journal of Occupational Therapy, 10*, 61–71.

Jacobs, B. L, Selby, S., & Madsen, M. K. (1996). Supporting academic success: A model for supported education in a university environment. *Occupational Therapy in Health Care, 10*(2), 3–13.

Johnsen, M., Samberg, L., Caslyn, R., Blasinsky, M., Landow, W., & Goldman, H. (1999). Case management models for persons who are homeless and mentally ill: The ACCESS demonstration project. *Community Mental Health Journal, 35*, 325–346.

Kelly, S., McKenna, H., Parahoo, K., & Dusoir, A. (2001). The relationship between involvement in activities and quality of life for people with severe and enduring mental illness. *Journal of Psychiatric and Mental Health Nursing, 8*, 139–146.

Kielhofner, G. (2002). *A model of human occupation: Theory and application* (3rd ed.). Baltimore, MD: Lippincott Williams & Wilkins.

Kielhofner, G., & Brinson, M. (1989). Development and evaluation of an aftercare program for young chronic psychiatrically disabled adults. *Occupational Therapy in Mental Health, 9*(2), 1–25.

Kohlman-Thomsen, L. (1992). *The Kohlman evaluation of living skills.* Rockville, MD: American Occupational Therapy Association.

Krupa, T., McLean, H., Estabrook, S., Bonham, A., & Baksh, L. (2003). Daily time use as a measure of community adjustment for persons served by assertive community treatment teams. *American Journal of Occupational Therapy, 57*, 558–565.

Krupa, T., Radloff-Gabriel, D., Whippey, E., & Kirsch, B. (2002). Reflections on. . .occupational therapy and assertive community treatment. *Canadian Journal of Occupational Therapy, 69*, 153–157.

Kuno, E., Rothbard, A. B., & Sands, R. G. (1999). Service components of case management which reduce inpatient care use for persons with serious mental illness. *Community Mental Health Journal, 35*, 153–167.

Lamb, H. R. (1976). An educational model for teaching skills to long-term patients. *Hospital & Community Psychiatry, 27*, 875–877.

Larimer, M. E., & Cronce, J. M. (2002). Identification, prevention and treatment: A review of individual-focused strategies to reduce problematic alcohol consumption by college students. *Journal of Studies on Alcohol Supplement* (14), 148–163.

Law, M. (Ed.). (1998). *Client-centered occupational therapy.* Thorofare, NJ: Slack.

Law, M., Baptiste, S., Carswell, A., McColl, A., Polatajko, H., & Pollock, N. (1998). *Canadian Occupational Performance Measure* (3rd ed.). CAOT Publications ACE.

Leonardelli, C. (1988). *The Milwaukee Evaluation of Daily Living Skills: Evaluation in long term psychiatry.* (Available from the author: C. Haertlein, Department of Occupational Therapy, University of Wisconsin-

Milwaukee, P.O. Box 413, Milwaukee, WI 53201 or chaert@uwm.edu)

Liberman, R. P., & Kopelowicz, A. (2002). Teaching persons with severe mental disabilities to be their own case managers. *Psychiatric Services, 53,* 1377–1379.

Lillie, M. D., & Armstrong, H. E. (1982). Contributions to the development of psychoeducational approaches to mental health service. *American Journal of Occupational Therapy, 36,* 438–443.

Lloyd, C., King, R., Lampe, J., & McDougall, S. (2001). The leisure satisfaction of people with psychiatric disabilities. *Psychiatric Rehabilitation Journal, 25,* 107–113.

Lloyd, C., & Samra, P. (2000). OT and work-related programmes for people with a mental illness. *British Journal of Therapy and Rehabilitation, 7,* 254–261.

MacDonald-Wilson, K. L., Nemec, P. B., Anthony, W. A., & Cohen, M. R. (2001). Assessment in psychiatric rehabilitation. In B. F. Bolton (Ed.), *Handbook of measurement and evaluation in rehabilitation* (3rd ed., pp. 424–445). Gaithersburg, MD: Aspen.

McGrew, J. H., Pescosolido, B., & Wright, E. (2003). Case managers' perspectives on critical ingredients of assertive community treatment and on its implementation. *Psychiatric Services, 54,* 370–376.

McGrew, J. H., Wilson, R. G., & Bond, G. R. (2002). An exploratory study of what clients like least about assertive community treatment. *Psychiatric Services, 53,* 761–763.

Mee, J., & Sumison, T. (2001). Mental health clients confirm the motivating power of occupation. *British Journal of Occupational Therapy, 64,* 121–128.

Mosher, L. (1999). Soteria and other alternatives to acute psychiatric hospitalization: A personal and professional review. *Journal of Nervous and Mental Disease, 187,* 142–149.

Moyers, P. A., & Stoffel, V. C. (2001). Community-based approaches for substance use disorders. In M. Scaffa (Ed.), *Occupational therapy in community-based practice settings* (pp. 318–342). Philadelphia: F. A. Davis.

Nagle, S., Cook, J. V., & Polatajko, H. J. (2002). I'm doing as much as I can: Occupational choices of persons with severe and persistent mental illness. *Journal of Occupational Science, 9,* 72–81.

NAMI. (n.d.). *People with mental illness enrich our lives.* Retrieved November 24, 2003, from http://www.nami.org/Content/ContentGroups/Helpline1/People_with_Mental_Illness_Enrich_Our_Lives.htm.

Neale, M. S., & Rosenheck, R. A. (2000). Therapeutic limit setting in an assertive community treatment program. *Psychiatric Services, 51,* 499–505.

Neistadt, M. E., & Cohn, E. S. (1990). *An independent living skills model for Level I fieldwork.* Rockville, MD: American Occupational Therapy Association.

Neistadt, M. E., & Marques, K. (1984). An independent living skills training program. *American Journal of Occupational Therapy, 38,* 671–676.

Oakley, F., Kielhofner, G., Barris, R., & Reichler, R. K. (1986). The Role Checklist: Development and empirical assessment of reliability. *Occupational Therapy Journal of Research, 6,* 157–169.

O'Farrell, T. J. (2001). In M. Hersen & V. B Van Hasselt

(Eds.), *Advanced abnormal psychology* (2nd ed., pp. X–X). New York: Kluwer Academic/Plenum.

Pitts, D. (2001). Assertive community treatment: A brief introduction. *Mental Health Special Interest Section Quarterly, 24*(4), 1–2.

Prince, P. N., & Prince, C. R. (2002). Perceived stigma and community integration among clients of assertive community treatment. *Psychiatric Rehabilitation Journal, 25,* 323–331.

Remien, R. H., & Christopher, F. (1996). A family psychoeducation model for long term rehabilitation. *Physical & Occupational Therapy in Geriatrics, 14*(2), 45–59.

Schaedle, R., McGrew, J. H., Bond, G. R., & Epstein, I. (2002). A comparison of experts' perspective on assertive community treatment and intensive case management. *Psychiatric Services, 53,* 207–210.

Smith, N. R. (1993). *Occupational Questionnaire.* Chicago: University of Illinois, Model of Human Occupation Clearinghouse.

Spaniol, L., & Koehler, M. (1994). *The experience of recovery.* Boston: Boston University, Sargent College of Allied Health Professions, Center for Psychiatric Rehabilitation.

Stein, L. I., & Santos, A. B. (1998). *Assertive community treatment of persons with severe mental illness.* New York: Norton.

Tsang, H. W. H., Ng, B. F. L., & Chiu, F. P. F. (2002). Job profiles of people with severe mental illness: Implications for rehabilitation. *International Journal of Rehabilitation Research, 25,* 189–196.

Tse, S. (2002). Practice guidelines: Therapeutic interventions aimed at assisting people with bipolar affective disorder achieve their vocational goals. *Work, 19,* 167–179.

Tse, S. S., & Walsh, A. E. S. (2001). How does work work for people with bipolar affective disorder? *Occupational Therapy International, 8,* 210–225.

Tse, S., & Yeats, M. (2002). What helps people with bipolar affective disorder succeed in employment: A grounded theory approach. *Work, 19,* 47–62.

Warren, A. (2002). An evaluation of the Canadian Model of Occupational Performance and the Canadian Occupational Performance Measure in mental health practice. *British Journal of Occupational Therapy, 65,* 515–521.

Waxler, N. E. (1979). Is outcome for schizophrenia better in nonindustrial societies? The case of Sri Lanka. *Journal of Nervous and Mental Disease, 167,* 144–158.

Weissenberg, R., & Giladi, N. (1989). Home economics day: A program for disturbed adolescents to promote acquisition of habits and skills. *Occupational Therapy in Mental Health, 9,* 89–103.

Wisconsin Blue Ribbon Commission on Mental Health. (1997). *The Blue Ribbon Commission on Mental Health: Final report.* Madison, WI: Office of the Governor.

Ziguras, S. J., Stuart, G. W., & Jackson, A. C. (2002). Assessing the evidence on case management. *British Journal of Psychiatry, 181,* 17–21.

Ziv, N. (2000). Application of the psychoeducational therapy approach in an occupational therapy group for women with depression. *Israel Journal of Occupational Therapy, 9,* E64.

Chapter 16

Living With Vision Loss

DON GOLEMBIEWSKI, MA

DON GOLEMBIEWSKI, MA

KEY TERMS

braille

cataracts

central vision loss (CVL)

diabetic retinopathy

eccentric viewing

glaucoma

legal blindness

macular degeneration (AMD)

no light perception (NLP)

peripheral vision loss (PVL)

photophobia

self-protection techniques

severe visual impairment

sighted guide technique

Snellen chart

OBJECTIVES

Upon completion of this chapter, the reader will be able to

- Describe the challenges to occupational performance (everyday living) experienced by people with each of the major age-related eye conditions;
- Describe the functional visual impact of each of the major age-related eye conditions;
- Describe the terms used to classify the levels of vision loss;
- Describe the phases of adjustment to a severe loss of vision;
- List the factors that improve the potential for increased independence in occupational performance;
- Describe adaptive strategies, equipment, and environmental modifications for optimal performance in daily activities for people with vision loss;
- Describe the impact lighting, texture, and color contrast have on the occupational performance of people with severe visual impairments;
- Describe the importance of texture and color contrast in successful occupational performance;
- List the benefits of early service intervention for people with a severe vision loss; and
- Describe the protections of the Americans With Disabilities Act for people with vision loss.

This chapter describes the visual impairments, short of total blindness, most commonly associated with aging. It details strategies that allow people with these conditions to function with confidence and independence. Many of the strategies, tools, and approaches also apply to younger people and those who are congenitally blind, who comprise a relatively small percentage of the population who have difficulty seeing (Kirchner & Schmeidler, 1997).

A severe vision loss will negatively affect virtually all activities of daily living (ADL) of people living with low vision (Carroll, 1961; Buettner, 2002). This functional impact will be different for each person and will vary in an intensity that may not be in proportion to the severity of the loss. Thus, the information presented in this chapter only touches on the full range of adaptive strategies and aids available to this highly diverse population. The chapter focuses on modifying the environment for activity limitations in the crucial performance areas of communication, mobility ADL, leisure, and work.

Definitions of Visual Acuity

Visual acuity levels neither dictate nor necessarily limit one's ability to function; they may be used to explain performance problems. Eye care providers (i.e., ophthalmologists and optometrists) report visual acuity levels using the following designations (Corn & Koenig, 1996):

- *No light perception* (NLP) means total blindness. People with NLP are totally blind and must use a variety of compensatory sensory skills to function. Hearing, the only other long-distance sense, must be used for mobility and to gather critical information about the environment. A person with NLP should be encouraged to learn braille, a tactual means of reading and writing, and the use of assistive technology (AT) for compensatory purposes.
- *Light perception* (LP) is the ability to perceive light only. LP can be useful in determining whether household appliances or lights are on, whether it is daytime, or whether window shades are open.
- *Light projection* (L. Proj.) is the ability not only to see light but also to determine the direction of the source. L. Proj can be essential in aiding mobility and in spatial orientation.
- *Hand movement* (HM) designates the ability to see movement or gross forms, such as a doctor's hand moving in front of the patient. HM ability is useful in orientation and safe travel and in observing other environmental activity. HM is an unreliable predictor of function but is a recordable level of vision when an eye chart is not distinguishable.
- *Counts fingers* (CF) or *finger counting* (FC), often used in conjunction with "at two feet" or another distance, also is an unreliable and seldom used designation of vision. This designation is neither truly objective nor exact, but it occasionally may be seen on medical reports. People with CF may be able to see a coffee cup on their desk or read newspaper headlines.
- *Snellen notation* is the tested level of vision that coincides with each line of progressively smaller print letters a patient is able to read on a Snellen chart. The use of the Snellen eye chart with the familiar large capital "E" or "O" on the top line is the standard tool for the measurement of distance acuity. Depending on the chart, the top line with large type may measure vision of 20/400 or 20/200. As each line of type decreases in size, the acuity level increases. The bottom line on most charts represents vision of 20/15.

Legal Blindness and Severe Visual Impairment

Clinical legal blindness is defined as having vision of 20/200 or less (using the Snellen eye chart measurement) in the better eye with best spectacle-corrected visual acuity (BSCVA), or having a visual field that encompasses (or *subtends*) an angle of 20 degrees or less. The first part of this definition states how clearly one can see (i.e., acuity), and the second part states how much area of the potential visual field one sees. 20/200 means the person sees at 20 feet what someone with 20/20 (i.e., "normal" or "perfect") vision sees at 200 feet. The "normal" visual field with both eyes (i.e., *binocular* vision) will approach 180 degrees (Jose, 1983). The National Center for Health Statistics defines severe visual impairment as a self- or proxy-reported inability to read standard newsprint (Nelson & Dimitrova, 1993).

Prevalence of Severe Visual Impairment and Blindness

The American Foundation for the Blind and Lighthouse International are general sources of information on visual impairments. Their contact information can be found in Appendix 16.B.

8.3 million (3.1%) Americans of all ages self-report some degree of vision impairment, defined as blindness in one or both eyes or any other difficulty seeing (Lighthouse International, 2003).

- 7.9 million people (approximately 3% of people 6 years of age and older) have difficulty seeing ordinary newspaper print, even when wearing corrective glasses or contact lenses (Lighthouse International, 2003).
- 3.9 million people (12% among people 65 years of age and older) report the same inability to read newsprint (Lighthouse International, 2003).
- More than 3 million people have low vision (Lighthouse International, 2003).
- About 12 million people have some degree of visual impairment that cannot be corrected by glasses (Lighthouse International, 2003).
- Approximately 1.3 million people (0.5%) report themselves to the Bureau of the Census as legally blind (U. S. Bureau of the Census, 2002).
- Approximately 20% of people who are legally blind (an estimated 260,000 people) have light perception or less representing (American Foundation for the Blind, 2002).
- Approximately 3.8 million people 65 years of age and older (11%) report a severe vision impairment. As baby boomers age, that number will increase to 4.3 million in 2010, 5.9 million in 2020, and 7.7 million in 2030 (Lighthouse International, 2003).

People with serious eye conditions cannot routinely expect their vision to remain stable. For most people, vision will likely change gradually over time. For some, vision may fluctuate on a daily or even hourly basis. Ophthalmologic reports provide specific measurements of components of vision, but they often do not tell the entire story of how those components affect a person's ability to function visually.

Impaired Visual Acuity

Whereas total blindness is a condition readily comprehended, people often misunderstand visual acuity in people who are severely visually impaired (Tuttle & Tuttle, 1996). Just as everyone has different physical abilities, each person with low vision can be expected to have a unique ability to see. Approximately 80% to 85% of all people who are legally blind have some level of useful vision (Flax, Golembiewski, & McCaulley, 1993).

Therefore, most people have the ability to see something, such as large print, the shapes of houses or furniture, trees or people, the action on television, or simply light and dark, and they are able to use their sight for purposeful activities. To complicate matters, however, many people with severe vision loss have visual abilities that fluctuate unpredictably. Physical or mental fatigue, poor lighting, glare, motivation, and other factors affect the ability to see. This uncertainty and variability can make service delivery challenging.

Each major eye condition causes a somewhat typical vision loss. Age at onset of condition, duration of condition, other eye conditions, other health concerns, personal motivation, and environmental factors will affect how well and how much each person sees and how they are able to use or process what they see. Regardless of the condition, however, anyone with a severe visual impairment may experience feelings of isolation, depression, inadequacy, and self-doubt.

Common Eye Conditions

Macular degeneration, diabetic retinopathy, glaucoma, and cataracts are the leading causes of age-related vision loss in the United States (Lighthouse International, 2003, Causes of Vision Impairment). Each of these conditions is described in the following sections.

Macular Degeneration

Macular degeneration, or age-related macular degeneration (AMD), is a condition that affects the central visual acuity, primarily in people 50 years of age and older. The vision loss may begin bilaterally or in one eye and later affect the other. Major concerns of clients with AMD include the inability to read small print, drive a car, see their grandchildren's faces, set their thermostat or stove dials, or see themselves in a mirror.

Many people with AMD find that using optical aids, such as magnifiers, telescopes, and video magnifiers, or closed circuit TVs (CCTVs), enables them to read and function at a much more satisfactory level. The use of *eccentric viewing* exercises and techniques also may help people with AMD use the viable area of their visual field (Flax et al., 1993). As one turns one's eyes, the central scotoma, or blind spot, moves with the visual field. To make best use of the remaining useful portion of the visual field, the person must not look directly at the object of concern but, rather, toward their best area of the peripheral field. Eccentric viewing is a means of locating and using the area of best visual function on the retina of a person with AMD.

People with AMD or other conditions affecting central vision must learn to use side or peripheral vision in a different way. The technique is to visualize an area that can be seen as though it were the face of a large clock showing only the 12, 3, 6, and 9, then imagine a central spot or target in the middle of the clock face. To use eccentric vision, a person must do the following to discover the location of the area of best remaining vision.

1. Sit comfortably about 10 feet from a familiar static object (e.g., a picture on the wall, the refrigerator, or a bookcase).
2. Use only the better eye, and cover the eye that has less acuity.
3. Look directly at the center of the target object. If done properly, the target should seem to disappear or get blurrier because it is being lined up with the central blind spot, or *scotoma*.
4. Next look slightly above the target, or at "12 o'clock." If the target becomes clearer or easier to see, practice the exercise several times.
5. Continue looking from the center of the target to each of the other clock times. The target will appear and disappear, but when the

best acuity spot is located, the person should look to that "time" for best vision.

Even if one position works, complete the exercise to find any other areas of useful vision. It is important to remember that to see the target most clearly, one must not look directly at it. Eccentric viewing techniques will not restore vision, but they can help get the most from remaining vision.

Diabetic Retinopathy

Diabetic retinopathy is a condition that affects the retinas of some people who are diabetic. The retina, or innermost layer of the eye, receives images transmitted through the cornea and contains rods and cones, which are sensory receptors. Diabetes may cause hemorrhages or blood vessel changes that affect the retina and thus interfere with vision (Figure 16.1). The entire visual field may become involved, causing severe functional limitations often characterized by episodes of highly fluctuating vision.

It is common for a person with diabetic retinopathy to say they feel as if they have cobwebs or lint on their eyes and they want to keep brushing it off or that everything has a reddish tint. They may

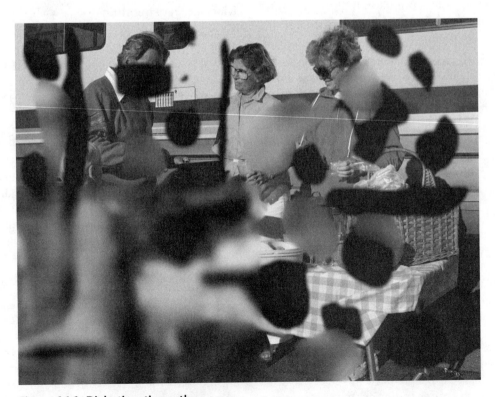

Figure 16.1. Diabetic retinopathy.

experience poor vision early in the day that improves through the morning, declines in the afternoon, and improves again late in the day. This fluctuation may be caused by blood sugar levels, the settling of vitreous debris, or the level of natural light.

People with diabetic retinopathy may need to adjust the timing of certain tasks, especially in the morning. Filling insulin syringes in advance or reading fine print may be better accomplished the night before or late morning.

A person with a recent hemorrhage may require stronger magnification, better color contrast, larger print, or the continual use of optical filters to reduce associated glare. A simple, low-cost adaptation to improve color contrast in reading material is to place a yellow acetate sheet over the printed page. The severity and location of the hemorrhage or scar tissue may require dependence on stronger magnification, computer speech output, auditory books, increased task lighting, and personal assistance to accomplish tasks.

Glaucoma

Glaucoma is another leading cause of blindness in the United States. Glaucoma is a buildup of pressure within the eye that damages the optic nerve. This increased pressure causes a decrease of vision in the peripheral field (commonly known as "tunnel vision"). As the term suggests, people with tunnel vision cannot see things on either side without turning their head. A person with glaucoma may have 20/20 vision in the central part of the visual field, but that area of vision may only be 10 degrees in size. People with glaucoma may find their reading ability relatively unchanged. Their ability to use their peripheral vision to negotiate steps, icy sidewalks, or to use their vision under dimly lit circumstances, however, is greatly diminished.

Cataracts

Cataracts are another common condition affecting the older population. A cataract is an opacity, or cloudiness, of the normally clear lens inside the eye. The lens is responsible for properly focusing light onto the retina. The aging process, disease, trauma, or other factors may result in cataracts, causing a person to have vision that is often described as "looking through a dirty windshield or a gauze curtain." The medical treatment for cataracts is surgery, most often the implantation of an artificial lens. Often people who have cataracts function well with optical aids, and they also may benefit from wearing special optical filter sunglasses (i.e., *absorptive lenses*) or broad-brimmed hats to reduce glare.

A person with cataracts will find increased problems with glare from the headlights of oncoming vehicles at night, adjusting to outside light after exiting a dark building, and at the beach or after a fresh snowfall on a sunny day. Some people use broad-brimmed hats and a variety of optical filter sunglasses for everything from sitting on the beach to washing dishes in front of a window to department store shopping under artificial lights.

Presbyopia

Presbyopia is the reduction in accommodative ability that occurs with age (Buettner, 2002). Accommodation refers to the ability of the eyes to adjust or focus. This condition, commonly beginning between the ages of 42 and 45, is characterized by the inability to focus on near objects, such as fine print in a book. Presbyopia is a normal consequence of aging and is not cause for alarm. It does cause functional complications, however, especially when combined with serious eye conditions.

Occupational Performance Consequences of Eye Conditions

For rehabilitation providers, the occupational performance consequences of eye conditions are of most concern. The following sections describe visual impairments resulting from central vision loss, loss of peripheral vision, and general vision loss.

Central Vision Loss

Central vision is often referred to as *identification* or *fine detail* vision because it is what we use to tell us at what we are looking. Central vision loss (CVL) will therefore cause a person to lose fine detail vision. CVL also affects color discrimination, which is located centrally on the retina. A simple analogy is to consider the normal circular visual field as a donut complete with donut hole. People with CVL will see the donut, but not the hole. Without the benefit of fine detail vision, the person will see better using eccentric or peripheral vision (see above). It is not unusual for a person with CVL to be unable to read newspaper headlines from inches away but able to see a fly in the corner of the ceiling or a bit of paper on the floor. Moreover, people with CVL often will complain of not being able to see photographs of grandchildren or recognize faces from across the table, but they may be able to see whether that person's shoes are shined. Figure 16.2 depicts a scene as viewed by someone with intact vision, and Figure 16.3 depicts the same scene as viewed by someone with CVL.

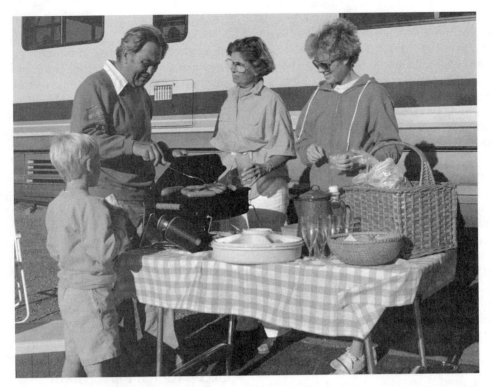

Figure 16.2. Clear or normal vision.

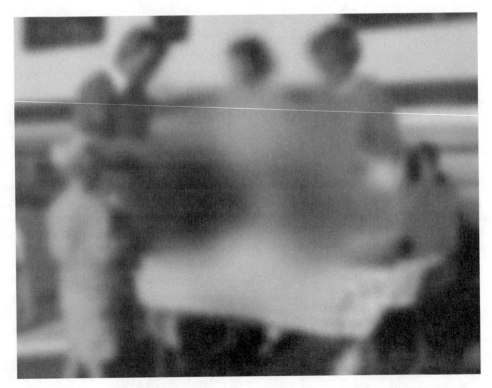

Figure 16.3. Central vision loss.

Case Study 16.1. Central Vision Loss (AMD)

R. L. is 83 and has a confirmed diagnosis of AMD. His wife is concerned about his vision and how it is limiting him. R. L. is unable to see newspaper headlines and contends that he cannot see well enough to do certain household chores. Yet, after his wife lost a sewing needle in a shag carpet and was unable to locate it, R. L. found it visually, thereby confusing his wife about his vision. Why couldn't he see well enough to help her but could find a tiny item for which she had searched at length? After the functional limitations of AMD were explained to her, she understood his inability to see fine detail while maintaining his ability to see peripherally.

Because doing dishes is a tactual job, the occupational therapist helped R. L. and his wife work out a compromise. He would do more housework, and she would be responsible for more of the visual tasks such as balancing the checkbook.

Peripheral Vision Loss

Peripheral vision loss (PVL) limits activities where peripheral or side vision is necessary. A person with PVL will have limitations with independent mobil-ity, especially in low-light situations. People with PVL have a narrow visual field and must continually scan their environment to view, in series, what people with a normal field see instantly (Figure 16.4). If an object is not immediately in the center field of vision, it appears to not exist. Often, low-lying objects such as coffee tables, steps, rugs, or uneven pavement cause serious difficulties.

Peripheral vision is sometimes referred to as "orientation vision" because we rely on it to tell us where we are in relation to objects in our environment. It also is the area of best vision in low-light environments. Many people with PVL function best when adequate task lighting, color-contrasting background, and centrally presented objectives are available.

General Vision Loss

Someone with general vision loss may experience a loss of vision in part or all of the field of vision (Figure 16.5). Cataracts or diabetic retinopathy may cause this general vision loss. Any portion of the visual field may be affected, and visual acuity will be variable.

Case Study 16.2. Central Vision Loss (AMD)

M. M. has AMD and misses seeing photographs of her grandchildren. She generally sees shapes of people sitting in front of her, but she cannot recognize them. Looking directly at someone's face, she can see rings on their fingers but cannot see whether they are wearing glasses or makeup.

One of her concerns is that her friends do not understand the impact of AMD. She can walk to the nearby grocery store and independently do her shopping with the assistance of a small, lighted magnifier, but she does not recognize or even see well enough to acknowledge friendly waves from across the street. In her neighborhood, this snub is considered serious and is not taken lightly. The occupational therapist encouraged M. M. to tell her friends about her inability to recognize people from a distance and to carry a white cane for identification purposes. She routinely offers friends a copy of a brochure on AMD she picked up from her ophthalmologist's office.

Case Study 16.3. Peripheral Vision Loss (Glaucoma)

P. T. has advanced glaucoma. He lives alone in a small home in a rural area and relies on a strong network of social supports. P. T.'s visual field is less than 10 degrees in his left eye, and he has no light perception in the right. His acuity is unknown. He is able to read some print quite slowly, usually one letter at a time when extremely bright task lighting is available. He has given up trying to walk alone outside except in bright sunlight, for which he uses sunglasses.

P. T. experienced his vision loss at least in part because he refused to follow his medication regimen. He told his occupational therapist that his uncle had glaucoma and lost all vision over a 10-year span despite taking drops to relieve the pressure. Because P. T. refused to take the proper medication, he had permanently lost his vision to glaucoma much faster.

Because optical aids are no longer an option, P. T. relies on talking books and volunteer readers and uses tactual markings for his appliances, medications, and household items. He uses a white cane for his daily walks.

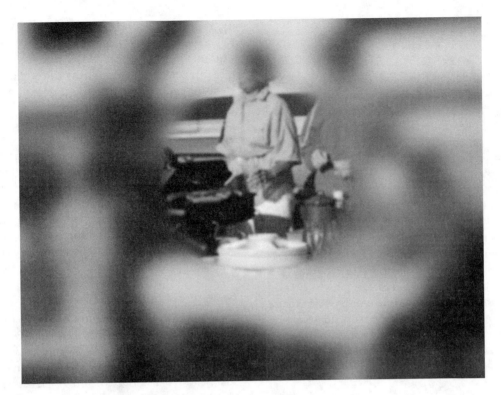

Figure 16.4. Peripheral vision loss.

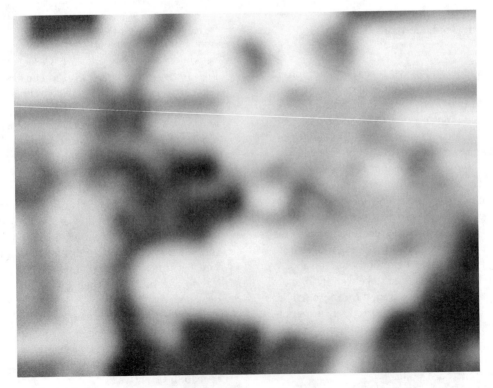

Figure 16.5. General vision loss.

Case Study 16.4. General Vision Loss (Diabetic Retinopathy)

B. A. is diabetic with greatly fluctuating vision. Her vision in the morning is cloudy, and everything appears dark. Turning on bright lights helps, but then B. A. sometimes needs to control the indoor glare by wearing optical filter sunglasses. When she reads, she tries to look around or past her numerous hemorrhages and retinal scars, which do seem to move about. By mid-morning, her vision seems to clear, so she tries to do her reading then, keeping her back to the brightest window. Later, her vision may become cloudy for a period before becoming relatively clear again during the evening hours.

Case Study 16.5. Severe Vision Loss

K. T. was despondent over his severe vision loss, which resulted in a self-imposed withdrawal from his "coffee club" group of fellow retirees at the nearby café. All were longtime friends who shared similar life experiences, sports allegiances, and sense of community connections. After K T.'s vision declined, he felt the others were being overly protective and treating him like a blind person, not as "good old K. T." For example, one friend apologized profusely after asking if everyone had seen the recent football game; the painful silence that followed made everyone uncomfortable. K. T. didn't feel they understood him at all, so he gave up his coffee group.

Eventually, K. T. heard of a support group for people with vision loss that met every month at the local senior center. Everyone was welcome, although most attendees were 70 years of age or older. No dues were collected, and the aging office provided transportation. After a few meetings that included discussions of dealing with the sighted world and living as a blind person, K. T. began to accept his vision loss and was able to better understand how he was misinterpreting his friends' comments. He resumed meeting with his coffee buddies and was able to Monday morning quarterback as he always had. He even told a joke about a dog guide for the blind that easily and permanently broke the ice.

Adjustment to Low Vision

Blindness shares much with other disabling conditions in the stages of the adjustment process. Seven phases of adjusting to life with blindness have been identified (Tuttle & Tuttle, 1996): (1) trauma, (2) shock and denial, (3) mourning and withdrawal, (4) succumbing and depression, (5) reassessment and reaffirmation, (6) coping and mobilization, and (7) self-acceptance and self-esteem.

Each person will feel the effects of blindness or low vision differently. For example, someone who has been highly active, has driven trucks for a living, or has been an outdoor enthusiast may have difficulty with a perceived need to adopt a more sedentary lifestyle. By the same token, an avid reader who develops AMD may feel much more loss than someone who has never enjoyed reading.

Social factors are an important part of adjusting to blindness. Because blindness limits ease of mobility, such as driving across town or walking to the corner coffee shop, people who have lost vision will not have the same freedom of movement they enjoyed previously. To avoid feelings of isolation, social contacts should be continued and new ones explored.

Evaluation of Occupational Performance

Because of the individualized nature of visual abilities, evaluation is necessary to help target service needs. This section describes two assessment tools. The first instrument, Assessment for Rehabilitation Teaching Services (Appendix 16.A; Golembiewski, 1998) is verbally administered to screen potential recipients of vision rehabilitation services. It is de-

signed for ease of use by professionals and nonprofessionals. The instrument assesses each functional area with three questions: (1) Can you accomplish the task? (2) If not, is it due to a vision loss? (3) Do you want assistance with the visually restricting task? Although assessments that are not performance-based have their limitations, this tool is designed to provide a simple means of identifying people who are truly appropriate for vision rehabilitation services and create a basis for formulating a plan of service.

The second assessment instrument is meant to be administered either in the client's home or in an institutional facility. This assessment, which is not standardized, identifies the need for adaptive aids and techniques that can be recommended by a person qualified to provide rehabilitation services for people with blindness or low vision. The areas of need that are identified form the basis for the individualized plan for services developed for the client.

Items included in this performance-based assessment are listed in Table 16.1.

Interventions for People With Vision Loss

Intervention options for people with vision loss can be organized according to the standard categories outlined in chapter 4: *remediation* (i.e., teaching and training), *compensation* (i.e., changing the task or environment), *disability prevention* (i.e., encouraging the performance of tasks that prevent health problems and encouraging safe task methods), and *health promotion* (i.e., encouraging engagement in meaningful, balanced, and healthy occupations and environmental interactions). This chapter focuses on compensatory strategies that permit accomplishment of ADL, including environmental modifications and specific procedures and techniques for accomplishing tasks using other sensory cues. The following sections describe compensatory strategies for lighting and color contrast changes in the environment, orientation and mobility, communication, household organization, food preparation, and personal management.

Environmental Lighting and Contrast

Proper lighting is critical to enable people with vision loss to best use residual vision (Jose, 1983). Too much, too little, or poorly directed light will hinder the ability to perform ADL (Tuttle & Tuttle, 1996.) The need for or tolerance to certain light levels is highly individual and must be assessed. Trials with various light levels are needed to establish the optimum visual environment that will improve performance and prevent fatigue.

Any work area should be illuminated with a general light source, adding focused task lighting as needed. The light source must be kept below eye level or be positioned behind or to the side of the person. Halogen standing lamps, gooseneck, or other types of flexible and portable lighting are an ideal source of extremely bright task lighting. Some lamps are available in portable models. Lampshades should be used to help eliminate glare and to direct light to the targeted work area. Improving household lighting is perhaps the least expensive but most beneficial of all adaptations that a person with visual impairments can make.

Many people use flashlights with ultrabright krypton or halogen bulbs for portable task lighting. These are useful for setting stove and laundry dials; adjusting thermostats; and seeing in dark areas of closets, drawers, or hallways.

Environmental light can be more useful if the work area is adjusted so the light streams from the

---

Case Study 16.6. Advanced Glaucoma

M. L. is 18 years old and has Down syndrome and advanced glaucoma. The visual acuity report is unreliable because of the communication limitations and questionable responses to standard tests. The special education teacher knew that people with glaucoma often find additional light to be useful. The teacher contacted the vision rehabilitation specialist for a consultation on a seemingly drastic and sudden functional decrease. When the classroom environment was reviewed, M. L.'s desk had been rotated so that he could look out of a large bank of windows facing an open area covered with snow. The teacher learned that turning the desk toward the light not only did not help but also caused severe problems with glare and photophobia. After rotating the desk so that M. L.'s back was to the windows, M. L. was able to resume visual tasks as before.

---

back or side of the task area. Rotating the task area or work surface from facing toward a window to a position facing away from a bright light source can often increase functional vision. Adjusting window shades or blinds also will minimize glare.

Photophobia is discomfort from abnormally increased sensitivity to bright sunlight or reflected light from water, snow, or even highly polished floors (Duffy, 2002). Some people with extreme photophobia experience discomfort even indoors, and especially from natural light on overcast days.

If glare is a problem, sunglasses with *absorptive lenses* or *optical filters*, which block infrared and ultraviolet light, may be helpful. Sunglasses that control glare and absorb irritating light are available in different colors, shades, and percentages of light transmission. Many people with photophobia or unstable conditions need different lenses for indoor and outdoor conditions.

Color Contrast

To enhance visual abilities for accomplishing ADL, one should widely incorporate the practical use of color contrast into all environmental features. The use of light dishware that stands out clearly against dark, solid-color tables or tablecloths is recommended. Two cutting boards should be available: a light-colored one for dark foods and a dark one for light foods. Contrasting or brightly colored items should be strategically placed to help locate furniture such as coffee tables and the backs or arms

Table 16.1. Functional Assessment of People Who Are Blind or Visually Impaired: Performance Items

Category	Performance Items
Vision	Near vision
	Intermediate vision
	Distance vision
	Current optical aid use
	Illumination
	Absorptive lenses
	Clinical low-vision exam
Orientation and Mobility	Sighted guide
	Self-protective techniques
	Doorways
	Indoor travel
	Room familiarization
	Outdoor travel
	Automobiles
	Searching techniques
	Cane
	Orientation and movement specialist
Communications	Braille
	Script writing
	Typing and keyboarding
	Using the telephone
	Using a tape recorder
	Telling time
	Library service
Personal Management	Grooming and hygiene
	Clothing care and identification
	Money handling
	Table etiquette
	Diabetic concerns
	Medication management
	Knowledge of eye disease
	Acceptance of eye condition
Home Management	Cleaning
	Laundry
	Household organization
	Minor repairs and tool use
	Safety
Food Preparation	Safety
	Labeling
	Reading and saving recipes
	Shopping
	Timing
	Pouring and measuring
	Cutting, peeling, slicing, and spreading food
	Using appliances
	Addressing dietary and nutritional concerns
Leisure Activities	Social and support groups
	Crafts and hobbies
	Table games
	Sewing
	Sports
Community Resources	Aging network

Case Study 16.7. Photophobia

C. D. had a combination of eye conditions and severe photophobia. She had trouble in bright outdoor conditions, on overcast days, and even indoors. After a few trials with optical filters, she realized that all three situations required different levels of light transmission and tints for her to be most comfortable. A high-light-transmission (40%) amber lens allowed her to use her vision best indoors for some reading; a medium-level (10%) gray was best for overcast days; and a dark green, low-transmission (2%) was necessary on bright days. The best environment for reading print was in natural light, so she positioned her reading desk by the brightest window available. Because the light was also irritating, however, C. D. used the amber lenses for reading.

of chairs. Colored tape strips can be added to countertop edges, doorsills, and steps to improve contrast. High-contrast electrical outlet switchplate covers and cabinet handles can make them easier to find. Contrasting or bright fluorescent tape added to tool handles will make them easier to locate on dark work surfaces.

Because some people have a decreased ability to distinguish color, especially in low-light conditions, high contrast is especially important for environmental landmarks. A simple cafeteria tray may be used not only to keep craft supplies from rolling away but also to increase color contrast. If possible, have a dark and a light tray available to contrast with the predominant color of the supplies. If only dark trays are available, consider applying white or light contact paper or electrical tape to one side to provide better contrast as needed.

In most instances, solid colors are best for background surfaces. Floral or festive "holiday" patterns or other busy backgrounds for tablecloths or other work surfaces act as camouflage (Figure 16.6). Avoid boldly patterned wallpaper or tabletop work surfaces. Electric outlets, eating utensils, and tools are difficult to locate on those types of backgrounds.

Orientation and Mobility

Orientation is a term for knowing where one is, where one is going, and how one is going to get to one's destination; *mobility* is the means of actually getting there. The most comfortable, widely used, safe, and efficient way to assist people who are blind or have low vision in traveling is use of a *sighted guide*. Certified orientation and mobility specialists are professionals trained in providing travel instruction to people who are blind. State and private agencies for the blind can provide information on obtaining services.

For outdoor or more advanced independent travel, clients may require instruction in the use of telescopic aids, a white cane, electronic mobility devices, or a dog guide. State agencies for the blind and private agencies can provide information on white cane safety laws and the regulations governing the legal use of a white cane.

Sighted Guide Technique

In this technique, the blind person holds the arm of the guide just above the elbow and is a half-step be-

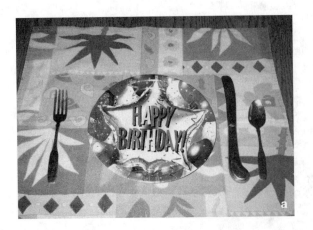
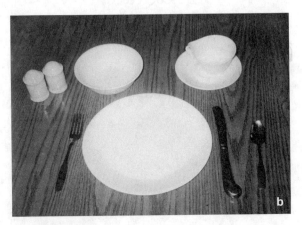

Figure 16.6. Avoid busy backgrounds and use solid colors to enhance contrast.

hind and to the side of the sighted guide. In this position, someone who is blind or has low vision can safely follow the guide's body movements as they walk (Figures 16.7 and 16.8).

To begin the sighted guide technique, the guide and the person to be guided first make contact with their arms. The guide verbally offers assistance. The person needing sighted assistance will move his or her hand up above the guide's elbow, keeping his or her thumb on the outside of the guide's arm. The four fingers should be on the medial side of the guide's arm and should maintain a firm and comfortable grip. The opposite shoulders of the traveling partners should be one behind the other (Hill & Ponder, 1976).

The question of which side is best for the process is based on a number of factors, most notably personal preferences. Strength, hand dominance, the need for a support cane, hearing loss, the need to carry a package or purse, and other factors affect this decision. Most experienced travelers find they are able to travel equally well on either side of a sighted guide. Also, with experience, most sighted guide partnerships require less verbal input about the travel environment. Travel companions

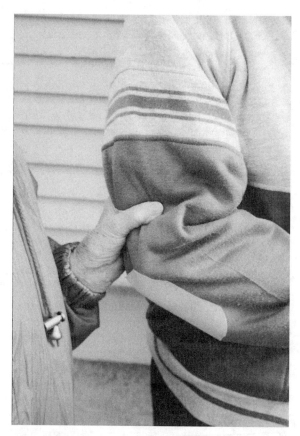

Figure 16.8. The proper grip of the sighted guide technique.

can safely carry on conversations just as other friends do.

Sighted guide techniques are adapted for specific situations, as follows:

- *Room Familiarization.* Room familiarization begins at the primary entrance to a room. The blind person should be guided around the perimeter of the room. The guide should emphasize locating all permanent or semipermanent landmarks, such as light switches and electric outlets, windows, furniture, closet doors, and hanging plants.
- *Narrow Spaces.* To negotiate narrow spaces, the guide moves his or her arm to the middle of the guide's back as a sign for the blind person to walk directly behind the guide. With arm extended, the increased space will prevent the blind person from walking on the heels of the guide and enables single-file travel through narrow or congested areas.
- *Curbs and Stairs.* At each change of elevation, whether at a curb or a flight of stairs, the

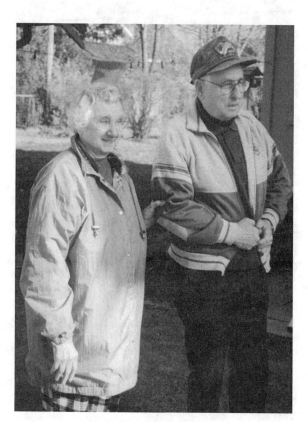

Figure 16.7. Sighted guide technique.

sighted guide should pause and describe the change. It is generally safer for the guide to keep his or her weight forward when ascending and backward when descending.

- *Seating*. The guide should lead the blind person to the chair so that his or her body comes in contact with the chair. The guide then places the blind person's hand on the back of the chair to provide a reference point.
- *Doorways*. After describing the direction in which the door opens (toward or away) and on which side it is hinged, the sighted guide always should go through doorways first. Revolving doors may cause problems for some slow-walking travelers; in those cases, the guide should use a different door, or the blind person should practice using revolving doors with the guide during less busy times.
- *Automobiles*. The guide should describe the direction in which the vehicle is pointing. After the passenger door is opened, the guide places one of the blind person's hands on the roof and the other on the top edge of the open door. It is neither safe nor efficient to attempt to guide a blind person by pushing him from behind. In this position, the guide will not readily see uneven pavement, patches of ice, water, or otherwise slippery surfaces. Moreover, sudden noises or safety concerns may cause a clumsy resistance to the guide's efforts. Finally, no one is in front of the blind person to act as a buffer or stabilizer should a stumble occur or an immediate stop become necessary.

Self-Protection

Self-protection techniques are necessary even in a familiar home environment. One technique involves holding one arm (usually the nondominant one) at shoulder height, palm out with the hand just below eye level (Figure 16.9). The dominant hand is held diagonally across the body, palm inward, in front of the opposite upper thigh. This positioning in front of the face and across the torso will provide safe coverage from open cupboards, closet doors, and narrow poles.

Systematic Searching Patterns

People with vision loss will find it useful to search for dropped objects in an organized or patterned way. Searching for a dropped object can involve listening for the sound of the object hitting the floor, turning to face that location, and searching for the

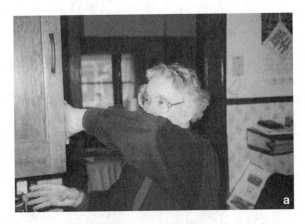

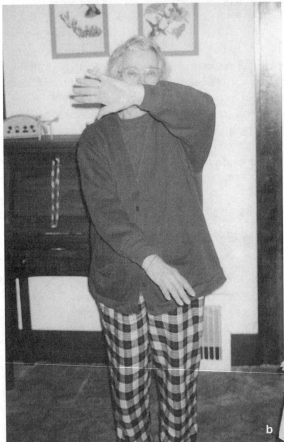

Figure 16.9. Two examples of self-protection techniques.

object in that direction using either a circular pattern with gradually increasing concentric circles radiating outward or a gridlike pattern. A methodical pattern will ensure complete coverage and reduce frustration.

Case Study 16.8. Glaucoma

M. T. is a widower living alone on the farm he has called home for more than 40 years. Despite his vision impairment, he thoroughly enjoys going to his workshop in one of his outbuildings. Glaucoma has reduced his visual field to a small tunnel, and his remaining vision does not work well in low-light conditions. M. T. placed a wind chime near his back doorway and strung a thin rope on posts from his house to the outbuilding. The rope gives him the guidance he needs, and the wind chime, given the right breeze, helps him locate the back door when he is elsewhere on his property. M. T. also uses a radio at his back door to provide an audible directional beacon for which to aim.

In his barn, M. T. must negotiate around a few low beams. He has strategically placed lengths of bailing twine about 3 ft in front of all low obstructions. These soft warning signs alert him and have saved him more than a few bumps on the head.

Case Study 16.9. Visual Field Cut

A stroke caused S. L. to become totally blind and confused about her location even in her own home. Her husband was concerned about helping her determine her location and the direction she must travel. A cuckoo clock with an audible tick-tock now provides the orientation to her current location and to the direction to the other rooms in her home.

Communication

Oral Communication

As with other disabilities, such as hearing loss, people with blindness and vision loss are sometimes treated inappropriately by people who do not understand their conditions. The following guidelines provide useful suggestions for polite, respectful, and appropriate interactions with people who have vision loss.

- When offering assistance, speak in a normal tone of voice (unless the person with visual impairment or blindness also has hearing loss). Speak directly to the blind person, not the sighted guide.
- Always introduce oneself; voice recognition is not always reliable, especially in a crowded or noisy environment.
- Inform the blind person when leaving. No one wants to appear foolish by starting to talk to oneself.
- Use words like *look* and *see* as in everyday conversations, because attempts to use substitutes are usually awkward and may make everyone less comfortable.
- When dining, use the "face of the clock" method of orientation to describe the location of food (e.g., "the peas are at 2 o'clock"; Figure

16.10). The same method can be used for locating utensils, condiments, and other items.
- Be specific when giving directions: Use directional cues such as right and left, behind or in front. Avoid gestures, pointing, and nonspecific statements such as "over there" and "that way" (e.g., "The blue candy dish is in front of you and to the right" or "It is at 2 o'-clock."
- Never move furniture without informing the blind person who is familiar with a particular arrangement.

Written Communication

Whenever possible, print size should be large and in clear block letters. Text should be black on either a white or yellow background, or vice versa. Avoid ornate, serif, and condensed typefaces. Most colored or patterned paper also should be avoided. Some people find that yellow paper offers better contrast for reading print and use a sheet of yellow acetate (e.g., a report cover) over black print on white paper.

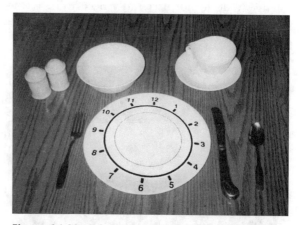

Figure 16.10. Orientation via "face of the clock."

Announcements and other notices should be posted in large print on bulletin boards in public places. One strategy used in senior centers is to post all headlines in large type, thereby allowing people with low vision to read the document with optical aids or request further assistance when indicated.

People with low vision face a variety of issues in written communications. The most basic hand-writing task is that of signing one's name. For some people, it is the single most important aspect of achieving a better sense of well-being and confidence. Everyone should be encouraged to sign his or her own name. Darkening the signature line with a bold pen can provide enough guidance for some people with low vision to sign their name.

Writing Guides and Templates

Signature guides may be as simple as a credit-card-sized piece of thin cardboard or plastic; they are usually black and have a rectangular cutout (Figure 16.11). Other guides may be metal, and some have an elastic band that allows the writer to easily make the tails of letters below the line. The guide is placed over the signature space creating a structurally rigid barrier or frame. With practice and encouragement, people can sign their names. Suggest using natural motions. Often, the faster one signs one's name after a long period of nonwriting, the better it looks.

Other important concerns with cursive writing include inability to stay on the line and writing on a slant, not crossing *t*s or dotting *i*s, and being uncertain of the need to correct mistakes. For people with relatively good vision, the first option is to use lined paper, which is available in various sizes of line width and boldness. This writing paper makes it easier to stay on the line. Some people use different paper of different line sizes for different purposes. Narrow-lined paper is suitable for writing personal letters that do not necessarily need to be reread. Very wide-lined paper is more useful for writing that

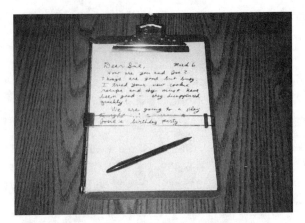

Figure 16.12. Marks script writing guide.

will be later referenced, such as an address book, a recipe, or a shopping list.

A black script-writing template of plastic or cardboard may be helpful for people with less vision. These templates force the writing to conform to the space available and ensure parallel lines. Paper clips hold the writing paper firmly. Using various widths of felt-tip pens makes it easier to see where the writing starts and stops.

A Marks writing guide is a clipboard-type device that holds writing paper in place and uses a line-sized frame that is moved down the page (Figure 16.12). As the writer reaches the end of each line, he or she moves the frame down to the next line. Envelopes also can be addressed using this type of guide. In addition, envelope templates, which have windows cut out for each line of the address, are available. Writing paper that is embossed with raised lines is available in 50-sheet pads.

Braille

Braille is a system of reading and writing using a configuration of six raised dots in a rectangular pattern resembling a muffin pan (Figure 16.13; Ashcroft & Henderson, 1963). Louis Braille, a blind Frenchman, developed the system for his own use. Prior to the development of braille, other systems of tactual reading were tried, but not until braille was developed did blind people have the ability to become truly literate by writing in addition to reading raised symbols.

In addition to reading and writing text, braille may be used for labeling items such as medicines, canned goods, or playing cards. Braille may be written with a *Perkins brailler,* which looks somewhat like an antique typewriter, or with a portable slate and stylus. Computer-embossed braille is becoming more readily available.

Figure 16.11. Black plastic signature guide.

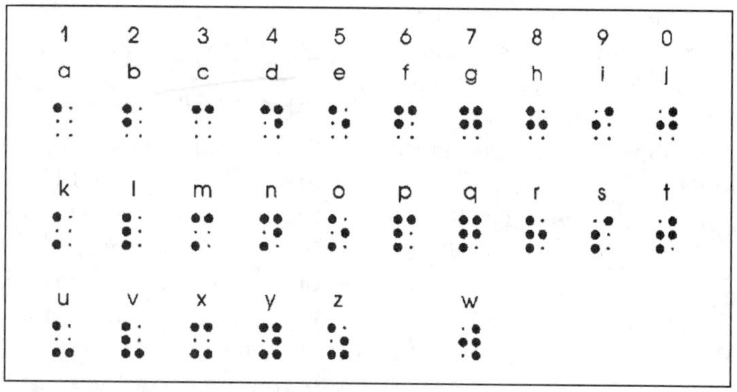

Figure 16.13. The Braille alphabet.

Electronic Communication and Other Helpful Devices

Telephones

Many styles of large-print telephones are available. Some have raised numbers in bold print, allowing easier location of each number. Many phones have volume controls for people with hearing loss. Voice-recognition telephones are available for people who have physical limitations in addition to vision loss. Speed-dial buttons may be tactually or visually marked for easy location. It is possible to adapt older rotary telephones with large-print dial overlays or tactual markers, and large-print push-button adapters may be applied to standard push-button telephones.

Standard push-button telephones can be dialed with a three-finger technique. The person using the phone places the three longest fingers on a row of numbers. For example, on the top row of a standard push-button phone, the pointer finger pushes the one, the index finger pushes the two, and the ring finger pushes the three. To reach the second row of four through six, one simply moves the three fingers down one row and so forth.

Most telephone companies offer exemptions from directory assistance charges for assistance calls made by people who are blind or visually impaired. Each company may have different regulations and eligibility policies. Check with local providers for details.

In 1996, the United States Congress amended the Telecommunications Law (Section 255) to ensure that telephone services and telephones, both traditional wireline and wireless, are accessible to people with disabilities. The Federal Communications Commission (FCC) oversees communication law, including the Section 255 disability provisions in the Telecommunications Act of 1996.

How to Get an Accessible Telephone is a pamphlet with step-by-step instructions about shopping for a phone and filing complaints with the FCC. It is available in standard print, large print, or braille from the American Foundation for the Blind at www.afb.org/section255.asp.

Tape Recorders

Cassette tapes and digital recordings are other options for storing and retrieving information. Peo-

---

Case Study 16.10. AMD

L. B. moved from her small town in South Carolina to northern Wisconsin to die. She came to live with her daughter because of an inoperable condition that caused her physician to predict only a 2-month life expectancy. The local rehabilitation teacher from the state services for the blind persuaded L. B. to enroll in the talking-book program to help pass the time. L. B.'s signature was required to receive services, but she told the teacher that she had been unable to sign her name for a few years because of AMD. The teacher showed her a black plastic signature template and assigned her a practice regimen. With time and encouragement, L. B. progressed to writing letters to her relatives and friends in South Carolina. After more practice, she was able to write telephone messages for her daughter's home-based business; this improved customer service, saved the cost of call-forwarding to an answering service, and boosted L. B.'s self-confidence as well. Because of her charming personality and wonderful South Carolina accent, she was a true asset to the business. And, happily contrary to her doctor's prognosis, L.B. continued working in this role for many years.

ple can mail taped letters to friends using special cassette mailers while qualifying for "Free Matter for the Blind or Physically Handicapped" mailing privileges. "Free Matter," as it is commonly known, allows matter to be sent "free of postage if mailed by or for the use of blind or other persons who cannot read or use conventionally printed materials due to a physical handicap." (See the U.S. Postal Service *Domestic Mail Manual* Web site for eligibility details and limits: http://pe.usps.gov/cpim/ftp/-manuals/ Dmm/E040.pdf.) A letter is recorded, placed in a special mailer, and dropped in the mailbox. Most mailers have double "from" and "to" labels, which reverse addresses on each side and are designed for repeated use. Other mailers contain a reversible, postcardlike label that is placed in a clear window.

Digital voice recorders are convenient and portable note-taking devices. Digital recordings can be sent via email and archived on home computers or recordable CDs.

Volunteer Reader Services

Perhaps the single most frequently used means of reading is to secure the services of a sighted volunteer or paid reader. Volunteers may be coordinated through religious organizations, aging units, government offices, and private agencies.

Computers

Job Access With Speech (JAWS) and Zoom Text are two types of adaptive technology software for computer access by people with low vision. JAWS enables voice output, and Zoom Text enlarges text on computer monitors. Section 508 requires that Federal agencies' electronic and information technology be accessible to people with disabilities.

In 1998, Congress amended the Rehabilitation Act to require Federal agencies to make their electronic and information technology accessible to people with disabilities. Inaccessible technology interferes with an individual's ability to obtain and use information quickly and easily. Section 508 was enacted to eliminate barriers in information technology, to make available new opportunities for people with disabilities, and to encourage development of technologies that will help achieve these goals. The law applies to all Federal agencies when they develop, procure, maintain, or use electronic and information technology. Under Section 508 (29 U.S.C. 794d), agencies must give disabled employees and members of the public access to information

that is comparable to the access available to others. (508 law)

Personal Digital Assistants and Braille Notetakers

Personal digital assistants (PDAs) have become the organizational tool of choice for many people, and they are now available for blind and low-vision users. BrailleNote from Pulse Data International and Braille Lite Millennium from Freedom Scientific are the two most common accessible PDAs. Both devices have a refreshable braille display and voice output in a portable package. The devices can send and receive Windows-style e-mail accounts using Microsoft's Outlook or Qualcomm's Eudora.

Basic and Instrumental ADL

Grooming and Hygiene

Techniques for shaving can be discussed and practiced with a razor (initially without the blade) or with an electric shaver. Using an electric shaver relies simply on touch. If a client is familiar with shaving and is comfortable with a specific type of shaver, he or she should practice with that type. Magnifying mirrors, some of which have lights, may help with makeup and shaving. For brushing teeth, many people simply dispense toothpaste onto a finger or directly into their mouths (if they are not sharing the tube of toothpaste).

Medication Identification

Rubber bands can be affixed around medication bottles to identify different prescriptions (Figure 16.14). Large-print index cards also can be used to identify medications. A 7-day pillbox can help manage medication use.

Household Organization

Organization is especially important for people with vision loss. Every household item should have its place and be in it when not in use. Cleaning supplies and toxic substances must be labeled in large print or by tactual means. The standard array of commercially available organizational aids, including assorted bins, pocket folders, files, and large-print or tactual labels, can be used to keep household items in their place. Textures, smells, colors, shapes, sizes, sounds, and other properties of objects all can be incorporated into organization techniques.

Marking and Labeling

People with vision loss can choose from a wide variety of marking and labeling aids. Textures, bright colors, high-contrast markings, and various shapes

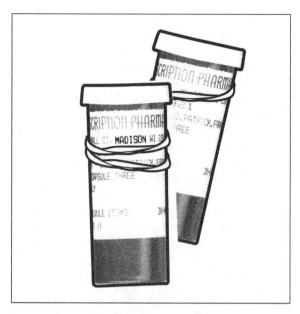

Figure 16.14. Medications are marked by the number of rubber bands.

can be used to mark and distinguish like-shaped items, dial settings, controls, clothing, tools, and other items. Following is a sampling of available aids:

- Hi-Marks is a bright orange, gluelike material that comes in a tube. Dots, bumps, letters, and lines can be drawn to provide both visual and tactual marks. Stoves, thermostats, microwave ovens, laundry equipment, radios, and virtually any dial on any appliance can be easily marked. Spot-N-Line is a similar tactual marking aid available in black or white. Both materials are durable and inexpensive, but they may be difficult for a blind or severely visually impaired person to independently apply as precisely as needed.

- Bump Dots (in black or white) are soft foam dots with sticky backing.

- Beads may be glued in place as tactual landmarks.

- Bright nail polish may be used for marking dials.

- Bold felt-tip pens are ideal for labeling purposes. Index cards may be marked in bold letters and attached to canned goods by rubber bands. After the item is used, the index card can be placed in an envelope, thereby creating the next shopping list. Index cards also are useful for labeling colors of clothing, medicines, and other items. Simply use a hole punch, add a rubber band, and attach the index card to the item.

Simplicity is usually the best approach to marking appliance dials. One or two temperatures are all that may be needed to mark an oven. If 325 degrees is the most common oven temperature, with practice, 350 degrees may be reliably estimated from the known 325-degree mark. Many manufacturers supply tactually marked dials or overlays for their products.

Clothing may be identified in a number of ways. Braille tags may be sewn into clothing in a nonvisual spot away from the skin. Some people use different sizes of buttons in different locations to distinguish between similar items. One way to keep socks in pairs is to use plastic disks with star-shaped cutouts in different shapes in which the socks are always kept when not being worn. The disks can remain attached through washing and drying and are stored that way. When the socks are being worn, the disks are kept in a spot where they are easy to locate. Simply attach the disks to the socks as they are put into the laundry hamper. The shapes allow easy identification. Different sizes of safety pins can be used to distinguish colors.

Some people organize closets into sections of "go together" clothes or group outfits together on the same hanger. Using the "simpler is better" approach, clothing details such as textures, buttons, or other distinguishing features can suffice for many people.

Money Management

Coin identification is taught by tactually exploring the rim or edges of coins with a thumbnail. Pennies and nickels, the two least valuable coins, have smooth edges; dimes and quarters have a milled or ridged edge (Figure 16.15). The size differences between smooth and ridged coins make correct

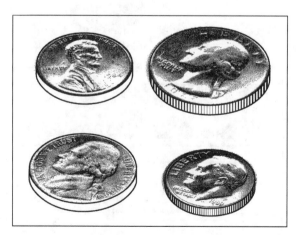

Figure 16.15. The edges of coins make identification easy.

Case Study 16.11. Appliance Marking

The purchase of a new stove precipitated M. P.'s referral to the vision rehabilitation specialist. She had a severe loss of vision but was trying to be independent. An avid baker, M. P. needed to be able to accurately set oven temperatures. With the application of Hi-Marks, she could feel and, at times, even see the location for her most common settings.

identification simple. Coin purses with separate channels for each denomination of coin are helpful in organizing change. Thirty-five mm film canisters or prescription bottles in various sizes also may be used to keep coins separated (Flax et al., 1993).

Paper money can be organized by folding the different denominations in various ways (e.g., $1 bills are unfolded, $5 bills are folded in half so that they are almost a square, $10 bills might be folded in half lengthwise, and $20 bills can be folded like $10 bills and then folded over a second time (Figure 16.16). Another common way to handle paper

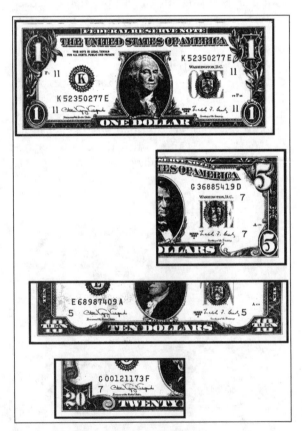

Figure 16.16. Paper money folded for quick identification.

money is to put the different denominations in different compartments of a wallet or purse. Still another method to simplify the identification of bills is to limit the paper money to just $1 bills and $5 bills and keep them in separate compartments or pockets.

Using checks for purchases or paying bills often is the only option. A number of approaches can be effective, including large-print checks, raised-line checks, or one of the many available check templates. Black plastic check templates have window cutouts to match the information fields. One brand, the Keitzer Check Guide, has an especially thick border to restrict the writing. Some people use markers to highlight the lines on personal checks. Large-print check registers can make financial recording easier for people with low vision. Banks generally can provide information on the availability of accessible checks.

Credit cards, of course, are a convenient way to make purchases. The card also can function as a signature guide by having the clerk place it under the signature line on the receipt.

Telling Time

Large-print, braille, and talking watches all are available from specialized catalog suppliers (Figure 16.17). Some people adapt existing equipment using tactual means or large print.

Meal Planning and Shopping

Food preparation includes many activities and skills that must be mastered in sequence. Menu development, shopping, reading recipes, identifying ingredients, peeling, chopping, slicing and dicing, pouring and measuring, setting oven and stovetop temperatures, timing, and safely handling hot utensils all are part of the task. Below are techniques that can help people with low vision accomplish this important ADL:

- Large-print, braille, or taped cookbooks can help develop menu items. Recipes also may be stored in large print or braille, or on cassette tape.
- Shopping is easier when a list of items to be included in a weekly menu is planned in advance. Index card labels from canned goods can be used in addition to a standard shopping list. Shopping assistance can usually be secured from store personnel, or optical aids can be used. Many communities offer online grocery shopping and delivery.
- Canned goods may be identified by shape, label designs, and by the sound when shaken.

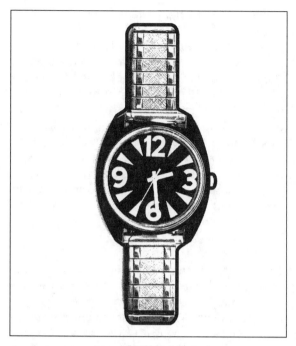

Figure 16.17. A large-print watch.

Some people write labels on index cards and attach them to cans with a rubber band (Figure 16.18). Others mark the cabinet and place all like items behind that label. Small bins may be used to organize items.

- Light-colored squares of flexible magnetic sheets can be marked with bold permanent

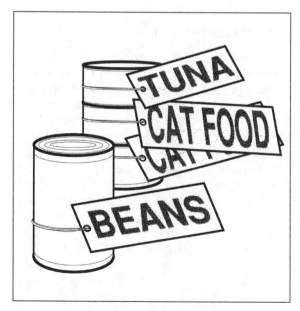

Figure 16.18. Large-print labels for food identification.

pens in large print or in braille. These can be affixed and easily reused. Some people with low vision can recognize certain brands of products by their logo or coloring but cannot read the print label.

- Labels, whether on index cards or magnetic, can be recycled into a "shopping list" envelope after the item is used. Spice containers, while appearing similar, may often be identified by smell, large print, or tactual labels.

Food Preparation

People who are blind or have low vision may find the following techniques of help in preparing food:

- Rinsing vegetables may make it easier to distinguish between peeled and unpeeled sections of foods.
- Dual-colored cutting boards—which are dark on one side and light on the other—or two different cutting boards can provide color contrast. Cutting boards with a funnel-shaped end enable easier transfer and placement of chopped foods.
- Kitchens must have sufficient task lighting or under-the-counter lights. Knives with adjustable slicing-width guides make uniform slices in meats, breads, vegetables, and other foods an easy task.
- Liquid-level indicators emit an audible signal when the poured liquid reaches the twin electrodes. Pouring and measuring can be practiced using cold water over a sink. Pouring colored liquids into a clear glass can be made easier if the glass is held against a contrasting background color (e.g., a dark wall or backsplash for pouring milk or a white background for pouring dark liquids). White coffee cups provide better contrast for pouring black coffee.
- By hooking an index finger over the edge or lip of a glass, one can determine when the level of the liquid reaches that point. Clients can practice over a sink or cafeteria tray to build confidence.
- Individual measuring cups or scoops are recommended and can be marked tactually or in large print. Large-print designations are available on some measuring spoons. Others may be marked with permanent bold-line pens or by filing grooves into the handles.
- Many types of large-print, audible, and braille timers are available (Figure 16.19). Some may be marked with additional tactual or large-print embellishments to ensure ease of use.

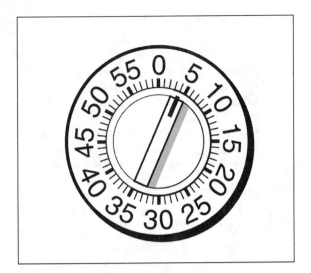

Figure 16.19. Large-print timer.

Safety around hot areas is always a concern for people with visual impairments. Large oven mitts are recommended to protect arms when removing hot dishware from ovens. Every kitchen should have an operable fire extinguisher in a handy location.

Leisure Participation

Leisure and recreation are important ADL. This section describes adaptations of common leisure activities for people with visual impairments.

Table Games

Playing cards are available in various large-print sizes, raised-line print, and in both standard- and jumbo-dot braille. Cribbage boards with raised borders around the pegging holes allow easy counting of points. Checkerboards with indented squares, round red, and square black checkers make the game accessible for totally blind players.

Braille dice are produced with raised dots on indented sides; large-print dice are simply large-sized dice. Large-print and braille bingo cards allow people to continue playing these games. Other board games are available from the catalog suppliers listed at the end of this chapter. Many people also tactually mark in braille (or other means) selected pieces of their favorite board games.

Crafts and Hobbies

Using wire-loop needle threaders is an almost automatic way to thread sewing needles. The threader is first put into the eye of a needle using the sense of touch. Because it is difficult to put the limp thread through the loop, it should first be wrapped around a toothpick. This rigid arrangement can easily be put through the loop. After that, it is quite simple to withdraw the wire loop and pull the thread through the eye of the needle. Wire-loop needle threaders also can be used to put fishhooks onto fishing line.

"Chimney-like" needle threaders also work quite well. Spread-eye needles are flexible needles that have a long eye that runs nearly the entire length of the needle. Self-threading needles have a tiny gap just above the eye; to thread them, the user places the sharp end of the needle in a bar of soap or a cork, locates the notch in the top, places the thread lengthwise into the notch, and firmly pops the thread into the eye.

Reading

The Library for the Blind and Physically Handicapped provides talking books on records, cassettes, or in braille for people who cannot read standard-print books. Accessible reading materials are mailed to people and are returned postage free. Applications and eligibility criteria are available from local libraries and state and private agencies for the blind.

Other Pastimes

Senior centers often provide a rich array of services, including exercise therapy, craft classes, computer-user groups, reading clubs, travel opportunities, nutrition programs, and recreation and peer support groups. "Touch me" exhibits in museums, "scent walks" in botanical gardens, and audio-described

---

Case Study 16.12. Playing Cards

S. S. always had a close relationship with her granddaughter and enjoyed playing cards with her. Low vision, however, severely affected S. S.'s ability to continue card playing. After she purchased a deck of large-print cards, she was able to continue regular card games with her granddaughter. Her vision was often good enough for her to identify the cards in good light, and with sufficient time, but she did not want to slow down a heated game of war with her granddaughter. A rehabilitation teacher from the state agency for the blind helped S. S. develop proficiency at writing braille using a slate and stylus. S. S. put the 15 braille symbols needed for playing cards on a deck of large-print cards so that as she lost more vision, she was able to learn to play cards using braille symbols.

historical tours are available in many locations. Organizations of blind athletes compete in sports including golf, soccer, weight lifting, beep baseball (played using an audible ball), diving, bowling, downhill and cross-country skiing, and windsurfing.

Social and Community Participation

Local peer support groups for people with visual impairments are available in many communities. Information is available through local agencies, state services for the blind, and local private agencies. The Lighthouse National Center on Aging and Vision is a leader in information on peer support groups (see Appendix 16.B).

Community programs and resources play an important role in the service plan for people with severe vision loss. Federally mandated Older Americans Act of 1965 (amended in 2000) services include transportation, nutrition (both home delivered and in congregate settings), and benefits counseling, which are available to everyone 60 years of age and older. These and other in-home support services are administered through local aging units or Agencies on Aging.

The American Foundation for the Blind, the Lighthouse National Center on Aging and Vision (see Appendix 16.B), consumer groups, and special interest groups in support of specific eye conditions can provide a wealth of information and referral to local services.

Work

Nationally, among people 21 to 64 years of age who have a visual impairment, only 41.5% are employed; among people unable to see words and letters, only 29.9% work. In contrast, an estimated 84% of people in this age group without any kind of disability are employed (McNeil, 2001). The Americans With Disabilities Act of 1990 (ADA) prohibits discrimination and ensures equal opportunity for people with disabilities in employment, state and local government services, public accommodations, commercial facilities, and transportation. The U.S. Department of Justice provides free ADA materials (see Appendix 16.B).

Summary

Acquired visual deficits can be caused by health conditions such as diabetes and stroke, normal aging, and injuries to the eye. These deficits can affect vision generally or produce limitations affecting central or peripheral vision, resulting in a variety of functional consequences. Assessing the needs of people with low vision requires a thorough consideration of their living environment and lifestyle. Many adaptive devices and techniques can help people adapt to the functional challenges of vision loss.

Study Questions

1. What is the definition of legal blindness?
2. What is the definition of severe visual impairment?
3. What is the impact of each of the four major age-related eye conditions on functional vision?
4. Which eye condition will have the greatest impact in low-light situations?
5. Describe adaptive strategies for cooking and housework for people with vision loss.
6. What are the most practical ways to control light and glare?
7. When and why should a person with low vision be referred to a self-help group?
8. What is the position and responsibility for a sighted guide?
9. What protections for people with visual impairment are afforded by the ADA?

References

508 Law. (2002, August 15). Retrieved April 1, 2004, from http://www.section508.gov/index.cfm?FuseAction= Content&ID=3.

American Foundation for the Blind. (2002, April 18). How to get an accessible telephone. Retrieved April 1, 2004, from http://www.afb.org/section255.asp.

Americans With Disabilities Act of 1990, Pub. L. 101–336, 42 U.S.C. § 12101.

Ashcroft, S. C., & Henderson, F. (1963). *Programmed instruction in Braille*. Pittsburgh PA: Stanwix House.

Buettner, H. (Ed.). (2002). *Mayo Clinic on vision and eye health: Practical answers on glaucoma, cataracts, macular degeneration, and other conditions*. Rochester, MN: Mayo Foundation for Medical Education and Research.

Carroll, T. J. (1961). *Blindness: What it is, what it does, and how to live with it*. Boston: Little, Brown.

Corn, A. L., & Koenig, A. J. (1996). *Foundations of low vision: Clinical and functional perspectives*. New York: AFB Press.

Duffy, M. A. (2002). *Making life more livable*. New York: AFB Press.

Flax, M., Golembiewski, D., & McCaulley, B. (1993). *Coping with low vision*. San Diego, CA: Singular.

Golembiewski, D. (1998). Asking the right questions. *RE:view: Rehabilitation and Education for Blindness and Visual Impairment, 30*(1), 29–30.

Hill, E., & Ponder, P. (1976). *Orientation and mobility techniques: A guide for the practitioner*. New York: American Foundation for the Blind Press.

Jose, R. T. (Ed.). (1983). *Understanding low vision*. New York: American Foundation for the Blind.

Kirchner, C., & Schmeidler, E. (1997). Prevalence and employment of people in the United States who are blind or visually impaired. *Journal of Visual Impairment and Blindness, 91*, 508–511.

Lighthouse International. (2003, December). Prevalence of vision impairment. Retrieved April 1, 2004, from http://www.lighthouse.org/research_nationalsurvey.htm.

McNeil, J. M. (2001). *Americans with disabilities: 1997* (Current Population Reports P70-61). Washington, DC: U.S. Government Printing Office.

Nelson, K. A., & Dimitrova, E. (1993). Severe visual impairment in the United States and in each state, 1990. *Journal of Visual Impairment and Blindness, 85*(5), 80–85.

Older Americans Act Amendments of 2000, Pub. L. 106–501.

Telecommunications Act of 1996, Pub. L. 104–104, 47 U.S.C. §§ 255.

Tuttle, D., & Tuttle, N. (1996). *Self-esteem and adjusting with blindness.* Springfield, IL: Charles C Thomas.

U.S. Bureau of the Census. (2000, June 29). *Disability data from the survey of income and program participation (SIPP).* Retrieved April 1, 2004, from http://www.census.gov/hhes/www/disable/dissipp.html.

Appendix 16.A.

Assessment for Rehabilitation Teaching Services

Name _____

Address _____

City _____

Phone _____

Birth Date _____

Zip _____

Are you able to read your mail, your recipes, or the newspaper?
Yes _____ No _____

   If "No" due to vision loss, check if help is needed. _____

Are you able to identify and properly take your medications?
Yes _____ No _____

   If "No" due to vision loss, check if help is needed. _____

Are you able to accurately tell time by reading your watch or a wall clock?
Yes _____ No _____

   If "No" due to vision loss, check if help is needed. _____

Can you tell a nickel from a quarter? A $1 from a $10?
Yes _____ No _____

   If "No" due to vision loss, check if help is needed. _____

Can you set the correct temperature on a thermostat or oven?
Yes _____ No _____

   If "No" due to vision loss, check if help is needed. _____

Are you able to write letters or a grocery list or sign your name?
Yes _____ No _____

   If "No" due to vision loss, check if help is needed. _____

Are you able to identify friends from across the room or table?
Yes _____ No _____

   If "No" due to vision loss, check if help is needed. _____

Are you able to follow the action or see characters on TV?
Yes _____ No _____

   If "No" due to vision loss, check if help is needed. _____

Can you handle your own household cleaning?
Yes _____ No _____

   If "No" due to vision loss, check if help is needed. _____

What are your favorite leisure activities? Can you still do them?
Yes _____ No _____

   If "No" due to vision loss, check if help is needed. _____

Are you able to prepare your own meals?
Yes _____ No _____

   If "No" due to vision loss, check if help is needed. _____

Can you handle your own shopping?
Yes _____ No _____

   If "No" due to vision loss, check if help is needed. _____

Are you able to identify traffic signals from across the street?
Yes _____ No _____

   If "No" due to vision loss, check if help is needed. _____

Do any magnifiers you use for your reading work well enough?
Yes _____ No _____

   If "No" due to vision loss, check if help is needed. _____

When did you last go to your eye doctor for a checkup? _____

When did you last have your eyeglass prescription changed? _____

Do your eyeglasses work well enough to read, watch TV, and see in the distance?
No _____ Yes _____

Has anyone from an agency for the visually impaired or blind been out to see you?
No _____ Yes _____ When _____ Who _____

Do you want someone to contact you to help you with any of the above?
Yes _____ Not Yet _____

Referral Source _____ Date _____

Phone _____

Comments:

Appendix 16.B.
Resources

Products

BrailleNote, 18- and 32-cell
U.S. Distributor:
　HumanWare
　6245 King Road
　Loomis, CA 95650
　800-722-3393 or 916-652-7253
　E-mail: info@humanware.com
　Web site: www.humanware.com
Manufacturer:
　Pulse Data International Limited
　64-3-384-4555
　E-mail: sales@pulsedata.com
　Web site: www.pulsedata.co.nz

Braille Lite Millennium M20 and M40
Manufacturer:
　Freedom Scientific Blindness and
　　Low Vision Group
　11800 31st Court
　North St. Petersburg, FL 33716
　800-444-4443 or 727-803-8000
　Fax: 727-803-8001
　E-mail: Sales@freedomscientific.com
　Web site: www.freedomscientific.com

Organizations

American Foundation for the Blind
Information Center
11 Penn Plaza, Suite 300
New York, NY, 10001
800-232-5463
Web site: www.afb.org

Federal Communications Commission
Consumer Information Bureau
445 12th Street, SW
Washington, DC 20554
888-225-5322
E-mail: access@fcc.gov
Web site: www.fcc.gov/cgb/

Lighthouse International
Lighthouse National Center on Aging
　and Vision
111 E. 59th St.
New York, NY 10022-1202
800-829-0500
212-821-9200
TTY: 212-821-9713
Fax: 212-821-9727
Email: info@lighthouse.org
Web site: www.lighthouse.org

U. S. Department of Justice ADA
　Information Line
800-514-0301 (Voice)
800-514-0383 (TDD)
Automated service is available for recorded
　information and to order publications.
Web site: www.usdoj.gov/crt/ada/publicat.htm

Chapter 17

Sexuality and People With Physical Disabilities

MARY ELLEN YOUNG, PHD, CRC

KEY TERMS

counseling

functional effects on sexual activity

sexual activity

sexual orientation

sexual response cycle

sexual rights

OBJECTIVES

Upon completion of this chapter, the reader will be able to

- Describe the occupational therapist's role in dealing with the sexual needs of clients;

- Describe common barriers to meeting these needs;

- Identify skills and knowledge needed by occupational therapists in addressing issues related to sexuality and sexual function;

- Describe the effects of specific disabilities, disorders, and diseases on sexual function; and

- Identify practical strategies in dealing with the effects of disability on sexual function.

We are all sexual beings: "Adult sexuality is an essential component of our identity and self image" (Freda, 1998, p. 364; Neistadt, 1986). Sexual, sensual, or flirtatious behavior occurs frequently in social interactions. Sexual activity is the way in which we share this part of ourselves with a "significant other." "Sexual activity is our most intimate way of expressing and receiving affection" (Neistadt & Freda, 1987, p. ix). The World Health Organization (WHO) has defined intimate relationships as an important part of social participation that contributes to the quality of life for people with disabilities (WHO, 2001). Sexuality for people with disabilities also has been defined as emotional, physical, or both, expressed alone or with a partner (White, Rintala, Hart, Young, & Fuhrer, 1992; 1994). An intimate relationship may or may not include a physical relationship, whereas a physical relationship may "take many different forms, including, for example, kissing, touching or sexual intercourse" (White et al., 1994, p. 56).

Sexual images abound in the media—songs on the radio, magazine articles, TV shows, movies, news, advertisements, music videos, novels, billboards, and, most recently, the Internet—inundate the daily lives of people in Western culture. People who happen to have disabilities or chronic medical conditions also live in this society and see all the images.

The perceived importance of sex and sexual activity is highly individual. Some people place a high value on this aspect of a relationship; for others, it may take a "back seat" to companionship and friendship. Whatever the case, neither age nor disability changes one's basic sexual nature (Figure 17.1; Freda & Rubinsky, 1991). The importance of sexuality to perceived well-being, quality of life, and even physical health has been demonstrated in many studies (McCabe, 1997; Ventegodt, 1998). Research has shown that sexual activity may reduce the risk of heart disease in men (Davey Smith, Frankel, & Yarnell, 1997) and may increase life satisfaction in elders (Spector & Fremeth, 1996). Other studies have shown that satisfactory adjustment to disability is also accompanied by greater satisfaction with and participation in sexual activity (Bianchi, 1997; Kreuter, Sullivan, & Siosteen, 1996). The importance of sexuality and sexual function to well-being makes it important for occupational therapy practitioners to include this aspect of daily life in their intervention planning for people with disabilities. Although physical disability may challenge "the usual way we think about sexuality" (Spica, 1989, p. 56), intervention plans that fail to consider this aspect of every-

> *As a human being, one is sexual from birth to death. Although acute, chronic, or disabling conditions and aging may necessitate certain adaptations in the way one expresses sexuality, one does not cease to be a sexual being.* (Spica, 1989, p. 58)

day living are incomplete. Through knowledge, providing information, and practical problem solving, occupational therapy practitioners can make important contributions to clients with disabilities.

Sexual Counseling and Sex Therapy

Sexual counseling and sex therapy were developed in the 20th century on the basis of knowledge gained through psychotherapeutic and medical practice. Freud (1962) provided an understanding of the psychological aspects of sexuality, but Masters and Johnson (1966) provided the observational and experimental studies to understand the physiological response to sexual stimulation. Sex therapists have devised specific techniques for helping people with specific sexual dysfunction (Kaplan, 1974) and

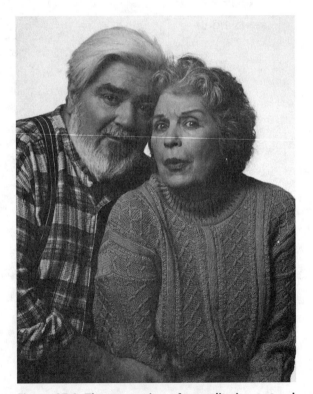

Figure 17.1. The expression of sexuality is a natural part of daily living for everyone, regardless of age or disability status. Photo © PhotoDisc, Inc.

have developed a model for deciding the level of intervention needed (LoPiccolo & LoPiccolo, 1978). This model, whose acronym is PLISSIT, has four levels of intervention:

1. *Permission* simply involves acknowledging the right of people to try different forms of sexual behavior without concern or embarrassment.
2. *Limited information* is provided about the condition affecting sexual performance.
3. *Specific suggestions* are positions, assistive devices, techniques, compensatory strategies, and adaptations that clients might not know about and might benefit from trying.
4. Only *intensive therapy* offers specific clinical interventions that occupational therapists would not usually perform within the realm of their professional practice.

Understanding Sexuality Counseling Within Current Views of Occupational Therapy Intervention

As viewed within the current framework for occupational therapy services, therapists provide four major categories of intervention: remediation, compensation, disability prevention, and health promotion. The provision of information regarding sexual function falls mainly within the categories of compensatory and health promotion strategies, although some intervention recommendations focus on disability prevention. Occupational therapists may provide interventions at all levels of the PLISSIT model, except for intensive therapy. Therapists may help their clients simply by listening and giving them permission to try different techniques or strategies. They may provide limited information or specific suggestions related to a particular disability or functional limitation. Many conditions require a modification of the manner in which sexual activities are performed or can benefit from modifications in the environment. These strategies are compensatory. Similarly, some devices that might be recommended also represent compensatory approaches or may assist in promoting *safe performance* of the activity. Used here, safety is a broader concept than that implied in the common expression "safer sex." Enabling participation in activities that express sexuality in a manner satisfying to the client is also a means of promoting health and well-being. Box 17.1 summarizes the skills and knowledge occupational therapists need to provide sexuality education and counseling.

Box 17.1. Preparing for Effective Sexuality Intervention

Practitioners need special skills and knowledge to provide sexuality education and counseling to their clients. To be effective, practitioners should have training in sexuality that addresses the following four components:

1. **Knowledge.** Practitioners need a sound and comprehensive information base about human sexuality, including human development, relationships, personal skills, sexual behavior, sexual health, marital and family dynamics, and society and culture. Practitioners should know their own limitations. They should know when and where to refer clients who have special problems and needs.
2. **Attitudes.** Practitioners should have an awareness and understanding of their own sexuality to increase their comfort level in addressing the sexual concerns of others. They should demonstrate an acceptance of the diversity of values, beliefs, and lifestyles in the communities they serve.
3. **Skills.** Practitioners should have communication and counseling skills to address sensitive and controversial subjects. Training should include opportunities for practice, and initial efforts should be supervised by more experienced practitioners.
4. **Personal Characteristics and Motivation.** Effective sexuality education and counseling require personal qualities such as emotional stability, patience, flexibility, and a sense of humor. Practitioners should possess the maturity and self-control to avoid imposing personal viewpoints and values on clients. They should have the motivation and commitment to address the sexual health needs of all clients needing such intervention.

Counseling From a Functional Perspective

Occupational therapists are not trained to provide intense psychological counseling on any topic. Their role lies in the occupational performance domain because the profession is firmly rooted in occupation and meaning. In this role, occupational therapists are qualified to deal with the sexual issues that arise as they relate to disability. Occupational therapists routinely deal with people who have had their lives disrupted by a chronic illness or disability. Treatment interventions are geared toward returning clients to productive and meaningful lives by helping them regain appropriate roles within their families and their communities. Occupational therapists are concerned with their clients' functional independence in all aspects of life, including supporting their return to an active, healthy sexual life.

Occupational therapists counsel, educate, or advise clients from an occupational performance perspective. Knowing how a disability limits activities provides a foundation for practical suggestions for managing sexual activity through alternative positions and adaptations. The therapist's assistance may be as simple as helping a couple think about changing a favorite position to better accommodate the disability. Occupational therapists may use the knowledge of adaptation to help clients and partners see the possibilities.

The occupational therapist can share sexual information verbally, with written materials, and through videos or DVDs in group or individual education sessions. He or she may use a combination of methods. What is comfortable for and most acceptable to the client will determine the appropriate choice. The information must be understandable, provided at an appropriate educational level with familiar vocabulary, and shared in a manner that is straightforward yet responsive to individual needs.

During a counseling or education session, it is important that the occupational therapist stay within the comfort zone of the client. Clients who are embarrassed, anxious, or concerned about privacy or other issues will not be able to benefit from the information. It is best to start out in a basic and simple way; check with the client frequently to determine the level of comfort and understanding of the material as well as to confirm its usefulness. The therapist may ask if the information being given is what the client needs or expects. Effective counseling and educational intervention require that the therapist be able to quickly change approaches to meet the informational needs of the client. A warm, yet professional tone should be maintained throughout the session.

Occupational Therapist as a Nonjudgmental Information Provider

Occupational therapists should give information and suggestions in a nonjudgmental fashion. Doing so, however, can sometimes be difficult when speaking about sexual issues. Therapists have attitudes and values that have been shaped by their families and personal experiences. It is important to acknowledge those feelings and put them aside during counseling sessions. Clients come in different shapes, sizes, and sexual orientations. They come

from different ethnic groups, cultures, and religions. It is certainly possible that therapists will encounter clients whose sexual practices are divergent from their own or, in some cases, even conflict with their own values and beliefs. As professionals, they must learn to set aside their own biases to give their clients the appropriate information while maintaining a solid therapeutic relationship.

Therapists who are involved in discussing sexual issues with clients must be comfortable with the topic of sexuality and have an open mind. A beginning is to be comfortable with one's own sexuality and to recognize that different viewpoints are not wrong, just different. Eckland and McBride (1997) suggested that the first step in increasing comfort level in discussions about sexual issues is to examine beliefs about sexuality through values clarification and discussions with other professionals. They also noted that one's values are one's own and should not be imposed on clients (Figure 17.2).

Because of the effective therapeutic relationship that often develops between the occupational therapist and the client, clients frequently turn to occupational therapists when they have questions about sexual functioning and activity. "Generally, it is the

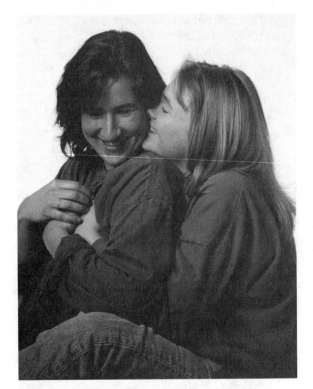

Figure 17.2. Practitioners must recognize that sexual expression takes many forms and avoid imposing their values or lifestyle preferences on their clients. Photo © PhotoDisc, Inc.

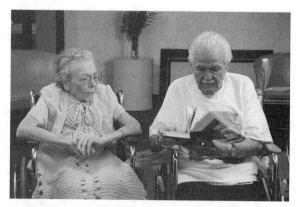

Figure 17.3. One common and incorrect assumption is that older people do not need to express their sexuality. This assumption represents a type of barrier to effective intervention that practitioners should strive to avoid. Image © PhotoDisc, Inc.

professional who has a good interpersonal relationship with the patient who is cast in the role of counselor" (Neistadt & Freda, 1987, p. 10).

Barriers to Meeting the Sexual Information Needs of Clients With Disabilities

Two major obstacles can interfere with providing effective intervention regarding sexual function: inhibitions within the professional community and client boundaries.

Barriers From Health Professionals

As mentioned earlier, many people, including health professionals, have a basic discomfort with the subject of sex. This discomfort alone is enough to prevent many health professionals from ever introducing the topic with a person in their care who has a disability. Some clinicians assume that it is someone else's responsibility; they will not deliberately ignore the need, but they truly believe that another member of the care team will handle the situation. In some cases, health professionals who are uncomfortable with sexuality assume that the client also is uneasy. As a result, no communication occurs.

Ageism (i.e., prejudices against older people) can be a barrier. Some health professionals do not address the issue of sexuality with geriatric clients because they assume that elderly people are not interested in sex. They often make this assumption before they have any idea what role sexual activity has played throughout that person's lifetime. In making such assumptions, they perpetuate a common mis-

understanding and may be revealing their own attitudes or prejudices about the sexual interests, needs, and capabilities of people during the later years of their lives.

Another barrier occurs when a health professional believes that sexual issues would not be of concern to someone with a particular disability. The health professional may assume that severe physical limitations make sexual activity impossible or too much trouble for the client. Again, that assumption is inappropriate and probably incorrect.

Ignorance and personal biases also may be a problem. Many health professionals simply do not know what the possibilities are for sexual activity within the framework of a particular disability. A health professional may believe that it is somehow wrong or inappropriate for a person with a particular physical or developmental disability to engage in sexual activity. Their beliefs may prevent them from offering information on sexuality. Ideally, the therapist should recognize and hold beliefs consistent with those embodied in the Valencia Declaration on Sexual Rights (Box 17.2). The declaration identifies rights and principles for all people to be able to express their sexuality. The presence of disease and disability should not compromise the sexual rights of occupational therapy clients.

Barriers From Clients

Clients themselves often create barriers to receiving information about sexuality or sexual activity; these barriers include embarrassment, cultural taboos, and emotional issues.

Sometimes an older person with a disability may be embarrassed to bring up the subject of sexual activity. Sometimes it is uncomfortable for an older person to discuss such personal issues with a younger person; moreover, people from a different generation often were raised to keep certain topics private and find it difficult to discuss them freely with virtual strangers.

Cultural barriers also exist. People from some cultures may not believe in sharing their concerns about sexual activity with anyone. Once a conversation about sexual activity is started, the occupational therapist must understand any cultural taboos regarding sex so as not to offend the person with an "inappropriate" suggestion.

Clients may be depressed immediately following the onset of a disabling condition or during a flareup of a chronic condition; their depression may hinder them from discussing sexual issues at that time. They may fear a reoccurrence of the condition or may worry about being hurt during sex. These

---

Box 17.2. Valencia Declaration on Sexual Rights

The 13th Annual World Congress on Sexology (i.e., the scientific study of sex), held in Valencia, Spain, adopted a declaration on sexual rights. The declaration declared that sexual health is a basic and fundamental human right and that human sexuality is essential to the well-being of individuals, couples, families, and society. It concluded that respect for sexual rights should be promoted through all means. Sexual rights include the following:

1. **The right to freedom,** which excludes all forms of sexual coercion, exploitation, and abuse at any time and in all situations in life. The struggle against violence is a social priority. All children should be desired and loved.

2. **The right to autonomy, integrity, and safety of the body,** which encompasses control and enjoyment of our own bodies, free from torture, mutilation, and violence of any sort.

3. **The right to sexual equity and equality,** meaning freedom from all forms of discrimination, paying due respect to sexual diversity, regardless of sex, gender, age, race, social class, religion, and sexual orientation.

4. **The right to sexual health,** including availability of all sufficient resources for development of research and the necessary knowledge of HIV/AIDS and STDs as well as the further development of resources for research, diagnosis, and treatment.

5. **The right to wide, objective, and factual information on human sexuality** in order to allow decision making regarding sexual life.

6. **The right to a comprehensive sexuality education** from birth and throughout the life cycle. All social institutions should be involved in this process.

7. **The right to associate freely,** which refers to the ability to marry or not, to divorce, and to establish other types of sexual associations.

8. **The right to make free and responsible choices regarding reproductive life,** the number and spacing of children, and the access to means of fertility regulation.

9. **The right to privacy,** which implies the capability of making autonomous decisions about sexual life within a context of personal and social ethics. Rational and satisfactory experience of sexuality is a requirement for human development.

---

and other emotions may inhibit a person from discussing sexual issues with a health professional. Additionally, the client may have had previous negative or harmful misconceptions about sexuality and disability, adding to their fear and discomfort regarding their own situation.

Like women without disabilities, women with disabilities are at risk for abuse (Young, Nosek, Howland, Chanpong, & Rintala, 1997). Abusive relationships have a significant impact on sexuality and healthy sexual functioning (Nosek et al., 1996). Occupational therapists should be aware of the signs of abuse and be prepared to intervene when necessary to protect their clients.

Knowledge Needed to Address Issues of Sexual Function Related to Disability

Occupational therapists must have a solid knowledge base regarding the diagnoses of clients in their practice environment. Before attempting any functional sexual counseling or education, the therapist must thoroughly understand the disability or disease process affecting the client. To apply the principles of typical sexual functioning, the therapist must realize what differences exist due to the specific disability or disease process, including central nervous system, cardiovascular, pulmonary, musculoskeletal or orthopedic, and developmental disorders.

Knowledge of Anatomy and Physiology

To adequately address issues of sexual function related to disability, therapists must understand male and female sexual anatomy and typical sexual functioning and be able to apply that information to their knowledge of disability and diseases processes. For example, it would be difficult for a therapist to discuss the changes caused by a specific disability if he or she did not fully understand the functioning of a normal system. This knowledge base includes the male and female genitalia and reproductive organs, human anatomy, physiology, and neuroanatomy.

It is extremely important for occupational therapists to understand the body's physiologic response during sexual activity, as identified by Masters and Johnson (1966). Therapists must know the difference between the ordinary physiologic effects of sexual activity and changes that occur for other, possibly problematic, reasons. For example, an autonomic dysreflexia response following sexual arousal in a person with higher level tetraplegia could cause a dangerous elevation in blood pressure.

Masters and Johnson (1996) identified four phases in the sexual response cycle:

1. *Excitement:* Breathing, pulse, and blood pressure begin to increase; muscle tension increases; breast and genital tissue begin to swell; vaginal lubrication in women and erection in men occur.
2. *Plateau*: The physical changes continue and intensify.
3. *Orgasm:* Men ejaculate; women experience contractions in their vagina and uterus; heart rate, breathing, blood pressure, and muscle tension all reach a peak.
4. *Resolution*: All the physiologic changes return to their pre-excitement levels.

Interpersonal Communication Skills

Dealing with the topic of sex can be a challenge because it is a sensitive and private matter. Therapists must have excellent interpersonal skills and be able to have open communication with their clients. The therapist may be cast in several different roles: facilitator, educator, counselor, and, sometimes, confidante. Each role requires effective communication skills and the ability to maintain a trusting therapeutic relationship.

Providing effective sexuality education and counseling is a challenging endeavor, one that requires good listening skills, compassion, and the ability to maintain a delicate balance between sensitivity and assertiveness. The occupational therapist must know when to listen and when to offer suggestions; when to push a bit and when to back off; when to offer comfort; and when to point out potential problems. An ability to read the clients' nonverbal messages is a necessary skill for successful counseling. The therapist must be able to recognize when the client has heard enough during a specific session and when the client wants and needs more information but may not quite know how to ask for it. The therapist must always listen for unspoken questions that are important to the client.

It is the therapist's responsibility to create the appropriate environment for the counseling session, one that is both comfortable and professional. The therapist's empathy should be evident, but he or she should maintain enough professional distance to provide the necessary information in the most therapeutic manner. It is most important for the therapist to provide appropriate, accurate information in a manner that the client finds comfortable and nonthreatening.

Additionally, the therapist must have information on prevention and recognition of sexually transmitted diseases. He or she should be able to provide information on recommended measures of prevention, including hygiene; discretion in partner selection; and the use of protective barriers, such as male and female condoms (Crooks & Baur, 1999). Knowledge of the impact of disabling conditions on fertility and birth control options and limitations also is essential (Crooks & Baur, 1999)

Impairments and Suggested Approaches During Sexual Activity

Before beginning intervention sessions with clients, the therapist should be fully informed about all aspects of the specific condition as well as other health problems that may affect sexual activity. Inexperienced practitioners can benefit from role-playing, extensive reviews of the literature, and discussions with more experienced colleagues. It is also advisable to coordinate plans for sexual counseling with other members of the care team to ensure that information provided to the client is consistent with the plan of care.

Joint Inflammation

Clients who suffer from diseases or conditions resulting in joint inflammation frequently have symptoms that include pain, stiffness, fatigue, and decreased range of motion. Any of these conditions can be a detriment to sexual activity. Kraaimaat and colleagues (Kraaimaat, Bakker, Janssen, & Bijlsma, 1996) stated that pain and limited range of motion may "interfere with sexual pleasure by distracting patients from pleasurable sensations, sexual thoughts and fantasies" (p. 121). The most common barriers to enjoyment of sexual activity are the fear of causing severe pain and anxiety about hurting the affected joint. Certainly, the same principles that apply to other daily living tasks apply to sexual activity. Occupational therapy practitioners should include the topics of energy-conservation and joint-protection techniques when discussing how to approach sexual activity (Box 17.3).

Spinal Cord Injury

Clients with a spinal cord injury (SCI) may have tetraplegia, paraplegia, or a combination of motor

---

Box 17.3. Specific Suggestions for Sexual Adaptations for Clients With Joint Inflammation

- Use joint protection techniques when deciding on positions for sexual activity. Positions that stress the affected joints should be avoided.
- Clients who adhere to a pain relief regimen should time the sexual activity for when pain relief is at its maximum (e.g., after taking medication or heat treatments) in order to enjoy the activity a bit more.
- If pain and stiffness are worst at the beginning of the day (as is typically the case with some types of joint inflammation), the client should delay sexual activity until the stiffness has relaxed and the joints move more freely. Conversely, if pain, swelling, and stiffness are problems later in the day, the client should arrange to have sexual activity earlier in the day.
- Clients should use positions that take advantage of unaffected joints for support and motion (e.g., if the shoulders and elbows are affected, the person should not use the superior position).
- Lying on one's side is a position that may be fairly nonstressful for most joints.
- Pillows can help create a comfortable position.
- When mobility is a problem on a given day, the client should try sexual activities other than intercourse that may be less stressful on the body, such as oral sex or mutual masturbation.
- Experimentation with assistive devices, such as a dildo (strapped on or with a built-up handle) or vibrator may be recommended if the client's hands are severely affected.

---

and sensory loss due to an incomplete injury. Functional problems associated with SCI include mobility loss, sensory loss, bowel and bladder problems (including the use of catheters), spasticity, erectile dysfunction, and loss of vaginal lubrication in women (Box 17.4). Clients with lesions above the fourth thoracic level may experience autonomic dysreflexia in response to sexual stimulation. Both the client with the SCI and his or her partner should be educated about this phenomenon and the actions to be taken to relieve it.

Although sexual functioning varies among people with SCI (even among those with the same level of injury), men with a cervical lesion are more likely to retain the ability to have erections and women with cervical lesions are more likely to retain the ability to produce vaginal lubrication. Ejaculation capabilities are most frequently seen in men with lesions at the thoracic level. Additionally, reflexogenic erections and lubrication can occur if the reflex arc is left intact, as frequently seen in people with an injury at the cervical level (Smith & Bodner, 1993).

Although people with SCI may not experience orgasms after injury in the same manner as prior to the injury, many report some feeling of pleasure, a building of excitement, or any number of bodily reactions (e.g., muscle spasms and flushing; Mooney, Cole, & Chilgren, 1975).

Fertility is not permanently affected in women with SCI. If a man with SCI is found to have viable sperm but cannot ejaculate, he may elect to have an electroejaculation procedure to collect sperm, followed by insemination of his partner (Freda, 1998).

Traumatic Brain Injury (TBI)

Serious brain injuries most frequently occur in young people (primarily men) at a time when they are beginning to explore and develop their sexuality. In addition to the physical problems (such as paralysis or movement disorders) that often accompany serious brain injury, significant cognitive and interpersonal effects result. Depending on the site of the injury, TBI can reduce sexual drive or increase its inappropriate expression by reducing inhibitions, a situation that occurs as a result of damage to the limbic areas of the brain.

Because of the complexity of the brain, the structures affected can result in a wide variety of physical, cognitive, and emotional consequences. Therefore, each TBI survivor must be carefully evaluated, and appropriate sexuality counseling should be provided on the basis of an individual client profile. A study by Kreuter and colleagues (Kreuter, Dahllof, Gudjonsson, Sullivan, & Siosteen, 1998) found that many survivors of TBI living in the community after rehabilitation experienced sexual problems, including an inability to achieve an erection, the inability to achieve orgasm, decreased sexual desire, and a reduced frequency of sexual intercourse. Factors related to satisfactory sexual adjustment included better physical independence and the absence of sexual dysfunction. The researchers concluded that improved efforts at sexual counseling could improve outcomes.

Stroke (Including Cognitive Deficits)

People who have had a stroke (cerebral vascular accident [CVA]) may have hemiplegia or hemiparesis, sensory loss, bowel and bladder problems, proprioceptive deficits, visual problems, communication disorders, swallowing problems, perceptual problems, and cognitive deficits. Fertility usually is not affected by a stroke; however, some decrease in libido has been reported. Men may experience decrease in ejaculatory function and erection (Monga, Lawson,

& Inglis, 1986; Zasler, 1991). People who experience CVA also may be depressed and suffer moderate to severe fatigue. Because many people who have a stroke are older, they may have other health problems that may be intensified or made worse by the stroke. Sometimes, the normal consequences of aging may also be magnified by the stroke (Box 17.5; Freda & Rubinsky, 1991).

Upper-Extremity Amputations

Upper-extremity amputations may result from trauma, disease, or congenital problems. Physiologically, upper-extremity amputations do not affect

---

Box 17.4. Specific Suggestions for Sexual Adaptations for Clients With Spinal Cord Injuries

- Clients with spinal cord injury (SCI) should let their partners know their functional limitations: where sensation is absent, whether erections are possible, which mobility deficits exist, and other relevant factors.
- The client's partner should concentrate touching and fondling on the intact areas of sensation on the client's body.
- When touching a body part without sensation, partners of clients with SCI should either tell the client what area they are touching or be sure the area is within the client's visual field so that enjoyment may occur on a level other than touch.
- Clients and their partners should experiment to find new "erogenous" areas (frequently, this occurs at the level of the last intact *dermotone,* or surface area of sensation; Neistadt & Freda, 1987).
- Two solutions may work for men with SCI who have an external catheter: (1) securing the tubing to the shaft of the penis and engaging in sexual activities or (2) if the man knows when he has to urinate, removing the catheter for short periods of time and engaging in sexual activities during those intervals (Neistadt & Freda, 1987).
- Clients with SCI who are on an intermittent catheterization schedule should adjust the timing of sexual activity accordingly.
- If a *reflexogenic erection* (i.e., one achieved by manual stimulation of the nerves in the perineal region) is possible, it can be achieved by direct manual stimulation of the testicles, penis, and

surrounding area. If an erection is not possible, several options are available:
   - Engaging in sexual activities other than intercourse, such as oral sex or manual stimulation
   - Using a vibrator or dildo if penetration is important to the couple
   - Using vacuum devices that can facilitate a short-term erection (a urologist must be consulted for this)
   - Obtaining surgical implants that can mimic an erection or partial erection (consult a urologist)
   - Exploring the possible benefit of pharmacological agents that can cause an erection (consult a urologist).
- If a woman with SCI has an indwelling catheter, the tube can be taped to the abdomen and the collection bag can be positioned away from the body. It is safe to engage in intercourse or digital stimulation while the tube is in place (Neistadt & Freda, 1987).
- Clients with SCI who have decreased or absent vaginal lubrication can use K-Y jelly or other water-soluble agents to assist with lubrication; their male partner can use a lubricated condom (Neistadt & Freda, 1987).
- Clients with tetraplegia can use a vibrator or another assistive device strapped onto the hand for manual stimulation; they also may use the heel or the side of the hand.
- Clients with SCI should be advised to use positions that take advantage of the movement and control that exists, such as being on the bottom; sitting on the bed, supported against the wall or headboard with pillows; sitting in the wheelchair or another chair; or lying on one's side.

Box 17.5. Specific Suggestions for Sexual Adaptations for Clients Following Stroke

- If the client experiencing stroke has receptive aphasia (i.e., the inability to understand spoken language), the partner may want to physically guide him or her to the part of the body that the partner wishes to be touched.
- If the client experiencing stroke has expressive aphasia (i.e., the inability to use spoken language), the couple may want to try incorporating a specific sexual activity communication board into their routine.
- Partners of clients with communication problems must be sure to observe their facial expressions and be perceptive to the body language to gauge a positive or negative response to a specific activity or position.
- If a functional communication problem exists, sexual partners should use familiar hand signals or develop a "safe" routine to decrease fear of the unknown.
- If the client experiencing stroke has a visual field loss, his or her partner should initiate the sexual activity within the intact visual field. If the client has severe visual problems, the couple may enjoy the use of verbal sharing and fantasies (Freda & Rubinsky, 1991).
- In cases of severe hemiplegia with a sensory loss, the partner will want to concentrate touching and fondling on the intact or uninvolved side of the body.
- In cases of motor loss, the couple should experiment with positions that allow the uninvolved side of the body to be active (i.e., lying comfort-

ably and safely on the involved side, allowing the uninvolved side to be free for touching and fondling).
- Depending on the severity of the motor loss, the unaffected partner may want to take a more active role and be in the superior or more supporting positions (Freda & Rubinsky, 1991).
- If fatigue is present, couples should plan the appropriate time of the day for sexual activity, when a lot of other energy has not already been expended. (Energy conservation techniques following stoke enable participation in many types of valued activities.)
- If the client experiencing stroke has difficulty focusing attention for an appropriate amount of time, sexual activity should be planned for a quiet time of the day that involves few or no distractions; incorporate attention *cues and assistance* into the sexual activity.
- If the client experiencing stroke has a cognitive sequencing deficit, his or her partner may want to verbally guide the person through the desired steps of a specific sexual activity (Freda & Rubinsky, 1991).
- Clients with short-term memory deficits may incorporate use of a memory log if that strategy has worked in other daily life tasks (Freda & Rubinsky, 1991).
- Clients with multiple cognitive issues should begin with simple, familiar activities for short periods of time (Freda & Rubinsky, 1991).
- If achieving or maintaining an erection is difficult, the client should consult his urologist to discuss the use of a vacuum device, penile implant, or drug therapy.

---

sexual functioning or fertility. Certainly, someone with an amputation may experience changes in body image and self-esteem, which can sometimes result in negative psychological consequences that can affect sexual interest and drive. Depression is more likely to be a problem if the amputation is traumatic and recent (Box 17.6).

Low Vision

It may not occur to a therapist to address the sexual needs of a client with visual impairments, especially if he or she has ordinary movement abilities. Loss of sensation, including vision, can have a significant

effect on sexual functioning, however, and adaptations are required (Box 17.7).

Summary

Sex counseling and education from a functional perspective is an appropriate role for an occupational therapist to assume with clients who have a disability. It is an important and challenging responsibility, but one that can be handled as long as the occupational therapist has the proper knowledge and competencies. Given the health-promoting benefits of the ability to express sexuality, help-

Box 17.6. Specific Suggestions for Sexual Adaptations for Clients Following Limb Amputation

- Clients with a unilateral amputation can use the amputated side for support (depending on the level of the amputation) and use the intact hand and arm for stimulating the partner.
- The stump may be used for sexual touching and stimulation if it is not tender or painful.
- A man with bilateral amputations may still use a superior kneeling position (kneeling precludes the need for upper extremity support) for intercourse.
- Oral sex is usually a viable option for men and women who have one or both arms amputated.
- A woman with bilateral amputations can take the bottom position with her partner on top, as long as the partner is aware of how much weight is on the woman, because she may not be able to "push" her partner off.
- Another option for a woman with bilateral amputations is to sit on her partner's lap for intercourse. Similarly, a man with bilateral amputations can sit on a bed or in a chair with his partner sitting on top for intercourse.
- Clients can attach sexual aids attached to a prosthesis or to the stump.

Box 17.7. Specific Suggestions for Sexual Adaptations for Clients With Low Vision

- Emphasize all the senses: Incorporate taste, smell, and hearing into the sexual activity.
- The partner must be aware of the client's exact visual acuity and whether central or peripheral vision is affected. Activity should remain within the intact field of vision to maximize the pleasure for the person with low vision.
- Strategies that have worked in other daily life tasks may work in the sexual area as well (e.g., specific lighting and distances).
- The partner may physically guide the client with low vision to a desired part of the body.
- The partner may want to talk about what he or she is about to do or is actually doing to increase the total experience for the client with low vision as well as not to surprise him or her with an unexpected touch or stimulation.
- Clients with low vision may want to use specific optical aids that have been helpful for other activities.
- Clients with blurred vision may need some assistance in localizing touch to a specific part of the body.

ing clients realize their fullest potential and participation in this aspect of life is a goal worth attaining.

Study Questions

1. Why is it appropriate for occupational therapists to handle questions related to sexuality following a disability?
2. What is the occupational therapist's role in dealing with issues related to sexuality and disability?
3. What knowledge is needed for occupational therapists to effectively deal with issues related to sexuality and disability?
4. What barriers exist within a health care environment that prevent adequate attention from being given to the issues of sexuality and disability?
5. What barriers within people with disabilities often prevent them from asking questions related to sexuality?
6. List some specific strategies someone with SCI might use for sexual activity.
7. List some specific strategies someone with low vision might use for sexual activity.

References

Bianchi, T. L. (1997). Aspects of sexuality after burn injury: Outcomes in men. *Journal of Burn Care & Rehabilitation, 18*(2), 183–186.

Crooks, R., & Baur, K. (1999). *Our sexuality.* Pacific Grove, CA: Brooks/Cole.

Davey Smith, G., Frankel, S., & Yarnell, J. (1997). Sex and death: Are they related? Findings from the Caerphilly Cohort Study. *BMJ, 315*(7123), 1641–1644.

Eckland, M., & McBride, K. (1997). Sexual health care: The role of the nurse. *Canadian Nurse, 93*(7), 34–37.

Freda, M. (1998). Sexuality and disability. In M. E., Neistadt, & E. Crepeau (Eds.), *Willard and Spackman's occupational therapy* (pp. 364–369). Philadelphia: Lippincott.

Freda, M., & Rubinsky, H. (1991). Sexual function in the stroke survivor. *Physical Medicine and Rehabilitation Clinics of North America, 2,* 634–658.

Freud, S. A. (1962). *A general introduction to psychoanalysis.* New York: Washington Square Press.

Kaplan, H. (1974). *The new sex therapy.* New York: Brunner/Mazel.

Kraaimaat, F. W., Bakker, A. H., Janssen, E., & Bijlsma, J. W. J. (1996). Intrusiveness of rheumatoid arthritis on sexuality in male and female patients living with a spouse. *Arthritis Care and Research, 9*(2), 120–125.

Kreuter, M., Dahllof, A. G., Gudjonsson, G., Sullivan, M., & Siosteen, A. (1998). Sexual adjustment and its predictors after traumatic brain injury. *Brain Injury, 12*(5), 349–368.

Kreuter, M., Sullivan, M., & Siosteen, A. (1996). Sexual adjustment and quality of relationship in spinal paraplegia: A controlled study. *Archives of Physical Medicine and Rehabilitation, 77,* 541–548.

LoPiccolo, J., & LoPiccolo, L. (1978). *Handbook of sex therapy.* New York: Plenum.

Masters, W. H., & Johnson, V. E. (1966). *Human sexual response.* Boston: Little, Brown.

McCabe, M. P. (1997). Intimacy and quality of life among sexually dysfunctional men and women. *Journal of Sex & Marital Therapy, 23*(4), 276–290.

Monga, T. N., Lawson, J. S., & Inglis, J. (1986). Sexual dysfunction in stroke patients. *Archives of Physical Medicine and Rehabilitation, 67,* 19–22.

Mooney, T., Cole, T., & Chilgren, R. (1975). *Sexual options for paraplegics and quadriplegics.* Boston: Little, Brown.

Neistadt, M. E. (1986). Sexuality counseling for adults with disabilities: A module for an occupational therapy curriculum. *American Journal of Occupational Therapy, 40,* 542–545.

Neistadt, M. E., & Freda, M. (1987). *Choices: A guide to sex counseling with physically disabled adults.* Malabar, FL: Robert Krieger.

Nosek, M. A., Rintala, D. H., Young, M. E., Howland, C. A., Foley, C. C., Rossi, C, D, et al. (1996). Sexual functioning among women with physical disabilities. *Archives of Physical Medicine and Rehabilitation, 77,* 107–115.

Smith, E. M., & Bodner, D. R. (1993). Sexual dysfunction after spinal cord injury. *Urology Clinics of North America, 20,* 535–542.

Spector, I. P., & Fremeth, S. M. (1996). Sexual behaviors and attitudes of geriatric residents in long-term care facilities. *Journal of Sex & Marital Therapy, 22*(4), 235–246.

Spica, M. M. (1989). Sexual counseling standards for the spinal cord-injured. *Journal of Neuroscience Nursing, 21*(1), 56–60.

Ventegodt, S. (1998). Sex and the quality of life in Denmark. *Archives of Sexual Behaviour, 27,* 295–307.

White, M. J., Rintala, D. H., Hart, K. A., Young, M. E., & Fuhrer, M. J. (1992). Sexual activities, concerns, and interests of men with spinal cord injury. *American Journal of Physical Medicine and Rehabilitation, 71*(4), 225–231.

White, M. J., Rintala, D. H., Hart, K. A., Young, M. E., & Fuhrer, M. J (1994). A comparison of the sexual concerns of men and women with spinal cord injuries. *Rehabilitation Nursing Research, 3*(2), 55–61.

World Health Organization. (2001). *International classification of functioning, disability and health* (ICIDH-2). Geneva, Switzerland: Author.

Young, M. E., Nosek, M. A., Howland, C. A., Chanpong, G., & Rintala, D. H. (1997). Prevalence of abuse of women with physical disabilities. *Archives of Physical Medicine and Rehabilitation, 78*(12, Suppl. 5), S34–S38.

Zasler, N. (1991). Sexuality in neurologic disability: An overview. *Sexuality and Disability, 9*(1), 11–27.

Chapter 18

Using Assistive Technology to Enable Better Living

ROGER O. SMITH, PHD, OT, FAOTA

MARGIE BENGE, BS, OTR

KEY TERMS

ABLEDATA

assessment

assistive technology device

assistive technology service

ATP

ATS

open market

RESNA

RET

OBJECTIVES

Upon completion of the chapter, the reader will be able to

- Describe the prevalence of assistive technology and the historical use of assistive technology in occupational therapy;

- Illustrate how assistive technology can be used as a key intervention strategy within the frameworks of various models of practice;

- Describe key steps in the assistive technology intervention process and appreciate the importance of each step;

- Describe examples of the roles of the assistive technology consumer in the delivery of assistive technology service;

- Identify various mechanisms of assistive technology service delivery and describe the advantages and disadvantages of each mechanism; and

- Appreciate the growth, need, and challenges associated with assistive technology in the U.S. health care system.

An observation Benjamin Franklin made in 1778 still applies in explaining how assistive technology (AT) contributes to better living: "Man is a tool-making animal" (*The Oxford Dictionary of Quotations*, 1980, p. 218). More than ever, we benefit from the unique and fortunate relationship between humans and tools. High- and low-technology tools enable everyone to maximize independence and efficiency in daily living. For people with disabilities, available technologies promote better living along a continuum. Mass-market technologies, such as garage-door openers and telephone voice dialing, are on one end of the continuum; a whole class of devices, specific to disabilities and defined as assistive technologies, are at the other end.

The vast number of assistive devices available today reflects the prominent contribution they make to independent living and improved quality of life. ABLEDATA (www.abledata.com), a federally funded database of assistive and rehabilitation technologies, catalogs more than 30,000 products. Of these devices, a significant percentage is classified as specific to self-care, and an even larger number could be described as tools for better living. Table 18.1 lists the types of products in the ABLEDATA database.

The assistive devices addressed in this chapter tend to focus on personal and home management. As can be seen, however, virtually all categories of assistive technology relate to better living. Significantly, occupational therapists take a central role in helping to link people with disabilities to the technologies that will benefit them. Accordingly, this chapter focuses on the use of assistive technology as an intervention strategy.

The *Occupational Therapy Practice Framework* (American Occupational Therapy Association [AOTA], 2002) all but ignores the role of assistive technology as an integral part of intervention used by occupational therapists. Although the federal government uses the term *assistive technology* in virtually every law related to disability, it is mentioned only once in the *Framework*. Similarly, the *Framework* uses the word *device* 11 times, but never in the context of an intervention. By contrast, early literature in occupational therapy—even going back to the journal *Archives of Occupational Therapy* in the 1900s or the first edition of Willard and Spackman's (1947) *Principles of Occupational Therapy*—reveals that assistive technology and adaptive devices have played a long and pervasive role in occupational therapy intervention.

The lack of overt discussion of assistive technology in the newest *Framework* (AOTA, 2002) may reflect that it has become so integral to daily prac-

Table 18.1. ABLEDATA Counts of Assistive Technology Devices, 2004

Product Function	No.
Architectural elements	1,309
Communication	2,561
Computers	2,569
Controls	1,738
Education	1,980
Home management	1,319
Orthotics	1,152
Personal care	4,638
Prosthetics	80
Recreation	2,250
Seating	1,401
Sensory disabilities	3,209
Therapeutic aids	2,501
Transportation	492
Walking	1,071
Wheeled mobility	1,608
Workplace	701

Note. ABLEDATA is a prominent, nationally funded database on assistive technology products that catalogs more than 30,000 devices. This list depicts the scope of the database and its quantities across its major product function types. Data retrieved January 9, 2004, from http://www.abledata.com/.

tice that it hardly stands as a distinct intervention strategy. This may be true in occupational therapy, but it is contrary to experience in disability- and rehabilitation-related professions. Assistive technology has become a specialty among professions serving people with disabilities. Today, the Rehabilitation Engineering and Assistive Technology Society of North America (RESNA) certifies practitioners as assistive technology practitioners (ATPs), assistive technology suppliers (ATSs), or rehabilitation engineering technologists (RETs). Occupational therapists comprise a large percentage of the credentialed professionals on the RESNA (2004) list. Extending beyond RESNA's certification process, however, many hundreds of occupational therapists have specialized in assistive technology by devoting a substantial portion of their professional time to the application of technology- and device-based interventions. This chapter describes a number of assistive technology practice concepts, many of which evolved from core philosophies and best practices of occupational therapy.

Legislation in the United States recognizes assistive technology as an effective intervention for people with disabilities. The terms *assistive technology devices* and *assistive technology services* appear in many federal laws and subsequent regulations. Definitions of these terms can be found in the following laws:

- The Rehabilitation Act of 1973 Amendments of 1998 (Pub. L. 105–220) and the Education for All Handicapped Children Act of 1975 (Pub. L. 94–142, 20 U.S.C. § 1400 *et seq.*), updated in the Individuals With Disabilities Education Act Reauthorization of 1997 (IDEA; Pub. L. 105–17, 20 U.S.C. § 1400 *et seq.*)
- The Americans With Disabilities Act of 1990 (ADA; Pub. L. 101–336, 42 U.S.C. § 12101)
- The Developmental Disabilities Assistance and Bill of Rights Act of 1975 (Pub. L. 94–103) and the Developmental Disabilities Act Amendments of 1984 (Pub. L. 98–527)
- The Older Americans Act (Pub. L. 89–73).

All of these pieces of legislation incorporate assistive technology requirements.

Examining the definitions of these terms yields perspective on an extremely important aspect of technology-based interventions. When we think about assistive technology, we often think only about the devices. When an assistive device does not work, however, the failure may occur not because of the device but, rather, because of a problem in the services that surround the device. For example, a client may have been provided an inappropriate device or received inadequate training for using it. Perhaps no follow-up plan was executed to evaluate the success of the intervention or address any problems the client might encounter with the device.

Occupational therapists must be vigilant in the methods they use as purveyors of assistive devices. As a factor affecting the success of an intervention, assistive technology services may be more essential than the devices themselves.

Assistive technology applications continue to blossom. Innovations in technology have created more device options, and in the past 10 years the ADA has changed how the public views people with disabilities. Use of assistive devices has become publicly acceptable. "The graying of America" also has changed how people understand disability and assistive technology. As the population of older people continues to grow, more family members and friends affiliate with people with disabilities and learn about available services and options. Members of the public have been increasingly exposed to the importance of assistive technology in enabling people with various disabilities to participate fully in everyday life.

Clearly, the need for and acceptance of assistive technologies has never been greater. A few years ago Vanderheiden (1990) explained that the potential user base for assistive technology and related interventions approximated "30-something million." Data from InfoUse (2003) substantiate the growing need for and importance of assistive technology.

The pervasive use of technology by elderly people in particular is well documented and is a global phenomenon. Parker and Thorslund (1991) surveyed a rural municipality in Sweden with a population of 20,000 people. They identified people ages 75 years and older who required technical aids or who had significant functional limitations. The 57 participants randomly selected for their study reported a total of 422 technical aids in their homes. Each person used an average of slightly more than 7 devices. Mann and Tomita (1998) interviewed 508 home-based seniors and found that older people own a mean of 13 function-related devices. A recent special report by the AARP Public Policy Institute (2003) estimated that almost one-third of people 50 years of age and older who had one limitation in activities of daily living (ADL) or instrumental activities of daily living (IADL) are users of assistive technology. The proportion rises to almost two-thirds for people with multiple disabilities, who cited use of multiple devices within and across categories. The AARP study demonstrated increasing use of special equipment or technology with age.

Assistive technology offers an inexpensive and quick method for people with disabilities to compensate for impairments and achieve or maintain independence in self-care activities. Effective use of an assistive device, however, involves more than pulling it off a storage shelf and handing it to the client. The appropriate device must be carefully selected on the basis of functional need, environmental setting, and available resources. Decisions must be made about whether the device is really necessary, how long it will be needed, and many other matters when providing even the simplest assistive technologies.

The consequences of failing to follow principles for making correct decisions about assistive technology can be costly. Poor outcomes can result from

- Providing unnecessary or inappropriate equipment,

- Providing the right equipment but not teaching the client how or why to use it, or
- Failing to recommend a device because of lack of knowledge about its existence.

When these problems occur, useful devices may never reach the clients who need them, or they may be purchased and delivered but never used. For either reason, functional abilities may be limited unnecessarily, possibly leading to secondary disability.

In the best situations, the practitioner makes decision in consultation with the client, and delivery of the assistive technology results in successful long-term use of the device. Making sound decisions about assistive technology may seem like an intuitive process to experts, but following appropriate principles can enable practitioners to make effective decisions about assistive technology regardless of their level of experience.

Overview of Assistive Technologies for Self-Care and Daily Living

A diverse set of assistive devices and services help clients in daily living. Devices range from low-technology tools, such as a swivel spoon, to futuristic, high-technology items, such as a robot that can feed a person who is completely dependent. The terms *low technology* and *high technology* represent one way to think about the range of assistive technologies. Assistive technologies can be classified in many ways, however. Technology can be appliances or tools that are minimal or maximal, custom or commercial (Smith, 1991). A helpful way to review the scope of these technologies is by organizing them according to the functions they perform.

This section highlights a representative cross-section of assistive devices and services used in self-care and daily living to illustrate some broad issues that relate to assistive technology interventions. More specific applications of assistive technology are discussed in diagnosis-specific chapters of this text. Important in this overview is to recognize the variety of technologies that occupational therapists need to track. Also worth considering is which other professions share the mandate to stay abreast of the latest developments in assistive technology.

As the World Wide Web has exploded in size, links to thousands of pictures of assistive technology devices have become available. Many of the photos available on the Internet show devices as they are being used.

Table 18.2 presents the results of an Internet search on www.google.com. Conducting an image search using the terms *assistive technology* and *adaptive equipment* resulted in 7,120 and 1,020 hits, re-

Table 18.2. Google™ Image Search Terms and Sample Hits, 2004

Category	Search Term	Hits
General assistive technology	Assistive technology	7,120
	Adaptive equipment	1,020
Basic activities of daily living	Swivel spoon	38
	Bath brush	1,650
	Suppository inserter	2
	Dressing stick	309
	Long-handled shoehorn	26
	Buttonhook dressing	33
Instrumental activities of daily living	Key-holder arthritis	5
	Adaptive driving controls	41
Leisure	Sitski	666
Seating and personal mobility	Wheelchair	66,500
	Ibot wheelchair	61
Orthotics and prosthetics	Prosthetics	6,280

Note. Data retrieved March 22, 2004, from http://images.google.com.

spectively. It is important to remember, however, that the publication of a photograph on the World Wide Web, or even the number of times a device is displayed, does not necessarily indicate whether the device is available or recommended by professionals for widespread use. Wise device selection requires careful deliberation and the consultation of comprehensive resources. At this writing, a number of prominent assistive technology distributors do not have Web-based stores.

Devices for Self-Care and Basic Activities of Daily Living

Assistive devices often are used to increase independence in eating and drinking. Special forks, knives, spoons, bibs, dishes, cups, glasses, and straws can help people with mild motor impairments eat more independently. Mealtime aids, a more high-tech intervention, can help people with severe disabilities.

Products that address dental care, hair care, nail care, and shaving, along with eyeglasses, can enable self-reliance in cleanliness, hygiene, and grooming. Independent toileting and bathing may require the use of special methods and devices for many people with disabilities. Toileting devices include catheters and accessories; ostomy supplies; devices dealing with incontinence; and commodes, toilets, and urinals. Brushes and scrubbing devices, seating devices, and equipment for helping a person move in and out of the bathtub or shower also are available. Products to enhance independence in dressing and undressing include adaptive clothing for all ages and needs along with shoes, helmets, dressing devices, shoe aids, stocking aids, and button aids (see Table 18.2).

Although smoking is clearly identified as a hazardous activity, devices are even available to help people be more independent in smoking. Health care professionals, including occupational therapists, may be placed in an ethical quandary when considering helping clients to become more independent in smoking. As a professional, one may express values for healthy living, but it is inappropriate to impose those values on other people. If the client has chosen to smoke, the therapist may be asked to obtain and provide an assistive device for smoking, in which case it is important for the practitioner to provide consultation, professional opinions, and assistance in identifying and selecting a product from among the available alternatives.

Some assistive devices for self-care enable reaching, carrying, holding, dispensing, and transferring objects. Several of these devices attach to wheelchairs or walkers, functioning as generic carrying devices like pouches and baskets. By design, other products hold specific objects, such as telephones or drinking glasses.

Self-care assistive devices that support a person's ability to maintain his or her health and well-being include arm supports, scales, thermometers, medication storage systems, and restraint devices. Other devices in this category have specific uses, such as sexual devices for people with disabilities or products designed to assist with child care activities, such as diaper changing.

Devices for IADL

Another category of assistive devices includes products that maximize a client's independence while at home or in the community. Home management devices include a wide variety of

- Kitchen appliances, cooking tools, and food preparation tools;
- Housekeeping items; and
- Specially designed furniture, including beds, tables, chairs, and steps.

Community participation devices often relate to driving and may include key-grip holders for car and house keys and adaptive steering, acceleration, and brake controls. Cognitive aids, such as palmtop computers, can be used as an active alarm clock for reminding a person about what he or she needs to be doing, when, and where he or she needs to be.

Devices for Work, Play, and Leisure

Hundreds of assistive devices are available to help people with disabilities accomplish tasks beyond basic ADL. Workplace-oriented devices range from computer access systems and utilities to telephone adaptations to ergonomic workstations and industrial tools. In the area of play and leisure, virtually every avocation—from bowling to downhill skiing, throwing snowballs, playing cards, needlepoint, and computer gaming—includes an associated set of assistive devices.

Historically, avocational technological interventions often required custom designs. Recently, however, engineering developments in leisure assistive technology design have brought many recreational products to the market, enabling people with disabilities to participate in more activities than ever before.

Some assistive devices are activity-specific, but other devices apply across many activities and occupational areas. The following sections briefly highlight a few of these areas.

Seating and Personal Mobility

Seating, positioning, and mobility form the core of the largest special interest group in RESNA. Wheeled mobility devices include manual and power wheelchairs (Table 18.2). Related devices include wheelchair accessories, wheelchair alternatives, transporters, carts, and stretchers. Walking mobility devices include canes, crutches, walkers, and standing equipment. Seating devices include inserts for wheelchair bases and support systems for use in other places where people sit, including

- Classroom desks,
- At work,
- Automobiles, and
- Public areas, including public transportation.

Seating devices can support parts of the body and help reduce seating pressure (e.g., with seat cushions). Seating experts often adjust seating systems, regularly using a variety of tools to ensure customized selection and fit. Seating monitors track pressure points to prevent pressure ulcers.

Communication

Communication is an important self-care task that can be aided by a variety of assistive devices. Mouth wands, head wands, reading aids, book holders, writing utensils, writing guides, typing systems, telephone adaptations, and communication systems for people who are nonvocal or have speech impairments all allow a person to communicate his or her needs.

Signaling equipment is a particular type of assistive device designed to notify certain people about specific circumstances or conditions. For example, many signaling products are designed for use in emergency situations. Advancements in this area during the past several years have included monitors for people who wander or who may be at risk for disorientation. Triggered by specified conditions that define emergencies, the devices are designed to notify sources of help. Centralized communication systems linked by radio can monitor or track the conditions and signal the need for assistance.

Orthotics and Prosthetics

Orthotics and prosthetics are critical categories of assistive technology. They can provide a person with disabilities independence or optimal efficiency that may not be possible otherwise. People who use prosthetic or orthotic devices have an additional special need. They must maintain and care for their equipment. It is easy to forget that putting on, taking off, and cleaning orthoses and prostheses often require special techniques and considerations. A wide range of orthotic and prosthetic devices are available (Table 18.2).

Architecture

Poor building and landscape designs create numerous problems that can be resolved through the use of assistive technology. Elsewhere, this text includes a more detailed discussion of universal design. In the context of assistive technology, however, it is notable that architectural elements and assistive technology often work together to optimize functional use of spaces and places. For example, doors and doorways can allow or prevent entrance or exit in key areas, and carefully selected appliances and fixtures in a kitchen or bathroom can make these environments functional for people with disabilities.

Assistive technologies pertaining to architectural elements include bathroom fixtures, door handles, door locks, flooring, hinges, kitchen fixtures, public restroom accommodations, special windows, and storage units or accommodations. Lighting, safety devices, security devices, and vertical lifts also enable or improve independent living for many people with disabilities. This area of intervention addresses the ability of a person to control his or her personal environment. Switching lights off and on, managing room temperature and humidity, and controlling consumer products in the home can be essential activities for independence. To this end, assistive technologies may include specific switches, remote switches, or switch interfaces that allow a person with a disability to maintain a safe environment.

This quick overview illustrates the wide range of available assistive devices. Given the breadth of choices available, the important role of the practitioner may not always be apparent. If a practitioner fails to provide information about a product or set of products, however, the client may not reach his or her full functional potential. As consumers, clients certainly must take responsibility for obtaining information about products they purchase, but health care professionals have a corresponding duty to stay fully informed about the availability and features of assistive devices. Practitioners must ensure that a person who needs assistive technology receives *all* the information necessary to make the best possible decisions. Reassuringly, resources are available to help practitioners meet this responsibility. The next section of this chapter reviews the process for choosing the most appropriate assistive technology.

Intervention Approaches, Including Assistive Technology

By themselves, assistive devices are not interventions. They are tools that must be integrated into a total intervention plan to optimize clients' daily living independence and efficiency. Providing a piece of equipment is not an outcome. Rather, it is one part of a strategy employed to achieve a clearly identified goal. When a piece of equipment is recommended, the specific goal it supports should be clear to all parties involved, including the client, reimbursement agency, and the therapist.

Occupational therapy practitioners use assistive technology with the entire range of intervention options to help people with disabilities overcome self-care problems. Assistive technology practice must be implemented as part of an integrated strategy. This chapter reviews the context of eight approaches in which assistive technology provides an essential component of the overall intervention:

1. *Reduce the impairments* that result in the self-care deficits. For example, if a person is extremely weak and is dependent for self-care, solving the weakness problem would solve the self-care deficit. This first approach requires no assistive technology. Remediating the impairments alleviates the need for further intervention. Total remediation of impairment is not always possible, however.

2. *Compensate for the impairments.* For example, a person with hemiplegia secondary to stroke may be unable to perform standard tasks bilaterally. Activities such as tying shoes may require new techniques, such as one-handed tying. This strategy also does not depend on assistive technology; rather, it depends primarily on tapping and further developing the potentials of the person's remaining skills.

3. *Use assistive technology* to modify tasks, making them easier and more efficient. A simple example is a rocker knife, which can make cutting food easier for someone who uses only one hand.

4. *Redesign the activity* so the person can perform the necessary functions. For example, a person who has trouble with closures and fasteners during dressing can wear clothing that does not require them. Pullover shirts often have no buttons, and pants with elastic waistbands allow the client to avoid zippers and buckles.

5. *Adjust the environment.* For example, a client who cannot use his or her conventional oven because of its design or location might switch to cooking with an accessible microwave oven.

6. *Use partial or full assistance from others* to accomplish necessary tasks. For example, designated caregivers may prepare table settings, provide occasional verbal cues and reminders, put on orthoses, and provide assistance with other tasks, such as placing a bath bench. These actions by the caregiver can facilitate a client's independent actions in various areas of occupation. Although this approach seems least "independent," it can allow a person to make the most use of assistive technology and to make the most of those activities or parts of activities that he or she can perform independently.

In addition to the six interventions, occupational therapists can make use of two preventive approaches. Health promotion can prevent impairment, and universal design can foster continual and seamless functioning, regardless of the existence of a disability that may limit a client's activity or social participation.

Figures 18.1 and 18.2 illustrate how each of these strategies for self-care, including assistive technology, might be applied to the activity of opening a wide-mouth jar of spaghetti sauce.

Several valid approaches exist for developing solutions to self-care problems. As just one approach, technology must be viewed in concert with other intervention strategies. Technology should always be considered, but only as one of several possible approaches that might be used to solve problems related to daily living skills (Smith, 2002a).

History of Self-Care and Technology

Occupational therapists have used assistive devices to help clients with ADL for many decades. Hundreds of journal articles and dozens of textbooks and monographs have been published dealing with this topic. Generally speaking, these publications have highlighted do-it-yourself approaches, described existing commercial devices, or focused on product comparisons.

Do-It-Yourself Assistive Technology

Occupational therapists have been proponents of do-it-yourself fabrication of assistive devices and adaptations for a long time, as is demonstrated by the historical "New and Brief" feature in the *American Journal of Occupational Therapy*. Many occupational therapy texts and monographs have contained fabrication notes and construction ideas for

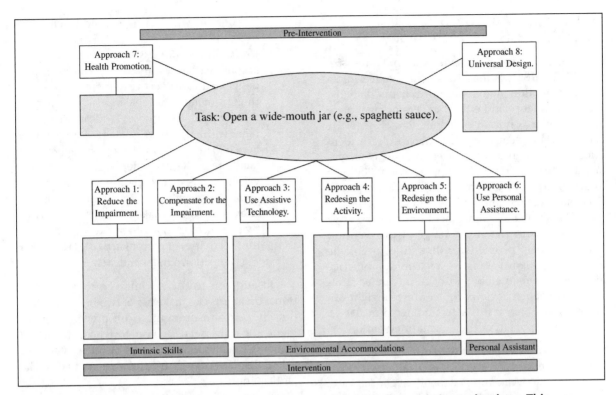

Figure 18.1. Approaches to occupational therapy intervention, including assistive technology. This worksheet provides a blank chart of the eight approaches to occupational therapy intervention described in the chapter. For each category, identify a specific strategy for the task of opening a stubbornly tight wide-mouth spaghetti sauce jar.

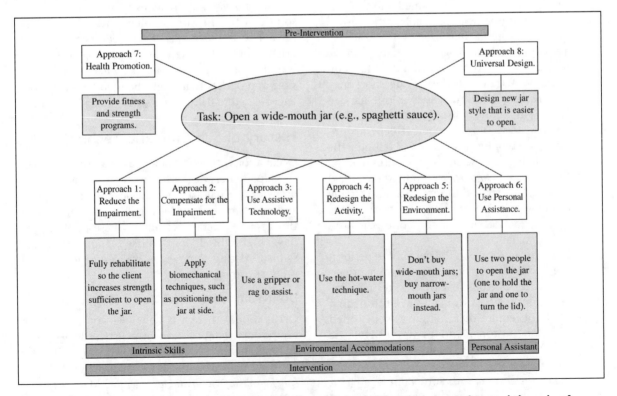

Figure 18.2. Completed worksheet. This figure illustrates each of the eight approaches and the role of assistive technology.

assistive devices. Still, publications that focus on do-it-yourself techniques often are viewed as "fugitive literature," published in small print runs, and not cited in mainstream bibliographical sources. Unfortunately, many good ideas never are disseminated beyond their inventors. Fortunately, commercial manufacturers sometimes see potential in do-it-yourself devices, and eventually commercial devices supersede them.

Commercial Assistive Technology Devices

Computers and electronic databases have improved the ability of therapists to stay current with information about developing technologies. Electronic sources can go beyond printed books, which quickly become dated. Using modern electronic databases, therapists and clients alike can obtain, update, and maintain information about assistive technology more easily and more comprehensively.

ABLEDATA is an important database that has been supported for more than two decades by the National Institute for Disability and Rehabilitation Research (NIDRR) of the U.S. Department of Education. ABLEDATA organizes devices using a thesaurus of terms. Combinations of keywords allow users to conduct more focused searches. For example, entering the keyword *spoons* provides a list of more than 100 products. By adding the keywords *pediatric* and *swivel* to the search definitions, a user can narrow the list to include only those products that might be suitable for a child with limited voluntary movement. Lists generated by searches on ABLEDATA include specific brand names for devices, prices, and the addresses of distributors and manufacturers. By comparing the listed information for a variety of devices, the therapist can begin to create a list of options suitable for further investigation or evaluation with a client.

In the early 1990s, the National Rehabilitation Hospital coordinated several product evaluation projects that resulted in published reports on assistive devices, including bath aids, canes, crutches, walkers, lifts, transfer aids, scooters, wheelchair cushions, and toilet aids (Irvine & Siegel, 1990; National Rehabilitation Hospital & ECRI, 1992). Such product-comparison reports offer a useful consumer's guide to the devices reviewed. For example, a report titled *Independence in the Bathroom* contains 173 pages of reviews of toilet and bath aids. The reviews identify product features and specifications, such as type of seat (hard or padded), shape, dimensions, inclusion of lid, adjustability of support legs, type of tip on the support legs, pail capacity, and other information.

Product evaluation and comparison volumes are valuable resources for therapists. Unfortunately, so many types of technologies now exist that it is becoming impractical to maintain up-to-date and exhaustive evaluative reports for available products.

Recently, the need for comparing and understanding the effectiveness of assistive devices has prompted NIDRR to support two major research projects. The Assistive Technology Outcomes Measurement System Project (ATOMS Project) and Consortium of Assistive Technology Outcomes Research (CATOR) investigate outcome measurement questions and work toward developing new techniques and instruments for documenting the outcomes of assistive devices and assistive technology services (ATOMS Project, 2003; CATOR, 2003).

Historical Application of Assistive Technology in Occupational Therapy

Over the years, several changes have occurred in the way practitioners apply assistive technologies. The literature has documented a slow shift from a do-it-yourself orientation to a commercial product orientation. At one time, occupational therapists needed to learn how to identify self-care problems, design assistive devices, and fabricate them; today, however, the more pressing need is for the therapist to know what commercial products are available and how to select the most appropriate devices. An occupational therapist's ability to design, create, and modify devices remains an important part of his or her expertise, but the need to effectively manage the large volume of available information has become an additional required skill for service providers.

Today's wider availability of mass-marketed self-care products promotes consumer empowerment. Years ago, therapists and other professionals assumed a prescriptive role in selecting assistive devices for people with disabilities. Consumers usually were thought of as "patients," and they rarely took an active role in the process of selecting assistive devices. Today, however, the situation has changed. Therapists now think of clients as consumers who need accurate information to make their own decisions. Consequently, approaches that help therapists select assistive devices have become more client centered. For example, practitioners often use the Matching Person and Technology instruments, which are designed to include the client's perspective (Institute for Matching Person & Technology, 2004).

The role practitioners play in delivering assistive technologies also has shifted over the years.

Most devices available today for people with activity limitations were developed for and are available either as special rehabilitation products, through rehabilitation distributors, or as mass-market consumer products, sold in department stores or from catalogs. As clients choose their assistive devices, assistive technology specialists have become a key resource, providing information, instruction, and recommendations. Later parts of this chapter examine this new role for occupational therapists.

Selecting Assistive Technology

Therapists work with each client to select the most appropriate assistive devices by matching his or her individual needs to the specific features of the available devices. The environmental and task-specific contexts in which each device will be used are critical factors in the choice. The process of appropriately matching the technology to the client's needs can incude as many as 19 steps (Rodgers, 1985). The basic process involves seven steps (Figure 18.3; Smith, 1991). By keeping these seven steps in mind, the therapist can minimize decision-making errors.

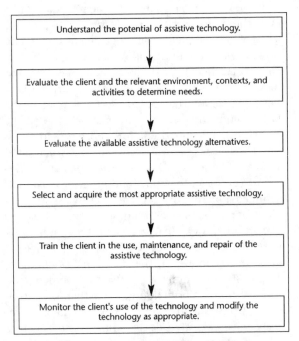

Figure 18.3. Process for selecting assistive technology to meet specific activity needs. From "Technological Approaches to Performance Enhancement," by R. O. Smith, in *Occupational Therapy: Overcoming Human Performance Deficits* (pp. 747–786), by C. Christiansen and C. Baum (Eds.), 1991, Thorofare, NJ: Slack. Copyright © 1991 by Slack. Reprinted with permission.

Assessing Individual Needs and Performance

Once the therapist has recognized the potential of assistive technology, the process of selecting the most appropriate assistive technology for a client begins with a comprehensive review of a client's skills and environments. This baseline assessment has several components (Enders, n.d.). First, all of the activities the person performs must be carefully assessed to determine the degree of independence and proficiency the person has without the help of assistive technology. New assistive devices will be helpful only for tasks the client does not already function independently or for which efficiency is low or effort is high. Second, the therapist must discern the client's priorities. How independent does the person want to be in each of the specific activities? If a client does not share the therapist's values about increased independence or efficiency in functional tasks, then assistive technology will likely be a useless intervention. Third, the helpfulness of assistance for each activity must be examined in terms of the type of assistance provided (e.g., assistive device, attendance, or setup) and the amount of time the task requires given that type of assistance. As a value, independence often competes with the time required for performance of a task. Being able to do a task completely by oneself may not be worthwhile if the cost in time is too burdensome. Finally, some activities, such as self-care activities, normally are repeated throughout the day. Therapists must not assume that self-care tasks like hygiene and grooming are limited to a morning routine. In work or community settings, people without disabilities carry combs and brushes, which they use in various locations throughout the day. People with disabilities, therefore, should not be limited to using combs or brushes only during the morning routine. The same is true for tasks such as going to the toilet or getting a drink of water. To summarize, the person's level of independence, his or her priorities, the benefits of the technology, and the frequency of its use must all be considered. Without evaluating all four components, it is difficult to select self-care assistive technology.

The instrument the therapist uses to assess the client's level of independence in self-care activities must be acceptable from an occupational therapy frame of reference. It should be capable of measuring both the need and the outcome. First, the therapist must be able to use the assessment tool to assess the client's performance without using the technology. After the technology has been acquired and the client has learned how to use it, the therapist must then be able to use the assessment tool to

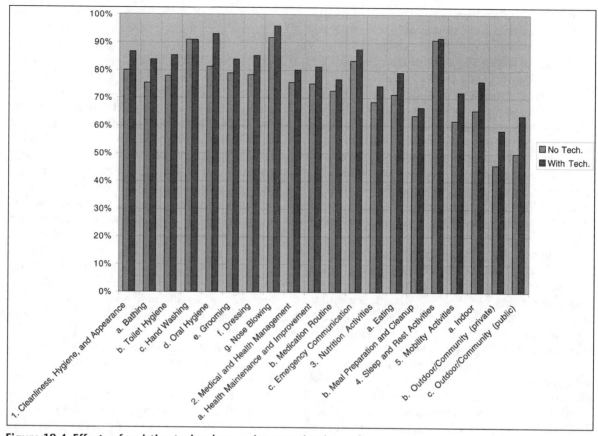

Figure 18.4. Effects of assistive technology as intervention in stroke.

reassess the client's performance using the assistive technology. This process makes comparisons possible and allows the therapist to ascertain the difference made by the assistive technology. The functional assessment instrument also must avoid penalizing function because a client uses assistive technology. Some assessment scoring systems inherently build the use of assistive devices into their scaling. This limits scores on independence and imposes an implicit and unwarranted value into the assessment process, in effect penalizing the client for performing a task in a different manner.

OT FACT (Smith, 1998, 2002b) provides an example of an assessment process that can tease out the impact of assistive technology as an intervention. OT FACT measures the effects of assistive technology on a client's total level of function by using a double scoring protocol (Rust & Smith, 1992). OT FACT distinguishes among environment-free scoring, environment-adjusted scoring, and environment-assisted scoring. Environment-free scoring measures how a person performs activities without any assistance or outside intervention and reflects only intrinsic abilities. This scoring is then repeated as necessary to observe the client's abilities over time and

evaluate changes in performance. As intrinsic scores are assessed, the parallel environment-adjusted scores are observed. Environment adjustments involve using assistive technology and other interventions, such as adapting the task. Environment-assisted scoring includes assistance from an attendant, cueing from a spouse, or hand-over-hand facilitated functional movement. In this way, OT FACT helps monitor the specific needs of a person, not only measuring the impact of occupational therapy interventions on his or her intrinsic performance but also reflecting the ability of the solutions to supplement the person's intrinsic attributes and skills. Figure 18.4 shows OT FACT data comparing performance in various activities following stroke with and without the use of assistive technology.

Identifying Assistive Technology Options

The next step in the selection of assistive technology is to identify and evaluate the options available for the client in light of the assessed needs. This step involves gathering information about the specific devices and systems available through commercial and other sources and gauging the quality of the information. Decision making is facilitated if the therapist and client are able to use the information gathered to reduce the number of possible alternatives.

For finding information on assistive technology, many information-searching methods are available, but no single method is unassailable. No flowcharts or formulas exist to sequence questions or to define the most appropriate answer. Several computerized expert systems that apply artificial intelligence techniques have been attempted but, so far, none has become widely used. State-of-the-art methods remain based on problem solving and intuitive logic and depend heavily on combining skill, luck, imagination, and curiosity. The methods are the same whether the therapist or the client is paging through catalogs, examining files, using the library, or accessing electronic databases.

The multitude of assistive devices available on the market today and the constant changes in manufacturers' product lines make it virtually impossible for any one person to know about all the available technologies. Watching product databases from one year to the next shows that a large portion of product information regarding available technology changes each year. Many occupational therapists feel something is wrong if they cannot immediately provide all of the information needed to help a client with his or her technology needs. Few therapists, however, can truly do this, even in a focused technology specialty. The important thing is to know how to use appropriate information resources to obtain the most up-to-date information.

A focused search will help the therapist locate the most helpful information on an assistive technology topic. A broad request to an information source (a reference librarian, an expert in the field, or an electronic database) such as "Please give me everything you have on X, Y, and Z" usually yields a general overview of the range of information available on the topic. Or, dangerously, an information specialist may arbitrarily define the topic to narrow the search and end up providing an entirely wrong set of information. If the information seeker is not aware of how the information was collected and provided, he or she may mistakenly assume that it is the best information available. An information request that is too general also may yield everything the information source can find on the topic. Acquiring too much information may be unhelpful because combing through it to find what is needed can be time consuming and confusing.

Well-targeted questions about assistive technology are not always easy to formulate. Completing a comprehensive needs assessment before beginning the search helps provide necessary focus. The answers to the questions shown in Table 18.3 create a framework the therapist can use to focus and organize the search for appropriate assistive technologies.

The possibility of biased information is a critical factor to remember when a vendor provides information about products. Consciously or unconsciously, vendors frequently make recommendations that are based on business considerations such as what products are in stock, which manufacturers have established accounts, or even which product provides the highest profit margin. Many assistive technology product vendors are ethical, but even they cannot avoid the subtle bias that comes from knowing their own products the best. Even if they suspect there might be another, possibly better product that they do not stock, it is easiest for them to highlight the features of their own products. An occupational therapist must remain open-minded to alternative vendors and products and recognize that vendor-supplied information may contain bias.

As obvious as it seems, it is also important to remember that assistive technologies do not work the same way for every person or in every environment. For example, a grab bar may appear to be a good solution following a clinical simulation, but the device may not fit properly in the client's bathtub. When funding is unavailable for the therapist to perform on-site evaluations at the client's home or workplace, the client (or a friend or family member) should be enlisted to measure the environment. Remembering to consider the individual needs and environments specific to the client can help the therapist avoid unfortunate situations (see Box 18.1).

Evaluating the Quality of Available Information Resources

Before using an information resource, the therapist should scrutinize the type and quality of its content. The words used to advertise an information guide, directory, or database usually provide a strong indication of its developers' knowledge. Language intended to emphasize selling typically will include phrases such as

- "The most comprehensive,"
- "The only up-to-date resource,"
- "A single information resource for all of your needs," and
- "The complete directory available for the first time."

Truly knowledgeable and ethical information resource developers rarely make such sweeping

Table 18.3. Person, Task, and Product Considerations in Selecting Assistive Technology Intervention

Person and Task Considerations

- What are the major tasks the user wants to accomplish?
- What are the user's functional abilities and inabilities?
  - Motor: grasp endurance, range of motion, etc.
  - Sensory: visual, auditory, tactile, etc.
  - Cognitive: knowledge, memory, ability to learn, etc.
  - Psychosocial: willingness to try something new, gadget tolerance, frustration level, etc.
- Will the level of disability change?
- Is the person independent or attendant-assisted?
- Will the person need extensive training to use the equipment?
- Is the equipment intended for long- or short-term use?
- Are there environmental restrictions, like space or wiring?
- Is a portable product required?
- Will the user need accessories and other options in the future?
- What are cleaning, maintenance, and repair requirements?
- What resources are available for providing cleaning, maintenance, or repair of the product?
- What are the health and safety considerations?
- What funding is available, and are there budget limitations for purchase?
- What funding is available, and what are the budget limitations for future repair?

Product Considerations

- What are the motor requirements (range of motion, strength) required for use of this product?
- Is the product used independently by the consumer or with the help of an attendant?
- What are the size dimensions and environmental requirements of the product?
- What safety features are required for using this product?
- What are the power requirements of the product?
- What materials are used, and are they strong enough for the intended use?
- What is the weight of the device?
- Is the device portable, or does it require permanent installation?
- How difficult is the device to clean and repair?
- What is the process for getting the device cleaned or repaired?
- What is the warranty?
- Are other products needed in conjunction with this product for complete system function?
- What is the reputation of the distributor and the manufacturer of this product?
- Will this product soon be obsolete?
- Are there other effective alternatives besides this product?

Box 18.1. The Perils of Missing "The Big Picture"

Failure to consider the context in which an assistive device will be used can be an expensive mistake. One occupational therapy department ordered a particular bath bench for every client. In principle, the bench was an ideal device for a wide variety of people. However, this department had no real bathtub to set up the bench for trial use. When one of the therapists left to work at a hospital that had a real bathroom setting, the therapist noticed that the usual bath bench was rarely ordered. On investigat-ing, the therapist discovered why: The legs in the highest position of the seat were 4 in. below the standard wheelchair seat height with a seat cushion. At the old hospital, none of the wheelchair users who received the bench had ever complained about it—they just did not use it.

Failing to consider the context in which a device will be used creates practical and financial problems. Device funding usually is available only once in a given number of years. Many assistive technologies are not returnable, and if a device proves unusable, a facility has no way to obtain a second round of funding.

claims. They know that any information resource is just repackaged information about other programs or products. To collect information for a directory or database, the developer has to locate, abstract, enter, and edit it—a process that usually takes weeks to months. It is not possible for a single source to have all of the information available on even one assistive technology specialty. Similarly, because the information available on the World Wide Web constantly changes, it is not uncommon to find broken links in an assistive technology Web site. A database requires continual maintenance.

Therapists also should look at the number of entries provided in the resource. A listing of a few hundred products, facilities, or publications is not a comprehensive guide to assistive technologies. Some directories that claim to be comprehensive have relatively few listings.

Some information systems claim to match technologies to disabilities. For these systems, it is critical to know what decision-making processes are used. Although computerized decision aids, called *expert systems*, may be one of the major advances made in the next 10 years, current (2004) expert systems remain tentative or experimental. Occupational therapists should not take for granted any information system's claim that it can locate the products that are appropriate for a specific client. Automated device selection systems typically remain limited by the extent of the evaluation that has been performed. For example, every self-care activity requires a certain degree of strength, range of motion, and motivation. It is necessary to identify how the systems included these factors in the process of selecting devices. The knowledge base and credibility of the person classifying the products also must be taken into consideration. Increasingly, occupational therapists must be able to recognize the strengths and weaknesses of expert systems that claim to identify appropriate assistive technologies.

The assistive technology field changes rapidly. Databases that feed product selection systems require ongoing updates to reflect changes such as new manufacturer phone numbers or addresses, new prices, new product features, or discontinuation of obsolete products.

Because of this constant change, therapists should investigate how old the information is in a resource guide or database, how frequently it is updated, and how long the lag time is between when the information is collected and when it is published. If the lag time is more than 1 year, a large percentage of the information will likely be out of date.

Finally, it is helpful to know how the producer of the information system addresses quality control issues. For electronic information systems, quality control usually includes technical procedures, such as standards or policies for assigning search vocabulary or indexed keywords. Quality searches require consistency in keyword coding. Systems that are constructed without careful, consistent coding may identify some key products or information but fail to identify similar items that have been coded in a different way. At the least, therapists should be aware that this problem can exist and take it into consideration as when planning any information search. If comprehensive information is being sought, several searches with different search strategies might be required.

Refining the Alternatives

Catalogs, databases, and other information resources all can help the therapist identify assistive technology alternatives. This section presents information about a few specific worksheets that can help guide the search process.

An assistive device worksheet can help students or recent graduates formulate a problem-solving approach to identifying assistive device needs (Figure 18.5). Reviewing this worksheet from time to time also may help experienced therapists refine their own searching skills. Sometimes experienced therapists can fall into unproductive habits. Reconsidering that a particular client may find the aesthetics or durability of a device particularly important can be helpful. The worksheet is intended to stimulate thinking about clients' individual needs and to provide a helpful way of taking notes to document those needs.

Choosing an assistive device usually means involving the client and the client's family in the decision-making process. Ideally, before starting the search, the therapist provides an overview of the entire search and selection process to the person who will use the products. Once a variety of products have been identified, the client and the therapist can compare the options. For example, the therapist might select information about five or six bath benches from a database and provide it to a client to help him or her think through the advantages and disadvantages of each device. A comparison checklist (Figure 18.6) or similar worksheet can guide the therapist, the client, and involved family members or caregivers as they talk about the various devices, features, and options to help them make a considered choice.

Problem Identified:	**Size**
Proposed Assistive Device:	• Where will the item be used?
Consideration Factors:	• Where will the item be stored?
	• Will it need to be portable or transported?

Problem Identified:

Proposed Assistive Device:

Consideration Factors:

Cost
- Is insurance coverage available?
- What is the client's remaining cost?
- What is the client's budget?
- Do other funding options exist? (e.g. church, community service clubs, diagnostic associations)

Psychological Factors
- How does client feel about using the device?
- What considerations has the client expressed?
- How will the device fit into client's body image?

Physical Factors
Identify any special needs for using the device in the following areas:
- Range of motion
- Muscle strength
- Sensation
- Cognition
- Perception

Aesthetics
Note any client preferences:
- Color
- Materials
- Style
- General appearance

Size
- Where will the item be used?
- Where will the item be stored?
- Will it need to be portable or transported?

Durability
- Duration of proposed use
- Frequency of use
- Client factors (e.g., is the client hard on equipment?)

Maintenance
- Hygiene considerations
- Replacement parts
- Assistance requirements

Availability
- When is the item needed?
- Is trial use recommended?

Operation
- Will the device significantly improve client's performance?
- What is the method for retrieval, donning, and doffing?
- Is assistance available, if needed?

Miscellaneous
- Does client have a personal preference for purchase source?
- Are family or friends able to assist with any construction?
- Are there any other considerations?

Figure 18.5. Assistive technology device worksheet.

Ownership of the assistive device must transfer from the occupational therapist, who has the idea that it might solve a functional problem, to the client, who will actually use the device. As a consumer, the client needs to own the device not only physically but also psychologically. If the client does not recognize the need for or help to choose the assistive device, the selection may not be fully appropriate and the device may go unused.

Trial Use

When possible, a potential assistive device should be tested before its final purchase. Some devices can be purchased and designated for trial use and training in an occupational therapy department. Cooperative agreements between independent therapists and larger occupational therapy programs or agencies may allow individual therapists access to assistive equipment and devices for testing and training purposes. Equipment vendors often stock items that can be borrowed on trial if proper hygiene precautions are followed. If a product is not in stock, a vendor may be able to arrange a loan from a manufacturer's representative or directly from the company.

Clients sometimes can order devices directly through vendors with an option to return them if the items do not work (with the exception of some self-care devices). Delivery may take weeks, however, which can delay assistive technology device decisions, and clients risk the cost of return shipping.

Occupational therapists also use available resources to closely simulate items being contemplated for purchase. For example, the therapist might be able to borrow a similar product for the client to try. Using simulations and similar products, the therapist and client may identify potential problems before the final purchasing decision has been made. When a client tries a product similar to the one being targeted, the therapist and client should discuss how the targeted device differs from the particular one being examined.

Use this chart to indicate if a device meets a client's needs.

	Device A	Device B	Device C	Device D	Device E
Assistive Device Description					
Source					
Cost					
Psychosocial Factors					
Physical Factors					
Aesthetics					
Size					
Durability					
Maintenance					
Operation					
Comments (pros and cons)					

Figure 18.6. Chart for comparing assistive technology devices. In clinical decision making, the process of choosing a device often is implicit. This chart makes the process more explicit by allowing the occupational therapist to examine alternatives side-by-side.

Infection-control measures must always be considered before a client uses an item involving personal hygiene. Assistive devices that are stocked for training purposes should be cleaned after each use and routinely sterilized as necessary. Some items, however, cannot be returned, cleaned, or reused if personal contact is made. Disposable covers can be kept on some items when a client is simulating an activity. If questions arise regarding correct hygienic procedures, the infection-control unit of any hospital or health care organization is a good resource for obtaining answers. In today's health care environments, special procedures generally are prescribed for cleaning devices, especially when blood-borne pathogens are involved.

Every occupational therapist has observed low- and high-technology systems that clients leave unused. Home health practitioners routinely find equipment stored in closets, and clients often are unaware of all the devices they already have. An assistive device may be rejected for multiple reasons, and it is important to identify them. Whether the therapist thinks the item is successful or not is of little consequence. If the client perceives the technology negatively in any way, it probably will not be used.

Involving the client and his or her family in product selection helps avoid this problem. One way of doing this is to have the client participate in a trial use of the item. Usually after completing a trial, the client and the family are equipped to make a decision with the guidance and opinions of the therapist.

Training

Once the assistive technology decision has been made, training should begin immediately. If the item has been ordered, simulated training can sometimes be substituted while waiting for the actual device to be delivered. Ultimately, the user must understand the device thoroughly to use it successfully.

Training efforts should be directed primarily to the client but should also include other people in the client's environment who will use or deal with the device. For example, the client may use a particular eating utensil, but other members of the family may wash it. Both the client and his or her family members or caregivers need specific information about all relevant aspects of use and maintenance.

Training should always consider the contexts in which the client will use the assistive device. Occupational therapy does not usually occur in the person's home environment or other environments where self-care technology will likely be used. Some self-care tasks may be performed differently in different settings, such as the hospital, at home, at school, or at work. For such tasks, training should encompass performing the task in all of the client's likely settings.

The client may need to be able to teach other people how an assistive device works. The occupational therapist may need to help the client feel comfortable with training others, including providing the opportunity for the client to practice training. Clients often are the best conveyors of information and training to others who need to learn about an assistive device. It can be beneficial to have the client train another person in the use of the device under the supervision of the occupational therapist. If the client encounters difficulties, the occupational therapist can help point out missing information or suggest other ways to explain the features of the equipment.

Therapists sometimes find it helpful to design training assignments that clients complete independently. The client and therapist can then discuss the results of each assignment. Some complex assistive technologies cannot be learned through quick instruction. For example, augmentative and alternative communication systems and their interface technologies often require extensive training. With such assistive technologies, having the client test the device in the natural environments where it will be used and report back on the trial's success can be helpful. Effectively operating some devices requires practice, which also can be done in time spent outside of therapy sessions. The client can then report back on the progress of the practice sessions.

Training is extremely important for many devices, but the need for training often is overlooked by therapists, clients, and manufacturers. Training also may need to be repeated, reinforced, or updated depending on the particular needs of the client. If a therapist does not set up a follow-up system, however, such reinforcement training may not take place. Additionally, limited third-party reimbursement can constrain the ability of a practitioner to provide follow-up service on devices. In these situations, the practitioner must be innovative in how to provide follow-through.

Owner's Manuals

Relatively few assistive devices come with owners' manuals from the manufacturer. Much self-care technology seems too simple to require a manual, but even low-technology devices may be complex enough to confuse someone who has never seen or used such devices before. Assistive technologies also frequently require special care and maintenance. For example, many devices are made with plastics that can sustain only low levels of heat. Microwave ovens, automatic dishwashers, hot-air laundry dryers, and car dashboards can easily exceed the heat tolerance of the material. To the therapist, these kinds of details may quickly become familiar and seem obvious, but if they are not explained carefully to each client, many assistive devices may be inadvertently damaged.

Some situations may call for a therapist to create an "owner's manual" as an informational tool for the client or caregivers. Creativity and careful thinking are the keys to creating these training tools, which need not be restricted to a written format. For example, a home video of the client using, cleaning, and storing the product can be regarded as a type of owner's manual. Audiotape messages can supplement written instructions. When the therapist provides written instructions, illustrations or pictures often are helpful. Over the next few years, many more user manuals will likely be found on the Internet for public perusal.

Some topics that should be included in an owner's manual are proper use, maintenance, precautions, and replacement procedures. Educational and mass communication research has shown us for years that information targeted to the general public should be geared to a grade-school reading level. Occupational therapists should be sensitive to this and customize the owner's manual to the particular educational, social, and cultural needs of the client. In any case, wording should be concise. The client and family should review the instructions before taking the device and demonstrate that they understand the manual.

Follow-Up

After a client has begun to use an assistive device, follow-up is almost always helpful. Follow-up will be most effective if it is scheduled when the person initially receives the device. With clients who receive ongoing therapy, the therapist can easily incorporate a schedule for reevaluating the use of the equipment. If a client lives far away or if funding for follow-up visits is unavailable, however, repeat visits may be more difficult to schedule. Follow-up sessions on the client's use of assistive devices might be scheduled at 6-week, 3-month, 6-month, and 1-year intervals. During these sessions, the therapist usually can evaluate the success of a system and arrange for any necessary modifications, tune-ups, or replacements.

If scheduling follow-up sessions with the client is impossible, many creative options are available. Such options include

- Making periodic phone calls to get feedback and to provide support to the client at home;
- Asking for feedback on specific issues from other health care professionals who may be providing continuing service to the client;
- Using Web sites and e-mail to provide needed follow-up services;
- Tapping an involved case worker or advocate to provide feedback; and
- Instructing the client to report any problems to the occupational therapist, provided the client is capable of doing so.

Telling the client that it is his or her responsibility to stay in contact with the occupational therapist often works well, but therapists should not use this approach as an easy way to shift follow-up responsibilities to the client. Other follow-up mechanisms often are necessary. Although follow-up is an important part of maintaining a high quality of service, funding may constrain it. Occupational therapists must continually innovate and advocate for fundable ways to provide these important services.

Funding

Lack of adequate funding can be a major obstacle to improving functional performance through assistive technology. Funding availability sometimes depends on the setting in which the occupational therapist practices. Occupational therapists who charge their time directly to third-party payers (e.g., inpatient and outpatient clinics or home health services) can sometimes bundle inexpensive assistive technologies into the cost of their services. Occupational therapists who do not charge their services to third-party payers (e.g., therapists working in school systems) may have a more difficult time acquiring devices for their clients. It is beyond the scope of this chapter to address the different funding options and methods for obtaining resources, but therapists should be aware of some basic information, as described in the following paragraphs.

Therapists should know how much assistive technology costs, and cost should always be one of the variables considered when recommending a particular device. The best procedure is to make sure the client and family are aware of the various costs of assistive devices so that they can factor this in when making their decision. Clients should never be surprised when they receive the bill for an assistive device.

Many federal laws, such as the Individuals With Disabilities Education Act, have opened doors to funding sources for assistive technologies. Even funding agencies that have not yet agreed to pay for assistive technologies may someday concede that they are a cost-effective way of improving or maintaining the functional abilities of people with disabilities.

Therapists should also keep in mind that funding agencies provide payments only for specified reasons related to their mission. To authorize payment, a medical insurance provider typically will require documentation that a particular device was necessary because of a person's medical needs. Educational funding providers will require evidence that assistive devices are important for the education of a student within their system. Vocational funding providers will require evidence showing how the assistive technology will likely affect a client's vocational readiness, ability to seek employment, or ability to maintain employment. Occupational therapists may need to write letters of justification to funding agencies using language that describes the client's needs for assistive devices in terms of each agency's function.

Funding assistive technologies has always been an intricate issue tied to the mechanisms of service delivery and society's perception of the importance of assistive technology (La Buda, 1988; Rein, 1988). Currently, the funding situation for health care and rehabilitation services in the United States is extremely complex. For many years, therapists and clients assumed that health insurance would pay for all rehabilitative and assistive technology because it was designed to cover costs associated with health and medical needs. However, health insurance did not focus on services or equipment designed primarily to help a person live more independently. In affluent times, third-party payers began funding assistive equipment that could be categorized in a "gray area" between necessity and convenience. Today, a leaner economic situation combined with escalating equipment costs and the proliferation of assistive devices now available limits access to funding for assistive technology. To therapists and clients, the issue may sometimes seem to be how to make insurers pay for assistive technology, but medical insurers were never meant to cover self-care devices for independent living. Unfortunately, society offers no easy solutions to the funding dilemma.

Issues Surrounding the Application of Assistive Technology

Consumer Empowerment

The client's role as a consumer in selecting assistive devices cannot be overemphasized. Occupational therapists in medical settings have historically thought of assistive technologies from an orthotic or prosthetic perspective, with the therapist or physician prescribing a device for the person with a disability. This conceptual model is outmoded. During the past 20 years, many clinical and scholarly observations have shown that the client's "buy-in" is essential to the effective use of assistive devices. The therapist's role, therefore, is not to evaluate a client and select a device but, rather, to serve as a resource, helping the client assess his or her own activity limitations and participation restrictions. The therapist then provides options and suggestions for ways of overcoming barriers to optimal function.

Occupational therapists can take many opportunities to include clients in the process of obtaining and integrating assistive technologies into their lives (Enders, n.d.). When the client's disabilities and impairments are being assessed, the therapist and client also can work together to complete a technology needs assessment, identifying what devices are needed to assist the person in becoming more independent. Once the client's specific needs have been identified, the therapist and client can work cooperatively to rank them and set realistic goals. If the client is not cognitively or emotionally able to participate in this process, members of the client's family or other appropriate caregiver can act as advocates.

After the client's goals for independence and daily living have been developed and ranked, brainstorming with the client helps to identify the full range of possible solutions. The therapist can discuss available strategic approaches with the client (see Figure 18.1). As discussed earlier in this chapter, intervention strategies may focus on

- Remediating the impairment,
- Developing skills to compensate for the impairment,
- Using assistive technologies,
- Modifying essential tasks,
- Using assistance to complete specific tasks or task components, or
- Using combinations of these approaches to balance the client's needs and resources and maximize the effectiveness of the intervention.

Having selected an approach, the therapist and client can then develop a mutually agreed-upon plan that realistically organizes and prioritizes the steps to be taken. Should a question arise about the feasibility or availability of resources or skills, the therapist and client can agree on a back-up plan in case the first choice does not work. The plan should include a role for the client in the training and follow-up needed to integrating the technology into the client's life.

Independence vs. Efficiency

A significant trade-off often occurs when therapists and clients opt to use assistive devices to promote functional independence. Assistive devices often enable a person to perform activities independently. This independence can be of significant benefit to the client, both psychologically and financially. If a client would otherwise require personal assistance to perform necessary tasks, substantial savings can result from using the assistive technology. A frequent problem, however, is that even though an assistive device may make it possible for a person to perform a task independently, it may take 10, 20, or even 50 times longer to perform the activity independently than it would if someone simply assisted the person.

Early-morning activities offer common examples of the trade-offs between independence and efficiency. Assistive technology may enable a person to be totally independent in dressing, cleanliness, hygiene, and appearance-related activities, but if the person has a severe motor disability, performing all these functions may take 3 hr to 4 hr each day. By contrast, a personal assistant could help the person complete these tasks within 30 min to 60 min. For many clients, fatigue can be critical consideration. Expending energy each morning to complete such tasks independently may degrade the client's ability to function efficiently in other tasks later in the day. Considering the client's personal preferences is a vital part of resolving this dilemma. Some people value their independence more than their time, but other people reverse these priorities.

From a societal perspective, this is a difficult trade-off. Society can choose to fund the assistive technology, the wages of the personal assistant, or both. Balancing the priorities, goals, relative costs, and likely outcomes of various intervention strategies can place decision makers in an awkward position. Box 18.2 portrays this problem as a cost–benefit formula.

Prescriptions vs. Open-Market Purchases

The shift to consider clients as consumers raises another important question: If some assistive devices are available to consumers through mass market outlets, should all such devices be made available that way? Why involve occupational therapists at all? Paradoxically, an open-market system might not be any better than the old prescriptive system. When consumers buy laundry detergent or apples from a grocery store, they expect to have access to all the information they need to make effective purchasing decisions. Having access to all the necessary information is not so easy—or even always possible—for consumers who need assistive devices. Assistive technologies often are highly specific. The complexities and nuances of the available information and the appropriate applications of the devices involved can make comparison shopping difficult. For example, a person with rheumatoid arthritis may select a particular assistive device on the basis of price and purpose only to discover that the device is medically contraindicated for her condition and actually stresses her joints improperly, aggravating her condition. In an open-market situation, depending primarily on the advertising information provided by manufacturers or retailers, consumers could make many inappropriate purchases. Also, many assistive devices have options and features that consumers find difficult to evaluate, understand, or operate without training.

Box 18.2. Cost–Benefit Formula for Deciding When to Use Assistive Technology (AT)

In calculating the worth of a device, people have a tendency to consider only its purchase cost. However, inefficient use of AT may be more costly than having a paid assistant perform the task for the individual with a disability. The time it takes a person to be independent in a task is a cost that must be incorporated into the decision. A more balanced consideration of value is achievable by factoring these different types of costs into an equation. The elements of the equation are as follows:

- Value of being independent = **Value of Indep Benefit [Value]**
- AT device cost = **AT Cost [ATC]**
- Cost of a human assistant's time (e.g., an attendant's wages) = **Cost AW [AWC]**
- Lost time available of the person with the disability = **LT Available [Time]**
- Result = **Cost/Benefit**

Formula for Optimizing Independence

Val of Indep Benefit − AT Cost − Cost AW − LT Available = Cost/Benefit

If one cancels out the traditional thinking, **Val of Indep Benefit** and **AT Cost**, this cost–benefit problem reduces to being simply a comparison between the **Cost AW** versus the **LT Available**. Whose time is more important: that of the attendant or that of the person with a disability?

Ideally, this trade-off is not necessary. If a person can be efficient with the use of AT, then the costs reduce to being only the cost of the AT, which is clearly the optimal target.

Occupational therapists play two important roles in helping clients be effective consumers of assistive technologies. They serve as an information broker and as a scout to identify other related needs. As an information broker, the therapist can help the client consider his or her individual needs to compare different devices, even those devices that may not be in stock or visible to the client.

Secondly, a client who requires an assistive device for one aspect of self-care often has difficulties with other tasks that might benefit from another type of device or intervention. A knowledgeable occupational therapist can help the client sort this out. The therapist also can help the client recognize the hidden usefulness of many assistive devices that can help maximize his or her ability to function and promote overall better quality of life (Figure 18.7).

Compliance and Abandonment: Outmoded Concepts

Years ago, the medical prescriptive model of assistive technology used the word *compliance* as a measure of successful integration of assistive technology into the lives of people with a disability. The idea was that assistive devices wound up stored in clients' closets because the users did not comply with the direction of their health care providers. Thinking on this issue has changed, and the change is important enough to be highlighted here.

User satisfaction with assistive technology now serves as a primary indicator of successful integration. Evaluating how well a client complies with the prescription has become an outmoded idea. If a client does not use an assistive technology, it is likely that he or she was not adequately involved in the selection process.

The concept of *abandonment* also is being reassessed. The idea that people abandon devices because they were inappropriately provided has gained superficial credibility. Abandonment may be a good thing, however, so the negativity associated with this term is not always appropriate. Clients stop using assistive devices for many reasons, including that they no longer need them because of successful rehabilitation or lifestyle changes. *Discontinuance* is a preferable term because it cannot automatically be associated with poor assistive technology application.

Vendor Roles

Occupational therapy departments have sometimes taken on the responsibility of being direct vendors of assistive technology products, particularly in the area of self-care. Intuitively, it makes sense that occupational therapists working in inpatient or outpatient rehabilitation should be able to go to the closet and select a self-care device for use by a client currently receiving services. As a stock of inventory is developed, occupational therapists can take on roles as vendors. This approach has both advantages and disadvantages, however, and the therapist should weigh the convenience of maintaining an inventory of items with the costs of doing so in comparison to working with a preferred supplier or relying on the open market.

Occupational Therapy Vendor

An advantage of being a vendor of self-care devices is the convenience of being able to provide a device to the client on the spot. When an occupational therapy program can vend a product directly, third-party reimbursers sometimes pay for items more readily, as these costs are incorporated into the cost of occupational therapy services. A disadvantage of direct vending is the higher prices that can result from the department's increased overhead (purchasing, storing and managing the inventory, and billing). Departments may find it difficult to stock a wide variety of items and clients often perceive occupational therapists who have taken this role as salespeople. Clients may feel pressured to purchase specific devices on the basis of the therapist's recommendations or may purchase items because of their familiarity with the devices used in a therapy session. As vendors, occupational therapists may fall into the trap of recommending the items in stock primarily because these are the items that they know best. This bias can limit the client's options and thus may result in the client not getting the optimal device. Po-

tential ethical dilemmas also can be associated with direct selling to clients unless the items sold are sold at cost or less expensively than the client would be able to obtain them on the open market.

Use of Preferred Equipment Supplier

An alternative to direct selling is working with a durable medical equipment dealer or an equipment supplier who has a business in the community. Focusing on a particular supplier can be advantageous because the occupational therapist can become familiar with the supplier's inventory. Another advantage is that the occupational therapist has no direct responsibility for financing the equipment. Clients assume some responsibility for purchasing the device from the supplier, which may lead to greater integration of the device into the person's life. A third advantage is that the client becomes familiar with the process of obtaining equipment from a vendor in the community and may be more

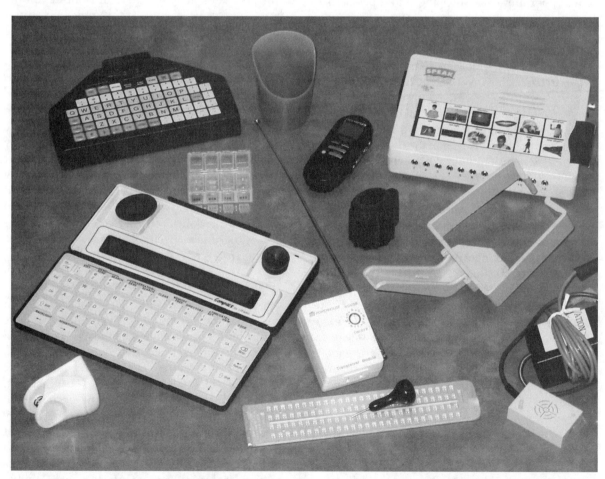

Figure 18.7. Examples of assistive devices whose functions are not transparent: mini-keyboard, cup with nose cutout, voice recorder, digitized speech augmentative communication device, weekly pill organizer, door-handle rubber grip, 1/2-gallon milk carton handle, portable TDD, environmental-control wireless receiver unit, adjustable proximity switch, paper stand, and Braille slate and stylus.

confident reusing this system in the future. Disadvantages to this model include some loss of convenience to the client, who may need to transport to different locations to obtain devices or equipment. Therapists also must be careful to work with or recommend only qualified, ethical suppliers who will stand by their products and not take advantage of clients.

Reliance on Open-Market Suppliers

A third option is for occupational therapists to stay out of product acquisition entirely and leave all of the procedures for acquiring the device up to the client. The therapist may provide a list of vendors or a variety of catalogs to the client, who then makes his or her own decisions. This option often works best in large metropolitan areas where clients can gain access to many different vendors. The client can then shop around to find the device from the vendor of his or her choice. The World Wide Web has broadened opportunities for shopping in the open market because clients who have access to the Internet now can access vendors throughout the world.

An advantage of this model is that the client becomes totally responsible for decision making about the purchase. This involvement likely will foster a high level of product use because the client will have made a substantial commitment by independently selecting and purchasing the device. One disadvantage of this model is that the client assumes all financial responsibility for the purchase. Additionally, some clients may be overwhelmed by the process and fail to follow through to purchase the assistive device. Lastly, when dealing with many different companies, some with extremely convincing marketing departments, clients can be persuaded to purchase inappropriate products. This model leaves the client responsible for evaluating the vendor. Clients who are primarily concerned about purchase costs may buy items from "fly-by-night" operations or from vendors who provide no supportive services. Finally, clients who depend on caregivers to acquire the devices may encounter problems if the caregivers do not understand the particular requirements for the device or do not take the time to obtain it.

Many vending options are available for assistive technologies. All the options have advantages and disadvantages, but the component that allows any system to work is the role chosen by the occupational therapist. Therapists who serve their clients as resources for acquiring assistive devices can take steps to avoid vendor bias and provide recommendations that are based on decisions made jointly with the client. When the therapist takes on this role, following any of the models described here can result in a positive outcome.

Purchase, Adapt, or Fabricate

If assistive technology has been selected as a component of a client's intervention, buying a device may not be the best answer. Another approach is to adapt an existing device to suit the particular needs of the client. For example, a standard table utensil might be adapted by building up the handle. A rehabilitation engineering technician or an experienced occupational therapist sometimes can design and fabricate an effective assistive technology device to match the client's needs.

Cost is an obvious variable when deciding to purchase, adapt, or fabricate a device. Two types of costs are involved in this assessment: the cost to purchase the assistive technology, or the parts and materials to fabricate it, and the time of the person who purchases, designs, adapts, or fabricates the device. These variables must be examined on a case-by-case basis. In some circumstances, such as school systems, hospitals run by the Department of Veterans' Affairs, or community agencies, paid professionals may be available to handle design and fabrication, but few financial resources are available to purchase materials or parts. In other settings, such as occupational therapy units in hospitals, home health agencies, or other medical programs, money may be available to pay for materials and parts, but the organization cannot withstand the personnel costs associated with the designing, adapting, and fabricating devices. When these costs are compared with the off-the-shelf price of a commercial assistive device, the prudent decision often is to purchase the equipment.

Family, Friends, and Clients as Experts

Clients, their family, and their friends also are an important but commonly overlooked resource available to occupational therapists. People with disabilities and their associates often begin to develop assistive devices on their own, long before they begin working with an occupational therapist. It is extremely important that the occupational therapist know what assistive devices are already integrated into the person's lifestyle and what strategies the client has already developed. In these circumstances, the therapist can best act as an advocate and adviser. Many clients and their families and friends have power equipment, innovative ideas, and much untapped ingenuity that can be a valuable part of the assistive technology formula.

Special Needs in Long-Term Care

Clients in long-term-care hospitals, nursing homes, day care programs, and community-based residential facilities have somewhat unique technology needs because they may not have consistent support available to them. In addition, the support personnel they encounter may have little education about assistive technologies and how they are used. Occupational therapists should help integrate the devices into the long-term-care agency for clients in these types of settings. The residential team must know when and how to use the assistive technology appropriately. If training is not provided, disuse can occur by default. Even worse than disuse, assistive technologies that are highly valued by the clients can sometimes be withheld as punishments, or teams may unthinkingly withdraw the use of the technology. Some clients in long-term-care facilities are incapable of being their own advocates because of cognitive or emotional limitations. In such cases, occupational therapists must examine the environment in which the assistive technology will be used and take steps to ensure that support personnel understand its importance and proper application.

Impoverished Settings

Socioeconomic status influences how easily clients gain access to assistive devices. Dealing with disabilities in developing countries, impoverished inner cities, or rural areas often requires unique interventions. In many cases, clients who are potential users of assistive technology have limited access to medical care, even less access to rehabilitative care, and no money to purchase assistive devices. Recognizing this situation, occupational therapists often must apply creative and innovative technology solutions to assist clients who do not have access to more conventional resources.

Useful strategies may include low-cost construction of assistive devices or purchasing devices or materials secondhand. For example, fabricating wheelchair-accessible work surfaces using triwall cardboard or surplus materials may be possible when commercial accessible furniture cannot be purchased. Self-fastening closures can be added to clothing or a wash mitt rather than ordering finished items from catalogs. Occupational therapists who work with clients in impoverished settings may more fully use their professional expertise and innovation in applying skills in splint making, sewing, and other fabrication technologies.

Occupational therapists will encounter social policies that prevent the appropriate application of assistive technology. Policies and regulations are often difficult and slow to change (Enders, 1988; Enders & Heumann, 1988). Occupational therapists innovate in the application of assistive technology, and they may also need to advocate for policy change.

Training Students

The field of assistive technology continues to change rapidly and dramatically. This dynamic state constantly challenges classroom teaching and fieldwork education. Assistive technology represents an area that has not yet been adequately addressed by occupational therapy curricula. Should there be an entire course in assistive technology? Should the information be embedded in all of the core disability-oriented courses in the curriculum? No clear best method has emerged for teaching assistive technology, but two options seem to make sense. First, assistive technology needs to be taught across the training curriculum. Technology needs to be discussed as an intervention option as each type of disability area is covered. This means technology should be deliberately taught in fieldwork education. Second, additional elective opportunities should be made available for students who desire more depth education in this area. The rapidly increasing complexity of assistive technology will likely continue for the foreseeable future. The occupational therapy profession must take great care to ensure that new students receive adequate information pertaining to assistive technology.

Teaming With Other Professionals

The role of the occupational therapist in assistive technology intervention seems evident. Occupational therapists comprehensively assess the needs of people with disabilities and help these client–consumers make efficacious and cost-efficient choices among the available technologies and intervention strategies. But occupational therapists cannot perform this function by themselves. Other professionals are immensely valuable members of the assistive technology team. Performance in ADL is highly dependent on mobility, and physical therapists have substantial information about technologies pertaining to walking and other mobility activities. Speech and language pathologists have expertise related to augmentative communication methods. Nurses often know more than most occupational therapists about self-care activities dealing with bodily functions, including bowel and bladder activities and milieu self-care activities, such as sleeping. Technologists can help adjust, adapt, troubleshoot, and even fabricate assistive technologies for particular needs and for complex cases. Engineers are particularly qualified for design when it is necessary to invent and fabricate a device that is not commercially available. This sampling of team members highlights that occupational therapists work best as members of a multidisciplinary team when applying assistive technologies.

Future of Assistive Technology for Better Living

Electronic technologies will continue to advance and provide new opportunities for people with disabilities. For example, wheelchairs that can stand up and climb stairs may solve many accessibility problems (Independence Technology, 2004). People with severe disabilities may find that more resources, such as robots, become available as cost-effective tools for self-care management. At the same time, the need will continue for improvements in and better applications of low-technology solutions. With thoughtful research, occupational therapists can apply assistive technology more wisely and efficiently. Therapists will increasingly be a key information source for clients, identifying and clarifying problems, pointing out available technological solutions, and describing how devices may be obtained. The information and assistance of the occupational therapist will be vital to helping clients make good decisions about assistive technology (see Mann & Lane, 1991).

Therapists cannot maintain a complete knowledge base of all available assistive technologies. The number of products and product features is increasing at an exponential rate. At the beginning of 2004, Apple Computer cataloged 23,173 computer-related assistive technologies. In the future, larger facilities may hire assistive technology specialists. If every clinic had one resource person with a focused knowledge base, other staff would not feel pressured to stay abreast of all the latest technology developments. In the United States and elsewhere, funding availability for assistive technologies will continue to be important. Awareness of the need for assistive technology is increasing, but the future direction of social policies—and the availability of resources to support those policies—remains a political and advocacy concern.

The growing emphasis on outcomes in health care and rehabilitation may influence societal decisions about which services can or should be provided to people with disabilities. Occupational therapists, whose models of practice blend traditional remediation and compensatory approaches within person–environment models of care, can and must demonstrate that many methods contribute to positive outcomes. Using assistive technology devices and services will continue to serve as a key strategy for occupational therapy practitioners.

Acknowledgment

Marian Hall contributed to earlier editions of this chapter. Her contributions are acknowledged with appreciation.

Study Questions

1. Identify and compare sources of information regarding assistive devices with respect to their value to therapists and clients.
2. Provide examples of assistive devices available to assist clients with activity limitations in ADL, IADL, work, leisure, play, and social participation.
3. Compare and contrast the terms *patient, client,* and *consumer* as they pertain to an understanding of assistive device selection, acquisition, and use.
4. Explain the trade-off between independence and efficiency.
5. Describe an assistive technology "owner's manual." What does it look like?
6. Identify examples of assistive devices that might be used by people without disabilities to enhance their efficiency or convenience.
7. Discuss the concept of universal design of environments as it may apply to assistive technology.

References

AARP Public Policy Institute. (2003). *Beyond 50.03: A report to the nation on independent living and disability.* Washington, DC: Author.

American Occupational Therapy Association. (2002). Occupational therapy practice framework: Domain and process. *American Journal of Occupational Therapy, 56,* 609–639.

Apple Computer. (2004). *Assistive technologies.* Retrieved January 9, 2004, from http://www.guide.apple.com/uscategories/assisttech.lasso.

ATOMS Project. (2003). Retrieved January 9, 2004, from http://www.atoms.uwm.edu.

CATOR: Consortium for Assistive Technology Outcomes Research. (2003). Retrieved January 9, 2004, from http://www.atoutcomes.com/.

Enders, A. (1988). Technology to assist physical function and aid independent living. *Proceedings of ICAART 88, the 1988 RESNA Conference, 11,* 568–571.

Enders, A. (n.d.). *Spinal Cord Research Foundation briefing paper: Rehabilitation/technology: Daily living.* Unpublished manuscript.

Enders, A., & Heumann, J. (1988). How adults with disabilities get the everyday technology they need. *Pro-*

ceedings of ICAART, the 1988 RESNA Conference, Washington, DC, 11, 580–583.

INDEPENDENCE™ iBOT™ 3000 Mobility System. (2004). Retrieved January 9, 2004, from http://www.independencenow.com/ibot/index.html.

InfoUse. (2003). AT Data: Assistive Technology Data Collection Project. Retrieved January 9, 2004, from http://www.infouse.com/atdata/csun_index.html.

Institute for Matching Person and Technology. (2004). Matching person and technology. Retrieved January 9, 2004, from members.aol.com/IMPT97/MPT.html.

Irvine, B., & Siegel, J. D. (1990). Product comparison and evaluation: Canes, crutches, and walkers. In Request evaluating assistive technology. Washington, DC: ECRI.

La Buda, D. R. (1988). Assistive technology for older adults: Funding resources and delivery systems. In Proceedings of ICAART 88, the 1988 RESNA Conference, Washington, DC, 11, 572–575.

Mann, W. C., & Lane, J. P. (1991). Assistive technology for persons with disabilities: The role of occupational therapy. Rockville, MD: American Occupational Therapy Association.

Mann, W. C., & Tomita, M. (1998). Perspectives on assistive devices among elderly persons with disabilities. Technology and Disability, 9(3), 119–148.

National Rehabilitation Hospital & ECRI. (1992). Independence in the bathroom. In Request evaluating assistive technology. Washington, DC: Author.

The Oxford dictionary of quotations (3rd ed.). (1980). London: Oxford University Press.

Parker, M. G., & Thorslund, M. (1991). The use of technical aids among community-based elderly. American Journal of Occupational Therapy, 45, 712–718.

Rehabilitation Engineering and Assistive Technology Society of North America. (2004). Credentialing. Retrieved January 9, 2004, from http://www.resna. org/.

Rein, J. (1988). Technology to assist physical function and aid independent living for children 0 to 21. Proceedings of ICAART 88, the 1988 RESNA Conference, Washington, DC, 11.

Rodgers, B. L. (1985). A holistic perspective: An introduction. A future perspective on the holistic use of technology for people with disabilities. Madison, WI: Trace Research and Development Center.

Rust, K. L., & Smith, R. O. (1992, October). Use of functional outcome measures to assess covariate dimensions of function [Abstract]. Archives of Physical Medicine and Rehabilitation, 73, 982.

Smith, R. O. (1991). Technological approaches to performance enhancement. In C. Christiansen & C. Baum (Eds.), Occupational therapy: Overcoming human performance deficits (pp. 747–786). Thorofare, NJ: Slack.

Smith, R. O. (1998). OTFACT Software System for Integrating and Reporting Occupational Therapy Assessment (Version 2.03) [Computer software]. Bethesda, MD: American Occupational Therapy Association.

Smith, R. O. (2002a). Assistive technology outcome assessment prototypes: Measuring "ingo" variables of "outcomes." Proceedings of the RESNA 25th International Conference, Technology & Disability: Research, Design, Practice and Policy, Minneapolis, MN, 25, 239–241.

Smith, R. O. (2002b). OT FACT: A multi-level performance-based software instrument with an assistive technology outcomes assessment protocol. Technology and Disability, 14(3), 133–139.

Vanderheiden, G. C. (1990). 30-something million: Should they be exceptions? Human Factors, 32, 383–396.

Willard, H. S., & Spackman, C. S. (1947). Principles of occupational therapy. Philadelphia: Lippincott.

Chapter 19

Environmental Adaptations: Foundation for Daily Living

MARGARET A. CHRISTENSON, MPH, OTR, FAOTA

KEY TERMS

accessibility

accessible design

barrier-free design

functional capacity as a basis for design

home evaluations

home modifications

reverse mortgages

transgenerational design

universal design

visitability

OBJECTIVES

Upon completion of this chapter, the reader will be able to

- Discuss the legislation and movements that were the precursors to the Americans with Disabilities Act (ADA),

- Explain why the ADA has had only minimal effects on home design,

- Explain how functional capability can be used as a basis for design,

- List age-related adaptations for the sensory and physical changes of aging and describe how compensating for those changes will benefit a broad population,

- Describe various home evaluations and ways in which they might be applied,

- Explain ways in which home modifications may be financed for low-income households, and

- Discuss how a reverse mortgage can make it possible for people to obtain home modifications to enable them to live in their own home.

Note. Portions of this chapter have been adapted from *PresentEase: Compensations for Age-Related Physical Changes,* by M. A. Christenson, 2002, New Brighton, MN: Lifease, Inc. Copyright © 2002 by Lifease, Inc. Adapted with permission.

One's environment is a major component of living well and being able to care for oneself. This fact is so logical that its significance often is overlooked. The environment should allow one to rest, complete daily tasks, conduct work, move about, and play with as few limitations as possible. Yet, the environment is a "hidden modality," a treatment technique that is available but not utilized (Kiernat, 1982). The people using a space should be the major consideration in discussions of its design. This chapter discusses how one's environment relates to one's ability to carry out activities of daily living and how that environment can be adapted to changes that occur over time as a result of aging or disability.

Setting the Stage: Questions to Ask When Building a New Home

When someone is building or remodeling a home, he or she must make many decisions:

- Where is the home, or where will it be located?
- How much will the construction cost?
- How many people will live there, and how old are they? What are their ages?
- What hobbies need to be accommodated?

If an occupant of the home is in a wheelchair or has obvious visual difficulties, an additional set of questions must be answered: How wide must the doorways be? How will the person move over the threshold when entering the home? Can tactual markings be installed to help distinguish the function of various knobs, buttons, or switches?

When the latter questions are asked, the focus switches from design considerations to compensating for a disability. Such situations have led to the development of an entire set of specialized ideas and building approaches for people with disabilities. When people with disabilities become segregated from the rest of society, however, accommodating a disability is sometimes perceived as something less than desirable. The use of special language in the design field sometimes contributes to this stigma; for example, terms such as "accessible," "barrier-free," "assistive technology," and "assistive devices" all indicate designs and features considered "outside the norm."

Historical Perspective

In the first half of the 20th century, civilians with disabilities were largely uncounted by the government. After World War I, only about 2% of veterans with spinal cord injuries (SCI) survived longer than 1 year. After World War II, the survival rate for veterans with SCI increased to 85%, an improvement that prompted major legislation to address the care of veterans. Subsequent amendments to that legislation broadened national recognition of people with disabilities and created rehabilitation benefits for civilians as well.

The polio epidemics of the early 1950s also drew attention to the needs of civilians with disabilities. In 1954, the government allocated grant funds for research and demonstration projects on rehabilitation.

Through the first part of the 20th century, legislative and scientific advances focused primarily on the clinical impairments of people with disabilities (Welch & Palames, 1995). In 1961, however, the American National Standards Institute (ANSI) published *A117.1 Making Buildings Accessible to and Usable by the Physically Handicapped.* The new voluntary standards described minimal requirements for eliminating major barriers that prevent people with disabilities from using buildings and facilities, including parking spaces, elevators, and toilet stalls. However, since these recommendations were voluntary, they were often ignored and changes were made.

During the mid-1960s, a national commission found that the greatest single obstacle to employment for people with disabilities was the physical design of the buildings and facilities they used. In response to those findings, Congress passed the Architectural Barriers Act of 1968 (Public Law 90–480). The act required that all buildings designed, constructed, altered, or leased with federal funds be made accessible. Following amendments in 1970 and 1976, the act began to have an effect on the accessibility of public buildings.

Public attitudes toward accessible building design have changed slowly. For significant change to occur, social and political perspectives on this issue must shift from a focus on overcoming the functional and vocational limitations of people who are labeled as "different" to emphasizing the environment's role in promoting full participation by everyone. This shift requires recognizing the role environment often plays in a person's disability (Hahn, 1988). One agent for change has been the disability rights movement, which had its roots in the civil rights movement and began to have its agendas recognized in legislation during the 1970s (Welch & Palames, 1995).

Sections of the Rehabilitation Act of 1973 (Public Law 93–112) provided the first regulatory defini-

Pendelter Chapter 19 Notes

occupation-based functional motion assessment
    ROM, strength, motor control
    observation while performing task/occupation

→ identify performance problems & plan client-centered
                      interventions

① functional motion assessment
② dynamic performance analysis
      < person
        task
        environment
③ clinical observation
      (a) client have adequate ROM?
      (b) enough strength
      (c) motor control?
      (d) client's understanding?
      (e) sensory/perceptual/cognitive deficits?

④ meaningful goals for client

tion of discrimination toward people with disabilities. The Rehabilitation Act of 1973 shifted disability issues from the realm of social services and therapeutic practice to the context of political and civil rights.

In 1975, Congress passed the Education for All Handicapped Children Act (Public Law 94–142), which mandated free, appropriate public education for children with disabilities. To accomplish "mainstreaming," public schools had to remove accessibility barriers.

The Architectural and Transportation Barriers Compliance Board (ATBCB; 1981) issued its "Minimum Guidelines and Requirements for Accessible Design." The guidelines established the basis for the Uniform Federal Accessibility Standards (UFAS) issued jointly by the U.S. General Services Administration, U.S. Department of Defense, U.S. Department of Housing and Urban Development, and U.S. Postal Service. The Air Carriers Act (1986) focused on expanding the rights of people with disabilities to participate in all aspects of society, in this case, the right to air travel.

In 1988, people with disabilities participated in lobbying for civil rights legislation, a process that resulted in Fair Housing amendments that included people with disabilities and families with children, and the initial version of the Americans with Disabilities Act (ADA). An examination of the democratic tradition of equal rights was the focus (Welch & Palames, 1995).

In 1990, the ADA was passed. This legislation has been responsible for many positive changes for people with disabilities. The intent of the law was to extend civil rights protection to people with disabilities and to prohibit discrimination against this group in employment, state and local government services, public transportation, telecommunications, and public accommodations (Perry, Jawer, Murdoch, & Dinegar, 1991). Many of the guidelines associated with the ADA have focused on accessibility and concentrate primarily on public buildings, including lobbies, dining rooms, restrooms, and admitting offices. It was hoped that through responsively designed environments and assistive technology, billions of dollars could be saved in institutional care that is largely underwritten by federal programs.

Anyone, at any moment, may benefit from the opportunities ADA provides should an accident or illness result in a disability. This legislation fostered public awareness that people with disabilities are not only people to be cared for but also viable members of and contributors to society. Today, places

and products are being designed for use by a broad range of people, not just those with disabilities.

Assistive Technology

Developing products to meet the needs of special populations is not a new concept to occupational therapists. Occupational therapy has been involved with providing assistive devices to clients almost from the inception of the profession. Assistive technology encompasses the research, development, and provision of services associated with assistive devices (Mann & Lane, 1995). The term also applies to devices created specifically to enhance the physical, sensory, or cognitive abilities of people with disabilities and to help them function more independently.

In the middle of the 20th century, assistive technology emerged as one of the domains of rehabilitation engineering, a specialty that applies scientific principles and engineering methodologies to the problems of people with special needs. During the 1950s, new engineering research centers sponsored by the Department of Veterans Affairs (VA) and other federal organizations addressed other technological problems of rehabilitation, including communication, mobility, and transportation. Now, decades later, ADA has helped awaken the American conscience to the fact that a broad sector of the population can benefit from more accessible and usable spaces and products.

Various terms have come into use to express such possibilities. *Accessibility* means free and normal movement throughout the environmental setting (Pirkl, 1994). An accessible environment minimizes obstacles and provides adequate, clearly defined cues for users with specific disabilities. The term *barrier-free* came into use during the 1950s as developing legislation responded to the demands of veterans and other people with disabilities and their advocates.

Early advocates of barrier-free design and architectural accessibility recognized the legal, economic, and social power of addressing the common needs of people with and without disabilities. As architects began to wrestle with the implementation of new standards, they realized that segregated accessibility features typically were more expensive to build or produce and were usually unsightly. They also noticed that many environmental changes made to accommodate people with disabilities actually benefited everyone. Today, architects and designers are beginning to recognize that many such features can be commonly provided, making them less expensive and stigmatized and more attractive and marketable (Welch & Palames, 1995).

Perceptions about the scope of assistive devices also are changing. For example, some manufacturers have changed the marketing of their products. Nowhere is this approach better exemplified than with the way the OXO Company markets its "Good Grips" line of cooking tools. Promotional materials never mention the tools' usefulness for people with weak grasp. Rather, OXO's entire advertising has focused on the tools' ease of use and comfort. "Good Grips are designed by a fellow cook; they are easier to use, easier to hold, and easier to care for" (Farber, 1992). People like to hear "can-do" messages, and by evoking positive images, OXO's marketing approach directs consumers' attention to their products' universal appeal.

Most people who have difficulties with daily tasks still see themselves as active and healthy (Yeung, 2003). Just because a person has a need for a specific adaptation or adaptive product does not mean that he or she will purchase or use it. People have a natural aversion to change. Also, a primary reason people resist adaptations that are "assistive" in nature may be the desire to continue to be perceived as active and healthy. Using the word "assistive" to describe a device implies a need for help, even though many such devices actually promote greater independence. As a result of these perceptions, people often choose to "make do" until an overwhelming crisis forces them to adapt.

One way for these tools of living to become an accepted part of everyone's home is to change the focus from creating items that people "need" to items that they "want." The OXO example illustrates an approach that can be useful in marketing the benefits of using assistive tools, particularly to older people. Also, because most people prefer items that are attractive rather than utilitarian, the aesthetics of assistive devices and adaptive settings cannot be overlooked.

During the past 20 years, as people with disabilities have rebelled against being labeled "different," a movement to reduce the separation created by "special needs" environments and products has taken hold. As professionals with and without disabilities in architecture, housing, interior design, medicine, nursing, physical and occupational therapy, and other allied fields have joined this movement, the trend toward greater inclusion has accelerated.

Universal Design

Pivotal to this change in thinking was the work of the late Ron Mace, an architect at the University of North Carolina. Mace coined the term *universal design,* and in 1988 he clarified the definition as "the concept of designing all products and the built environment to be aesthetic and usable to the greatest extent possible by everyone, regardless of their age, ability, or status in life."

Accessible or adaptable design codes and standards primarily have targeted people with mobility restrictions. By contrast, universal design has become an umbrella term that encompasses designs that meet the needs of a wide range of people. These designs include accessible and adaptive designs but target people of all ages, sizes, and abilities (Mace, 1988).

Universal design integrates rather than segregates. It focuses on the widest possible applicability of products and spaces, does not restrict its focus to people with disabilities, and avoids potentially stigmatizing labels such as "special" or "different." Nonetheless, concepts of universal design have not been wholeheartedly embraced by the public. Some of that reluctance may come from the embedded notion that "universal design implies it could happen to me" (Leibrock & Terry, 1999).

Modifications that work for everyone and allow us to function at our maximum capacity can be seamless and totally inconspicuous. They may be as simple as an electronic switch or push button that allows us to automatically open and close a drape, a window, a door, or a garage door. Without the button, each of these tasks requires a different amount of strength and positions of the body and hands. Some people may give no thought to opening a curtain, door, or window but find it challenging to open a garage door. Other people would find it difficult to open any of those items without assistive devices.

A variety of tools and devices used on a wide scale reduce physical effort and make everyday tasks easier for everyone. For example, no one relishes carrying garbage and trash to the curb for pickup, but the task has been made easier by the introduction of wheeled trash containers. Having used a wheeled container, few people prefer to return to lifting heavy trash cans. Labor-saving electrical devices also have become common; few kitchens lack an electric mixer, blender, toaster, microwave oven, and coffeemaker. The tasks these appliances perform make cooking considerably easier. These tools and devices make every home environment easier and more accessible.

Principles of Universal Design

With major funding provided by the National Institute on Disability and Rehabilitation Research (NIDRR) of the U.S. Department of Education, the Center for Universal Design developed seven principles of universal design (Center for Universal Design,

1997). The seven principles cover a wide range of design disciplines, including environments, products, and communications, and provide criteria that can be used to evaluate existing designs, guide the design process, and educate designers and consumers about the characteristics of more usable products and environments (Table 19.1). The principles are intended to offer guidance so that designs will better meet the needs of as many users as possible.

A Convergence of Design Trends

Although they evolved from different starting points, universal design and assistive technology often converge in practice. Assistive technology attempts to meet the specific needs of individuals, and universal design strives to integrate people with disabilities into the mainstream of society, laying a foundation whereby environments and products meet the needs of a broad segment of society. At the intersection of the two disciplines, products and environments are neither clearly "universal" nor "clearly assistive;" rather, they have characteristics of both types of design. An attractive, properly placed grab bar, for example, acts as an assistive device to help a person get in or out of a bathtub. When towels are hung on it, it blends into the decor and becomes another component of universal design (Figure 19.1).

Professionals in many fields come together to wrestle with this task of creating environments that everyone may use to the greatest extent possible. The potential benefits of this cooperation are exciting but are mostly unrealized. Consider the collaboration between interior designers and occupational therapists. Designers can learn much from occupational therapists' understanding of the functional needs caused by disability and aging. At the same time, occupational therapists and their clients can benefit from designers' expertise in creating products and environments that work well, are safe, and are attractive for users.

Sometimes conflicts occur. When curb cuts were first introduced, little thought was given to the difficulty they might present for people with visual problems. The focus was strictly on making sidewalks wheelchair accessible. Before the advent of curb cuts, people with severe visual impairments had used the tactual cue of feeling the edge of the curb with their canes. With no curb, this cue was lost.

Curb-cut design progressed to include textured surfaces on the slope of the cut to restore a tactual cue. This was an improvement, but people with partial sight and who did not use canes still needed a cue to alert them that the end of the curb had been reached. To accommodate this need, color contrast has now been incorporated into the textured slope (Christenson, 1999).

Functional Performance as the Framework for Design

When a living space is built or a tool is made for performing a task, it makes sense that the design of the space or tool should allow as wide a range of people as possible to accomplish the desired task. Because designers, contractors, and manufacturers do not always understand specialized needs, however, environmental features and products often are created that do not work for everyone. A design framework needs to be created that provides guidelines for making products and spaces usable by as many people as possible. To focus this effort, we need to identify a group for whom

- A well-designed space or tool makes it possible for them to function at their maximum capacity;
- The performance components lost or impaired include physical, sensory, and cognitive capabilities;
- Addressing multiple functional needs will allow more activities to be possible in the setting; and
- Modifications allow tasks to be done relatively easily, so that any continued difficulties clearly arise from intrinsic problems directly related to the person's diagnosis or condition rather than from deficiencies in the environment.

The population of older adults constitutes such a group. When features of products or built environments maximize physical, sensory, and cognitive capabilities, we are on the road to universal design. Developing adaptations for the physical, sensory, and cognitive change of aging will create a broad base of tools and environments that are usable by a wide range of people.

Transgenerational Design

Basing design on the compensations needed by an older population is not a new idea. Introduced about 10 years ago by James Pirkl, transgenerational design uses age-related needs as a basis for design. Transgenerational design is the practice of making products and environments compatible with the aging-associated physical and sensory impairments that limit activities. It insists that "products and environments be designed at the outset to accommodate a transgenerational population, which includes the young, the middle-aged, and the elderly—with-

Table 19.1. Principles of Universal Design

Principle 1

Equitable Use: The design is useful and marketable to people with diverse abilities.

Guidelines:
1a. Provide the same means of use for all users: identical whenever possible; equivalent when not.
1b. Avoid segregating or stigmatizing any users.
1c. Provisions for privacy, security, and safety should be equally available to all users.
1d. Make the design appealing to all users.

Principle 2

Flexibility in Use: The design accommodates a wide range of individual preferences and abilities.

Guidelines:
2a. Provide choice in methods of use.
2b. Accommodate right- or left-handed access and use.
2c. Facilitate the user's accuracy and precision.
2d. Provide adaptability to the user's pace.

Principle 3

Simple and Intuitive Use: Use of the design is easy to understand, regardless of the user's experience, knowledge, language skills, or current concentration level.

Guidelines:
3a. Eliminate unnecessary complexity.
3b. Be consistent with user expectations and intuition.
3c. Accommodate a wide range of literacy and language skills.
3d. Arrange information consistent with its importance.
3e. Provide effective prompting and feedback during and after task completion.

Principle 4

Perceptible Information: The design communicates necessary information effectively to the user, regardless of ambient conditions or the user's sensory abilities.

Guidelines:
4a. Use different modes (pictorial, verbal, tactile) for redundant presentation of essential information.
4b. Provide adequate contrast between essential information and its surroundings.
4c. Maximize "legibility" of essential information.
4d. Differentiate elements in ways that can be described (i.e., make it easy to give instructions or directions).
4e. Provide compatibility with a variety of techniques or devices used by people with sensory limitations.

Principle 5

Tolerance for Error: The design minimizes hazards and the adverse consequences of accidental or unintended actions.

Guidelines:
5a. Arrange elements to minimize hazards and errors: most used elements, most accessible; hazardous elements eliminated, isolated, or shielded.
5b. Provide warnings of hazards and errors.
5c. Provide fail-safe features.
5d. Discourage unconscious action in tasks that require vigilance.

Principle 6

Low Physical Effort: The design can be used efficiently and comfortably and with a minimum of fatigue.

Guidelines:
6a. Allow user to maintain a neutral body position.
6b. Use reasonable operating forces.
6c. Minimize repetitive actions.
6d. Minimize sustained physical effort.

Principle 7

Size and Space for Approach and Use: Appropriate size and space is provided for approach, reach, manipulation, and use regardless of user's body size, posture, or mobility.

Guidelines:
7a. Provide a clear line of sight to important elements for any seated or standing user.
7b. Make reach to all components comfortable for any seated or standing user.
7c. Accommodate variations in hand and grip size.
7d. Provide adequate space for the use of assistive devices or personal assistance.

---

out penalty to any group" (Pirkl, 1994, p. 228). Examples of transgenerational design are no-step thresholds at entry doors and placement of handrails on both sides of a staircase.

Visitability

In an attempt to incorporate some of the benefits of universal design into single-family housing, the concept of *visitability* took root in the suburbs of Atlanta in 1986. Visitability seeks to ensure basic access for people with disabilities in newly constructed private homes. The total cost of incorporating visitability features when a home is being constructed is approximately $200 per single-family home. Visitability focuses on all homes, not just homes for people with special needs. The rationale behind visitability is that no one should be barred from visiting a home because of the structure's inaccessible design. The Inclusive Home Design Act was introduced in Congress in 2003. It calls for "ba-

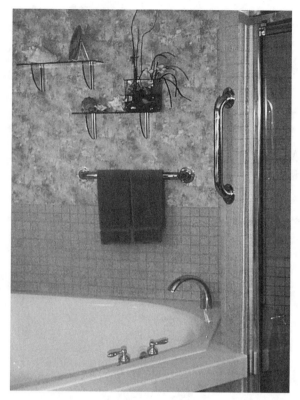

Figure 19.1. Grab bar.

sic access''—at least one step-free entrance, wider interior doors, and a bathroom everyone can get into and use—in all homes built or otherwise assisted with federal assistance. The bill is the latest effort of the burgeoning "visitability" movement in the United States. At the same time of this chapter's writing, the bill had not been adopted.

Visitability features include no-step entrances, hallways at least 36 in. wide, and one bathroom with a 32 in. doorway in each home or apartment. An advantage of visitability features is that they remove barriers for many groups of people, not just older adults; they work just as well for a child's school friend who may have a disability, parents, aging grandparents, anyone with a broken leg, users of wheeled luggage, parents with strollers, and people with wheelchairs.

Visitability allows a home to be welcome to all people. More information about visitability is available at www.concretechange.com, the Web site of Concrete Change, the founding organization (Clausen, 2002).

Designing for Children

Children with physical disabilities that affect mobility, stability and balance, hand and arm functions, and other capabilities share some of the same needs

as adults with disabilities. Children with disabilities also benefit from no-threshold entrances, automated openers, and ease-of-use items. Significantly, the needs of children with physical disabilities change as they progress through the major developmental stages; infancy, toddler, preschool, school age, adolescence, and early adulthood each bring different challenges and demands. Spaces designed and built with considerable flexibility work the best. Major concerns in addition to accessibility include limiting damage from wheelchairs, controlling access to danger zones, and solving toileting problems. The home design also must consider the child's needs for independence, socialization, and privacy (Olsen, Hutchings, & Ehrenkrantz, 2000).

Adaptations for children with disabilities will be diminutive and feature additional components to accommodate caregivers. For example, carrier seating that brings a child to eye level with peers aids in socialization. In the bathroom, a bath chair should be of the correct proportions. A reclining bath chair is appropriate for children who are unable to maintain balance.

The needs and desires of other family members also must be considered. A properly designed home makes tasks easier for all family members. For example, if the child with a disability is unable to bathe independently, a raised bathing and changing table can eliminate the need for caregivers to bend when they bathe or assist the child with bathing (Olsen, et al., 2000).

Of particular interest to occupational therapists are Olsen's design suggestions for children with sensory integrative disorders. Olsen describes such children as either "avoiders" or "seekers." For children who generally try to avoid sensory stimuli, the sight of a vacuum cleaner may cause panic because they associate the loud noise from the vacuum cleaner with pain. These children also may avoid other stimuli, such as rough materials. By contrast, seekers do not respond to sensory stimuli presented to them, so they tend to seek greater tactual contact. Design suggestions for the homes of seeker children include lots of texture, such as rock walls, rattan chairs, pillows, and carpeting. Seekers will enjoy the vestibular stimuli afforded by a front porch swing. Homes of avoider children could include small prints, less dramatic color, and smooth flooring. A recessed nook with a curtain for privacy provides a perfect hideaway for an avoider. White boards can offer beneficial outlets for all children (Olsen et al., 2000).

Baby Boomers: Becoming the Older Population

Throughout their lives, the "baby boom" generation has been a driving force for change in the United

States and other industrialized societies. In 2010, the baby boomers will begin to reach the age of 65 and officially join the population of older adults. If they affect society's attitude on aging as much as they have affected other trends, the idea that an older person must be seen as a person first and then as someone who is old will no doubt become society's standard (Comfort, 1990).

As baby boomers reach their older years, the standards that have been established to determine "appropriate design criteria" will likely change. In the past, recommended dimensions have been based on the measurements of 18- to 25-year-old male military personnel. The standards were based on this group because, some time ago, the federal government committed the necessary resources to compile the data it needed to properly equip and clothe its military personnel. Because few comparable civilian studies existed, the anthropometric measurements of these young men were extrapolated to the population at large (Panero & Zelnik, 1979). As the U.S. population shifts in age, however, the measurements will likely cease to be the basis for design criteria.

Focusing on the functional needs of the older population has a sound basis. In the United States, 70 million people are older than 50 years of age, a group that represents 25% of the adult population (U.S. Census Bureau, 1999). Older adults are the fastest growing demographic group. In 2010, a projected 5.7 million people will be more than 85 years of age (U.S. Census Bureau, 1993).

The United States is not alone in its recognition that the needs of older adults should play a key role in the development of new approaches and techniques for designing products and environments. The Centre for Applied Gerontology at the University of Birmingham in the United Kingdom was established in 1999 to gather information about what older people think about the products of modern industry, what their unmet needs are, and how industry can best provide for these needs. The Centre's motto is, "Design for the young and you exclude the old; design for the old and you include the young" (University of Birmingham, Centre for Applied Gerontology, 1999; www.bham.ac.uk/gerontology). Coined by the late Bernard Isaacs, this motto reflects the philosophy of people everywhere who seek to make environments more accessible and products more usable by a much wider segment of the population.

Older adults tend to have not one severe disability, but many minor ones. They may have impairment of mobility, vision, hearing, strength, dexterity, balance, and memory to different degrees. They may neither need nor want specially designed products, but they may both need and want some modifications of existing products to make them easier to use. Widening the appeal of future products and environments for this market also will mean making them aesthetically pleasing.

Modifications for Age-Related Changes

Modifications for common age-related changes can be divided into three categories: physical, sensory, and cognitive. This section provides a few examples of specific applications and considerations in each category. Many additional possibilities exist. Occupational therapists must incorporate this knowledge so that they can find and recommend products and environments that go beyond meeting the basic needs of the client. "Being an occupational therapist is more than being a clinician. It is about scanning your environment and determining how your present skills, combined with clinical knowledge, can meet the needs of a population" (Yeung, 2003).

Age-Related Physical Changes

The physical challenges that result from aging can be grouped into 10 areas: stability, mobility, carrying items, climbing stairs, sitting, rising, bending, reaching, grasping, and pinching. Injuries or illness at any age can cause similar limitations. Modifications can be suggested to address each type of age-related physical concern.

Maintaining Stability and Mobility

Stability is the ability to stand upright and move about without losing one's balance. The degree of the client's problem with stability determines the kind and amount of support used or needed. *Mobility* is the capacity to move over a variety of surfaces by walking or rolling; it includes lifting the foot up and over a rise or an obstacle. Surface resistance, degree of incline, and, for people with wheelchairs, the turning radius of the wheelchair also are factors in mobility.

A front entry door should have no threshold and a protected overhang. A small, wood or metal wedge-type ramp can be placed over an existing threshold. Similar inserts can be used for sliding doors. When ramps are needed, they should have a 1:20 pitch (the ramp must extend 20 ft. for each foot of elevation). Nonslip wood, vinyl, or limestone floors provide surfaces that are easy to roll on. Removing scatter rugs from smooth floors or using nonslip material between the floor and rug en-

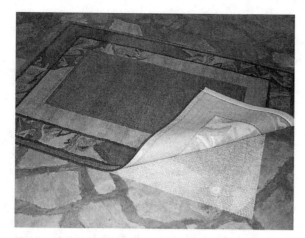

Figure 19.2. Nonslip rug pad.

hances safety (Figure 19.2). Outdoors, ground surfaces should be kept free of ice, snow, moss, and wet leaves to prevent slipping. Ice grippers worn on shoe bottoms can reduce the possibility of slipping. Moss inhibitors can be applied to walkways.

Stable furniture and handrails provide support. Handrails should contrast in color with the wall, have a diameter of 1¼ in. to 1½ in., and be placed no more than 1½ in. from the wall. In ramped areas, an additional lower rail helps people with wheelchairs pull themselves along.

For wheelchair access, doorways need a minimum width of 32 in. If more clearance is needed, an offset hinge will add 2 in. Ideally, doors should be 36 in. wide. Wheelchairs require a turning radius of 5 ft.; motorized chairs require a turning radius of up to 7 ft.

In bathrooms and kitchens, floor coverings should extend to the back wall under the sink so that people with wheelchairs can access the sink, counter, or cooktop.

Grab bars should be installed for use when entering and exiting bathtubs so that clients will not use unsafe towel bars for support. Grab bars must be mounted into studs, into 2 in. by 6 in. supports placed between the studs, or on wall surfaces covered with ¾ in. plywood. Mounted plywood will allow the grab bars to be installed at any point on the wall. A patented fastener called the WingIt (www. wingits.com) also can be used to install grab bars on walls without structural backing. Towel bars are not sufficiently sturdy and should not be used as grab bars, but grab bars can be used as towel bars. Available in a variety of colors and textures, grab bars can be attractive bathroom accessories. If a grab bar is also used as a towel holder, the number of towels hung on the bar should be limited to preserve an open place for the client to grasp. A vertical grab bar should be installed for support when exiting a tub.

Curbless showers allow access for a shower chair. Doors on curbless showers should be installed with a tight seal on the door. A long, narrow shower built with glass blocks and a sloped floor to drain eliminates the need for a shower door. The drain should be located toward the back of the shower floor with a drop to the drain of no less than 1¼ in.

Public buildings present distinct challenges. Elevators are not always easily available to people with wheelchairs. A mechanism that accommodates people moving between floors is the Travelator, an angled escalator without steps (Figure 19.3). The surface of the Travelator is smooth, which allows wheeled luggage, strollers, or wheelchairs easy access from one floor to another.

Carrying

Carrying is the ability to lift an item and move it from one place to another. A variety of carts, trolleys, and other wheeled devices can help older people move items at home. For example, a small plant trolley on casters can be used to move heavy trash bags or boxes from one area to another.

Climbing Stairs

Climbing stairs requires a combination of endurance, balance, and leg strength as well as arm and hand strength to use handrails. In public buildings, handrails on stairways often have a horizontal extension to provide support on the landings. This feature should be included in the home. Stair gliders provide a means for a person with limited climbing ability to move between floors. Some gliders are designed with tracks that go around landings.

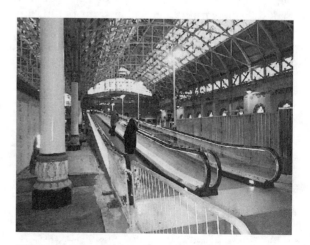

Figure 19.3. Travelator.

When a new home is built, placing identical closets one above the other on each floor can make future installation of a home elevator much easier. The dimensions of the closets should reflect the fact that most elevators are deeper than they are wide. Additional closet space on the bottom floor can be converted to a mechanical room.

Sitting and Rising

Sitting and rising are the combined capabilities of getting up or down from a raised surface such as a bed, toilet, or couch and standing up from the floor, a tub bottom, the ground, and so forth. Designers should consider both the amount of support needed and how that support can be obtained, such as by providing handholds or stable surfaces that can be grasped or leaned on.

Chairs should have wide, solid arms, provide good neck support, and allow ample space under the chair for an older person to place his or her feet for ease in getting up and down. Chairs with a sled base are easier to move but compromise safety because canes or walkers can become caught between the base and the area under the chair.

Tables that are high enough to accommodate wheelchairs can be uncomfortable for non-wheelchair users because they must have at least 29½ in. of clearance from the floor to allow space for wheelchair arms. As a result, ambulatory residents and residents in wheelchairs tend to sit at separate tables—an example of how environments can separate people rather than bring them together. One way to provide common table seating at mealtimes is to insert a leaf into a square table. The person with a wheelchair can be seated in front of one of the apronless leaves.

Round pedestal tables also can be problematic because wheelchair foot pedals often touch the pedestal, preventing the person from pulling up closely enough to use the table. Tables with legs work better and are more stable. Tables with legs often are discouraged in long-term-care facilities, however, because the table legs can become nicked by the foot pedals.

Higher toilets make it easier for some older people to sit down or get up but can create problems for shorter people. It may be preferable to leave the toilet at the lower height but add grab bars. If the toilet is positioned next to a wall, one grab bar can be installed on the wall and a fold-down grab bar installed on the opposite side. If the toilet is not near a wall, fold-down grab bars can be used on each side. If placement of a grab bar is not possible, a grab pole may be installed.

Former tub bathers who need bath chairs will benefit by using transfer benches that have an extension over the side of the tub. Replacing a shower door with a shower curtain allows maneuvering room when getting in and out of the tub and while bathing. A two-paneled curtain that draws toward the middle will close around the bench, reducing water splashes on the floor. Showers may be adapted with handheld shower devices.

Bending and Reaching

Reaching is the extension of the arms and hands away from the body at or above shoulder level, at or below knee level, or away from the body directly in front or to the side. *Bending* is the ability to lean forward and bring the shoulders and arms down to the level at which the hips would be when standing. The definitions of bending and reaching include the ability to use these motions to complete tasks. Bending and reaching can be facilitated by several design features.

In the kitchen, installing open shelves instead of cupboards will make it easier to reach items. Revolving corner shelves can make accessing items in corner cupboards easier. Installing pullout shelves in place of stationary shelves can eliminate some of the need for bending. A raised dishwasher reduces the need to bend. If the appliance is placed under a counter, 6 in. to 8 in. is usually the maximum it can be raised (Figure 19.4). If the dishwasher is built into a cabinet, it often can be raised up to 18 in. This height allows a person in a wheelchair to reach the inside to the back of the dishwasher; it also is beneficial for anyone standing to load or unload the dishwasher. Reaching over burners to get at the back controls of stoves is dangerous. Look for appliances that have the control knobs at the front. Recent safety innovations include knob covers that can prevent small children from turning the knobs. Alternatively, the knobs can be removed when the stove or cooktop is not being used.

Elsewhere in the house, lowering the rods in bedroom closets or placing them in the open in the bedroom makes accessing clothing easier. Shoes can be stored for easy retrieval on a bedroom closet shelf. In the laundry room, washers and dryers with front controls can be raised by placing the appliances on a platform. A long-handled dustpan can reduce the need to bend when sweeping. Varieties of reachers (sometimes called grabbers) are marketed through many sources.

Grasping and Pinching

Grasping is the ability to move the hand into a variety of positions and to manipulate an object with

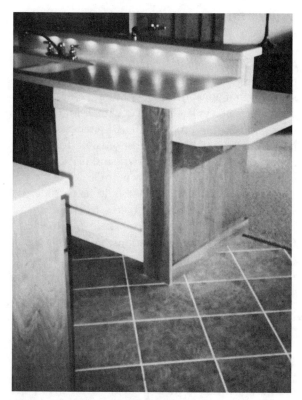

Figure 19.4. Raised dishwasher.

one or both hands; manipulation requires adequate strength to grasp, release, or squeeze the object. *Pinching* is the ability to bring the thumb and fingers in opposition and requires adequate strength to remove or close objects such as bottlecaps or to pick up small items. A criterion for making a decision about an assistive device is whether it can be manipulated easily with a closed fist without the need for grasping or pinching.

A number of accommodations and devices can help older adults maintain independence in tasks that involve grasping or pinching. For example, rocker-style light switches may be turned on with the fist, palm, or even the elbow. Stable lamps with rocker switches near the base are available, or lamps can be converted to touch-control lamps by plugging them into a control unit that is then plugged into the electrical outlet. Both types of switches eliminate the need to reach overhead or fumble for the lamp switch. Lever door handles are much easier to turn than door knobs because they virtually eliminate the need for grasping. The backs of door handles should be filled or enclosed because an open back often has a rough, uncomfortable surface. Similarly, lever faucets require less grasping ability than do round knobs. Lever-handled shower controls that allow temperatures to be preset are

easy to operate. In the kitchen, glassware styles can facilitate or hamper hand function. Textured plastic drinking glasses will not slip out of a person's hands as easily as smooth plastic or glass styles.

Age-Related Sensory Changes

Age-related sensory changes affect a person's vision, taste, smell, touch, temperature, hearing, and balance.

Vision

Low-vision concerns can include difficulties with acuity, accommodation, lighting, glare, sight recovery, color perception, depth perception, and upward gaze. Aging results in decreased *visual acuity,* the ability to see objects clearly. This occurs as

- The eyeball develops internal structural changes, small opacities, and vascularities;
- The muscles that surround and control the eye change;
- The lens of the eye becomes less elastic and gradually thickens at its center; and
- The changes collectively generate a scattering of light that blurs the retinal image.

A number of accommodations can improve visual acuity as well as support the older person whose visual acuity is diminishing. Major color contrasts can enhance acuity in distinguishing signs and symbols; cups, dishes, utensils, and table settings; and telephone or other appliance controls. In long-term-care settings, handrails should contrast with wall colors. In dining rooms, trays and tables should contrast, and dishes and napkins should contrast with the trays. Controls on appliances, telephones, and kitchen tools should have large numbers in contrasting colors from the background. Bath towels, bedspreads, and carpets also should be in contrasting colors.

Presbyopia. Sometimes called "far-sightedness," presbyopia is a decrease in the ability of the eye to accommodate and differentiate details. Presbyopia leads to diminished ability to focus on objects that are close at hand. It occurs because the lens of the eye becomes less elastic with age and the ciliary muscle is less able to adjust the curvature of the lens. Initially, corrective lenses for near vision will rectify difficulties in reading fine print, but correction may not be possible in later stages. When bifocal lenses no longer compensate for the inability to read fine print, switching to large-print newspapers, books, and magazines can be helpful. Published material increasingly is available on audiotape. Magnifiers can meet a variety of needs; they can be worn around the neck or handheld, and they come in lighted and nonlighted variations, including magnifying mirrors for the bathroom.

With aging, the lens of the eye gradually thickens and becomes less transparent, admitting less light to the retina. The pupil also becomes smaller. Both changes reduce the ability of the eye to function in low light. At 80 years of age, a person needs approximately three times more light to read than he or she did at 15 to 20 years of age. Window treatments can be adjusted to help control levels of sunlight. Many types of lightbulbs and lamp designs also are available to enhance artificial illumination (e.g., angled shades project direct light straight downward, and fixtures with incandescent bulbs create diffused light). Positioning lamps to direct light below eye level can be helpful (e.g., strip lighting can be placed under cabinets to provide task lighting; Figure 19.5). Night-lights and small, portable lights like those available on key chains can be invaluable.

Most standard lamps and shades are designed for use with incandescent or fluorescent bulbs rated at 60 watts. Be sure to select lightbulbs of the appropriate type and wattage for the lamp. Using high-wattage bulbs in fixtures that are not designed to handle them can create a risk of fire.

Glare. Glare is a painful and often disorienting problem caused by too much illumination. *Direct glare* occurs when light floods the eye directly from its source; *indirect glare* arises when the light reflects into the eye after rebounding off of another surface. To reduce problems with direct glare, position seating so that the older person does not have to look directly into sunlight. Torchère lamps with incandescent bulbs provide a good source of indirect

lighting. To reduce indirect glare, use lightly buffed sheet vinyl flooring rather than flooring that is shiny.

Color Perception and Depth Perception. With increasing age, the lens of the eye takes on a yellowish color that alters the quality of light entering the pupil. The perception of green, blue, and purple hues can become problematic. Differences among pastel shades often become impossible to detect, and dark shades of navy, brown, and black can become indistinguishable except in intense light. Changes in color perception should be considered when choosing contrasting colors to enhance visual acuity. Care also must be taken with medications, because many medications have similar colors and may be difficult for the older person to distinguish.

Depth perception depends on brightness and contrast; therefore, any age-related process that affects the amount of light reaching the retina also will affect a person's depth perception. Again, contrasting colors can help with age-related changes in depth perception. From a distance, any item that contrasts with its background will be easier to perceive (another reason why seating should contrast with the color of the floor). Providing color contrast between the edge of the bathtub, the floor, and the inside of the tub enhances safety by providing stronger visual cues. In long-term-care facilities, pictures, objects, and signs should be large and positioned about 20 ft. apart so that they can be easily distinguished.

Highlight the edges of steps, particularly top and bottom steps. Outdoor steps or stairs leading to a basement can be marked with tape or paint. On carpeted stairs, place stair lights along the steps, with switches at both the top and the bottom of the stairs. Carpet or rug colors and patterns also should be selected to minimize confusion: To an older person, sections of markedly darker color on the floor may appear recessed, which may prompt the person to try to step down. Lighter patterns may appear elevated, causing the person to attempt to step up.

In an older person, the amount of time required for the eye to adjust when moving from a dark area into a light area or vice versa is markedly increased. Light intensity also affects adjustment time: The greater the contrast is, the more time that is required. For those reasons, objects should not be placed in entryways, and lighting should be designed to avoid sudden changes in light levels.

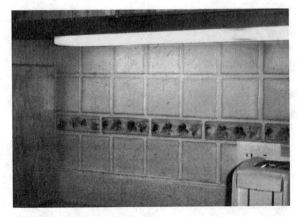

Figure 19.5. Strip lighting.

Areas should be illuminated before anyone steps inside.

Upward Gaze. The ability to see items that are placed above eye level often becomes limited as people age. This phenomenon may be caused by multiple problems, including increased age; the failure of the eyelid to open as widely as when the person was younger; a forward inclination of the head, reflecting weakened neck muscles; or a forward tilt of the entire upper body because of osteoporosis. To offset difficulties with upward gaze, place important signage, like directional signs or numbers, within the person's field of vision. Ideally, signs should be placed about 3½ ft. to 5 ft. above the floor. In some situations, placing directional signs on the floor itself may be helpful.

Taste and Smell

A person's taste buds distinguish sweet, salty, bitter, and sour flavors. The taste buds for those flavors are located from front to back on the tongue, and they lose sensation in that order (i.e., the first taste buds to lose their sensitivity are the sweet taste buds). Two thirds of our response to taste lies in our sense of smell. Food aromas can change mere acceptance into appreciation of flavor. The sense of smell affords both protection and pleasure and often generates associations with past experiences.

Older adults may lose sensitivity to body and household odors. A reduced ability to smell smoke or gas fumes can become a safety concern, as can difficulty in distinguishing spoiled food. Visual signaling devices can be installed to enhance smoke detectors and natural gas leak detectors for older people who also have difficulty with hearing. Other helpful accommodations related to smell include reprinting expiration dates on food packaging with a marking pen using large numbers or labeling refrigerator shelves for each week of the month and placing food on the designated shelves. Check perishable items every 2 weeks to be sure expired items are being discarded.

Tactual and Temperature Cues

Sensory input conducted through the skin is subdivided into the touch and tactual systems. Touch is used for awareness and protective responses. Tactual input is used to interact with the environment. Tactual input has implications for environmental design. In long-term-care environments, familiar themes such as wood carvings and wall hangings can incorporate textures into the environment. Any textured wall decoration should be cleanable and fire retardant. Temperature sensitivity also decreases with age. Because an older person's responsiveness to heat and cold is diminished, accidental scalding can become a danger. Settings for hot water heaters should not exceed 120 degrees.

Hearing

As people age, their ability to hear high-frequency sounds, as well as sounds in general, diminishes. Hearing aids have been developed that amplify sound at different frequencies, but many hearing aids also transmit confusing background noise. A variety of signaling devices are available to alert people with hearing impairments to sounds in the environment. In-depth information about hearing loss and hearing aids can be obtained from the National Institute on Deafness and Other Communication Disorders (www.nidcd.nih.gov).

Older people may find discerning consonant sounds more difficult than distinguishing between vowel sounds. When speaking to an older person with hearing impairment, it can be helpful to

- Move closer to the person,
- Speak more slowly,
- Allow a longer separation between words,
- Use a slightly louder voice, and
- Consciously lower your vocal tone.

Carpeting in corridors and other noisy areas helps reduce distracting ambient noise. Acoustical panels placed around small groupings of tables in a dining room also can make it easier for older adults to hear each other when conversing (Figure 19.6).

Kinesthesia

Kinesthesia, the position sense of muscles, tendons, and joints, includes proprioceptive and vestibular

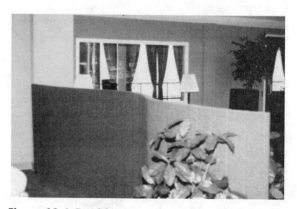

Figure 19.6. Partition.

input and is affected by the aging process. Proprioception is discussed under "balance" in the modifications for age-related physical changes section of this chapter. *Vestibular input* relates to the way a portion of the inner ear helps a person determine the position of his or her head in space. With age, this internal orienting mechanism can become less reliable. Problems with kinesthesia can contribute to difficulties with falls and, in subtle ways, with a person's sense of orientation in space. Environmental adaptations can compensate for certain losses in these senses (Birren & Schaie, 1977). For example, when a person's detection of vertical movement has become compromised, signage or other cues indicating the identity of the exact floor must be obvious when he or she gets off an elevator.

Age-Related Cognitive Changes

Specific interventions are crucial for clients with dementia as well as their caregivers. Everyone, however, can benefit from adaptations that assist memory, such as automatic shutoff switches on small appliances and effective directional cues in corridors.

People with dementia most likely experience certain sensory and physical changes, but in dealing with the specific manifestations related to the dementia, other age-related changes often are overlooked. Before specific environmental adaptations are made for people with dementia, the environment should be assessed and changes made that compensate for general age-related changes. When modifications for age-related changes are made, behaviors associated with the cognitive difficulties often are reduced. When modifications or additions to the environment reduce problematic behavior, they also make the role of the caregiver easier.

Adaptations recommended for people with dementia include safety awareness, way finding, reducing confrontation, visual cues, promoting memory and reminiscing, medication management, providing reassurance and support, avoiding confrontations, creating a calm environment, and addressing wandering.

Basic Safety Issues

Always the first consideration in any home modification, basic safety includes the security of the person as well as general security from outside forces. Trim foliage near windows and add prickly bushes, such as holly, fire bush, roses, Russian olive, bougainvillea, or similar plantings to eliminate hiding places for burglars. Always select nonpoisonous plants for outdoor and indoor locations. In the kitchen, remove flammable items that might be placed on the stove or

stored in the oven. If possible, select appliances with automatically timed shutoff switches.

Orientation

Everyone relies on signs and landmarks to find one's way through unfamiliar territory. For the person with cognitive difficulties, consistent cues become crucial and should be thoughtfully incorporated into the daily environment. For example, in long-term-care facilities, landmarks (any building design, item, or picture that helps identify a specific place) should be placed in conspicuous places on the corridor walls, where they can be used for cuing. Architectural configurations might include the barber shop, coffee shop, library, and so on. Interior landmarks may include specific items, such as a grandfather clock, a mailbox, or a jukebox. Ideally, large pictures should be of familiar scenes. All landmarks should have distinctive, easily recognized colors and offer good contrast with the surroundings.

In multifloored residences, determining which floor one is on can be challenging, particularly to someone with cognitive or kinesthetic challenges. From inside an elevator, the space immediately outside the elevator should appear markedly different on each floor. Signs by the doors of residents' rooms should be positioned at their eye level. Signs should provide effective contrast between the numbers or letters and the background colors, and numbers should be at least 2 in. high. It also can be helpful to provide space on the signs for small personal mementos or allow wall space on which such mementos can be placed.

Importance of Visual Cues

Beyond adapting for age-related visual changes, arrangement of items helps the person with dementia with activities of daily living. Planning and organizing the environment with this in mind can reduce some frustrations. For example, grouping items that are used together in the same place, such as placing a shirt and pants for one outfit on the same hanger, can help with functioning. Similarly, a person's toothbrush and toothpaste can be grouped on a vanity counter, a water glass and water pitcher can be grouped on a table, and so forth. Another strategy is to put clothing of one type in a drawer, which can be labeled if the person still understands the meaning of written words. A third strategy may be to place clothing in open baskets, where it can be readily seen.

Products and ideas that compensate for short-term memory loss can be helpful. Some items also may stimulate long-term memory. To help clients with orientation to people, time, and place, use photograph albums with labels of people and places to stimulate long-term memory. Provide maps for residents to use to show where they were born or where significant events in their life took place. A calendar on which days are marked off can help orient a person to time. Sometimes clients will retain the meanings of certain symbols, such as flags or items of ethnic significance. Such items can be used to elicit discussion.

People with cognitive difficulties like dementia may have problems with taking (and not taking) medications. Consider a variety of tools and techniques to ensure proper adherence to medication regimens, from simple reminders and organizers to measures designed specifically to prevent overmedication.

Reassurance and Support

Products and measures that provide reassurance can increase peace of mind for clients with dementia as well as their caregivers. Interventions may be as simple as compiling information about where to go or whom to call for information or establishing procedures to ensure that help will be available in an emergency. People and technology can help in preparing emergency plans. For information about the emergency response system, the best source is the client's local hospital. Soon, cell phone technology will help monitor people with dementia. Telephones in which picture inserts replace the speed dial buttons provide photo cues and links to significant people when even programmed numbers might be forgotten.

It is possible to identify and avoid many situations that might lead to major confrontations. In a confrontation, a client's responses may escalate to what are referred to as "catastrophic reactions." Each person with dementia may respond differently to a set of circumstances. Attempting to view the environment from the perspective of the client can be helpful. Whenever a potential problem is identified, eliminate it if at all possible, as in the following examples:

- Some clients inappropriately remove their clothes; in response, caregivers often reverse regular clothing to make it more difficult to remove. Doing so, however, may be irritating to the client and thus worsen the problem, because the clothing will not fit properly. Instead, caregivers should purchase clothing designed with zippers in back.
- Bed rails may not be practical for every person in a long-term-care facility. If the client attempts to crawl over them, the mattress can

be placed on the floor. It may be necessary to obtain a waiver to do this.

- If the client uses objects for different purposes (e.g., mistaking a water fountain for a urinal or a wastebasket for a toilet), consider removing the items or making changes that reduce the likelihood that the client will encounter the objects. For example, rather than have the client walk to the water fountain to get a drink and risk becoming confused, place a plastic pitcher of water and glasses in a convenient place.
- The resident's inability to discern colors that do not contrast may allow you to camouflage doors to storage and linen closets by making the signs and the wall the same color.
- Install magnet locks on doors to cupboards where harmful or fragile items are kept. Magnet locks keep the door locked until a magnet is placed on the door opposite the lock to release the catch mechanism.
- Design the environment with calming colors and include tranquil motifs. Moving water has a calming effect. If an artificial pond or stream will be part of the landscaping, the depth of the stream should be less than 1 in., and pebbles should be embedded in the concrete bed of the pond or stream. Large, immovable stones also may be added.

Movement and Wandering

The client with dementia often has an ingrained need for movement. This need may play itself out as wandering. Providing a place where the client can expend excess energy therefore can be beneficial. Ideally, an enclosed, safe outdoor area will allow the client to move about freely. A circular path is best, with no dead ends or points where decisions must be made about which way to go. The walkway shown in Figure 19.7 goes around the house to another door.

The Alzheimer's Association makes available a variety of person identifiers, including pendants, bracelets, key chains, and clothing labels. Identification is available for caregivers as well as for the person with dementia.

Home Evaluations

When chronic health conditions coexist with age-related changes, the therapist must work with the client or family to identify the specific home modifications needed. When accidents or other major health problems result in disability, a client-focused directive to make the correct design changes should take place. To accomplish this task, a thorough

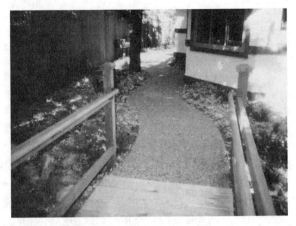

Figure 19.7. Walkway.

home evaluation is crucial to determine the best course of action for treatment and discharge. The home evaluation provides a means of communicating with the client and incorporating his or her specific wants and desires. Effective communication skills are critical in understanding clients' needs and priorities (Duncan, 2002).

A home evaluation should include an assessment of the needs of the caregiver. A survey by the Administration on Aging (2002), identified more than 7 million caregivers in the United States. Environmental coping strategies not only support the older person but also ease the demands on the caregiver. Many home modifications and assistive devices can provide this additional assistance (Overton, Pynoos, & Sabata, 2003).

The occupational therapist is a valuable member of the assessment team. Occupational therapy expertise can lead to an assessment that more thoroughly accounts for the complexities of the client's functional concerns. Many client homes were built more than 40 years ago and do not compensate for lifestyle changes. Most such homes were built without universal design principles, so they have features such as steep stairs, poor lighting, raised thresholds, and doorknobs. Living independently involves two key variables: physical function and environmental barriers. Fixing either variable mitigates barriers to independence. When products and spaces are based on universal design principles, they meet the broadest range of individual needs as possible.

A thorough assessment of the home is necessary to determine the exact needs of the person and any caregivers (see chapter 3). The client's needs must drive the decisions about environmental design. The key to effective design is to develop a plan that can grow and change with the needs of the client and the family (Duncan, 2003).

The type of home evaluation depends on several factors, including time and funding available; detail required; expertise of the builder, remodeler, or designer; and client diagnosis, health complications, and prognosis. To encompass as many of these factors as possible, the ideal home assessment team includes the building contractor, designer, occupational therapist, client, and, when appropriate, client's family (Duncan, 2002).

Performing a home evaluation historically has been a part of occupational practice, and many therapists have created their own forms. Most home evaluations created by various organizations are in a paper-and-pencil format. These checklists ask questions about the home, but they do not ask questions about the client. The resources listed in the following section are intended to provide the reader with additional ideas for home evaluation.

Home Evaluation Checklists

"The Accessible Home," a pocket-sized checklist in booklet form, organizes information about what features must be addressed immediately and what may be considered in the future when buying or remodeling a home may improve accessibility. This checklist includes useful information about the various areas of the home and which items should be considered. Each recommendation is followed by a brief rationale stating why the suggestion has been included (Lasoff & Lorentzen, 2003).

Many organizations have created their own home evaluation checklists. The following Web sites provide home environment checklists or resources for developing a customized checklist. If a paper-and-pencil checklist is adequate for your needs, these checklists may provide you with ideas upon which you can expand.

- **Safety for Older Consumers Home Safety Checklist (www.cpsc.gov/cpscpub/pubs/ 701. htm).** In 1981, the U.S. Consumer Product Safety Commission (CPSC) developed a checklist. Researchers had estimated that more than 622,000 people over the age of 65 were treated in hospital emergency rooms for injuries associated with products they lived with and used every day. CPSC believed that many of these injuries resulted from easily overlooked hazards in the home and that finding and fixing some of those hazards might prevent many injuries. CPSC developed the consumer checklist to help spot possible home safety hazards.
- **AARP's Rate Your Home Checklist (www. aarp.org/life/homedesign/ratehome).**

Following the principles of universal design, AARP has developed an easy-to-use online checklist organized by areas of the house. Although simple alterations can prevent home accidents, the changes suggested enhance comfort and can increase the likelihood of an older person remaining independent in his or her home and community. Questions about each room prompt the user to identify ideas for improvement and match these with lifestyle. Following the sections on each room is a section on challenges that many people face. This section includes possible solutions that incorporate universal design features. The AARP Web site has other information related to universal design, including an interactive tour of a home.

- **Center for Universal Design (www.design. ncsu.edu/cud).** The Center for Universal Design has guidelines for home modifications and universal design and offers information packages on ADA-related issues. The organization's "Technical Assistance Packs" are a source of home modification information. Assistance packs have been developed on each area in and around the home, including decks, porches, patios, and balconies; doors and doorways; bathrooms; and kitchens. The packs include definitions, standards, design elements, materials, and furnishings and incorporate detailed and dimensioned drawings. They show how to make housing more accessible, whether a single- or multifamily residence or new or existing construction. The information packs are invaluable for anyone involved in designing in-depth home modifications.
- **Practical Guide to Universal Home Design (www.wilder.org/research/reports/pdf/ude sign6-02.pdf).** This online guide lists commonsense features that can make a home a more pleasant place to live. A hard-copy version of the guide also is available (SAIL, 2002). Including these features in a home when it is built can help the homeowner avoid unnecessary changes later. The checklist provides room-by-room options.
- **Home Modifications Assessment and Solutions Checklist by Rebuilding Together® (1998; www.rebuildingtogether.org/home_ modifications/house_assessment_check list.shtml).** This online checklist focuses on accessibility issues that face homeowners and their families, including fall hazards. Button

links connect to possible solutions that can help the homeowner prioritize tasks.
- **GEM (available at www.cornellaging.org/ gem/assessments_environmental.html).** Gerontologic Environmental Modifications (GEM; Cornell University, Weill Medical College, 2000) is a downloadable checklist that provides a comprehensive walk-through of the home environment. GEM includes questions about various potential obstacles and hazards along with questions to prompt a return visit to indicate whether the problem has been corrected.
- **The National Resource Center on Supportive Housing and Home Modification at the Ethel Percy Andrus Gerontology Center at the University of Southern California (www.homemods.org).** This organization plays a role in research and education on housing and maintains a clearinghouse for reports, guides, and fact sheets on supportive housing and home modifications. The Web site has links to hundreds of other resources in this topic area.

Beyond Home Evaluation Checklists

The following assessment tools provide more directions and information than typical paper-and-pencil checklists. They are available in hard copy as well as online. Some of the tools are downloadable, others are interactive, and still others are available as software. Comprehensive Assessment and Solution Process for Aging Residents (CASPAR™) is software designed to assess homes and specify modifications. Health care professionals such as occupational therapists or nurses (or sometimes a knowledgeable family member) can use this tool to gather information about clients. CASPAR includes a training guide, forms, and a videotape on measuring and taking photographs. When the assessment has been completed, the information is returned to the CASPAR developer and a set of recommendations are prepared. The recommendations include suggestions and rationales for the best possible solutions, alternative solutions, architectural drawings (if necessary), product specifications, comparative costs, installation specifications and drawings, and vendor information. The CASPAR user then works with the client, family members, and home modification provider (e.g., local contractor) to bring the project to completion. In some areas, government-administered or nonprofit organizations make modifications (Brown, 2002).

The Client Assessment Sheet and Client Measurement Sheet developed by ADAptations Inc.® expand on the traditional home evaluation checklist. The Client Assessment Sheet asks for general information about the person, the home, and the functional ability of the client. The Client Measurement Sheet provides for measurements of critical places in the home as accessed from both a standing or sitting position. Together, the assessment sheets create a thorough evaluation that is particularly suited to the person doing extensive home modifications. The assessment sheets accompany the video *Up Close and Personal,* which describes the importance of measuring and ways to measure to plan for a client's needs (Duncan, 2002).

Ease®3.2 software offers a computerized functional assessment tool to provide solutions for daily living. The software works with a database of solutions and product information. The assessment reviews personal needs and abilities and uses that data to identify potential home environment problems. It then lists the best possible solutions in a customized report (Christenson, 2004).

LivAbility™

LivAbility™ is an Internet-based software program that provides information about solutions to meet various needs in one easily accessible place. It is modeled after the Ease software and is driven by the same Ease Search engine. A self-assessment questionnaire that makes it possible for anyone to access solutions, LivAbility facilitates information gathering about products and ideas that can help seniors or people with disabilities find modifications to help them remain independent in their homes (Christenson, 2001).

The major difference between Ease software and LivAbility lies in how solutions are chosen. Users of the Ease software select the products and ideas that appear in the report; LivAbility selects the solutions in advance by matching them to responses in the self-assessment questionnaire. LivAbility is available on the Lifease Web site (www.lifease.com).

Financing Home Remodeling

One's home is usually one's largest single investment. Borrowing against the equity in the home while continuing to live in the home can pay for necessary home modifications. Grants and other types of funds may also be available for people with low incomes.

Housing and Community Development Grants

A type of funding known as "Section 504" loans is available to homeowners in rural areas. This U.S. Department of Agriculture program helps low-income households remove health and safety hazards. To be eligible, homeowners must live in a community with a population smaller than 20,000. Loan length is from 10 to 20 years, and interest is set at 1% for people who can repay the loan. If the home is sold within 3 years of receiving the assistance, the loan must be repaid. Local Rural Development offices process Section 504 applications. The central Web site for these offices is www.rurdev.usda.gov.

Federal loans with a lifetime maximum of $7,500 are available for homeowners older than 62 years of age who do not qualify for a Section 504 loan. More information is available at www.usda.gov/services.html.

Funds From Organizations

Many types of organizations may provide funds for housing renovations for people with disabilities, including local businesses, community groups, religious organizations, building supply companies, housing rehabilitation agencies, and neighborhood associations or planning councils. Public agencies, foundations, and other donors may provide funds that are administered through nonprofit housing and community development agencies.

Social Services and Health Waivers

When a person's medical condition requires accessibility modifications to enable him or her to continue living independently at home, Medical Assistance Waivers may provide funds. This option is for people who would be institutionalized if changes were not made. Information on waivers is available from the state or local department of human services.

Veterans' Specialty Housing Grants

If a U.S. veteran has major service-related disabilities, grants from the Veterans' Administration (VA) are available to build or purchase an accessible home or to remodel the home the veteran currently owns. For information about eligibility, contact the VA field office where the veteran's records are located. The VA Web site is www.va.org. The VA also offers home improvement loans to assist veterans with non-service-related disabilities.

Funding Through Vocational Rehabilitation Centers and Independent-Living Centers

If a person cannot function at home, it may be impossible for him or her to work. Vocational rehabilitation centers provide advocacy, skills training, counseling, information, and referral services. Some staff members have expertise in home assessment, construction, and financing.

Workers' Compensation

Compensation for work injuries may include home modifications. To be eligible for compensation, the alterations must be required for the person to function.

Crime Victims' Services

Crime victims, family members, or dependents may be eligible for home modifications funding through the Office of Justice Programs. Maximum awards are $50,000. Information on funding is available from their Web site: www.dps.state.mn.us/OJP/funding/index.htm#VOCA.

Civic, Advocacy, and Trade Groups Projects

Many community groups provide money, volunteer labor, or materials for home accessibility projects. Local options vary greatly but might include

- Organizations raising funds from certain types of gambling;
- Civic groups, churches, and synagogues;
- Community groups that specify a period of time for home repair projects;
- Groups that work on repair projects for low-income households;
- Building industry product retailers or professionals; or
- Advocacy agencies and vocational technical schools.

Private Loans

Refinancing of a home mortgage may provide additional funds for remodeling. The lender evaluates factors relating to repayment of the refinanced loan and current value of the property to determine whether and how much it will lend. If the homeowner has other outstanding loans, they may be consolidated into the new mortgage.

- Long-term-care insurance may cover the cost of purchasing or installing home accessibility features. Long-term-care insurance is a supplement to health care insurance that offers both institutional and in-home coverage for people who are partially or completely disabled. Some policies include a benefit for accessibility modifications.
- Over time, homes increase in value; *equity* is the term used to refer to the difference between the purchase price of a home and its current value. An equity line of credit is like a credit card, allowing dollars to be borrowed up to a certain amount, based on the equity in a home, for the life of the loan and a time limit set by the lender. Amounts can be paid back in a lump sum or in periodic payments.
- A reverse mortgage is a special type of loan used primarily by older Americans to convert the equity in their homes into cash. In a reverse mortgage, the payment stream is "reversed." Instead of a homeowner making monthly payments to a lender, as with a regular first mortgage or home equity loan, the lender makes regular payments to the homeowner in return for a share of the equity in the home. While a reverse mortgage loan is outstanding, the homeowner continues to hold the title to the home.

To qualify for a reverse mortgage, a person must be at least 62 years of age and own his or her home. No income or medical requirements are involved. A person may be eligible for a reverse mortgage even if he or she still owes money on a first or second mortgage. The most popular way of receiving money is through a line of credit. Other homeowners may select a lump-sum or fixed monthly payment (National Reverse Mortgage Lenders Association, 2002).

The size of the reverse mortgage depends on age when applying for the loan, the type of reverse mortgage, the value of the home (the amount of any outstanding debts against it), current interest rates, and neighborhood market conditions. The costs associated with getting a reverse mortgage are similar to those for regular mortgages.

The money provided from a reverse mortgage is tax-free. It does not affect regular Social Security benefits, but it may affect certain other types of government aid, such as Medicare. Specific information is available from local Area Agency on Aging offices (see www.eldercare.gov). A meeting with an approved financial counseling agency must precede the application for a reverse mortgage. The U.S. Department of Housing and Urban Development has posted a list of approved counseling agencies by state at http://www.hud.gov/offices/hsg/sfh/hcc/

441

Case Study 19.1. Mr. C.

Mr. C. developed a neurological condition that created severe pain in his lower right leg and generated mobility difficulties. He also had limited arm range of motion, particularly above his shoulders. He was forced to retire and spent his day lying on a bed that had been placed in the family room.

The family home consisted of multiple levels, but Mr. C. could not use the stairs. The family room was the only living space on the ground level, and the entrance was from the garage. A laundry room with a sliding door adjoined the family room. A small bathroom with a shower was located off the laundry room. Mr. C. was not able to stand up to shower.

To provide room to help her husband shower, Mrs. C. had the door between the bathroom and laundry room) removed and had a shower chair installed. For Mr. C. to sit, however, it was necessary to remove the shower door. Because of his limited range of motion, he could not use a handheld shower himself. Mrs. C. donned a raincoat and assisted him with showering.

The couple's children were married, and two of them lived in the same city. Including Mr. C. in family gatherings was virtually impossible because he could not go to either the living room or the basement entertainment area, and meeting in the family room was too crowded. Therefore, Mr. C. could not be a part of the family activities. His life, as well as that of the entire family, had been compromised by his disability.

Mr. and Mrs. C. decided that finding a house to remodel was the best solution. They bought a new house, and extensive remodeling began. They decided to incorporate a universal design perspective in the home design and furniture. As a result, their house is on a single level and has wide doorways and hallways, a no-threshold entry, decorator grab bars, rocker light switches, lever door handles, and a raised dishwasher and dryer. Mr. and Mrs. C. furnished it with sturdy furniture, including dining room chairs with arms. All the features are inconspicuous, add to a sense of openness, and increase the house's ease of use. A deck with ramped areas and handrails goes around the house.

The new house provides ample room for Mr. C. to move around, whether walking or in a wheelchair. The bathroom includes an open wet room and a stationary shower seat with a regular shower, so he can once again be independent in bathing.

Mr. C. had a change in medications and received pain management interventions. Because of his poor physical condition, he underwent an intensive period of rehabilitation that included both occupational and physical therapy. He now can walk and is no longer limited to lying on a bed. The floor plan of the house, with its wide hallways, handrails, and stable furniture, allows Mr. C. to continue to gain independence. The exterior promotes outdoor exercise. Family gatherings again include him.

Any limitations Mr. C. now experiences are an integral part of his disease process, but the home environment presents no obstructions to his independence. He believes the design of the house was significant in his recovery.

---

hccprof14.cfm. The counselor's job is to provide information about reverse mortgages and alternative options and to help people determine which reverse mortgage product may best fit their needs.

The home need not be sold to pay off the loan. Homeowners and their heirs can pay off the reverse mortgage and keep the home. The amount owed on the reverse mortgage can never exceed the value of the home at the time the loan must be repaid. If the home is sold and the sales proceeds exceed the amount owed on the reverse mortgage, the excess money goes to the person or his or her estate (Minnesota Housing Finance Agency, 2003).

Tax Benefits

Modifications to an existing home can be deducted from federal income tax when they are made to accommodate a resident with a disability. The IRS distributes resource booklets with information on medical capital deductions. More information is available at the IRS Web site at www.irs.org.

A portion of capital expenses is deductible for a home used for business. The business also can deduct the cost of improvements needed to make the business accessible. The design standards are the same as those for public and commercial space.

Some states offer a sales-tax exemption on materials purchased for installing stair glides, platform lifts, or elevators. For the purchasers to qualify for the exemption, a physician must authorize the need for those features.

If accessibility improvements will increase the value of an older home, a portion of the increase may be excluded from the property value of the home for a limited time. Check with the local government for more details.

Summary

Adapting a home to create an environment where people can remain independent is not only doable, but also can be accomplished in a way that is attractive and creates a place where anyone would like to live. The ideas and resources that have been included in this chapter will help occupational therapists look at their clients' home environments in a new way.

Study Questions

1. What group of people were the initial driving force behind legislation in the United States that focused on people with disabilities?
2. What are three essential components in visitability?
3. What is the ADA, and when was it passed?
4. List the seven principles of universal design, and explain what they mean.
5. List modifications that will adapt a home for a client with age-related physical changes.
6. List five modifications that will adapt a home for a client with age-related sensory changes.
7. Identify three modifications that will adapt a home for a client with cognitive issues.
8. What resources are available for financing modifications to a home?

References

AARP. (1995). *Rate your home.* Retrieved April 5, 2004, from www.aarp.org/life/homedesign/ratehome/.

American National Standards Institute. (1961). *Making buildings accessible to and usable by the physically handicapped.* Washington, DC: Author.

Architectural Barriers Act of 1968. Pub. L. 90–480, 42 U.S.C. § 415 *et seq.*

Birren, J., & Schaie, K. (1977). *Handbook of the psychology of aging.* New York: Van Nostrand Reinhold.

Brown, A. (2002). *CASPAR*™ [Computer software]. Chicago: Extended Home Living Services.

Center for Universal Design. (1997). *Principles of universal design.* Retrieved September 24, 2003, from www.design.ncsu.edu:8120/cud/univdesign.

Christenson, M. A. (1999). Embracing universal design. *OT Practice, 4*(9), 12–15, 25.

Christenson, M. A. (2001). *LivAbility*™. New Brighton, MN: Lifease.

Christenson, M. A. (2002a). *PresentEase*™: Age-related physical changes. New Brighton, MN: Lifease.

Christenson, M. A. (2002b). *PresentEase*™: Age-related sensory changes. New Brighton, MN: Lifease.

Christenson, M. A. (2002c). *PresentEase*™: Cognitive issues. New Brighton, MN: Lifease.

Christenson, M. A. (2004). *Ease®3.2* [Computer software]. New Brighton, MN: Lifease.

Clausen, A. (2002, June). Eleanor Smith looks to affect concrete change. *Goshen College Bulletin.* Retrieved October 31, 2003, from www.goshen.edu/news/bulletin/02june.

Comfort, A. (1990). *Say yes to old age: Developing a positive attitude toward aging.* New York: Crown.

Cornell University, Weill Medical College. (2000). *Gerontologic Environmental Modifications (GEM): Welcome.* New York: Author. Retrieved October 25, 2003, from www.cornellaging.org/gem.

Duncan, S. (2002). *Up close and personal* (The ABCs of Accessibility Part 2) [Videotape]. Bellevue, WA: ADAptations Inc.®

Duncan, S. (2003, September). Universal design is good design for everyone. *Housing Washington,* pp. 8–9.

Education for All Handicapped Children Act of 1975. Pub. L. 94–142, 20 U.S.C. § 1400 *et seq.*

Farber, S. (1992). *Good Grips Tools.* New York: OXO International.

Hahn, H. (1988). The politics of physical differences: Disability and discrimination. *Journal of Social Issues, 44*(1), 39–47.

Kiernat, J. (1982). Environment: The hidden modality. *Physical and Occupational Therapy in Geriatrics, 2*(1), 3–12.

Lasoff, S., & Lorentzen, L. (2003). *The accessible home.* Minneapolis, MN: Fairview Press.

Leibrock, C. A., & Terry, J. E. (1999). *Beautiful universal design.* New York: Wiley.

Mace, R. (1988). *Housing for the lifespan of all people.* Washington, DC: U.S. Department of Housing and Urban Development.

Mann, W. C., & Lane, J. P. (1995). *Assistive technology for persons with disabilities* (2nd ed.). Bethesda, MD: American Occupational Therapy Association.

Minnesota Housing Finance Agency. (2003). *Home accessibility design and guidelines.* Retrieved October 27, 2003, from www.mhfa.state.mn.us./homes/Access_Financing_Grid.pdf.

National Reverse Mortgage Lenders Association. (2002). *Just the FAQs: Answers to common questions about reverse mortgages.* Washington, DC: Author.

Olsen, R. V., Hutchings, L., & Ehrenkrantz, E. (2000). *A house for all children.* Newark, NJ: New Jersey Institute Press.

Overton, J., Pynoos, J., & Sabata, D. (2003). Environmental coping strategies can help reduce the stress of caregiving. *Maximizing Human Potential, 11*(2), 1, 6.

Panero, J., & Zelnik, M. (1979). *Human dimension and interior spaces.* New York: Whitney Library.

Perry, L. G., Jawer, M. A., Murdoch, J. R., & Dinegar, J. C. (1991). *BOMA International's ADA compliance guidebook: A checklist for your building.* Washington, DC: Building Owner's and Manager's Association.

Pirkl, J. J. (1994). *Transgenerational design: Products for an aging population.* New York: Van Nostrand Reinhold.

Rebuilding Together. (1998). *Home modifications assessment and solutions checklist.* Washington, DC: Author. Retrieved October 6, 2003, from www.rebuildingtogether.org/home_modifications/house_assessment_checklist.shtml.

Rehabilitation Act of 1973. Pub. L. 93–112, 29 U.S.C. § 701 *et seq.*

Rosenblum, J. (1999). *A reader's guide to Shakespeare.* New York: Salem Press/Barnes & Noble.

SAIL. (2002). *Practical guide to universal home design.* St. Paul, MN: East Metro Seniors Agenda for Independent Living.

U.S. Census Bureau. (1993). *We the American elderly*. Washington, DC: Author.

U.S. Census Bureau. (1999). *Federal Interagency Forum on Age-Related Statistics*, Data Base News in Aging. Washington, DC: Aging Studies Branch, U.S. Census Bureau.

U.S. Consumer Product Safety Commission. (1981). *Safety for older consumers home safety checklist*. Washington, DC: Author.

University of Birmingham, Centre for Applied Gerontology. (1999). [Applied Gerontology home page]. Birmingham, England: Author. Retrieved October 15, 2003, from www.bham.ac.uk/gerontology.

Welch, P., & Palames, C. (1995). A brief history of disability rights legislation in the United States. In P. Welch (Ed.), *Strategies for teaching universal design*. Berkeley, CA: Adaptive Environments Center and MIG Communications.

Yeung, Y. (2003). Educating older adults in AT. *OT Practice, 8*(15), 12–15.

Chapter 20

Therapeutic Partnerships: Caregiving in the Home Setting

MARGARET A. PERKINSON, PHD

PATRICIA LAVESSER, PHD, OTR/L

KERRI MORGAN, MSOT, OTR/L

MONICA PERLMUTTER, MA, OTR/L

KEY TERMS

ethnographic approach

explanatory model of illness

family caregiver

family-centered care

personal assistant services

personal care attendant

OBJECTIVES

Upon completion of this chapter, the reader will be able to

- Understand the scope of formal and informal caregiving services currently provided;

- Describe the characteristics of a family-centered approach to occupational therapy practice;

- Define an explanatory model of illness;

- Identify the family caregiver's values, needs, and priorities as part of the occupational therapy evaluation process for any person with disabilities;

- Describe the contributions that a family caregiver can make to the planning and implementation of treatment;

- Identify the three stages of a caregiving career and the ways the occupational therapist can work with the family caregiver at each stage; and

- Recognize the occupational therapist's role in working with a person to develop the instrumental activities of daily living skills of an attendant care manager.

amily caregivers frequently play a pivotal role in developing strategies for daily living for people with disabilities. In addition to assisting with actual activities of daily living (ADL), family caregivers act as gatekeepers to the health and social services system for relatives requiring more extensive assistance with ADL. For people who cannot manage health decisions alone, family caregivers usually interpret the illness, decide how symptoms should be managed, and eventually decide when and how professional health care providers should become involved. Family caregivers are most often "informal" (i.e., unpaid relatives providing assistance), although that is not universally the case (LaPlante, Harrington, & Kang, 2002; Nosek, Fuhrer, Rintala, & Hart, 1993). "Formal" caregivers are paid personal care attendants who are directly employed by the person or family requiring assistance. This chapter explores how occupational therapists can best work with formal and informal caregivers of people with disabilities.

Importance of Family Caregiving

Family caregivers provide at least 80% of the care received by older adults (Doty, 1995). Although most recipients of home care are elderly people, more than one third are people younger than 60 years of age (Marks, 1996). Family members provide care for people who have a variety of physical or mental disabilities or chronic conditions, ranging from cerebral palsy and Down syndrome to cancer, AIDS, diabetes, dementia, arthritis, multiple sclerosis, and heart disease.

For several reasons, the family's role in caregiving is especially important now. Hospitals discharge patients to the community earlier in their recovery, thereby placing greater responsibility on the family to provide posthospital care. Higher survival rates for previously fatal injuries and conditions, the AIDS epidemic, and policies favoring deinstitutionalization also contribute to the increase in home care (Baum & LaVesser, 1994). Perhaps most significant to the rise in family caregiving, however, is the rapidly growing number of older adults in our population. Less than 100 years ago, people older than 65 years of age represented only 4% of the U.S. population. By 2000, this group had grown to 35 million, or 12.4%, and by 2050 they are projected to represent 79 million people, or 20.6% of the total population (U.S. Bureau of the Census, 2001). People age 85 and older represent the fastest growing segment of the population; in the 1990s this group increased by 38% (U.S. Bureau of the Census, 2001).

Aging does not inevitably lead to disability, and most older adults do not require help with ADL (Zedlewski, 1990). Nevertheless, activity limitations tend to increase over time as a result of underlying disease states (Kunkel & Applebaum, 1992). The need for assistance with ADL rises rapidly as aging progresses: Less than 3% of people younger than 65 years of age require help with ADL, compared with

- 9.3% of people 65–69 years of age,
- 10.9% of people 70–74 years of age,
- 18.9% of people 75–79 years of age,
- 23.6% of people 80–84 years of age, and
- 45.4% of people 85 years age and older (U.S. Bureau of the Census, 1990).

Most adults with disabilities continue to live in the community (Day, 1985), and they are able to do so because of the informal care they receive from family members (Doty, 1995). Caregivers' attributes, such as level of perceived burden and self-rated health, are important predictors of early institutionalization of people with disabilities (Gaugler, Kane, Kane, Clay, & Newcomer, 2003).

Research on family caregiving shows that maintaining people with disabilities in the community is challenging (Pruchno, 1999; Schulz & Quittner, 1998). Family caregiving can be disruptive and stressful and can have significant negative effects on the mental and physical health of care providers (Pinquart & Sorensen, 2003; Wright, Clipp, & George, 1993). Family caregiving also can provide positive and uplifting experiences (Beach, Schulz, Yee, & Jackson, 2000; Ohaeri, 2003). As a group, caregivers do not receive sufficient support from family and friends, and health and social services providers generally do not offset this need for assistance (Aneshensel, Pearlin, Mullan, Zarit, & Whitlatch, 1995). How can occupational therapists more effectively aid family caregivers; that is, how can they ameliorate the negative aspects of providing care and enhance its positive dimensions?

Therapist–Family Caregiver Relationship

According to the *Occupational Therapy Practice Framework* (American Occupational Therapy Association [AOTA], 2002), both the person referred for occupational therapy services and the people involved in supporting or caring for that person may be considered clients. Client-centered practice therefore supplements information received from the person with disabilities with information provided by his or her caregivers. As noted above, family caregivers typically experience a significant amount of stress, which often leads to physical and mental distress. Signs of depression, such as emotional exhaustion, listlessness, inability to sleep (or sleeping too much), loss of appetite, loss of interest in favorite activities, and feelings of guilt or sadness are signals that the family caregiver requires some form of intervention (Morris & Gainer, 1997). Suggestions for coping with stress, such as time-management techniques and the use of respite care, may help family members who are approaching caregiving burnout.

Although the caregiver-as-client approach is useful in certain situations, it still defines the relationship between the occupational therapist and the family caregiver as one between an expert and a person in need. This type of relationship implies an imbalance of power in which the client is expected to submit to the authority of the expert (Lawlor & Mattingly, 1998; Perkinson, 1992). By definition, clients have a dependent status; they are encouraged to rely on experts to define their problems, assess the causes of those problems, and determine the proper treatments. Clients are expected to comply with the plans proposed by experts and provide little active input into solutions. Such relationships frequently lead to "unilateral dependency" (Estes & Binney, 1991), in which clients give up their responsibility for active involvement in decision making and passively accept the expert's advice.

A different model of care, one that is based on a philosophy of "helping people to help themselves," emphasizes the development of self-reliance and empowerment. Advocates of this empowerment model encourage clients to take an active role in resolving their problems and needs. The goal is to encourage caregivers and people with disabilities to discover and develop their own strengths and talents, thus improving their likelihood of success in dealing with their situations (Perkinson, 1992).

Therapists using this model approach family caregivers (and the person with disabilities, to the extent possible) as partners in care and work to develop a collaborative therapeutic relationship. The result is a "therapeutic alliance" that is based on mutual understanding, respect, and cooperation among the therapist, the family members, and the referred client or patient (Brown, 1998). The trend toward a family-centered partnership approach has evolved throughout the field, from pediatric to geriatric occupational therapy (Baum, 1991; Case-Smith & Nastro, 1993; Hasselkus, 1991). It is the fundamental intervention model promoted in the Educa-

tion for All Handicapped Children Amendments of 1986 (Pub. L. 99–457), 20 U.S.C. § 1401, Part H, Section 677 (Schultz-Krohn, 1997).

Family-centered care acknowledges that family members know their relatives in ways that the therapist does not and that they are well qualified to make decisions regarding their relatives' care (Law, 1998; Perkinson, 2002; see Figure 20.1). Unlike health care professionals, who come and go, family members are a permanent and vital part of the life of a person with disabilities (Weinstein, 1997). With family-centered care, the focus is on the care recipient as part of a family (rather than on the care recipient alone). Rather than use their professional expertise to control and direct intervention, therapists provide information, knowledge, and options to the family and respect the decisions made by the family (Allen & Petr, 1998). In a collaborative relationship, both the family and therapist participate in the evaluation, problem-solving, and decision-making processes. The family has significant input in deciding the extent, type, and priorities of therapy. The traditional therapist-as-expert thinking is supported by a strict medical model but may affect the caregiver in ways the therapist does not anticipate (Case Study 20.1).

A collaborative partnership represents a fundamental shift in the way therapy is defined and delivered (Toth-Cohen, 2000). Lawlor and Mattingly (1998) noted that this model presents challenges such as understanding issues confronting the person with disabilities and his or her family from the family's point of view and sharing decision-making power. The following section suggests ways to deal with some of those issues to achieve an effective partnership with family caregivers.

How to Work in Partnership With Family Caregivers

An effective partnership between caregivers and therapists depends on a shared view and understanding of the illness or disability involved and how it should be treated (Hasselkus, 1988; Le Navenec & Vonhof, 1996). The first step toward achieving that goal is to identify what anthropologists call the *explanatory model* of illness held by the caregiver. Explanatory models are sets of beliefs and knowledge that people use to explain sickness and treatment. The models provide a way of thinking about illness that influences its meaning and guides choices among various therapies (Kleinman, 1988; Krefting & Krefting, 1991). An explanatory model can include beliefs about an illness's cause, seriousness, and prognosis; the possibility of a cure; the ap-

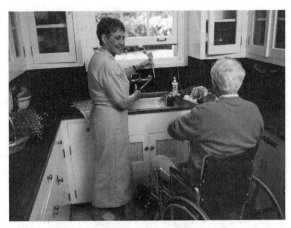

Figure 20.1. Family-centered caregiving is a philosophy that encourages partnerships between therapists and family members. It recognizes that family members bring important knowledge and are essential to the caregiving process. Photo © PhotoDisc, Inc.

propriate treatment; and legitimate sources of help. The model influences whether a person even recognizes or believes a problem exists. The explanatory model underlies decision making about the illness; it guides decisions about treatment and help seeking and defines sources of help and caregiving goals.

People understand the health care information and messages given to them within the context of their own beliefs. In effect, information and suggestions from the therapist are filtered through the explanatory models of both the person with disabili-

ties and the caregiver. Aspects of the message that are most compatible with a person's explanatory model are more likely to be heard, accepted, and remembered. Elements of the message that conflict with the model are more likely to be tuned out or dismissed. For example, if a family caregiver of a cardiac patient sees the heart as a machine that has been fixed by the patient's bypass surgery, the caregiver may believe that the heart problem has been resolved and treatment is over. The caregiver may not understand the need for ongoing attention to lifestyle changes, such as modification of diet or maintenance of a permanent exercise plan. Therapists need to recognize the role of the explanatory model in caregiver behavior.

To develop a collaborative partnership with the family caregiver, the therapist must identify the caregiver's explanatory model and recognize potential points of conflict or differences in understanding between that and the therapist's explanatory model. In conducting the initial assessment with the family caregiver, the therapist might include questions to elicit the caregiver's explanatory model (as well as that of the person with disabilities, when appropriate). Therapists include the following questions:

- What do you think caused the problems of the person with disabilities?
- Why do you think this illness happened at this particular time?
- How serious do you think this illness or condition is?

Case Study 20.1.
Carrie: Example of the Medical Model Applied to Dealing With a Family Caregiver

Twelve-month-old Carrie was diagnosed with cerebral palsy, moderate right hemiplegia. She was referred for early intervention services, including occupational therapy. Carrie was living with her mother, father, and three older siblings in a one-story, ranch-style house on a farm owned and operated by her parents and grandparents.

Even with years of experience parenting Carrie's two brothers, ages 5 and 7 years, her mother was having tremendous difficulty dealing with Carrie's needs and emerging developmental delays. At the time of referral, Carrie was not using her right hand at all, was demonstrating asymmetrical posture, and used scooting in a sitting position as her primary

means of mobility. Her drooling and difficulty handling table foods made mealtimes difficult. The occupational therapist assigned to the case quickly established a home program emphasizing neurodevelopmental treatment techniques to address the identified motor difficulties. Although she could find time in her schedule to see Carrie only once a week, the therapist spent considerable time teaching the home program she had designed to Carrie's mother.

Carrie began to show progress, so the occupational therapist was greatly surprised when the mother informed her that she was no longer in need of occupational therapy services through the early intervention agency. Instead, she was going to drive 50 miles roundtrip to the nearest children's hospital to have Carrie receive outpatient occupational therapy services twice a week.

Case Study 20.1. *Continued*

An interview with the family at this time revealed some interesting information. It was learned that, although the occupational therapist had always been professional and friendly, she was always rushed and seemed never to ask Carrie's mother for her opinion of what was needed. The home program instructions were always written out and reviewed, but the tasks involved were more complicated and took more time than the mother thought she could handle. She reported feeling inadequate and guilty that she could not accomplish everything, frustrated with her attempts, and angry with the therapist for not being aware of her difficulties. When routinely asked "How are you doing with the exercises?" she felt chastised for not doing more. She also had mixed feelings about the direction the therapy was taking. She agreed that Carrie's motor skill development was important, but what really worried her was that Carrie was not getting enough nutrition because of her feeding difficulties, and she just wanted to have a pleasant mealtime with the entire family. Finally, she believed that more therapy on a regular schedule was desirable and that she could handle the drive better than she could handle being a surrogate therapist for her daughter.

Case Analysis: What Should Have Happened?

Had the occupational therapist approached this case from a family-centered perspective, the results may have been different. On the very first visit, a family interview could have identified and ranked family strengths, needs, and goals. Collaborating with the family on an ongoing basis most likely would have moved things along a different course, resulting in progress for Carrie and better satisfaction for her mother and the family.

- What worries you the most about this illness or condition?
- What kind of treatment would you like your family member to receive?
- What are the most important results you expect to achieve with treatment? (Kleinman, 1980; Krefting & Krefting, 1991)

During the initial assessment, the therapist also should determine the meaning of the caregiving role to the family member and how he or she makes sense of the caregiving role. Additional questions might include the following:

- What motivates you, and what is the significance of caregiving to you?
- What influences how you provide daily care?
- What do you find most burdensome about caregiving?
- What do you find most satisfying about caregiving?
- What are your major concerns? (Gubrium & Sankar, 1990; Hasselkus, 1988, 1989)

The assessment should include a joint evaluation by the caregiver and therapist of the family's problems and resources in addressing caregiving needs. The caregiver and therapist can then collaborate on the basis of the joint assessment to develop goals and procedures that are acceptable to all the people involved.

The Canadian Occupational Performance Measure (COPM; Law et al., 1998) is an assessment tool that can be used to establish occupational profiles of people with disabilities as well as their caregivers (AOTA, 2002). This tool is an interview-based rating scale that asks the person with disabilities or the family member to identify problem areas and priorities for intervention. Another tool, the Functional Behavior Profile (Baum, Edwards, & Morrow-Howell, 1993), asks caregivers to report the frequency of various behaviors that they have observed during recent interactions with the person with disabilities and provides valuable information for case planning. The Burden Interview (Zarit, Reever, & Bach-Peterson, 1980) and the Memory and Behavior Problems Checklist (Teri et al., 1992) provide therapists with insight into the factors that contribute to feelings of burden by family members.

The therapist may supplement traditional assessment techniques with an ethnographic approach to information gathering about caregiving. Ethnographic methods offer ways to understand the family caregiver's perspective and techniques for achieving a joint appraisal of the situation and the client's needs (Gitlin, Corcoran, & Leinsmiller-Eckhardt, 1995; Hasselkus, 1990, 1997). Using an ethnographic approach, the therapist attempts to understand a way of life as it is viewed by another person (in this case, the family caregiver). An ethnographic interview focuses on values, meanings, beliefs, and how the person providing the information makes sense of his or her situation. Conducting the interview in a nonjudgmental manner, the therapist suspends his or her own beliefs and values as to the appropriate course of treatment in an attempt to discover what actually goes on (Gitlin et al., 1995). The interview is semistructured; it consists of open-ended questions and appropriate probes, in which the therapist attempts to elicit and understand the caregiver's (or, when appropriate, the care recipient's) point of view.

Weinstein (1997) designed an interview for therapists to conduct with family members or principal caregivers to discover the caregiver's level of knowledge and comfort with this role. Weinstein's semistructured interview format invites caregivers to

- Identify their opinions, personal goals, and needs;
- Describe their perceptions of the care recipient's problem;
- Describe a typical day at home;
- Describe the effect of the situation on themselves and other members of the family; and
- Identify what kind of information or support they personally would like from the occupational therapist.

This type of interview can lay the groundwork for establishing the collaborative partnership that is central to the philosophy of family-centered care. As the therapist takes the time to understand the caregiver's perspective (including the meaning ascribed to caregiving, how care is provided in the home, and what is perceived as problematic), the therapist also builds rapport with the family member. This rapport establishes a measure of trust and enhances the level of comfort with future discussions in which the therapist can share perspectives on the caregiving situation (Hasselkus, 1997).

After identifying the caregiver's views and his or her understanding of the care recipient's condition and needs, the therapist may want to discuss any differences in perspective that could lead to misunderstandings or points of disagreement. Respect for the caregiver's and care recipient's points of view should always be maintained during this process.

Often, family caregivers and therapists use different explanatory models for the condition of the person with disabilities. Medical anthropologists have developed a therapeutic approach to enhance cross-cultural communication between patients and health care providers (Berlin & Fowkes, 1983) that

can be useful when this occurs. Structured around the acronym LEARN, this set of guidelines helps therapists and family caregivers with initially different points of view to "get on the same wavelength" and take the first step toward developing a therapeutic alliance. The steps of the LEARN approach are as follows:

1. *Listen* with sympathy and understanding to the caregiver's perception of the illness and caregiving situation. After the family caregiver's perspective has been recognized and good rapport has been developed with the caregiver, the therapist can then share a personal point of view.
2. *Explain* the therapist's perceptions of the problem.
3. *Acknowledge* and review the areas in which the therapist and the caregiver agree, and work to resolve major conceptual conflicts.
4. *Recommend* a treatment plan that involves both sides as full partners in deciding what to do.
5. *Negotiate* to reach a treatment plan that is agreeable to all parties and that takes the perspective of each person (the person with disabilities, the caregiver, and the therapist) into account.

The ethnographic approach and the LEARN techniques can help therapists work with family caregivers to develop treatment strategies that fit the values and beliefs of each family but remain rooted in the theory and practice of occupational therapy. Viewing the family caregiver as a partner and taking the values and beliefs of the family into account will increase the likelihood that the jointly developed treatment plan will be successfully integrated into family routines (Corcoran & Gitlin, 1992; Gitlin, 1993). In acknowledging the family caregiver as a partner who has much to contribute, the therapist encourages the family to assume and maintain responsibility for long-term care.

What Family Caregivers Can Contribute

A family caregiver has much to contribute as a partner in the planning and execution of treatment (Perkinson, 2002). As a mediator between the person with disabilities and the therapist, the family caregiver can

- Assist the family member with disabilities in voicing his or her own needs and concerns,

- Communicate those needs and concerns to the therapist, and
- Communicate or clarify treatment plans and goals to the family member with disabilities.

Family caregivers typically have a wealth of information that can help therapists better understand the clients, their needs, and how best to address them. Usually, caregivers are attuned to the nuances of behavior and physical states of family members with disabilities. The caregiver knows what is "normal" for the person and can help the therapist define more realistic treatment goals. Caregivers also can advise the therapist of significant changes in the health status of people with disabilities. A caregiver typically has knowledge of the person's ability to conduct ADL (including self-care tasks) that may affect treatment plans.

The family caregiver can give the therapist tips for interacting with the person with disabilities and for interpreting his or her reactions to the therapist or to treatment suggestions. Caregivers often can sense how receptive the family member will be to a given treatment plan and may suggest ways to present the plan to maximize the likelihood that he or she will accept it. For example, the caregiver might present the plan to the care recipient or, to the extent possible, enlist him or her in contributing to the development of the plan (thus enhancing the family's investment in it). Table 20.1 offers a checklist of useful client-related information that family members can share with the therapist to optimize intervention planning. Family caregivers also can assist in motivating people with disabilities by encouraging them to cooperate with the treatment plan.

Occupation is a critical factor in determining quality of life, no matter how ill a person may be or what disabilities he or she may have (Baum, 1995). With their knowledge of the family member's past history and preferences, family caregivers can play a vital role in identifying meaningful tasks and engaging the person with disabilities in those activities. They also can help identify the person's abilities and limits, what tasks or activities frustrate the person, and what tasks or activities give him or her satisfaction. This information helps the therapy team set realistic, appropriate, and challenging goals. Identifying and incorporating the preferences of the person with disabilities into the treatment plan should significantly improve his or her quality of life and the probability that he or she will find the plan acceptable. As the treatment plan is carried out, the family caregiver also can assist in its evaluation and modification by giving feedback to the therapist about what is working and what should be changed.

What Family Caregivers Need

As research on family caregiving has expanded to include longitudinal studies, researchers have begun to develop the outlines of various stages of the caregiving career (see Table 20.2; Aneshensel et al., 1995). Those stages include role acquisition, role enactment, and role disengagement. Each stage brings different challenges and needs on the part of the person with disabilities and the caregiver. The family-centered treatment plan should take into account these stage-related needs.

Role Acquisition Stage

Role acquisition occurs at the onset of the condition or illness or when the family member first assumes the role of caregiver. During this stage, the person with disabilities and the caregiver must learn to adjust to the new situation and plan for the future. The family caregiver typically has little knowledge about the illness (unless it tends to run in the family or the family caregiver has had experience in the health care field). Therapists can assist caregivers in this stage by providing information to help the family understand the illness, its possible causes, the various options for treatment, and what typically lies ahead.

The initial stage of a major illness represents a significant life transition for both the person with disabilities and his or her family caregiver. It often requires considerable adjustments in life goals, relationships, daily activities, and routines. Emotional support is essential at this stage (Meuser & Marwit, 2001; Pinquart & Sorensen, 2003), and the therapist may consider linking the family to appropriate counseling services. Interaction with family members and caregivers of people with similar conditions through support groups or peer counseling programs can be especially helpful. Peer caregivers can share strategies for dealing with everyday issues, including managing ADL, and they can provide encouragement rooted in empathy (Perkinson, 1995).

Therapists can provide much assistance at this stage by helping the family take steps to prevent future problems. Therapists can help family caregivers identify potential legal and financial issues, such as the need to obtain durable powers of attorney for asset management and health care if the family has not already addressed these issues. Therapists also can provide general information and referrals to legal or financial planning sources for help with other issues, such as writing advance directives and wills

Table 20.1. Checklist of Information About the Client to Assist in Planning Caregiver Intervention

Information Category	Information Useful to the Therapist and Caregiver
Client Characteristics	• What significant background information about the care receiver will help the therapist know the client as a person and better understand the care receiver's behavior and moods? For example, information on the care receiver's past occupation, hobbies, interests, significant life events, memberships in clubs or organizations, and travels will help the practitioner interact with the client on a more personal level. • What are known motivators (i.e., what pleases or excites the client)? • Does the client have particular idiosyncrasies (e.g., unusual modesty, aversion toward noise)? • What fears does the client have (e.g., fear of confined spaces, crowds, or being left alone)? • What special activities can be used to deal with emotions? When the client is upset or stressed, what are the habitual or effective ways of dealing with this (e.g., calming music, being left alone, diverting attention, touch, massage)? Is the client receptive to trying new routines or does he or she prefer an established pattern of activity? • What are the client's known allergies, pet peeves, and emotional triggers? • How well does the client typically cope with stress?
Activities of Daily Living/ Instrumental Activities of Daily Living	• Does the client prefer a shower or bath? • When is bathing preferred? • Are there bathing accessories that are customarily used (e.g., bath oils, loofah mitts, sponges, scrubbers, brushes)? • What dressing and grooming preferences does the client have (e.g., hairstyles, type of perfume or cologne, body lotions, clothing styles and colors, aversive reactions to fabrics)? • What are the client's food preferences and eating habits (e.g., eating a large breakfast, snacking throughout the day)? • Can the family caregiver assist in maintaining the client's proper diet or nutritional needs during meal preparation? • Can the family member identify a suitable bathing assistant with whom the client can be comfortable?
Leisure	• What are the client's favorite types of exercise or physical activity? • Is the client motivated to pursue an exercise program? • Does the client like to read the paper and/or magazines? Does he or she have favorite television programs? • Does the client have favorite hobbies or other pastimes (e.g., board games, crossword puzzles)?
Social Participation	• Does the client call friends and relatives regularly? • Does the client regularly receive and send mail or e-mail?

Table 20.2. Stages and Needs of the Caregiving Career

Stage	Family Challenges	Practitioner Role
Role acquisition	Must adjust to new demands Must learn about illness and what lies ahead	Provides information and reassurance Helps family anticipate future needs
Role enactment	May need training in direct care skills and behavioral management May need advice about institutional placement or community resources	Provides training as needed, such as in the use of assistive devices and transfer skills Provides information on placement options and resources
Disengagement	Adjustment to death of care receiver Adjustment to social isolation and burnout	Assists family with transition Makes referrals to resources that can help with grief or readjustment

and making financial arrangements to anticipate increased medical costs (Baum, 1991; Overman & Stoudemire, 1988).

Role Enactment Stage

Following role acquisition, the role enactment stage encompasses most of the caregiving experience. It includes the provision of home care and, in some cases, the decision for institutional placement. During this stage, family caregivers require continued education about the nature of the illness or condition of the person with disabilities, including its expected trajectory. Caregivers also may benefit from training in direct-care skills, especially those relating to helping the person with disabilities perform self-care tasks. Topics of interest might include

- Safely transferring or bathing the person with disabilities,
- Learning to cue various self-care tasks, and
- Setting up routines to promote the highest level of performance (Baum, 1991; Schulz, 2000; Sorensen, Pinquart, & Duberstein, 2002).

Therapists also can instruct the caregiver on the use of relevant assistive devices and conduct home assessments to suggest various environmental interventions that may make the home safer (Gallagher-Thompson, 1994; Gitlin, Corcoran, Winter, Boyce, & Hauck, 2001; Heagerty & Eskenazi, 1994).

When appropriate, coaching in behavior management techniques may be especially helpful to caregivers in dealing with disruptive behaviors (Teri et al., 2003; Zarit & Teri, 1991;). In some cases, such as the advanced stages of Alzheimer's disease or other forms of dementia, family caregivers may benefit from instruction in communication techniques. A growing literature offers suggestions on ways to preserve the sense of identity and personhood for people with severe cognitive impairments and how to communicate more effectively with them (Perkinson, 1999; Sabat & Harre, 1992).

Family caregivers may benefit from instruction in stress management (Steffen, 2000) and time management. They may need help in setting limits, developing realistic standards, and prioritizing goals (Aneshensel et al., 1995). Caregivers also may require help in dealing with changing family dynamics. Disagreements among family members often emerge as a result of differences in perceptions of the illness or condition and methods for managing it. Conflicts may arise in determining who will assume responsibility for tasks previously done by the person with disabilities and how the additional work and costs of caregiving will be shared. Care-givers also may need guidance on how to explain the family member's illness or condition to extended family and friends in such a way that they maintain continued supportive relations (Fortinsky & Hathaway, 1990).

Family caregivers often are unaware of available community resources and how to access them (Morris & Gainer, 1997). Therapists should develop a resource file to identify relevant resources, including payment sources. Such resources would include programs offering training and support, such as classes in caregiving and health education, support groups, e-mail discussion groups, and 24-hour hot lines. The therapist can identify a number of useful health newsletters, Web sites, and publications on caregiving, such as *The 36-Hour Day* (Mace & Rabins, 1994).

Therapists can provide advice to family caregivers regarding in-home services that offer help with self-maintenance tasks, such as home health aides who can help with bathing, dressing, grooming, and transfers (Figure 20.2). Homemaking services can be hired to help with specific household chores like cleaning, laundry, or even shopping. Nutritionists can instruct caregivers about special nutritional needs, and agencies providing home-delivered meals can assist with meeting those needs. Physical therapists and exercise or rehabilitation programs can assist in developing and maintaining an exercise regimen for the person with disabilities.

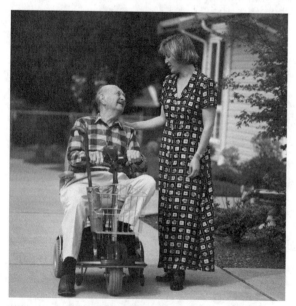

Figure 20.2. Occupational therapists can advise family caregivers on strategies to promote the well-being of their loved one while coping with stress and avoiding burnout. Photo © PhotoDisc, Inc.

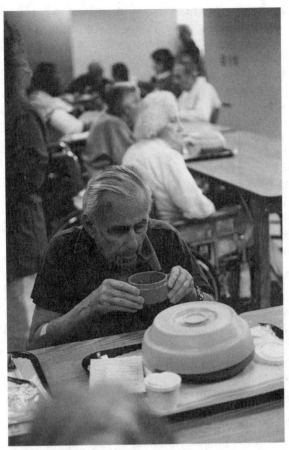

Figure 20.3. When caregiving burdens become too great for family members, therapists can assist in exploring alternate care options or can recommend temporary respite care. Photo © PhotoDisc, Inc.

Family caregivers must recognize the stressful nature of their role and take active steps to prevent burnout (Figure 20.3; Gitlin, et al., 2003). Therapists can assist caregivers by encouraging self-care and discussing community sources of respite care, such as

- Adult or child day care programs,
- Extended overnight respite programs (offered by some nursing homes), and
- Informal support systems that can provide respite (e.g., the caregiver's support systems of family and friends).

In addition to learning how to access community services and programs and how to locate appropriate sources of payment for these services, caregivers also can benefit from instructions on how to work effectively with health care providers. The following section offers suggestions for caregivers working with formal personal care attendants, a type of health provider especially relevant for peo-

ple with disabilities requiring outside assistance with ADL.

Caregiving and Personal Care Attendants

Personal care attendants are employees of people with disabilities; they are hired specifically to assist them with performing ADL that their employers cannot perform independently (Kahn, 1980). Attendant care is a service associated with the independent living (IL) movement that began in the early 1970s (DeJong & Wenker, 1983). The concept of independent living focuses on allowing people with disabilities to live as they choose in their communities, rather than confining them to institutions. Services provided by personal care attendants enable people with severe disabilities to live independently within the community.

A person with disabilities who is seeking formal personal assistance services (PAS) has two options: agency-provided services or consumer-directed services. Traditionally, the person with disabilities would be referred to a company or agency to arrange for the necessary assistance. Agencies hire and pay their own employees, who are trained and evaluated by the agencies' standards. The person with the disability works with that company to plan the assistance that he or she needs, not knowing if the specific assistant will be reliable, friendly, or efficient.

The shift toward the IL model in the disability community brought a shift toward greater consumer control and direction of PAS delivery. Under this model, the person with disabilities determines the services needed; their frequency and duration; and the selection, training, and retention of personal care attendants (DeJong & Wenker, 1983; Doty, Kasper, & Litvak, 1996; Flanagan & Green, 1994; Shapiro, 1993). The person with disabilities (or, sometimes, the family caregiver) is responsible for finding the needed assistance and setting the specifications for those services and actively recruiting, selecting, managing, and directing the personal care attendants or other service providers (Batavia, DeJong, & McKnew, 1991).

The population that requires PAS is vast and heterogeneous, as are the types of assistance needed. PAS recipients include people of all ages with various types of physical, sensory, cognitive, and psychiatric disabilities; older adults; and people with different chronic conditions. PAS provided by the attendant enable people with disabilities to live independently within the community and participate in major life activities in the home, in the community, and at work.

Occupational therapists play a crucial role in working with the person with a disability to identify tasks that can be adapted and performed independently and tasks that will need to be completed with a personal care attendant. Early in the course of rehabilitation, the therapist should help both the person with disabilities and his or her family begin the process of identifying specific PAS needs. This process starts with clarifying needs and expectations regarding relationships, work, and family. Encouraging the client to become assertive and to discuss his or her personal care needs facilitates this process. Consider the following questions in relation to specific ADL:

- What does the person with the disability value more—independence in performing a specific task, or conserving energy and time for other tasks?
- Who should provide the assistance for this task?
- What does the person with disabilities expect or want from the attendant?

Should a person with disabilities struggle for more than an hour getting dressed alone? If so, how much energy will be left for other tasks during the rest of the day? Some clients find it important to perform self-care tasks independently. Other clients find that the challenges of work and the pleasures of family or other relationships are enhanced when they receive assistance from someone whom they have personally chosen and trained to help with self-care and other daily requirements.

Once the necessity of a personal care attendant has been established, the responsibility of the occupational therapist includes assisting the person with disabilities and his or her family with developing skill as an "attendant manager." The exercise of this skill can be considered an instrumental activity of daily living (IADL). The relationship between people with disabilities and their attendants has been described as an employer–employee relationship (Lindley, 1995). Lack of management skills may be one of the most common problems encountered by the person with a disability in dealing with a personal care attendant. Necessary management skills related to personal care attendants include the ability to

- Communicate expectations in terms of standards of performance,
- Provide appropriate and timely feedback, and
- Terminate employment when necessary (Opie & Miller, 1989).

People with disabilities also must have the knowledge and communication skills necessary to train personal care attendants in how to complete the necessary tasks.

Recruitment, selection, and retention of PAS attendants can be difficult. Attendant turnover is a critical problem for PAS consumers. High turnover often can be attributed to employment disincentives such as low pay, few benefits, and lack of job status (Ulicny & Jones, 1985). Under the IL model, occupational therapists typically are not directly involved with this aspect of PAS. They can, however, help the person with disabilities by providing information to help guide the initial organization of PAS recruitment. The therapist can help the person with disabilities think through specific issues, such as how personal attendant chores should be defined and the times of day at which assistance will be needed. For example, someone who must leave for work early in the morning might need assistance with minimal self-care tasks (e.g., washing, dressing, and brushing teeth) in the morning. More time-consuming tasks (e.g., bowel care and showering) can be scheduled for the evening, when time is not at a premium. Similarly, housekeeping and environmental management tasks can be organized into specific time slots. For example, meals may be prepared ahead of time, cleaning tasks interspersed with cooking, and laundry started in the morning and finished in the evening.

Ulicny and Jones (1985) proposed using performance checklists to outline job tasks for the attendant. Specific work routines can be outlined to identify the frequency of each task, the materials needed to support the task, and the setup. Checklists provide specific instructions and help the employer monitor, evaluate, and provide feedback on the attendant's performance. Once training has been completed, checklists can be used for continued supervision. Checklists also can be used during interviews to help a prospective employee know what will be expected of him or her.

The process for developing a checklist is straightforward. First, self-care tasks that require assistance are defined. Then the identified tasks are analyzed to develop a written list of procedures to support and accomplish each task.

Another suggestion that can help potential employers of personal care attendants is to write an employment contract (De Graff, 1988). A contract can outline in great detail all the tasks to be performed and specify the expectations and obligations of both the attendant and the employers. Contracts cover items such as the hourly pay rate, the pay rate for portions of an hour worked, if and what the attendant will be paid if work is canceled, expectations if the attendant cancels, and any other potential problems. Occupational therapists should be aware of local community resources that can assist in the effective employment and management of personal care attendants. The therapist should be able to inform people with disabilities requiring PAS about these resources. For example, many independent living centers have PAS programs that can help recruit, interview, train, and provide funding options for personal care attendants. Local colleges may have a service program for students with disabilities or even a personal care attendant pool. Community organizations, such as the local Spinal Cord Injury Association chapter, American Heart Association, Multiple Sclerosis Society, and local rehabilitation centers, also may provide resources for people with disabilities requiring PAS. Finally, hiring through a home health agency may provide convenience and a higher level of training in exchange for some control, especially in terms of choice of providers.

For many people with disabilities, formal PAS are a vital part of living independently within their communities. Occupational therapists play an important role in determining the need for PAS, training people with disabilities in skills to manage their personal care attendants, and providing information on available resources.

Caregiving Options in Residential Facilities

If the demands of caregiving exceed the abilities and resources of family care providers even with the help of in-home and community services, the therapist can identify various residential options for placement of the person with disabilities. Options might include assisted living facilities, group homes, continuing care retirement communities, hospice, or nursing homes. The occupational therapist, working in conjunction with the client's physician, social worker, and physical therapist, can review the advantages and disadvantages of each option and suggest the level of care most appropriate for the care receiver. The therapeutic team also can offer suggested criteria for evaluating and selecting a residential facility.

Placement of a loved one in an institutional setting typically represents a difficult transition for the family caregiver and the person with disabilities. Many family members prefer to remain involved in their relative's care but are unsure what they can do or will be allowed to do (Perkinson, 2003). A growing body of evidence shows that family involvement in nursing home care is linked to lower levels of depression among family caregivers and higher life satisfaction among nursing home residents whose family caregivers remain involved (Bowers, 1988; Brody, Dempsey, & Pruchno, 1990).

Therapists can assist family caregivers at this stage of their caregiving career by helping them learn to negotiate the nursing home system. Therapists can identify daily routines within the facility, suggest how to voice concerns effectively to nursing home staff and administrators, and outline strategies to help the person with disabilities adjust to life in his or her new setting (Perkinson, Rockemann, & Mahan, 1996). For safety reasons, family members of nursing home residents generally are discouraged from assisting in the more physically demanding tasks of self-care, such as toileting, transferring, or bathing. Family members may be encouraged, however, to help with ADL tasks such as grooming and feeding. Besides helping with these kinds of self-care tasks, family members continue to offer companionship to their relative in the nursing home and, when necessary, may act as advocates for the resident (Figure 20.4; Perkinson, 2003).

Role Disengagement Stage

The death of the person with disabilities signals the final stage of the caregiving career, during which the family member must deal with bereavement and loss.

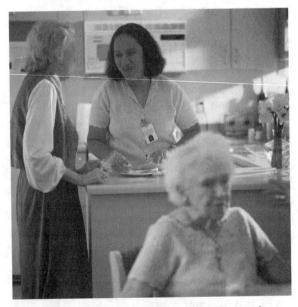

Figure 20.4. Therapists can assist family members to become advocates and maintain their caregiving roles when a relative is placed in an institutional setting. Photo © PhotoDisc, Inc.

The family caregiver typically undergoes a period of adjustment in which he or she must disengage and come to terms with the end of the caregiving role.

Caregiving during the later stages of an illness often is all consuming, and caregivers frequently cut out social activities and neglect friendships as they attempt to address the ever-growing needs of the family member with disabilities. When the person dies, the caregiver often finds him- or herself socially isolated. In addition to emotional support, he or she may need help developing new activities to restore balance to a life long structured by the caregiver role (Aneshensel et al., 1995; Mullan, 1992; Strang & Koop, 2003). Occupational therapists can assist family caregivers with these needs and help them make the transition to a new phase of life (Case Study 20.2).

Summary

Family-centered caregiving has limits. Some families may be uncomfortable with the new role of full participation in decision making and prefer to remain in the passive role traditionally assigned them by the health care system (Weinstein, 1997). With family-centered care, family caregivers should be able to select their own levels of involvement. This level may vary according to the age of the person with disabilities, the type of services available, the caregivers' comfort level with their own opinions, and their experiences as providers of care. They should not be pressured into taking on more than they can handle. Some family members may lack the necessary skills or knowledge to act as partners in the therapeutic relationship. Some practice environments may simply not support the implementation of a family-centered model.

To overcome these obstacles, various strategies can be implemented. One possibility is simply to make a personal commitment as a therapist to implement a more family-centered approach to intervention (Weinstein, 1997). Therapists can schedule in-service training on the topic to share ideas for increased collaboration with families. Therapists also can encourage family participation in the treatment process by modeling appropriate behaviors and recognizing that family resistance may need to be overcome gradually. To incorporate family-centered approaches into existing service delivery systems, these concepts should be taught in educational programs for occupational therapists. Expanding the family-centered model into practice with people at all stages of the life cycle should be a priority.

Finally, therapists should be mindful that the legal and ethical issues of care do not disappear when family-centered approaches are used. Personal safety issues take priority over family preferences. Occupational therapists will always be challenged to balance the best interests of the person with disabilities, respect for the family as a unit, and their own professional expertise in any situation (Allen & Petr, 1998).

Study Questions

1. List four reasons why the number of families providing care to family members has grown significantly in recent years.
2. Differentiate between the medical model and family-centered approaches to working with caregivers.

Case Study 20.2. Mrs. Kannon: Example of Stages of Caregiving

Background

Mrs. Kannon is 84 years of age and has macular degeneration, dementia, and depression. She has been deaf since she was 13 years old. Mrs. Kannon's primary caregiver is her daughter Carol.

Occupational Profile

Mrs. Kannon raised two children and enjoyed a happy 40-year marriage before her husband died. Throughout her adult life, she liked to garden, was active in her church, enjoyed reading, and loved to travel.

Carol is 66 years of age and lives with her husband William. Carol is a retired librarian. She loves to decorate her home, cross-stitch, and attend Bible-study classes. Carol is in relatively good health, although she has intermittent low-back pain.

Role Acquisition Stage

Mrs. Kannon began to experience memory problems about the same time she began to lose her central vision due to macular degeneration. She had difficulty remembering to pay her bills and forgot the names of acquaintances at church. Mrs. Kannon was living in her home of 60 years in a Kansas City suburb. Carol lived in Chicago, and her son John lived in Los Angeles. Carol began to visit her mother more fre-

Case Study 20.2. *Continued*

quently to accompany her mother to doctor's appointments and assist with transportation to the grocery store. Mrs. Kannon decided that this would be a good time to grant her daughter powers of attorney over her finances and health care in case this was needed in the future, and she and her daughter revisited her advance directive and updated her will with the assistance of an attorney. They also visited the local Low Vision Resource Center.

Role Enactment Stage

After a year or so of Carol making regular trips to help her mother, Mrs. Kannon began to experience increased confusion and memory loss. Her neurologist indicated that she had dementia, probably caused by Alzheimer's disease. She required more support from her daughter to plan meals and clean the house and could no longer monitor her finances. One weekend, Mrs. Kannon went out to get the mail and wandered off. That event prompted Carol to ask her mother to move to Chicago to live with her and her husband. Although she was reluctant, Mrs. Kannon agreed to the move.

Mrs. Kannon was able to participate in all self-care activities but needed supervision for cutting food, retrieving clothes, and bathing. Carol attempted to involve her mother in household chores and activities, but as Mrs. Kannon's cognitive status declined she was less able to participate.

Carol consulted the local Alzheimer's Disease Foundation and obtained information about making her home safe for her mother. Carol remained concerned about her mother's wandering. In addition, she consulted an occupational therapist who specialized in low vision. The therapist administered the Canadian Occupational Performance Measure, which revealed that Mrs. Kannon had difficulty with using her computer and text telephone (TTY) device and no longer could read standard print or garden. The therapist provided recommendations regarding self-care concerns: She suggested optimizing the lighting in the home; using large, bold keyboard labels for the TTY device; and implementing adaptive strategies so that Mrs. Kannon could pursue her leisure interests.

The occupational therapist also conducted an informal caregiver interview and administered the Memory and Behavior Problems Checklist. These caregiver assessments indicated that Carol was feeling overwhelmed with caring for her mother and was frustrated by her mother's repetitive behaviors and need for constant reminders. She expressed the need for a companion to stay with her mother so that she could run errands and attend her Bible-study class. Carol indicated growing resentment toward her brother because she was bearing most of the responsibility for her mother's care. The therapist contacted the local deaf communication program as a possible resource for students who might provide respite services. The therapist also provided information about the local chapter of the Alzheimer's Association, a support group, and an online chat room for caregivers of people with Alzheimer's disease. Carol and the occupational therapist discussed ways of approaching her brother to determine how he might assume some of the responsibilities for their mother's care.

Mrs. Kannon lived with her daughter and son-in-law for 2 years. During this time, a companion stayed with Mrs. Kannon two mornings per week, allowing Carol to attend Bible-study classes and run errands. Mrs. Kannon's son, John, made two to three trips to Chicago each year so that Carol and her husband could travel. As Mrs. Kannon's cognitive abilities declined, it became evident that she would be better cared for in a nursing home setting. This difficult transition for Mrs. Kannon and her children was made easier with the support of the occupational therapist, social worker, and nursing home staff. Mrs. Kannon visited her mother daily and, over time, developed a collaborative relationship with the nursing home staff.

Role Disengagement

Mrs. Kannon died after living in the nursing home for 5 months. Carol and her brother experienced a significant sense of loss. In addition, Carol found that she had become somewhat socially isolated and had to slowly rebuild her connections with her friends and volunteer activities. She attended several bereavement support group sessions, and the occupational therapist at the nursing home talked with her about identifying her priorities and restructuring her weekly routine.

3. Imagine yourself in the role of caregiver to an elderly relative or a child with special needs. Describe your explanatory model of the illness. How might your model differ from someone else's model of the same illness?

4. Identify one assessment tool that would be useful in identifying a family caregiver's values, needs, and priorities to use in a collaborative approach to intervention. Practice filling out this assessment with a peer or client.

5. A 35-year-old woman who was diagnosed with multiple sclerosis in her late 20s is referred to you for home health occupational therapy assessment and intervention. She lives with her mother and father. At what stage of their caregiving career are her parents, and how will you include them in your assessment and treatment plan?

6. You have been working with a young man who sustained a spinal cord injury and is an inpatient in a rehabilitation unit. He is ready for discharge to home and needs to consider hiring a personal care attendant. Plan a treatment session during which you will address this need.

References

Allen, R. I., & Petr, C. G. (1998). Rethinking family-centered practice. *American Journal of Orthopsychiatry, 68*(1), 4–15.

American Occupational Therapy Association. (2002). Occupational therapy practice framework: Domain and process. *American Journal of Occupational Therapy, 56*, 609–639.

Aneshensel, C. S., Pearlin, L. I., Mullan, J. T., Zarit, S. H., & Whitlatch, C. J. (1995). *Profiles in caregiving: The unexpected career.* San Diego, CA: Academic Press.

Batavia, A. I., DeJong, G., & McKnew, L. B. (1991). Toward a national personal assistance program: The independent living model of long-term care for persons with disabilities. *Journal of Health Politics, Policy and Law, 16*(3), 523–545.

Baum, C. M. (1991). Addressing the needs of the cognitively impaired elderly from a family policy perspective. *American Journal of Occupational Therapy, 45,* 594–606.

Baum, C. M. (1995). The contribution of occupation to function in persons with Alzheimer's disease. *Journal of Occupational Science: Australia, 2*(2), 59–67.

Baum, C., Edwards, D. F., & Morrow-Howell, N. (1993). Identification and measurement of productive behaviors in senile dementia of the Alzheimer type. *Gerontologist, 33*(3), 403–408.

Baum, C., & LaVesser, P. (1994). Caregiver assistance: Using family members and attendants. In C. H. Christiansen (Ed.), *Ways of living: Self-care strategies for special needs* (pp. 453–482). Rockville, MD: American Occupational Therapy Association.

Beach, S. R., Schulz, R., Yee, J. L., & Jackson, S. (2000). Negative and positive health effects of caring for a disabled spouse: Longitudinal findings from the caregiver health effects study. *Psychology and Aging, 15*(2), 259–271.

Berlin, E. A., & Fowkes, W. C. (1983). A teaching framework for cross-cultural health care. *Western Journal of Medicine, 139*(6), 934–938.

Bowers, B. J. (1988). Family perceptions of care in a nursing home. *Gerontologist, 28,* 361–368.

Brody, E., Dempsey, N., & Pruchno, R. (1990). Mental health of sons and daughters of the institutionalized aged. *Gerontologist, 30,* 212–219.

Brown, P. J. (1998). *Understanding and applying medical anthropology.* Mountain View, CA: Mayfield.

Case-Smith, J., & Nastro, M. A. (1993). The effect of occupational therapy intervention on mothers of children with cerebral palsy. *American Journal of Occupational Therapy, 47,* 811–817.

Corcoran, M. A., & Gitlin, L. N. (1992). Dementia management: An occupational therapy home-based intervention for caregivers. *American Journal of Occupational Therapy, 46,* 801–808.

Day, A. T. (1985). Who cares? Demographic trends challenge family care for the elderly. *Population Trends and Public Policy, 9,* 1–17.

De Graff, A. (1988). *Home health aides: How to manage the people who help you.* Fort Collins, CO: Saratoga Access Publications.

DeJong, G., & Wenker, T. (1983). Attendant care. In N. M. Crewe & I. K. Zola (Eds.), *Independent living for physically disabled people* (pp. 157–170). San Francisco: Jossey-Bass.

Doty, P. (1995). Older caregivers and the future of informal caregiving. In S. Bass (Ed.), *Older and active: How Americans over 55 are contributing to society* (pp. 97–121). New Haven, CT: Yale University Press.

Doty, P., Kasper, J., & Litvak, S. (1996). Consumer-directed models of personal care: Lessons from Medicaid. *Milbank Quarterly, 74*(3), 377–409.

Education for All Handicapped Children Amendments of 1986 (Pub. L. 99–457), 20 U.S.C. § 1401, Part H, Section 677.

Estes, C., & Binney, E. (1991). The biomedicalization of aging: Dangers and dilemmas. In M. Minkler & C. Estes (Eds.), *Critical perspectives on aging: The political and moral economy of growing old* (pp. 117–134). Amityville, NY: Baywood.

Flanagan, S., & Green, P. (1994). *Consumer-directed personal assistant services: Key operational issues for state CD-PAS programs using intermediary service organizations.* Cambrige, MA: SysteMetrics, The MEDSTAT Group.

Fortinsky, R. H., & Hathaway, T. J. (1990). Information and service needs among active and former family caregivers of persons with Alzheimer's disease. *Gerontologist, 30,* 604–609.

Gallagher-Thompson, D. (1994). Direct services and interventions for caregivers: A review of extant programs and a look to the future. In M. H. Cantor (Ed.), *Family caregiving: Agenda for the future* (pp. 102–122). San Francisco: American Society for Aging.

Gaugler, J. E., Kane, R. L., Kane, R. A., Clay, T., & Newcomer, R. (2003). Caregiving and institutionalization of cognitively impaired older people: Utilizing dynamic predictors of change. *Gerontologist, 43,* 219–229.

Gitlin, L. N. (1993). Therapeutic dilemmas in the care of the elderly in rehabilitation. *Topics in Geriatric Rehabilitation, 9*, 11–20.

Gitlin, L. N., Belle, S. H., Burgio, L. D., Czaja, S. J., Mahoney, D., Gallagher-Thompson, D., et al. (2003). Effect of multicomponent interventions on caregiver burden and depression. The REACH multisite initiative at 6-month follow-up. *Psychology and Aging, 18*(3), 361–374.

Gitlin, L. N., Corcoran, M., & Leinsmiller-Eckhardt, S. (1995). Understanding the family perspective: An ethnographic framework for providing occupational therapy in the home. *American Journal of Occupational Therapy, 49*, 802–809.

Gitlin, L. N., Corcoran, M., Winter, L., Boyce, A., & Hauck, W. W. (2001). A randomized, controlled trial of a home environmental intervention: Effect on efficacy and upset in caregivers and on daily function of persons with dementia. *Gerontologist, 41*, 4–14.

Gubrium, J. F., & Sankar, A. (1990). *The home care experience: Ethnography and policy.* Newbury Park, CA: Sage.

Hasselkus, B. R. (1988). Meaning of family caregiving: Perspectives on caregiver/professional relationships. *Gerontologist, 28*, 686–691.

Hasselkus, B. R. (1989). The meaning of daily activity in family caregiving for the elderly. *American Journal of Occupational Therapy, 43*, 649–656.

Hasselkus, B. R. (1990). Ethnographic interviewing: A tool for practice with family caregivers for the elderly. *OT Practice, 2*, 9–16.

Hasselkus, B. R. (1991). Ethical dilemmas in family caregiving for the elderly: Implications for occupational therapy. *American Journal of Occupational Therapy, 45*, 206–212.

Hasselkus, B. R. (1997). Everyday ethics in dementia care: Narratives of crossing the line. *Gerontologist, 37*(5), 640–649.

Heagerty, B., & Eskenazi, L. (1994). A practice and program perspective on family caregiving: Focus on solutions. In M. H. Cantor (Ed.), *Family caregiving: Agenda for the future* (pp. 35–48). San Francisco: American Society for Aging.

Kahn, P. (1980). Maintaining personal care attendant services. *American Rehabilitation*, pp. 24–26.

Kleinman, A. (1980). *Patients and healers in the context of culture.* Berkeley: University of California Press.

Kleinman, A. (1988). *The illness narratives: Suffering, healing, and the human condition.* New York: Basic.

Krefting, L., & Krefting, D. (1991). Cultural influences on performance. In C. Christiansen & C. Baum (Eds.), *Occupational therapy: Overcoming human performance deficits* (pp. 101–124). Thorofare, NJ: Slack.

Kunkel, S. R., & Applebaum, R. A. (1992). Estimating the prevalence of long-term disability for an aging society. *Journal of Gerontology, 47*, S253–S260.

LaPlante, M. P., Harrington, C., & Kang, T. (2002). Estimating paid and unpaid hours of personal assistance services in activities of daily living provided to adults living at home. *Health Services Research, 37*(2), 397–415.

Law, M. (1998). *Client-centered occupational therapy.* Thorofare, NJ: Slack.

Law, M., Baptiste, S., Carswell, A., McColl, M. A., Polatajko, H., & Pollock, N. (1998). *Canadian occupational performance measure* (3rd ed.). Toronto, Ontario, Canada: CAOT Publications.

Lawlor, M. S., & Mattingly, C. F. (1998). The complexities embedded in family-centered care. *American Journal of Occupational Therapy, 52*, 259–267.

Le Navenec, C., & Vonhof, T. (1996). *One day at a time: How families manage the experience of dementia.* Westport, CT: Greenwood.

Lindley, J. (1995). *Finding and keeping an attendant.* Puyallup, WA: Center for Independence.

Mace, N. L., & Rabins, P. V. (1994). *The 36-hour day* (2nd ed.). Baltimore: Johns Hopkins University Press.

Marks, N. F. (1996). Caregiving across the lifespan: National prevalence and predictors. *Family Relations, 45*, 27–36.

Meuser, T., & Marwit, S. (2001). A comprehensive, stage-sensitive model of grief in dementia caregiving. *Gerontologist, 41*, 658–670.

Morris, A., & Gainer, F. (1997). Helping the caregiver: Occupational therapy opportunities. *OT Practice, 2*(1), 36–40.

Mullan, J. T. (1992). The bereaved caregiver: A prospective study of changes in well-being. *Gerontologist, 32*, 673–683.

Nosek, M. A., Fuhrer, M. J., Rintala, D. H., & Hart, K. A. (1993). The use of personal assistance services by persons with spinal cord injury. *Journal of Disability Policy Studies, 4*(1), 89–103.

Ohaeri, J. U. (2003). The burden of caregiving in families with a mental illness: A review of 2002. *Current Opinion in Psychiatry, 16*(4), 457–465.

Opie, N. D., & Miller, E. L. (1989). Personal care attendants and severely disabled adults: Attributions for relationship outcomes. *Archives of Psychiatric Nursing, 3*, 205–210.

Overman, W., & Stoudemire, A. (1988). Guidelines for legal and financial counseling of Alzheimer's disease patients and their families. *American Journal of Psychiatry, 145*(12), 1495–1500.

Perkinson, M. A. (1992). Maximizing personal efficacy in older adults: The empowerment of volunteers in a multipurpose senior center. *Physical and Occupational Therapy in Geriatrics, 10*(3), 57–72.

Perkinson, M. A. (1995). Socialization to the family caregiving role within a continuing care retirement community. *Medical Anthropology, 16*, 249–267.

Perkinson, M. A. (1999). Family and nursing home staff's perceptions of quality of life in dementia. In R. Rubinstein, M. Moss, & M. Kleban (Eds.), *The many dimensions of aging* (pp. 116–128). New York: Springer.

Perkinson, M. A. (2002). *Nurturing a family partnership: Alzheimer's home care aide's guide.* Washington, DC: AARP Andrus Foundation.

Perkinson, M. A. (2003). Defining family roles within a nursing home setting. In P. B. Stafford (Ed.), *Gray areas: Ethnographic encounters with nursing home culture* (pp. 235–261). Santa Fe, NM: School of American Research Press.

Perkinson, M. A., Rockemann, D., & Mahan, L. (1996). *Families in nursing homes manual.* Washington, DC: AARP Andrus Foundation.

Pinquart, M., & Sorensen, S. (2003). Differences between caregivers and noncaregivers in psychological health and physical health: A meta-analysis. *Psychology and Aging, 18*(2), 250–267.

Pruchno, R. A. (1999). Caregiving research: Looking backward, looking forward. In R. Rubinstein, M. Moss, &

M. Kleban (Eds.), *The many dimensions of aging* (pp. 197–213). New York: Springer.

Sabat, S. R., & Harre, R. (1992). The construction and deconstruction of self in Alzheimer's disease. *Aging and Society, 12,* 443–461.

Schultz-Krohn, W. (1997). Early intervention: Meeting the unique needs of parent–child interaction. *Infants and Young Children, 10*(1), 47–60.

Schulz, R. (Ed.). (2000). *Handbook on dementia caregiving: Evidence-based interventions for family caregivers.* New York: Springer.

Schulz, R., & Quittner, A. (1998). Caregiving for children and adults with chronic conditions. *Health Psychology, 17*(2), 107–111.

Shapiro, J. (1993). *No pity: People with disabilities forging a new civil rights movement.* New York: Times Books/Random House.

Sorensen, S., Pinquart, M., & Duberstein, P. (2002). How effective are interventions with caregivers? An updated meta-analysis. *Gerontologist, 42,* 356–372.

Steffen, A. M. (2000). Anger management for dementia caregivers: A preliminary study using video and telephone interventions. *Behavior Therapy, 31,* 281–299.

Strang, V. R., & Koop, P. M. (2003). Factors which influence coping: Home-based family caregiving of persons with advanced cancer. *Journal of Palliative Care, 19*(2), 107–114.

Teri, L., Gibbons, L. E., McCurry, S. M., Logdon, R. G., Buchner, D. M., Barlow, W. E., et al. (2003). Exercise plus behavioral management in patients with Alzheimer disease: a randomized controlled trial. *JAMA, 290*(15), 2015–2022.

Teri, L., Truax, P., Logdon, R. G., Uomoto, J., Zarit, S. H., & Vitaliano, P. P. (1992). Assessment of behavioral problems in dementia: The Revised Memory and Behavior Problems Checklist. *Psychology and Aging, 4,* 622–631.

Toth-Cohen, S. (2000). Role perceptions of occupational therapists providing support and education for caregivers of persons with dementia. *American Journal of Occupational Therapy, 54,* 509–515.

Ulicny, G., & Jones, M. L. (1985). Enhancing the attendant management skills of persons with disabilities. *American Rehabilitation, 2*(2), 18–20.

U.S. Bureau of the Census. (1990). *The need for personal assistance with everyday activities: Recipients and caregivers.* Washington, DC: U.S. Government Printing Office.

U.S. Bureau of the Census. (2001). *The 65 years and over population: 2000* (Census 2000 Brief). Washington, DC: Author.

Weinstein, M. (1997). Bringing family-centered practices into home health. *OT Practice, 2*(7), 35–38.

Wright, L. K., Clipp, E. C., & George, L. K. (1993). Health consequences of caregiver stress. *Medicine, Exercise, Nutrition, and Health, 2,* 181–195.

Zarit, S. H., Reever, K. E., & Bach-Peterson, J. (1980). Relatives of the impaired elderly: Correlates of feelings of burden. *Gerontologist, 20,* 649–655.

Zarit, S. H., & Teri, L. (1991). Interventions and services for family caregivers. *Annual Review of Gerontology and Geriatrics, 11,* 287–310.

Zedlewski, E. A. (1990). *The needs of the elderly in the 21st century.* Washington, DC: Urban Institute Press.

Glossary

A

ABLEDATA: An Internet directory that provides a searchable database of assistive technology and rehabilitation devices

Accessibility: Free and normal movement throughout the environmental setting

Accessible design: Products and environments designed and constructed to be readily accessible to and usable by people with disabilities

Acquisition: The initial learning phase of an activity where learners may not be able to perform the target skill at all or may perform with limited competence

Activities of daily living (ADL): An area of occupation that includes activities oriented toward taking care of one's own body. Also referred to as basic activities of daily living (BADL) and personal activities of daily living (PADL).

Activity limitation: Previously referred to as "handicap"; loss or limitation of opportunities to take part in the life of the community on an even level with others

Adaptive equipment: Devices or materials used to allow engagement in an occupation for people with impairment in the performance skills, patterns, and/or client factors needed to complete the targeted occupation; these may include modifications to existing equipment, such as seat inserts, or the use of new devices or materials, such as use of reachers

Adaptive strategy: Any action taken by an individual to accomplish a task or meet an environmental demand; may involve equipment, techniques, or routines

Aesthetic anxiety: Fear of others whose characteristics are perceived as disturbing or unpleasant

Age appropriate: The temporal context of the client's chronological age

Alzheimer's dementia (AD): A progressive, degenerative disease of uncertain causes that manifests itself in damage to the brain

Alzheimer's dementia stages: The three stages of cognitive decline described as mild, moderate, and severe; used to describe and predict behaviors that are expected to emerge during the course of the disease that may span 17 years

Analysis of occupational performance: The step in the evaluation process during which the client's assets, problems, or potential problems are specifically identified, preferably in context in order to identify barriers and resources to occupational performance; skills and patterns of performance, contexts, activity demands, and client factors are considered, but not all may be individually assessed; desired (target) outcomes are identified

Ankylosing spondylitis (AS): A chronic systemic disease in which the primary sites of inflammation are the ligamentous, capsular, and tendinous insertions into the bone; primarily involving the sacroiliac, spinal apophyseal, and axial joints

Antecedent events: Those actions (e.g., environmental changes) that occur before the target behavior or goal

Aphasia: Absence or impairment of the ability to communicate through speech, writing, or signs due to dysfunction of brain centers

Apraxia: Inability to perform purposive movements although there is no sensory or motor impairment

ASIA Impairment Scale: Defines the level of injury as the last caudal segment with intact motor and sensory innervations; also referred to as the International Standards for Neurological and Functional Classification of Spinal Cord Injury

Assertive community treatment: Originated in Madison, Wisconsin, and called the PACT program (Program of Assertive Community Treatment); offers full-support case management services in the community with a team whose expertise informs the group decision-making; teams work with the community and families as a collaborative process

Assessment: The use of specific tools in the evaluation process

Assistive devices: Equipment or devices used to increase, maintain, or improve performance of occupations

Assistive technology device: A commercial, custom-fabricated, or homemade device used to assist in the performance of tasks involved in everyday living

Assistive technology practitioner (ATP): A certification credential recognized as the nonspecialized foundation level of competence identified by RESNA

Assitive technology service: An agency or unit that provides information or other assistance regarding the need, acquisition, modification, or maintenance of assistive technology devices

Assistive technology supplier (ATS): A certification of basic competence recognized by the Rehabilitation Engineeering Society of North America

Ataxia: Inability to perform coordinated muscle movements

Augmentative communication: A system, which can be personal, technical or electronic, that enhances communication abilities

Autograft: A graft of tissue taken from a different area of the person receiving the graft

Autonomic dysreflexia: A reflex action of the autonomic nervous system in response to noxious stimuli, such as a distended bladder, rectal mass, bladder irritation, rectal manipulation, painful stimuli, and visceral distention; a phenomena seen in people with spinal injuries above the T4–T6 level; symptoms may include pounding headache, anxiety, perspiration, flushing, chills, nasal congestion, paroxysmal breathing, hypertension, and bradycardia; a medical emergency and life threatening

B

Barrier-free design: Similar to accessible design but refers primarily to the environment

Baseline data: Level of a client's performance as measured before instruction begins

Biscapular abduction: Active motion of scapular abduction, which produces tension on a cable or switch to operate the terminal device and/or elbow unit

Body power prosthesis: The terminal device and/or elbow unit on the prosthesis operated by upper extremity or upper quadrant voluntary muscle movements

Boutonnière deformity: A deformity caused by disruption of the extensor apparatus at the proximal interphalangeal joint level resulting in proximal interphalangeal joint flexion and distal interphalangeal joint hyperextension when active finger extension is attempted

Boutonnière precautions: Avoidance of composite active flexion of the fingers with deeper partial or full-thickness dorsal hand burns; instead, isolated MP flexion is combined with IP joint extension to avoid stress to a possibly compromised extensor tendon mechanism

Braille: A system of reading and writing using a configuration of six raised dots in a rectangular pattern resembling a muffin pan

Brain cortex lobes: The part of the nervous system that is most significantly damaged by AD and TBI; the four main structures of the brain that are commonly affected by AD and TBI are the frontal, parietal, temporal, and occipital lobes

C

Case management: A service that assists clients in negotiating for services that they both need and want

Cataracts: An opacity, or cloudiness, of the normally clear lens inside the eye

Central vision loss (CVL): The loss of central or straight-ahead vision

Cerebral palsy: A disability resulting from a nonprogressive lesion of the central nervous system originating before, during, or shortly after birth that manifests as a muscular incoordination; intellectual, sensory, speech, seizure, and behavioral disorders may also be present

Clubhouse model: Also known as the Fountain House Model; model in which people with serious mental illness join together to support one another as they adjust to community living and help one another find jobs; rather than serving "patients," people join as "members" and work side-by-side with staff to run the psychosocial clubhouse and the many programs offered

Cognitive rehabilitation: Interdisciplinary interventions designed to remediate or compensate for cognitive function, activities, and participation; use cognitive and behavioral learning strategies to design programs for AD and TBI

Community support program (CSP): A model of psychosocial intervention in which the mental health practitioners go to where the client lives and works to provide the needed services

Compassion: A quality among caregivers of feeling kindly when faced with another person's sufferings and responding willingly and helpfully to their needs

Compensatory: Finding a new way to accomplish a task when performance capabilities are limited; occurs through modifying the task or environment

Consequences: The events (planned or unplanned) following a target response

Correlation: The extent to which two or more variables or tests are related

D

Developmental disability: A severe, chronic disability of a person that is attributable to a mental or physical impairment or combination of mental and physical impairments; developmental disabilities are manifested before the person attains age 22; are likely to continue indefinitely; result in substantial functional limitations in three or more of the following areas of major life activity: self-care, receptive and expressive language, learning, mobility, self-direction, capacity for independent living, or economic self-sufficiency; and reflect that person's need for a combination and sequence of special, interdisciplinary, or generic care, treatment, or other services that are individually planned and coordinated

Diabetic retinopathy: A condition that affects the retinas of some individuals who are diabetic; diabetes may cause hemorrhages or blood vessel changes that affect the retina and thus interfere with vision

Disability: Impairment, activity limitation, and participation restriction

Disarticulation: Amputation occurring through a joint, i.e., wrist, elbow, or shoulder

Discontinuance: Preferred term to describe the nonuse of an assistive technology device

Division of labor: A pattern of work roles linked to age and sex within a family and in the wider society

Donor site: Area from which the upper layer of the skin is taken for a skin graft

Dual diagnoses: Occurs when a person with a serious mental illness concurrently has a substance use disorder

Dysarthria: Difficult and defective speech due to impairment of the tongue or other muscles essential for speech

Dysphagia: Inability to swallow or difficulty in swallowing

E

Eccentric viewing: A means of locating and using the area of best visual function on the retina of a person with macular degeneration or a central vision loss

Ectropion: The turning outward or eversion of the eyelids or lips due to skin contractures

Electronic prosthesis: Prosthesis that is operated through external power of motor, which is activated through several means, such as a pull switch or toggle switch

Empowerment models: Also referred to as consumer/survivor models, in which consumers have much greater control over services and may actually provide them

Energy conservation: Using daily strategies that minimize fatigue, conserve energy, enhance safety, and foster adequate stability

Engagement: State of being involved with occupations that are meaningful to the person

Environmental factors: Social attitudes, architectural characteristics, legal and social structures, as well as climate, terrain, etc.

Epidermis: The outermost layer of the skin

Eschar: Nonviable, slough of necrotic tissue produced by a burn

Ethnographic approach: The attempt to understand another way of life from the informant's point of view; focuses on values, meanings, beliefs, and how the informant makes sense of his or her situation

Evaluation: An ongoing process of collecting and interpreting data necessary for planning intervention

Existential anxiety: An unconscious fear about loss of physical capabilities that able-bodied people often experience when in contact with people with disabilities

Explanatory model of illness: A set of beliefs and knowledge, explanations of sickness and treatment, which provide a conceptual framework to give meaning to a particular illness experience and guide choices among various therapies

Extended client care network: The group of individuals who have an interest in a client's well-being, including employers, group home supervisors, guardians, and others

F

Family caregiver: Any family member providing unpaid care to a person who, because of a physical, cognitive, or psychological impairment, would not be able to care for him- or herself

Family-centered care: A term used to describe a constellation of beliefs, values, and treatment approaches that recognizes the role of family members as full collaborators on the health care team

Fibromyalgia (FM): A chronic and painful disorder characterized by widespread discomfort and tenderness at anatomically defined points that are thought to be influenced by the neuroendocrine, biorhythmic, and nociceptive systems

Fluency: Phase of learning that concerns improving the accuracy, quality, and speed of performance

Full-thickness burn: A burn that extends through and causes necrosis of all three layers of the skin

Functional capacity as a basis for design: A decision framework that provides guidelines for the applicability of all products and home modifications based on the identified sensory, physical, and cognitive changes of aging

Functional effects on sexual activity: The effects of a disability that may impede sexual activity

Functional mobility: The use of wheeled devices such as strollers, transport chairs, or wheelchairs to enable transportation if disability restricts it

G

Generalization: Phase of learning that is concerned with how a skill is performed and improved under changing conditions (e.g., location, materials, time, task variation)

Glasgow Coma Scale (GCS): A commonly used scale measuring the severity of brain injury at the onset of the brain trauma, consisting of a 15-point scale used to rate eye opening, and motor and verbal responses; based on the duration of prolonged unconsciousness or deep sleep

Glaucoma: A leading cause of blindness in the United States, causes damage to the optic nerve and retinal nerve fibers due to a build up of pressure within the eye; increased pressure causes a decrease of vision in the peripheral field, commonly known as tunnel vision

Graduated guidance: System of prompts where the more intrusive physical prompts are applied initially, then faded out

Greifer: Prehensor that can be powered by a myoelectric or electronic prosthesis

H

Hand function: The ability to flex and extend the wrist and flex and extend the fingers in a coordinated manner with sufficient strength to grasp and release objects

Health condition: A disease, disorder, or injury as defined by medical science

Health promotion: An intervention approach "that does not assume a disability is present or that any factors would interfere with performance. This approach is designed to provide enriched contextual and activity experiences that will enhance performance for all persons in the natural contexts of life" (*Occupational Therapy Practice Framework*, AOTA, 2002, p. 627).

Hemipares/Hemiplegia: Paralysis affecting only one side of the body

Heterotopic ossification: Bone formation occurring at an abnormal location in the body

Home evaluations: A step-by-step method of reviewing pertinent aspects of a person's home

Home modifications: Preventative steps to make a home safe, particularly for the elderly and disabled communities; these steps are designed to allow elderly people to age comfortably in place and for disabled to live in safety

Homonymous/Hemianopsia: Blindness of nasal half of the visual field of one eye and temporal half of the other, or right or left-sided hemianopsia of corresponding sides in both eyes

Humeral flexion: Active motion of humeral flexion, which produces tension on the cable to operate terminal device and/or elbow unit

Hybrid prosthesis: Prosthesis with more than one style of component, such as a body power component and an electronic component

Hyperpigmentation: Excessive darkening of skin color due to overproduction of skin pigment, often accelerated by sun exposure

Hypertrophic scar: Excessive scar formation that rises above the level of the skin plane but does not extend beyond the original borders of the burn wound

Hypopigmentation: Lighter-than-normal skin color due to underproduction of skin pigment

I

Identity: An overall view of self

Illness: An individual's actual experience of disorder or suffering, whether or not caused by an identifiable disease

Impairment: Problems in body function or structure such as a significant deviation or loss

Independent living movement: A philosophy in which individuals are responsible for their decision making and performance of self-care and community activities within the limits of their capabilities

Infantilization: The tendency of some caregivers to treat to an adult who needs help with self-care as if he or she were a baby; an inappropriate manner of talking to and providing services to person with impairments

Instrumental activities of daily living (IADL): Area of occupation that includes activities oriented toward interacting with the environment

Intermittent catheterization: A method for bladder emptying in which a catheter is inserted into the bladder allowing urine to flow out; the catheter is removed after all urine is emptied; this process is performed several times during the day on a regular timed schedule.

International Classification of Functioning, Disability, and Health **(ICF):** Provides a unified and standard language and framework for the description of health and health-related states

Intervention plan: "An outline of selected approaches and types of intervention, which is based on the results of the evaluation process, developed to reach the client's identified targeted outcomes" (*Occupational Therapy Practice Framework*, AOTA, 2002, p. 632)

J

Joint protection and energy conservation principles: Active strategies related to lifestyle for reducing the progressive deterioration of joints in RA; emphasis is placed on principles such as proper body alignment, adequate rest, use of assistive devices, and alternate methods of task completion

Juvenile rheumatoid arthritis (JRA): A systemic joint disease characterized by three major types (systemic onset, polyarticular onset, pauciarticular onset) and seven subtypes based on symptoms after onset; all types involve fatigue, fever, and malaise

K

Keloid scar: Excessive scar formation that rises above the level of the skin plane and continues to extend, mushroom-like, beyond the original borders of the burn wound

L

Legal blindness: Having vision of 20/200 or less (using the Snellen Chart measurement) in the better eye with best standard eyeglass correction, or having a visual field that encompasses or subtends an angle of 20 degrees or less

Leisure: Freedom or opportunity to do something

M

Macular degeneration (AMD): A condition that affects the central visual acuity, primarily in those over age 50

Maintenance: Phase where a skill is used routinely and improved under fairly stable and familiar conditions

Mini-Mental Test: A commonly used measure designed to evaluate the cognitive impairment of clients with dementia

Modification: An intervention approach directed at "finding ways to revise the current context or activity demands to support performance in the natural setting...[includes] compensatory techniques, including enhancing some features to provide cues, or reducing other features to reduce distractibility" (*Occupational Therapy Practice Framework*, AOTA, 2002, p. 627)

Myoelectric prosthesis: The terminal device or other component of the prosthesis is operated by the electrical signal from a voluntary muscle contraction

N

Narrative: The personal story within which each individual constructs meaning through activity engagement over time

No light perception (NLP): The designation used to mean total blindness or the inability to distinguish light from dark

Norms: Performance scores or data gathered on reference groups to permit comparison with the score obtained by an individual

O

Occupational deprivation: A state of prolonged preclusion from engagement in occupations of necessity or meaning due to factors outside the control of an individual

Occupational disruption: A transient or temporary condition of being restricted from participation in necessary or meaningful occupations, such as that caused by illness, temporary relocation, or temporary unemployment

Occupational performance problem statement: Succinctly describes the occupational status of a person, identifying the problems amenable to intervention; focuses intervention on the occupations and activities, performance skills and patterns, underlying factors, and contexts needing change in order to resolve the performance problem

Occupational profile: The initial step in the evaluation process that provides an understanding of the client's occupational history and experiences, patterns of daily living, interests, values, and needs

Open market: Items available for purchase from the mass commercial market

Osteoarthritis (OA): The most common rheumatic disease, affecting both men and women equally during their middle age and beyond; It involves a progression of articular cartilage wear and bony build-up at the margins of a joint, leading to stiffness and limited range of motion rather than pain

Osteoporosis (OP): A condition, more common in women than men, in which bones become fragile and more susceptible to fractures because the density or amount of bone decreases

P

Paraplegia: An impairment of thoracic, lumbar, and sacral segments of the spinal cord resulting in functional impairments in the trunk, legs, and pelvic organs

Partial participation: Ability to perform part of an activity or a somehow modified activity rather than carrying out the entire task in a typical way

Partial-thickness burn: A burn injury extending through the epidermis and into the dermis

Participation: Involvement in a life situation

Performance failure: An inability of the body to perform activities that were once done automatically and taken for granted

Peripheral vision loss (PVL): The loss of side vision

Personal assistant services: The employment of an individual who assists a person with a disability in performing tasks; the person with a disability employs the personal assistant and provides direction on tasks to be performed

Personal care attendant: A paid employee who provides in-home assistance with essential activities of daily living to a person with a severe disability who is functionally dependent

Personal factors: Gender, age, coping style, social background, education, profession, past and current experience, overall behavior pattern, character, and other factors that influence how disability is experienced by an individual

Photophobia: Discomfort from the abnormally increased sensitivity to bright sunlight or reflected light from water, snow, or even highly polished floors

Play: An area of occupation that provides enjoyment, entertainment, amusement, or diversion

Positioning: The placement and alignment of a body part or the entire body to prevent abnormal or unnecessary movements, allow or enhance the engagement in occupations, and/or provide safety during engagement in occupations

Post-Traumatic Amnesia Scale (PTA): A measurement obtained by estimating the duration of memory loss from the moment of the brain trauma to the time of evaluation, at which point clients are able to demonstrate the ability to communicate about memory

Postural stability: The ability to maintain a desired bodily position, such as sitting, kneeling, or propping on elbows, while engaged in a meaningful occupation

Power mobility: Motorized devices for mobility, such as wheelchairs or scooters, which use switch-activated battery power and various steering mechanisms to enable movement

Pressure ulcer: Localized area of cellular necrosis characterized by an open wound in which tissue necrosis has occurred, usually in response to externally applied pressure

Prevention: An intervention approach designed to "address clients without a disability who are at risk for occupational performance problems. This approach is designed to prevent the occurrence or evolution of barriers to performance in context. Interventions may be directed at client, context, or activity variables." (*Occupational Therapy Practice Framework*, AOTA, 2002, p. 627)

Probe data: Information gathered regarding a client's progress once training has begun by monitoring progress using criterion or test conditions

Procovery: Attaining a productive and fulfilling life regardless of the level of health assumed attainable; an approach to healing based on hope and grounded in practical everyday steps that individuals can take to move forward

Psychoeducational approaches: Reflects an approach to teaching the basic skills of everyday living based on the goals of learning from the consumer's perspective, and in the environments in which they live, work, and play

Q

Quality of life: A person's dynamic appraisal of his or her overall satisfaction with the various domains of life

R

Rasch Analysis: A mathematical model for calibrating measurement scales that considers the relationship between the probability of success and the difference between an individual's ability and an item's difficulty

Reciprocity: A system of exchanging goods and services between individuals and groups that is a fundamental basis for social relations

Rehabilitation engineering technologist (RET): A certification of basic competence recognized by the Rehabilitation Engineeering Society of North America (RESNA)

Reliability: The consistency and precision with which an assessment measures a specific behavior or skill

Remedial: An intervention that is designed to improve or establish a skill or ability that has not yet been developed in order to meet the requirements of task demands

Remediation: An intervention approach "designed to change client variables to establish a skill or ability that has been impaired" (*Occupational Therapy Practice Framework*, AOTA, 2002, p. 627)

RESNA: Rehabilitation Engineering Society of North America

Response prompts: Those cues given by the therapist to facilitate a client's performance of an activity (e.g., gestures, physical touch, and modeling)

Reverse mortgages: A special type of loan used primarily by older Americans to convert the equity in their homes into cash; instead of making monthly payments to a lender, a lender makes payments to the homeowner in return for a share of the equity

Rheumatoid arthritis (RA): A systemic disease with inflammation of the synovium (or sac), which provides lubrication for the joint, as a primary symptom, and primarily affects the extremity joints and the neck

Routines: Behaviors that are repeated over time and organized into patterns and habits

S

Scar maturation: Progressive remodeling of a scar as demonstrated by a softening and flattening of scar texture and complete resolution of erythema, usually over a 12- to 18-month period following initial burn injury or surgical reconstruction procedure

Self-management principles: Knowledge related to reducing the adverse consequences of disease on lifestyle, including understanding the disease and its causes, awareness of medications and their side effects, and recognition of practical techniques and devices that can prevent or reduce disease progression and improve function and the quality of life

Self-protection techniques: Techniques involving holding one arm (usually the nondominant one) at shoulder height, palm out, with the hand just below eye level; the dominant hand is held diagonally across the body, palm inward, in front of the opposite upper thigh, thus protecting oneself

Sensory defensiveness (hypersensitivity): A negative reaction, motoric or emotional, to a sensory experience that most people would not consider to be harmful or unpleasant

Serious mental illness/psychiatric disability: Typically reflects conditions such as schizophrenia, bipolar disorder, mood disorders, and personality disorders, with or without substance use disorders, which result in reduced abilities to be fully engaged in meaningful occupations of everyday life

Severe visual impairment: The inability to read standard newsprint

Sexual activity: Activities aimed toward giving or receiving sexual pleasure

Sexual counseling: Giving information to patients and clients from a functional perspective *only* related to sexuality and disability

Sexual orientation: A person's erotic, romantic, and affectional attraction to people of the same sex (homosexuality), to the opposite sex (heterosexuality), or to both sexes (bisexuality)

Sexual response cycle: The physiologic responses to sexual stimulation/excitement as described by Masters and Johnson (1966)

Sexual rights: The rights of individuals to have the information, education, skills, support, and services they need to make responsible decisions about their sexuality consistent with their own values

Sick role: A temporary excuse from normal social responsibilities (such as going to work or doing housework) due to illness; involves giving up control over one's situation and status as a competent member of society until declared well by a medical authority

Sighted guide technique: The position a blind person uses to hold the arm of a sighted guide just above the elbow; the blind person will be a half step behind and to the side of the sighted guide. In this position, a blind person can safely follow the guide's body movements as they walk

Snellen Chart: A test chart of lines of letters or symbols of various sizes used for assessing visual acuity

Social role: A set of behaviors that has some socially agreed-upon function and for which there is an accepted code of norms

Specialized amputee team/clinic: Experienced physicians, therapists, prosthetists, and other clinicians who have practiced exclusively in the field of prosthetics and amputations; the specialized team provides consultants, assessments, and treatments for individuals with amputations, and meets and communicates on a scheduled basis

Spiritual: Pertains to experiences that inspire, motivate, or bring meaning to a person's life

Split-thickness skin graft: A skin graft containing the epidermis and the upper portion of the dermis

Stability: The consistency of a measure over time

Stages of learning: Four specific phases in which skills are learned during intervention, from acquisition through fluency, maintenance, and generalization

Standardized: Instruments that have a well-defined procedure, norms (if applicable), and standards for administration

Stigma: Prejudicial devaluing by a social group based on some characteristic or trait; negative social evaluations attached to (1) minority ethnic and racial groups, (2) morally disapproved behaviors, or (3) physical differences caused by chronic illnesses or disabilities

Stigma symbols: Aspects of appearance that others may unfairly use as evidence that someone is not a fully competent member of society

Stimulus prompts: Graded environmental cues that provide varying levels of support for an individual's performance

Superficial burn: A burn injury that only involves the epidermis

System of least prompts: Hierarchy of 2–3 prompts that are selected to "work" both for the client and the activity; they are used one at a time, starting with less assistance and moving to more assistance

Systemic lupus erythematosus (SLE): A systemic inflammatory disease usually occurring in women that is characterized by a diverse clinical picture involving small vessel vasculitis

Systemic sclerosis (scleroderma, SSc): The generalized form of a group of disorders that are mainly characterized by sclerosis of the skin

T

Tenodesis grasp: A natural action of the wrist and hand musculature as a result of the pull of the extrinsic finger flexor and extensor muscles across the wrist; the fingers tend to flex when the wrist is extended, forming a finger pinch; fingers extend when the wrist flexes, creating a release of finger pinch

Terminal device: The end device of a prosthesis

Tetraplegia: An impairment in motor and/or sensory function in the cervical segments of the spinal cord resulting in functional impairment in the arms, trunk, legs, and pelvic organs; the term *tetraplegia* has replaced the formerly used term *quadriplegia*

Time delay: Pause or delay period added before giving a prompt on each step of an activity; the client may either wait for assistance or try the response independently during these periods

Training data: Information on performance of a target behavior collected during intervention sessions

Transgenerational design: The practice of making products and environments compatible with the physical and sensory impairments that limit activities and are associated with human aging

Transhumeral amputation: Amputation occurring proximal of the shoulder joint

Transradial amputation: Amputation occurring proximal of the elbow joint

Traumatic brain injury (TBI): A non-progressive, persistent damage to the brain; usually caused by a blow to the head, either from an external object or due to internal forces caused by high-speed acceleration or deceleration

Traumatic brain injury stages: The three stages of cognitive function and/or progression described as mild, moderate, and severe; used to describe and predict behaviors that may emerge during the recovery of the brain trauma

U

Unilateral neglect: Impaired ability to attend, respond, or orient to stimuli presented unilaterally, frequently occurring across various sensory systems

Universal design: The concept of designing all products and the built environment to be aesthetic and usable to the greatest extent possible by everyone, regardless of their age, ability, or status in life

V

Validity: The extent to which one can have confidence in the results of an assessment

Visitability: The purpose of visitability is to ensure basic access for disabled people in newly constructed private homes; at least one exterior door is at ground level with no steps, and a bathroom on the main floor has a door with at least 32 inches of passage

W

Work: An area of occupation that includes activities related to remunerative employment or volunteerism

Index

References in *italic* refer to figures.
References in **boldface** refer to tables and boxes.

About the Editors

Charles H. Christiansen, EdD, OTR, OT(C), FAOTA, is dean and George T. Bryan Distinguished Professor at the University of Texas School of Allied Health Sciences in Galveston. He has been involved in the education of rehabilitation providers for the past 25 years and is an active researcher with an interest in lifestyle and health, occupational science, and functional assessment. Dr. Christiansen is a fellow of the American Occupational Therapy Association and a member of the Canadian Association of Occupational Therapists. He is the founding editor of *OTJR: Occupation, Participation, and Health* and the author and editor of several textbooks in occupational therapy.

Kathleen M. Matuska, MPH, OTR/L, is associate professor and graduate program director at the College of St. Catherine, St. Paul, Minnesota. She has more than 20 years of experience as an occupational therapist providing direct service and consultation in a variety of settings and 10 years of experience in undergraduate and graduate education. Ms. Matuska is author and project director of several community-based service-learning grants and co-investigator of past and current research in multiple sclerosis with Virgil Mathiowetz. She is treasurer of the Society for the Study of Occupation, USA. She is the author of several journal articles and book chapters.